Meet the editor

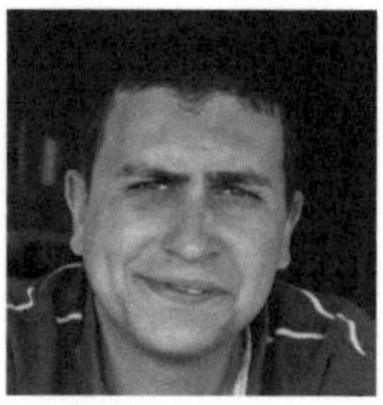

Dr. Jacob Lorenzo-Morales graduated from the Faculty of Biological Sciences at the University of La Laguna (ULL), Tenerife, Canary Islands, Spain in 2001. He was granted a PhD degree in Parasitology in the same University in 2006. Since then he has been working on water-borne and zoonotic diseases (mainly protozoa) in different institutions such as the University of the West Indies in Jamaica and the University of Edinburgh, Scotland, United Kingdom. Currently he is working as the Senior Researcher at the University Institute of Tropical Diseases and Public Health of the Canary Islands, ULL. His interests and areas of research are epidemiology, molecular biology and therapy against emerging pathogens such as free-living amoebae and zoonotic parasites. Dr. Lorenzo-Morales is the author of more than 30 papers and chapters in international journals and books.

ZOONOSIS

Edited by **Jacob Lorenzo-Morales**

Zoonosis
Edited by Jacob Lorenzo-Morales

Published by InTech
Janeza Trdine 9, 51000 Rijeka, Croatia

Publishing Process Manager Sasa Leporic

Technical Editor Teodora Smiljanic

Cover Designer InTech Design Team

Additional hard copies can be obtained from orders@intechopen.com

Zoonosis, Edited by Jacob Lorenzo-Morales
p. cm.
ISBN 978-953-51-0479-7

For EU product safety concerns:
IN TECH d.o.o., Prolaz Marije Krucifikse Kozulić 3, 51000 Rijeka, Croatia,
info@intechopen.com or visit our website at intechopen.com.

Contents

Preface

A zoonosis (derived from New Latin, *zoo-* animal -+ Greek *nosos* –disease-) is defined as an infection or disease that is transmissible from animals (vertebrates) to human beings. Sometimes there is also a vector involved in the transmission. Nevertheless, animals play a main role in maintaining the infections in nature. Zoonotic diseases are mainly due to bacterial, viral or parasitic agents although "unconventional agents "such as prions could also be involved in zoonotic diseases. Many of the zoonotic diseases are a public health concern but also affect the production of food of animal origin and thus they could cause problems in the international trade of animal-origin goods. A major factor contributing to the emergence of new zoonotic pathogens in human populations is the increased contact between humans and animals. This is mainly due to either by encroachment of human activity into wilderness areas or by movement of wild animals into areas of human activity due to anthropological or environmental disturbances. For all the described issues above, some zoonotic diseases are emerging or re-emerging worldwide, thus the importance of these diseases worldwide is gaining major concern within the clinical and veterinarian point of view. This book covers different aspects of zoonotic diseases from epidemiology to some of the major zoonotic bacterial, viral and parasitic agents worldwide.

The first part of this book covers one of the most important aspects of any zoonotic pathogen study which is the epidemiology and monitoring of these diseases. Different epidemiological approaches are covered in chapter I of this book. The other sections (chapter II) of this book are dedicated to bacterial (leptospirosis, brucellosis, anthrax) and viral zoonotic agents of high importance all over the world. Parasitic agents (protozoa and nematode) are discussed and reviewed in chapters III and IV including emerging and re-emerging zoonotic diseases affecting the world population and animal origin goods international trade.

Finally and taking into account the effect of zoonosis in the veterinary and farming field, the last section of the book is dedicated to zoonotic agents affecting pets and farm animals. These pathogens are causing enormous economical damages all over the world.

Therefore, the authors and the editor of this book hope that the work compiled in it would help to raise awareness and interest in this field and also help researchers, clinicians and other readers in their investigations, clinical usage and as a source of information for any other aspects that zoonotic agents could be affecting.

Dr. Jacob Lorenzo-Morales
Senior Researcher at the University Institute
of Tropical Diseases and Public Health of the Canary Islands, ULL
Spain

Part 1

Managerial Epidemiology

1

Managerial Epidemiology and Zoonoses: Application of Managerial Epidemiology in Control of Zoonotic Disease in Bosnia and Herzegovina

Semra Čavaljuga
The Faculty of Medicine, University of Sarajevo, Bosnia and Herzegovina

1. Introduction

1.1 How to define managerial epidemiology?

Managerial epidemiology is rather new subdiscipline of epidemiology defined by Fos and Fine (2005) as: the use of epidemiology for designing and managing the health care of populations—the study of distribution and determinants of health and disease, including injuries and accidents, in specified populations and the application of this study to the promotion of health, prevention, and control of disease, the design of health care services to meet population needs, and the elaboration of health policy.

In order to fully understand all benefits in using management knowledge, approaches and skills merged with knowledge and practice of epidemiology let us consider several most frequently used definitions of management:

- Management is an activity performed by people for organizations (Gram, 1991),
- Management is a process of getting things done through and with people (Liebler, 1999),
- Management is the planning, organizing, leading and controlling of resources to achieve organizational goals effectively and efficiently (Jones, 1998),
- Management is a process of modelling and sustaining of environment in which individuals work together in teams efficiently to reach targeted goals. (Weinrich, 1994)

If we were to simplify this, we would say that management is a process of making and implementation of decisions through and with people.

Similar to the case of definitions of term *management*, epidemiology is described in various terms,most recently as:

- a study of the distribution and determinants of diseases and injuries in human populations (Mausner and Kramer, 1985).
- a branch of medicine which deals with incidence, distribution and possible control of diseases and other factors relating to health (Oxford English Dictionary, 2011)

- a study of the distribution and determinants of health-related states or events in specified populations and the application of this study to the control of health problems (Last, 2001).

By the Last's definition (2001), »study« includes surveillance, observation, hypothesis testing, analytic research, and the experiments; »distribution« refers to analysis by the time, place and classes of persons affected; and »determinants« are all physical, biological, social, cultural, and behavioural factors that influence health.

Management science theory is a contemporary approach to management that focuses on the use of rigorous, quantitative techniques to help managers make maximum use of all resources to produce the best from them for the benefits of a company and its stakeholders. This approach includes various quantitative approaches to decision-making processes and is characterized by an interdisciplinary systemic approach. One of the examples is managerial epidemiology, which tries to combine epidemiology, with its main focus of interest in the population health control and disease prevention and application of management quantitative approaches. This is a challenge not fully answered yet. Having in mind the development of epidemiology – from merely observing and describing interesting health-related events having the status of epidemics or just having some common characteristics among all cases (e.g. cholera in London 1854; Measles on the Faroe Islands 1846; Studies of smoking habits of Doll and Hill, 1947 and 1951) and today we can speak easily on observational and experimental studies conducted respecting all rules of applied epidemiological methods and there developments in the last 50 years, one can expect some similar development of managerial epidemiology too.

It has been an undisputed fact for more than a century that epidemiology is a main public health discipline. There is hardly any population health status assessment or strategy or a policy developed and/or changed without use of basic epidemiology principles.

2. Basics of application of epidemiological principles in the assessment of health status of populations

Many epidemiologists throughout the globe will say when explaining their daily work that they are searching for answers to 5 simple questions: who, what, where, why and how.

First step in any managerial epidemiology activity is gathering information on population. It includes measurements of morbidity and mortality rates, particularly incidence rates (both cumulative and incidence rate) and prevalence rates. Disease frequency measurement is the basic point for any health status assessment. Absence of such data would make any proper assessment difficult, if possible at all.

Starting point of any situation analysis is application of descriptive epidemiology principles and its three primary objectives in order to find a spreading pattern, as disease does not occur randomly, but rather in patterns that reflect the mode of operation of underlying factors. Description of the pattern by each of the characteristics requires a description of the three categories: person, place, time. These characteristics may directly or indirectly relate to the occurrence of a disease or event. In investigation of zoonotic disease outbreaks among humans, important facts necessary to establish would be contacts with animals or animal products, or, for some illnesses, presence in some specific area.

An analytic study immediately and inevitably follows the descriptive study. Descriptive studies are used to identify health related problems and define number of cases and distribution of the disease within a population and serve to formulate a hypothesis of disease outbreak source and way(s) of transition. Analytic studies are concerned with disease determinants, and with very special methodology used in hypothesis testing, acceptance or rejection in order to confirm or reject the source or way(s) of transmission defined by the descriptive study. Case - control and cohort studies are particularly useful in zoonotic diseases outbreaks, such as food borne outbreaks.

Descriptive studies or both descriptive and analytic studies are used as a basis for any planning, monitoring and evaluation of a prevention and/or control activity.

In management of infectious diseases probably the most important epidemiological principle to observe is surveillance. It is an ongoing systematic collection, analysis and interpretation of outcome-specific data for use in planning, implementation and evaluation of public health practice (Thacker, 2000). All health care systems worldwide have established some kind of surveillance system for communicable diseases as structured systems for disease data collection. In order to meet its objectives, public health surveillance system, particularly surveillance of communicable diseases, should be legislated. It is very important to differentiate between monitoring and surveillance: unlike monitoring process, data obtained from surveillance system is considered information for action. Only with undertaking actions based on surveillance system findings of an event, such event can be modified. Modification usually means the end of disease transmission and outbreak or epidemic is called off.

Strict observance of all the above mentioned basic epidemiological principles not only that makes health managers daily life easier, but also contributes significantly to population health status. If managers use modern management techniques, practice and skills, they will help health care system in making the best use of its resources to fulfil goals, objectives and/or targets in disease prevention and/or control.

Having said this, we can also define managerial epidemiology application of basic epidemiological principles using modern management techniques, practices and skills in a disease prevention and/or control.

3. Application of managerial epidemiology in control of zoonotic disease in Bosnia and Herzegovina

3.1 Surveillance of communicable disease in Bosnia and Herzegovina

To understand the communicable diseases surveillance system in Bosnia and Herzegovina (B&H), the enduring consequences of the 1992-1995 war and of the Dayton peace agreement must be taken into account. These consequences include a substantial decrease in human population, massive outward migration and widespread social problems. B&H is also a country still in transition from a communist regime and suffers substantial weaknesses in public administration, taxation system, public services funding and general economy. The Dayton peace agreement provided neither the legal framework for constitution of the ministry of health or agriculture at the state level and instead delegated the responsibilities for most of governmental functions related to health, food safety and agriculture to the three state entities, the Federation of Bosnia and Herzegovina (FB&H) and Republic of Srpska (RS) and the independent district of Brcko (DB). This, coupled with a distinct lack of coordination between all involved stakeholders, has presented a major handicap to the country's overall development during the post war period (Čavaljuga et al, 2009a).

In addition, communicable disease surveillance, and/or public health surveillance in general, in developing countries such is B&H is marked by some specific issues:

- human health care system organization is as an integral part of government services,
- communicable diseases surveillance systems are independent for two branches-veterinary and human health medicine.

As described in that 2009 paper on the development of communicable diseases surveillance in Bosnia and Herzegovina through one health approach regarding reporting of communicable diseases in B&H nothing has being change significantly until present days: communicable disease reporting has being legislated throughout entire B&H for all administrative part: District of Brčko (DB), Federation of Bosnia and Hercegovina (FB&H) and Republic of Srpska (RS). In FB&H according to the Law on population protection against communicable diseases total of 84 diseases are mandatory for reporting; out of that almost 50% are zoonotic (Legislation FB&H 2005). In RS reporting of communicable diseases has being legislated by the Law on population protection against communicable diseases from 2010 (Legislation RS, 2010) - a total of 57 diseases and syndromes or diseases groups are mandatory for reporting. At the national - B&H level - there is no unified legislation or common list of communicable diseases required for reporting. Surveillance system is not based on case definition - there is no case definition standards implemented in the country, but case defining and reporting is done based on the clinical signs and symptoms according to the ICD 10th revision and is highly dependent on physician/clinician personal assessment and therefore variable. There is no laboratory-based surveillance and reporting to epidemiological departments; microbiological laboratories send their clinical results to the referral physicians only. This brings the question whether system of surveillance of communicable diseases exists at all. That is the reason why this paper we discusses reporting of a disease more than surveillance of diseases.

When in the second half of the last century a decrease in number of communicable diseases was reported in B&H as well as in the rest of the world, particularly „classic" zoonoses such as anthrax and rabies, an opinion was formed that prevention, treatment and, of course, control of communicable diseases, were not important or necessary anymore. However, such opinions were proved wrong when in Bosnia, like in the rest of the world, an increase in number of cases of unknown or hardly known diseases with no previous reports or sporadic reports has been recorded.

As opposed to the veterinary sector, there is no national mandate for human communicable diseases reporting and control in B&H. Consequently, there is no unified system of surveillance for communicable diseases for the country. Health care finance, management and organization are the responsibilities of each of the state entities and each of them operates a separate health care system under their own authority. Accordingly, B&H has thirteen ministries of health for an estimated population of slightly more than four million people (B&H Agency for Statistics, 2010).

3.2 A brief overview of the situation with zoonosis in Bosnia and Herzegovina

World Health Organisation (WHO) defines zoonosis as any disease and/or infection which is naturally "transmissible from vertebrate animals to man" (WHO, 1959), and emerging zoonosis as "a zoonosis that is newly recognized or newly evolved, or that has occurred previously but shows an increase in incidence or expansion in geographical, host or vector range" (WHO/FAO/OIE, 2004a). In paper of Čavaljuga (2008) the current situation on zoonotic diseases in Bosnia and Herzegovina was analysed with reflection to up-to-date knowledge on human pathogens and zoonosis.

There are many research publications discussing known number of human pathogens, their structure and level of emergence. The range of the total number of human pathogens, according to such publications (Taylor et al., 2001, Hart; 2008, Woolhouse and Gowtage-Sequeria, 2005) varies from 1,407 to 1,870 with similar percentage of zoonosis within: 58-69%. Publication on the research conducted 2005 by Woolhouse and Gowtage-Sequeria met all criteria Čavaljuga was researching in 2008 in order to study the spread in Bosnia and Herzegovina of diseases with known human pathogens - pathogens that can infect more than one host, matching the WHO definition of emerging diseases; human pathogens with taxonomic classifications, defined by the WHO and the Centers for Disease Control and Prevention (CDC) criteria. The study survey identified 1,407 recognized species of human pathogens (Woolhouse and Gowtage-Sequeria, 2005). Out of them, according to the same research, 816 - 58% - were proved to be zoonotic; with the interesting fact that of the total 177 were regarded as emerging or reemerging and 130 or 77% of them were found to be zoonotic.

The list of emerging diseases is massive and all predictions say it will continue to increase in the future. About 600 human pathogens were found in the last 30 years (Hart, 2008), as a result of science improvement and technological achievements. The grow this partly due to some other factors such as jumping from one species to another - like in the case of bovine spongiform encephalopathy (BSE) or Sin Nombre virus. Factors leading to such results are also mutations, natural selection and evolution processes, environmental changes, climate changes, increase in travel and transportation, but the role of the host factors cannot be neglected, particularly with behavioural and practice changes leading to immunity changes. It is not disputable that, regarding the growth of zoonotic diseases, growth in animal population for human consumption resulted in increase of animal zoonosis cases. Adaptability of microorganisms to various and changeable environmental factors should be taken into account as other contributing factor. The novel influenza strain virus - Influenza A(H1N1) 2009 pandemic should be seen as event already proving such hypothesis.

3.3 Zoonotic diseases in humans

Major animal diseases with zoonotic potential in B&H by Čavaljuga et al in 2009 and based in greater part on her previous researches (Čavaljuga, 2008, 2009a) according to the both human and animal health reports are: Anthrax, Brucellosis, Leptospirosis, Rabies, Q fever, Tuberculosis, and Trichinellosis, while consequent human cases were reported for Leptospirosis, Q fever, Brucellosis and Trichinellosis, with substantial number of contact/exposure to Rabies but without recorded clinical cases in humans. In addition several zoonotic diseases that are not covered by the national animal diseases reporting systems are occurring in human population in B&H (e.g., Hemorrhagic fever with renal syndrome (HFRS)). Many of these diseases may be considered as emerging according to the above given definitions since no or few cases of these diseases were reported for the area of B&H in period before 1995.

Table 1 contains reported frequency of human cases of zoonotic diseases for the period 2001-2010.

As the figures given in the Table 1 demonstrate, an increasing trend in case frequency is present for contact and exposure to rabies and Brucellosis, while the number of cases of Leptospirosis, Q fever, Trichinellosis and HFRS vary without presenting an obvious trend.

Disease \ year	2001	2002	2003	2004	2005	2006	2007	2008	2009	2010*
Leptospirosis	26	40	15	11	79	56	32	41	22	9
Q fever	18	250	29	314	60	71	69	30	30	15
Contact and exposure to rabies	59	16	173	151	141	140	140	151	145	156
Brucellosis	5	14	48	90	137	156	513	994	460	25
Trichinellosis	41	110	75	68	82	23	47	17	32	0
HFRS	8	143	9	6	17	10	10	16	5	2

Table 1. Reported frequency of human cases of Leptospirosis, Q fever, Brucellosis and Trichinellosis along with frequency for contact/exposure to rabies for period 2001 - 2010 (source: SFOR/EUFOR Communicable diseases bulletins, 2001 - 2010)

3.4 Zoonotic diseases in animals

B&H did not have the central level administration and national disease control and surveillance plan during the period from 1995 to 2003. This created a negative influence on the animal health situation and isolated the country from regional and international markets for animals and animal products. Reliable animal disease data were almost non-existent during the immediate post-war period (Cornwell et al, 2000). Initially, disease information was passively acquired. Collection was sporadic and most commonly initiated in response to public pressure. The usual response to a disease outbreak was implemented through a policy of test and removal of positive animals. This was hampered by a lack of sufficient funding for farmer's compensation resulting in limited reporting of disease suspicion by animal caretakers. The following zoonotic diseases were reported by sources from entity's and DB veterinary sectors: Anthrax, Brucellosis, Leptospirosis, Rabies, Q fever, Tuberculosis, and Trichinellosis; as shown in Table 2. The most remarkable are the figures on brucellosis cases both in large and small ruminant population, but also steady presence of rabies in domestic and wild animals (predominantly foxes). Other diseases listed in the table were present in animal population in B&H on sporadic or endemic levels. It is very important to point to the decline in number of Brucellosis cases among animals as well as in humans as direct result of all the prevention and control measure used by respecting application of both the epidemiological and management principles by all sectors and levels.

Disease \ year	2001	2002	2003	2004	2005	2006	2007	2008	2009	2010
Anthrax	-	3	1	-	3	-	-	2	-	11
Brucellosis-small ruminants	16	11	168	787	838	2.263	6.830	22.122	2.426	294
Brucellosis- cattle	28	47	4	28	48	32	76	260	214	99
Leptospirosis	106	93	18	34	10	15	24	1	1	1
Rabies - wild animals	68	55	60	39	35	64	51	85	44	36
Rabies - domestic animals	26	15	15	17	5	13	9	20	28	11
Q fever	448	98	220	184	122	166	11	21	2	411
Tuberculosis	3	1	4	2	1	-	-	2	45	4
Trichinellosis	180	158	164	156	146	146	202	91	58	66

Table 2. Data on frequency of zoonotic diseases in animal population in B&H from 2001 to 2010 (animal health data base, State Veterinary Office of B&H)

3.5 A common–one health–approach to the prevention and control of zoonoses in B&H

Improvements in functioning of the animal health sector became apparent after the State Veterinary Office of B&H was established in December 2000, under the Ministry of foreign trade and economic relations of the national government. Since then, measurable efforts have been implemented within country's veterinary administration with the aim to fulfil the requirements for accession to the World Trade Organization (WTO) and harmonization with animal health standards of the European Union (EU). However, one of the main goals still remains to reassess the current animal disease information system and adjust it to prevailing surveillance requirements.

Simultaneously, but independently, work has been done to strengthen surveillance of communicable diseases systems in the human health sector in accordance with WHO and EU standards. Even superficial comparations of the above zoonosis data in B&H collected independently from animal and human sectors proved the necessity of future coordination of activities between animal health and public health agencies. This has been underscored during the last decade situation with Avian Influenza and potential threat of a pandemic influenza new strains. Baring in mind that at least 61% of all human pathogens are zoonotic, and have represented 75% of all emerging pathogens during the past decade (Acha et al, 2003) prevention activities for Avian and Pandemic Influeza in B&H have shown possible that a common approach can and should be used. This is true not only for this particular disease, but also more widely on all zoonosis. This common approach fits the widely and globally propagated "one health" concept. This concept represents a more holistic approach to preventing disease for the benefit of humans and their domesticated animals.

The quoted studies Čavaljuga in 2008 and 2009 and updates until 2010 (presented in tables 1 and 2) indicate, as the most interesting, the data on brucellosis. Until 2000 only sporadic cases were reported (Gaon in 1952, described first 2 cases in BiH, and one more outbreak with about

40 cases was recorded in 1985 on mountain Manjača near Banjaluka (RS)) (Gaon et al 1989, Dautović-Krkić et al, 2006). Brucellosis outbreak investigation in 2000 proved that Brucellosis first appeared among persons who got the donated animals at the area of Zenica-Doboj Canton (Dautović-Krkić et al, 2006). Afterwards, due to mobility of small ruminants - commonly sheep as major hosts of brucelloses in B&H - outbreak slowly spread to the epidemic throughout entire B&H (FB&H & RS Bulletins, 2000-2010, CDC, 2007). Today, brucellosis in Bosnia and Herzegovina is considered endemic. In all outbreak investigations and analyses commonly made only in FB&H until 2007 and starting from 2007 in RS as well, the most dominant mode of transmission was direct contact with sick animals, found among more than 90% of cases (FB&H & RS Bulletins, 2000-2010). Number of brucellosis cases among both humans and animals was significantly increasing in the observed period, according to the findings of Čavaljuga in 2008 - particularly during 2006 and 2007, reaching their pick by the end of 2008: 994[1]. Morbidity rates (such as incidence) cannot yet not be calculated with relevant precision, as denominator - population number - is only estimated, and the last population census in B&H was done 1991. The data on brucellosis from 1996 to 2007 were extrapolated using Holt's linear trend method, as greater significance is given to the recent data for the most optimal period by this method, which was 4 years for all analysed diseases, based on the known data for 12 previous years. Trend for brucellosis among humans showed almost exponential growth. The original graph is presented as graph 1.

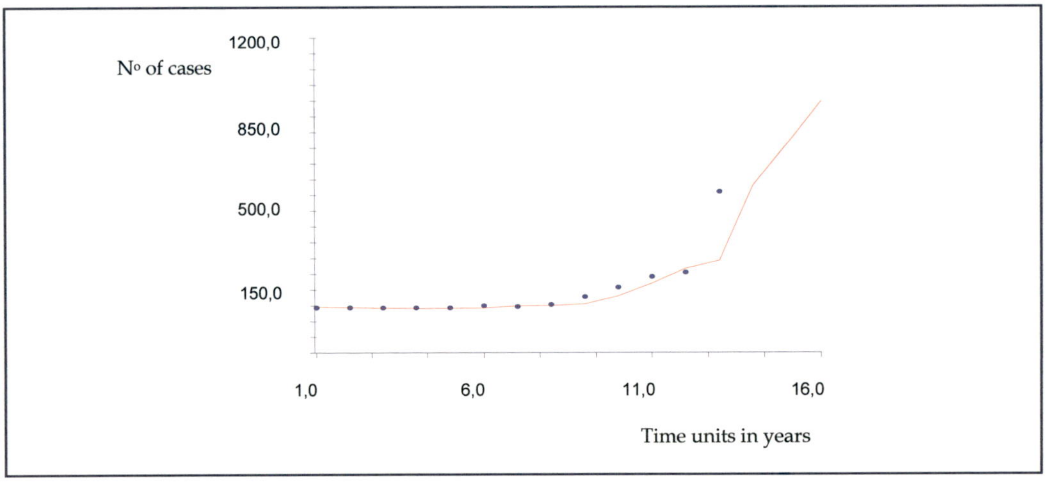

Source: Cavaljuga, 2008

Graph 1. Brucellosis human cases in B&H trend – based on data 1996-2007

Based on the presented numbers it is easy to conclude that adequate control and prevention measures were not undertaken. However, regardless of almost 500 cases in FB&H in 2007, and even more in first 6 months of 2008 (when the research was conducted and paper was submitted for publication) an outbreak/epidemic has never being called on for the

[1] This data was not included in the cited paper from 2008, as the paper was submitted for publication July 2008. Thus, 2008 number of reported cases was not included in the extrapolation.

Federation, but only for most attacked cantons. In order to undertake adequate control and prevention measures it was necessary to call the situation an outbreak. In her paper in 2008, Čavaljuga concluded: "...strategy of disrupting this pathogen transmission from sick animal to human with long term strategy of brucellosis elimination is something B&H still has not developed. Recommended steps for action are given, among other recommendations, in the report of the CDC team mission conducted in July 2007 (CDC, 2007): introducing standardized case definition for this (but to for the other diseases as well) implemented as recommended by WHO/EU Communicable Diseases Surveillance Guidelines (WHO, 2006); set laboratory criteria for classification of confirmed, possible and suspect cases according to the WHO and EU recommendations (WHO, 2006); introduce regular training for all physicians and all relevant heath workers for a case recognition and reporting, as well as additional training in use of analytical epidemiology and laboratory techniques; and, perhaps the most important: zoonotic diseases investigation should be conducted in both human and animal sectors. Some 1,200 cases of brucellosis in 2011 is not only a result of statistical extrapolation, but reality. Severity of clinical signs and symptoms indicate that each case costs, directly or indirectly, 1,000 BAM (B&H currency, about 510 Euros) at the minimum. The question is can we afford not to do anything despite the fact that at this moment brucellosis is the only emerging zoonosis at this moment in Bosnia and Herzegovina?"

The following is the story on brucellosis in Bosnia after 2008: the outbreak was admitted but never official proclaimed by the respective entity governments as by the end of 2008 the total number of reported cases was 994, and almost all the suggested measures were undertaken. Laboratory capacities were strengthened, all professionals involved in the brucellosis investigation, treatment, prevention and control were trained using different methodologies, and veterinarian sectors increased their efforts as well as level of activities in control the disease among animals. Major activities started in 2009. With the strong funding support by the Swedish Development Agency and the Swedish Embassy that enabled purchasing animal brucellosis vaccines through public procurement procedure as well as equipment and supplies required for implementation of sheep vaccination program activities. All competent agencies from the veterinary sector in B&H were actively involved in implementation.

The result of the described implementation of relevant managerial and epidemiological principles in human health protection is easily seen from table 1: number of registered human cases in 2010 was 25 and in sheep 294.

There are other examples on implementation of various epidemiological principles with managerial approach in health status assessment or strategy/policy developed or changed in disease prevention and/or control, such as the study on flock level risk factors for ovine brucellosis in several cantons of Bosnia and Herzegovina (Šerić-Haračić et al, 2009). It also contributed to the previously mentioned successful story on fight against brucellosis epidemic in Bosnia and Herzegovina.

Brucellosis reports in recent years indicated an increase in the number of reported outbreaks in ruminants, especially sheep. The objective of such studies was to investigate risk factors associated with the brucellosis status of sheep flocks in several cantons of Bosnia and Herzegovina. A cross-sectional study was conducted on 138 sheep flocks during the period of July-September 2005. The brucellosis status of the flocks was established through serological testing of serum samples using Rose Bengal and complement fixation tests applied in series. Data on risk factors were obtained through a study questionnaire. Risk factor analysis was performed using logistic regression analysis. The brucellosis risk factors identified were those usually associated with traditional management of small ruminant flocks in this region. It was concluded by the authors that the risk based approach to the disease surveillance would increase the overall sensitivity of the disease detection and allow more effective allocation of limited resources for disease containment. However, in order to reach comprehensive and scientifically based disease detection program, further investigation of disease epidemiology are needed. Following this study, future studies were suggested as needed to reliably establish small ruminant brucellosis prevalence and incidence in the country and investigate specific relationship between brucellosis in humans in animals. That would improve the market competitiveness of domestic sheep production by increasing consumer trust, and most importantly, help in prevention of human cases.

Another one is describing conducted case control study of food borne illnesses in humans in the central region of Bosnia and Herzegovina during 2006 (Čavaljuga et al, 2009b). As part of the feasibility study for the Regional center for food, agriculture and veterinary medicine, financed by the EU RED (Regional Economic Development) fund, a random survey of population sample in Srednjobosanski and Zeničko- dobojski canton, was conducted during 2006. In the overall sample of participants investigators identified cases (families with recorded cases of food borne illnesses in previous year) and controls. Cases and controls were matched one on one, according to the family size (number of adults and children), education level of adults and category of monthly income. Investigated outcome was recorded dichotomously and numerically, as well as the type and kind of the incriminated food source and severity of clinical symptoms. The study showed that nowadays, food represents much higher risk for human health despite increased attention given to the food safety by today's consumers, producers and food inspectors. The study was conducted to prove that integration and industrialization of food production chain and implementation of the surveillance system "form stable to table" has decreased frequency of outbreaks of food born diseases and concurrently increased magnitude of their consequences (number of cases, severity of clinical symptoms, antimicrobial resistance etc.). The lack of a uniform reporting system on food borne illnesses in humans, under- reporting and poor communication between veterinary and public health sectors in Bosnia and Herzegovina (B&H) additionally impair insight into the state and size of the problems in this area. Certain progress in forming and strengthening of the institutional capacities as well as recent frequent occurrences of "food poisoning" had have huge impact on reaffirmation of the needs for systematic epidemiological research in the area of food safety.

Although number of food borne illnesses cases was not quite high, there are not yet - by the end of 2011 - a uniform reporting system for both sectors – human and animals.

4. Instead of a conclusion

There are various risk factors which contribute to the emergence and spread of zoonotic diseases including social, technological, ecological and microbial. However, the greatest risk factor may be the existence of inadequately resourced and ill-prepared public and animal health systems, as well as the lack of a well-coordinated and effective global surveillance and response mechanisms (WHO/FAO/OIE, 2004b).

In B&H, the first step in overcoming any specific or general disease threat is strengthening the communicable disease surveillance systems and methodology for both human and animal sector at the national level. In addition, reliable surveillance systems in both sectors should serve simultaneously as an early epidemic warning system and provide the objective rationale for public health intervention. Early detection of communicable diseases and immediate public health intervention can curtail the numbers of communicable illnesses, deaths and negative effects on both national and international health, travel and trade (Čavaljuga et al, 2009a).

In the post-war period B&H, a country in transition has been dependent on international assistance given separately to both sectors by various international and development organizations towards meeting international standards for animal and public health. The most significant and sustainable contribution by international parties to both sectors was and still is the improvement of diagnostic capabilities and transfer of the most advanced knowledge on epidemiology principles with disease surveillance planning. In order to promote and strengthen linkages between animal and human health sectors in the country which proved by the cited publications and studies as very successful strategy to fight against zoonotic diseases, a more active role needs to be taken in learning and exploiting modern managerial techniques, knowledge, principles and skills and implementing those ones in realization of common priorities and goals.

If not done through merging all available resources including knowledge and experience in humans as the most powerful as well as the cheapest resource of all - team approach and work in systemic planning and complementary actions and in development of infrastructure and expertise around public health and veterinary system - one health -control and/or prevention of any communicable disease, particularly zoonotic diseases will fail to meet its general purpose of optimal, high-quality and cost-effective protection of human health and welfare.

To be proficient in a field of science is good, but to be proficient in many fields is an accomplishment!

5. References

(Bulletins) Bilteni o kretanju zaraznih bolesti, Institut za zaštitu zdravlja RS, 2000-2010.

(Bulletins) Bilteni o kretanju zaraznih bolesti. Zavod za javno zdravstvo FBiH, 2000-2010.

(Legislation)- Zakon o zaštiti stanovništva od zaraznih bolesti, Službene novine Federacije BiH, 18 May 2005; 29/05

(Legislation) Zakon o zaštiti stanovništva od zaraznih bolesti. Službeni glasnik RS, 25 Jan 2010; 14/10.

Acha, PN., Szyfres, B. (2003). Zoonoses and Communicable Diseases Common to Man and Animals, 3rd edition. PAHO Publications,.

CDC. (2007). Epidemiologic and Laboratory Capacity for Human and Animal Brucellosis, Q fever, and Salmonelloses: Bosnia and Herzegovina, Final Report. - by the author's personal correspondence

Cornwell, S., Ferizbegović, J., Fejzić, N. (2000) Veterinary Challenges in a Transitional Economy. In: the 9th Symposium of the International Society for Veterinary Epidemiology and Economics. Breckenridge, Colorado.

Čavaljuga S. (2008). Zoonoses in Bosnia and Herzegovina: Is there any emerging among humans. *Folia Medica Facultatis Medicinae Universitatis Saraeviensis,* 43, 2, 77-83

Čavaljuga, S., Šerić-Haračić, S., Vasilj, I., Fejzić, N. (2009a) Development of communicable diseases surveillance infrastructure for zoonoses in Bosnia and Herzegovina - A common approach? *HealthMED,* 3: 2, 183-189-

Čavaljuga, S., Šerić-Haračić, S., Fejzić, N., Smajlović, M., Gorančić, E. (2009b) Case control study of foodborn illneses in humans in the central region of Bosnia and Herzegovina durring 2006. *Veterinaria,* 58: 1-2; 29-37.

Gaon, JA., Borjanović, S., Vuković, B., Turić, A., Puvačić, Z. (1989) Specijalna epidemiologija zaraznih bolesti. Svjetlost, Sarajevo

Hart, CA. Zoonoses, University of Liverpool, Velika Britanija [*18 August 2008*]. Available at URL: http://www.sibthorp.org.uk/downloads

Krkić-Dautović, S., Mehanić, S., Ferhatović, M., Čavaljuga, S. (2006) Brucellosis epidemiological and clinical aspects (Is brucellosis a major public health problem in Bosnia and Herzegovina?), *Bosn J Basic Med Sci.* 6, 2:11-5

Oxford English Dictionary, [*15 Nov 2011*] available at: http://oxforddictionaries.com/definition/epidemiology

SFOR/EUFOR (2001 - 2010). Communicable diseases bulletins.

Šerić-Haračić, S., Salman, M., Fejzić, N., Čavaljuga, S. (2008) Brucellosis of ruminants in Bosnia and Herzegovina: disease status, past experiences and initiation of a new surveillance strategy. *Bosn J Basic Med Sci.;* 8,1:27-33.

Taylor, LH., Latham, SM., and Woolhouse, ME. (2001). Risk factors for human disease emergence. Philos Trans R Soc Lond B Biol Sci. 356, 1411: 983–989

Thacker, S. (2000). Historical development. In: *Principles and practice of public health surveillance. Second edition.* Teutch S, Churchill RE, editors. pp. (1-16). OUP, Oxford.

WHO/EU (2006). Communicable Disease Surveillance Guidelines for Bosnia and Herzegovina, WHO.

WHO/FAO/OIE. (2004a). Consultation on Emerging Infectious Diseases. May [*15 Nov 2011*] Available at: http://www.who.int/mediacentre/news/briefings/2004/mb3/en/

WHO/FAO/OIE. (2004b).Joint consultation on emerging zoonotic diseases. Geneva, Switzerland,

Woolhouse, MEJ., Gowtage-Sequeria, S. (2005) Host range and emerging and reemerging pathogens. *Emerg Infect Dis* 12, 11,

World Health Organization. Zoonoses. Technical report series no. 169. Geneva: The Organization; 1959

2

Health Adjusted Life Years (HALY) – A Promising Measure to Estimate the Burden of Zoonotic Diseases on Human Health?

Dietrich Plass[1], Paulo Pinheiro[1] and Marie-Josée Mangen[2]
[1]*University of Bielefeld,*
[2]*University Medical Centre Utrecht (UMCU),*
[1]*Germany*
[2]*Netherlands*

1. Introduction

Reliable, comprehensive and comparable information on the impact of (zoonotic) diseases on population health are important for policy decision making in Public Health to support allocation processes of scarce resources with best available evidence. Although the availability and quality of health data has increased in the recent past (Boerma et al. 2007, Murray, 2007), there are still relevant limitations when traditional health indicators are used to prioritize diseases and to allocate resources for intervention measures. Difficulties especially come up when comparisons over time, between sub-groups or even between diseases are intended.

In the past, major efforts have been made to describe adverse health effects on population level by using traditional epidemiological indicators such as mortality and the derivative life expectancies (e.g. Greenberg et al. 1989; Shi 1993). Infant mortality rates, life expectancies at birth and other indicators from this group are estimated using information on mortality and thus only reflect the fatal contribution to disease burdens. The morbidity of human populations is usually assessed by using incidence or prevalence measures, giving no information on the severity of the disease for human health. Comparability of disease impacts on the health of populations and health related quality of life is limited due to the characteristics and the large variety of indicators. Composite measures such as Health Adjusted Life Years (HALYs) aspire a comprehensive and comparable description of the burden of disease by integrating the impact of both, mortality and morbidity on population health. Especially for zoonoses which can significantly contribute to mortality as well as morbidity, the concept of HALYs can be a helpful technique to comprehensively assess the burden of disease. In addition HALYs can also be an useful metric for the intangible costs of morbidity and mortality to be used in economic analyses evaluating potential control programs for zoonotic diseases considering also their impact on human health.

Zoonoses were historically defined as diseases only affecting the animal species. In a postulate from 1959 the World Health Organization (WHO) defines zoonotic diseases as an "(...) infection that is naturally transmissible from vertebrates to humans (...)." Further, "(...)

zoonoses may be bacterial, viral or parasitic, or may involve unconventional agents (...)" (WHO, 1959). This definition, still in use, highlights that there is the need to concentrate on two major hosts (animals and humans) that can be affected by various types of agents. Currently, more than 200 zoonotic disease entities, with highly heterogeneous clinical and epidemiological characteristics are known and cause adverse health effects in both humans and animals (Krauss et al. 2004; Palmer et al. 1998). Zoonoses, as well as other infectious diseases play a major role in countries that are characterized by low- and middle income levels. But also so-called high-income countries are not free of threats by zoonotic diseases as has been shown in the recent epidemics of Q-fever in the Netherlands, with more than 999 reported cases in humans in 2008, the largest known Q-fever epidemic so far in the world (VWA, 2011). Inadequate hygienic conditions, close contacts with animals and raw animal products are potential transmission routes for zoonotic diseases.

Several epidemiologic indicators were used to describe the impact of zoonoses on population health (e.g tick-borne encephalitis in Russia; Tokarevich et al. 2011). However, a comprehensive and comparable assessment of zoonoses is a still ongoing effort. In the first Global Burden of Disease and Injury (GBD) Study the impact of 108 disease conditions was estimated for 192 WHO member states (Murray & Lopez, 1996) – a groundbreaking study estimating the health status of the world's population. The GBD study estimated the disease burden of highly heterogeneous disease entities including 27 disease entities defined as infectious diseases. Using the strict definition of natural transmission from animals to humans, 20 of these 27 disease entities can also be classified as zoonoses (Coleman, 2002). In the GBD study the Disability Adjusted Life Years (DALY) was used as the unit of measure to quantify the impact of diseases on population health. The DALY measure belongs to the family of HALYs and was thus considered qualified to comprehensively assess the global burden of disease.

Since the first GBD study, HALY measures and especially the DALY have increasingly been used in Public Health to inform about the overall health status of a population, and to support policy-decision-making processes and/or research priorities. The term HALY covers a broad range of measures that have the feature in common to quantify, both the impact of morbidity and premature mortality, due to diseases (e.g. zoonotic diseases) or other hazards on human population health (Lopez et al. 2006; Mathers et al. 2007). HALY measures have widely been used in human burden of disease (BoD) studies but have also been applied in cost-effectiveness analyses to assess human health-related outcomes resulting when evaluating intervention programs (Zinstag et al. 2007; Roth et al. 2003).

This chapter therefore aims at giving an introduction to the concept of HALYs and discussing their applicability for zoonotic diseases. The first part of the chapter (section 2) will introduce the main ideas and applications of burden of disease analyses and further provide an overview of HALYs. In section 3 major focus is put on the DALY measure. As the DALY was initially developed for the GBD study, a part of this section is dedicated to the main concepts and ideas of the GBD study and will introduce current estimates of zoonoses as presented by the WHO, using the latest estimates available for the year 2004. Section 4 will then give a short overview of studies that used DALY as an outcome-measure to present the disease burden of zoonotic agents and discuss the suitability and usefulness of the HALYs when used for estimating the burden of disease due to zoonotic pathogens. In section 5 we will present and discuss the use of DALYs in cost-effectiveness analyses.

2. Burden of Disease (BoD)

In this section we will introduce the main ideas and applications of burden of disease analyses. Also we will provide an overview of HALYs putting major focus on the DALY measure.

2.1 Burden of Disease – A rationale

In the field of Public Health there is no unambiguous definition and understanding of the term and idea of burden of disease. Burden of disease or the sometimes synonymously used phrase "burden of ill-health" are mainly used to describe heterogeneous concepts that have the idea in common to assess and quantify the impact of adverse health effects on human health (Connecticut Department of Public Health, 1999). Since the early 1990s the term "Burden of Disease" has become closely related and associated with the framework of the Global Burden of Disease and Injury project (GBD) that was jointly initiated and conducted by the WHO, the Harvard School of Public Health and the World Bank. This first and groundbreaking GBD study provided a first comprehensive and comparable overview of disease burden patterns for 192 WHO member states, included both disease and injury conditions, and allowed for stratification by age, sex and WHO regions. The main aims of the GBD study were to provide consistent, comprehensive and globally comparable estimates of the impact of mortality and non-fatal health outcomes on population health. In addition to the first estimates for the year 1990, the GBD project has introduced the public health community to a new conceptual and methodological framework to integrate, validate and analyze incomplete or fragmentary information on disease and injury consequences. The BoD concept as it was used in the GBD study was comprehensively defined by Colin Mathers as:

"a standardized framework for integrating all available information on mortality, cause of death, individual health status, and condition-specific epidemiology to provide an overview of the levels of population health and the causes of loss of health" (Mathers, 2006).

According to this definition BoD can be understood as a conceptual and methodological framework that aims at providing a consistent and comprehensive assessment of disease and injury consequences in humans by combining several sources (mortality and morbidity) of information on the health status of a population. The BoD framework further makes use of composite measures also known as Summary Measures of Population Health (SMPH) for comprehensive assessments of the disease burden (Field & Gold, 1998).

The results and concepts introduced by the first GBD study – though having been critically discussed - have increasingly been used in several countries to provide information for disease prioritizing and health policy decision making processes (e.g. Arnesen & Nord, 1999; Anhand & Hanson, 1997; Arnesen & Kapiriri, 2004). Since the first GBD study the results and methodology were disseminated throughout the public health community and updated results of the GBD study for the years 2000, 2001 and 2004 were generated and are publicly available (Mathers et al. 2003; Lopez et al. 2006; WHO, 2008a). Additionally to the GBD results, the concept was used in several national burden of disease assessments (USA, The Netherland, South Africa) and assessments related to specific disease entities (chikungunya, dengue, foodborne pathogens) (e.g. Melse et al. 2000; Bradshaw et al. 2003; Kemmeren et al. 2006; Michaud et al. 2006; Lier & Havelaar 2007; Krishnamoorthy et al.

2009; Luz et. al 2009). The majority of all these studies used the DALY measure to quantify the impact of various conditions on population health. The DALY is one of the most frequently used and increasingly accepted measure of the HALY family.

2.2 Health adjusted life years – Concepts and definitions

In the literature, three terms are used synonymously to describe population health measures that include both mortality and morbidity information: Health Adjusted Life Years, Summary Measures of Population Health and Composite Health Measures. HALYs are defined by Gold and colleagues as measures "(…) that allow the combined impact of death and morbidity to be considered simultaneously." (Gold et al. 2002). With this characterization HALY share their definition with the so called summary measures of population health (SMPH) which are systematically defined by Field and Gold as:

"Measures that combine information on mortality and non fatal health-outcomes to represent the health of a particular population as a single numerical index"
(Field & Gold, 1998)

According to the definitions both HALY and the more systematized SMPH, have the feature in common to include information on mortality and morbidity and to represent the health situation of a particular population by a complementary measure. These features enable HALYs for comparisons of populations, diseases and interventions and thus present HALYs as being qualified for disease burden assessments.

HALYs can be broadly divided into two major branches - health expectancies and health gaps. Health expectancy measures estimate the time span expected to live in full health taking the impact of disabling conditions on health related quality of life into account (Mathers, 2002). Health expectancies can be understood as an extended idea of the life expectancy indicator that additionally includes morbidity information. A wide of range of health expectancy measures are available and used to quantify healthy life expectancy patterns of various populations. Healthy Life Years (HLY), Disability Free Life expectancy (DFLE) and Disability Adjusted Life Expectancy (DALE) are exemplary entities that have frequently been used in the past. Technically, these measures are built upon the so called Sullivan method, which requires a period life table based on age- and sex- specific death counts in a population and the implementation of information on age- and sex-specific prevalence of people living in a state that is considered to be less than full health (Sullivan, 1966). The HLYs are e.g. used by the European Union as a structural indicator to describe the health situation of the European population (Jagger et al. 2008). Using the same underlying method, DFLE and DALE mainly differ in their definition and quantification of disability. The DFLE uses a dichotomous definition presenting as disability or no disability. In contrast, the DALE measure uses a graduated valuation of severity and includes so called disability weights. The DALE was introduced as a component of the GBD study to elucidate the life expectancies of populations when considering the underlying prevalence of disability (Murray & Lopez 1997; Mathers et al. 2001).

Another well-established member from the group of health expectancies is the Quality Adjusted Life Year (QALY) that is frequently used in the field of health economics. The QALY was developed by economists, operations researchers, and psychologists and is mainly used in cost-effectiveness analyses to quantify the intangible costs of bad health and premature mortality. Using the QALY in cost-effectiveness analyses allows for assessing the effect of a certain intervention measure (e.g. preventive or curative) by calculating the QALYs gained resulting from positive intervention effects. One QALY can be seen as one year lived in perfect health. Quality of life in the QALY concept is defined as "utility", a measure of preference that people assign to health outcomes. The quality scale of the QALY ranges from death (0) and a state of perfect health (1) (Gold et al. 2002). The QALY has been used as outcome measure in numerous cost-effectiveness and cost-utility analyses all over the world and is mainly associated with the field of health economics. But in particular in high-income countries QALYs, which are data-intensive, has become a standard tool in health technology assessment studies (Belli et al., 1998). QALYs are widely used for diseases like cancer, whereas for infectious diseases there no, or only poor QALYs available, and in particular for infants and children (WHO, 2008b).

In contrast to health expectancies, health gaps measure the time of healthy life lost due to certain disease or injury conditions. The health gaps as a normative measure use a predefined (arbitrarily set or observed) health goal that is expected to be reached by a certain population. Having this normative feature, health gaps then can be used to quantify the difference between the ideal health and the current patterns observed in a population. Figure 1 shows the conceptual framework of health gap measures. In this figures a survivorship curve of a hypothetical initial birth cohort is presented. The x-axis shows age in years and the y-axis the percentage of the hypothetical population surviving over a lifespan of 100 years. The upper curve in the figure indicates for each age along the x-axis the proportion of the hypothetical cohort that will remain alive at that age and includes people living in an ideal health state as well as people living in a state worse than perfect health.

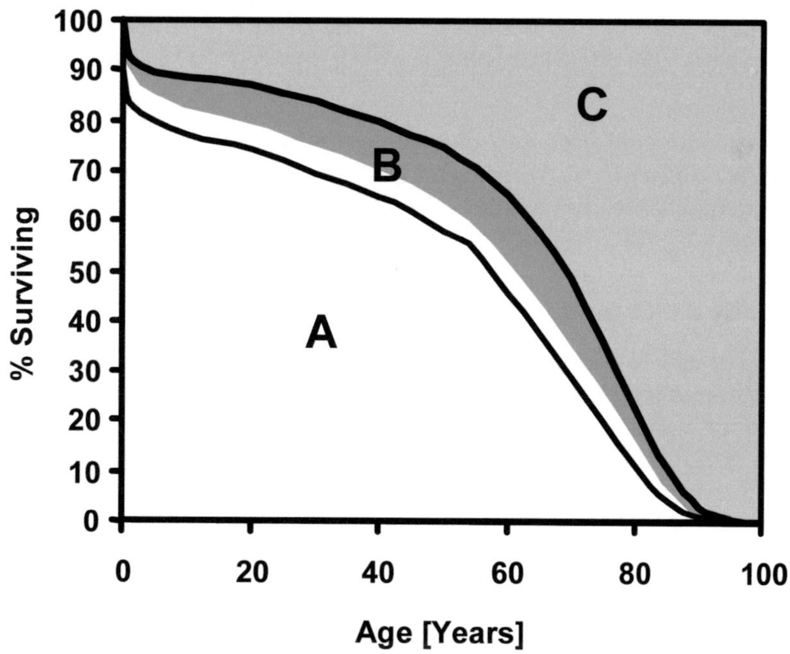

Fig. 1. Basic understanding of the complementary measures - health gaps and health expectancies (modified according to WHO, 2001)

Having identified the percentage of people living in optimal health and people living in health states less than full, an additional second curve (in this example indicated by the lower curve) can be drawn in order to allow for estimates of the burden due to non-fatal health outcomes. Also, setting the health goal and identifying the population in health states less than full will result in the delineation of three areas. While areas A and B under the survivorship curve can be used to derive e.g. life expectancy at birth, health expectancies can be derived from these areas by taking into account some lower weights for area B, i.e. the years lived in health states worse than perfect. As health gaps measure health losses, additional information on the normative health goal is needed to assess the difference between the current health of the population and the potential goal for population health. In figure 1, the health goal is represented by the upper horizontal line enclosing area C. Thus, it is in this particular case assumed that every person in this hypothetical cohort lives in ideal health until the age of 100 years. By adding this health goal, health losses due to both mortality and morbidity can be derived. In figure 1, the losses due to mortality are represented by the area C. Health losses due to living in health states worse than perfect are assessed by adding the upper part of area B to the losses in area C due premature mortality. The size of the part of area B is estimated by using weighting factors, the so called disability weights that estimate the severity of the impact of a certain disease or injury condition. The weights are anchored on a scale from scale between 0 and 1, with zero indicating a state of full health and 1 associated with a state that is comparable to death.

Summing up both health expectancies and health gaps are qualified to present the health status of populations. Health expectancies are using a positive quantification of expected years in full health and health gaps are using a normative description to inform about health losses due to mortality effects and additional impacts of non-fatal health outcomes. For the health expectancies the QALY measure is the one most frequently used in the field of economics to assess the cost-effectiveness of e.g. preventive or curative interventions measures.

One of the most commonly used and globally accepted members of the health gap family are the Disability Adjusted Life Years developed and used as the core measure in the first and all sub-sequent GBD studies to assess the disease burden of a wide range of disease and injury conditions.

3. The Disability Adjusted Life Year (DALY)

The DALY as a member of the health gap family quantifies losses of healthy life years according to a normative health goal. This measure provides estimates of the burden of disease by using a single number reflecting the comprehensive negative impact of heterogeneous conditions on human health. Understanding and interpreting DALY estimates requires having a look beyond the DALY's methodological curtain. The DALY offers several optional inputs, when calculating the disease burden and thus requires to be well informed about how the particular DALY is constructed. Therefore, the following section aims at a) providing detailed information on the DALY concept and b) presenting the complexity of the measure that is needed to comprehensively understand and correctly interpret the DALY estimates. In addition, this chapter will also provide a critical discussion on the use of the DALY for estimating the disease burden of infectious diseases and zoonotic diseases in particular.

The DALY measure as it was used for several regional, national and local burden of disease assessments was initially developed to meet the GBD study objectives (Begg et al. 2007, Michaud et al. 2006 , Murray, 1994). Tailored according to this needs the DALY was introduced as a measure that allows for incorporating effects of mortality and morbidity on health and thus for comprehensively and comparably quantifying health losses globally in one single measurement unit (Murray & Lopez, 1996). One general assumption that was met in the GBD study to allow for e.g. cross-national comparisons was to treat like events occurring in different settings (e.g. countries, socio-economic environments, living conditions) equally. Considering this e.g. an amputation of a leg in Zimbabwe should result in the same disease burden as an amputation of a leg in Turkey (Murray, 1994). Different circumstances e.g. living conditions may have effects on how people can cope with a certain disability. An amputation of a leg that requires the use of a wheelchair may have a smaller disabling effect on an individual who is living in developed nation where facilities are handicapped accessible. Irrespective of e.g. the living conditions both events should contribute equally to the overall disease burden and thus need to be treated equally (Murray, 1994). Thus, to assure comparability of different groups or of a certain group over time it was decided to construct the DALY detached from socioeconomic or environmental conditions (Murray, 1994). Technically, the DALY quantifies the disease burden in terms of years of healthy life lost either due to premature death or due to the impact of non-fatal disease outcomes on population health. Time was chosen as the unit of measure in burden of disease assessments because time, as a general unit of measure is qualified for use in a composite health measure as it presents a simple and intuitive method to subsume effects of mortality and morbidity.

The DALY as a summary measure is calculated by combining complementary information from Years of healthy Life Lost due to premature mortality (YLL) representing the fatal component and from Years of healthy Life lost due to Disability (YLD) reflecting the impact of non-fatal health outcomes.

3.1 Years of Life Lost due to premature death (YLL)

The YLLs basically inform about health losses due to impact of fatal disease and injury conditions. Measuring time lost due to premature mortality, the YLLs can be estimated by the use of different approaches that result in different estimates for the numbers of years lost. Before calculating the YLLs, it is therefore needed to define which approach fits best with the underlying research objectives. To calculate the YLLs, it is further essential to define the health goal that then can be used as a reference value to calculate the difference between the ideally expected and the truly observed values and patterns. There are at least two concepts of life-expectancies that can be used for setting up health goals. On the one hand, there is the idea of a potential life expectancy which sets a potential limit to life at e.g. 65 years of age. People who die before having reached this potential limit would then contribute to the YLLs. E.g. a death of a person at 40 years would contribute to 25 years of healthy life lost. These so called Potential Years of Life Lost (PYLL) are e.g. used by the Organization for Economic Co-operation and Development (OECD) as an indicator for the mortality related disease burden. The OECD uses a potential limit of 70 years and estimates lost years according to this reference value (OECD, 2009). In literature, it was argued that the concept of PYLLs neglects deaths beyond the chosen age limit and thus does not take into account mortality patterns of the elderly population. Further, interventions focusing on health of the elderly population would result in no benefit when using PYLLs as primary outcome measure (Murray, 1996).

On the other hand, there is also the idea of using concepts that focus on remaining life expectancies. Calculating remaining life-expectancies requires for setting up life tables. Life tables include information on previously observed mortality patterns and trends in populations and thus are qualified to estimate the life expectancy at a certain age. Having arranged the life expectancies allows for estimating the lost remaining life expectancy for a death at a certain age. Technically, there are different techniques to derive life tables that can be used to estimate Period Expected Years of Life Lost (PEYLL), Cohort Expected Years of Life Lost (CEYLL) or Standard Expected Years of life Lost (SEYLL). PEYLLs are based on a period life table, CEYLL on a cohort life table and SEYLL are based on a standard life table, respectively. The DALYs as used in the GBD study follow the concept of Standard Expected Years of Lost and calculate health losses based on the West Level 26 standard life table (WHO, 2001). This life table was derived for a hypothetical cohort using the highest life expectancy at birth observed for Japanese women at the time of the first GBD study. Thus, life expectancy at birth for women and men was set to 82.5 and 80 years, respectively. The two and a half years difference between men and women does not represent the empirically observed, but was chosen in order to only account for the life expectancy differences that can be explained by biologic factors. It was decided not to include lifestyle related, gender-specific differences such as occupational risks, or increased high risk behavior (alcohol, smoking, injuries) (Murray, 1994). Even though this assumption was discussed in literature, the authors of the GBD project postulated, that using the biological sex difference allows for more balanced estimates of YLLs especially when observing the narrowing of the gender gap in low-mortality, high-income countries (Murray, 1994). Technically, the YLLs in the GBD study are calculated as shown below in the formula by multiplying the number of death cases (N) at a certain age of death with the remaining life (L) expectancy at age of death (x) as taken from the standard life table.

$$YLL = N \times L_x$$

Thus e.g. three female neonatal death would contribute to 3 x 82.5y = 247.5 YLLs. As the SEYLL concept uses remaining life expectancy values even deaths at high ages still contribute to the disease burden and interventions aiming at the elderly population would still possibly result in measureable benefits. The values of the West Level 26 standards life table were used to calculate the disease burden for all 192 WHO member states. It can be argued that using this standard set of values sometimes may over- or underestimate the true and observed life expectancy in a certain country, but having the idea of burden of disease in mind this feature enables the estimates to be compared over time, and between age, sex and country (Murray, 1994).

3.2 Years of Life Lost due to Disability (YLD)

As the main idea of the DALY measure was to comprehensively assess and comparably quantify the disease burden, a second and complementary measure, the Years of Life Lost due to Disability (YLD) was used to describe the impact of disabling conditions primarily non-fatal conditions on population health. There are different concepts of how to describe and quantify the effects of non-fatal health outcomes. The understanding of non-fatal outcomes implemented in the GBD studies is based on the concept of disability as it was defined by the International Classification of Impairments, Disabilities and Handicaps (ICIDH). In the ICIDH of the WHO, disability is described as the lack of ability to perform certain activities in a manner that is normal for human being (WHO, 1980). Using this general definition of disability as a proxy for the impact of conditions on health related quality of life allows for excluding social and environmental aspects. This feature ensures that disabling conditions in different circumstances are measured equally. This narrow definition of disability was used to meet the need for globally comparable information on the impact of disabling conditions.

Further, to assess the impact of diseases and injuries on human health the GBD study provided a set of so called "disability weights" reflecting and quantifying the severity of a disabling condition. Basically, disability weights describe the impact of a disease or an injury on health related quality of life arranged on a scale from zero to one. Zero is representing a status of full health and no disability. In contrast the value one represents life-threatening disability comparable to death. There are different approaches to derive disability weights. Common techniques used are visual analogue scales, methods of standard gambling, person trade-off or time trade-off to derive disability weights in panel settings. These panel settings again may differ in their composition (experts, lay-men and/or patients). Therefore, in literature it was argued that using different panels may result in varying disability weights (Anand & Hanson, 1995). For the GBD study the disability weights were derived for 22 indicator conditions using the person trade-off (PTO) exercise in a group of health professionals who were asked to trade of the life extension of individuals living in different hypothetical health states (Murray & Lopez, 1996). A comprehensive list of disease and injury specific disability weights was presented by Lopez and colleagues (Lopez et al. 2006). Since the first GBD study several additional studies aimed at improving disability weights and resulted in complementary sets of weighting factors (Stouthard et al. 1997; Haagsma et al. 2008; Haagsma et al. 2009). Though, methodological differences do not allow for ad hoc comparisons between the different disability weight sets the studies provide additional (missing) disability weights and introduce methods that allow for more adequate assessment of disability weights. The currently ongoing 2005 update of the GBD study, which is coordinated by the Institute for Health Metrics and Evaluation (IHME) will provide new disability weights based on global panel using an online questionnaire. For more details see (www.globalburden.org).

To calculate the years of life lost due to disability for a particular disease, it is needed to have information on the number of incident cases and the duration of the disease/injury as well as information on the severity of the disease/injury is needed. Technically, the YLDs are calculated using the following simplified formula:

$$YLD = I \times DW \times D$$

In this formula, *I* describes the number of incident cases, *DW* the disability weight (on a scale from 0 to 1) and *D* the duration of the disabling state. According to the formula, e.g. five female cases of mental retardation after a bacterial meningitis with disease onset at 10 years of age would contribute to 5 x 0.483 (DW for mental retardation) x 72,99 y (remaining life expectancy at 10 years from the West Level 26 standard life-table) = 176,3 YLD.

3.3 Calculating DALYs

Having estimated the YLLs and YLDs for a particular disease/injury and a given population, DALYs are then estimated as the sum of both measures.

$$DALY = YLL + YLD$$

3.4 Social value choices

Apart from the disability weights that are used to provide condition-specific preference values, there are two other features of the DALY that can optionally be used to introduce social value choices into the DALY estimates - age-weighting and time-discounting. Both concepts can be incorporated to weigh DALYs reflecting certain preferences about societal concepts.

The time-discounting concept has its source in the field of economics. Basically, time-discounting reflects that most of the people if asked about, prefer benefits today rather than in the future and thus discount the value of future goods (Murray, 1996). It was argued that these preferences can also be applied for health when it is considered as a good. From an individuals' perspective, it was concluded that being healthy today is more worthy then being healthy somewhere in the future. To implement this concept, a 3% time-discount rate was applied in the GBD study to discount future health losses, a rate that is also recommended in the field of economics (Tan-Torres Edejer et al. 2003).

The age-weighting concept is based on the theory of human capital (Drummond, 1997). Human capital describes the value of people for the society they are living in. The main idea of an age-weighting is to provide higher weights to people that are in productive ages (high value for the society because of their roles for economic and social welfare) and lower weights to very young and old people as they are somehow dependent on care and financial support (e.g. pension) of people in productive ages.

In general, the inclusion of social value choices into the DALY has critically been discussed in literature. The main criticism to both of these concepts arises from the ethical perspective. Both age-weighting and time-discounting attach different weightings to years of life lost. Thus for age-weighting e.g. the value of life of an 80 years old person is seen as not of same worth as compared to a person who is 25 (Anand & Hanson 1997). Murray counters this thinking with his view that "unequal age weights (…)" is "(…) an attempt to capture different social roles at different ages " and further, "higher weights for a year of time at a particular age does not mean that the time lived at that age is per se more important to the individual, but that because of social roles the social value of that time may be greater" (Murray, 1994). Thus it is not the worth of a year of an individual, but more the value for society (Murray, 1994). Murray describes the very young and old as being dependent on the rest of society for physical, emotional and financial support. When using both time-discounting and age-weighting one should be aware of possible double counting for certain age groups.

The DALY calculation for the first GBD study used a 3% time discount and non-uniform age-weighting (Murray & Lopez 1996). Since a lot of criticism was expressed the estimates of 2001 and also the most recent update for 2004 were provided using different scenarios with age-weighting and discounting, with age-weighting and no discounting, with discounting but no age-weighting, or even without the inclusion of these social value choices. However data on the scenarios is only publicly available for WHO regions. Country, age and sex specific data for 2004 is only available with non-uniform age-weights and a 3% time discount rate. DALY measure and especially the social value choices were discussed critically. The main results as presented in the WHO's 2004 update document still use a 3% time-discount rate and non-uniform age-weighting (Arnesen & Kapiriri, 2004; Anand & Hanson, 1997; Anand & Hansen, 1998).

3.5 Incidence versus prevalence

DALYs can be based on both incidence and prevalence data. Since the first GBD study, there is an ongoing debate whether to use the incidence or the prevalence approach. For fatal conditions and the calculation of YLLs it is obvious that using incidence data is obligatory. But for YLD both prevalence and incidence data can be used to estimate the impact of non-fatal health events. Using the prevalence approach and thus assuming a steady state for diseases may result in inaccurate DALY estimates. It was further argued, that the dynamic nature of populations and diseases is more adequately reflected by the use of the incidence approach. For the GBD study it was decided to use the incidence approach to provide estimates being more sensitive to changes in disease trends (Murray, 1994).

3.6 DALY estimates of zoonoses in the GBD estimates of 2004

The GBD studies provide comprehensive and comparable estimates on the current burden of disease for the 192 WHO member states and for 108 disease and injury conditions. The most recent estimates published in 2008 present the burden of disease results for the year 2004 (WHO, 2008a). To get a comprehensive overview of the disease burden, a particular disease classification system was compiled for the GBD study. The GBD disease classification system disentangles in a tree-structure with up to four levels of disaggregation. At first level the disease burden is split up by group I, II, and III conditions. Group I conditions represent communicable, maternal, perinatal, and nutritional conditions and thus, include the entities from the zoonotic disease group. Group II conditions include all non-communicable disease entities (e.g. malignant neoplasms, neuropsychiatric conditions). Group III conditions further incorporate all intentional and unintentional injuries. Single disease conditions such as measles or tetanus are arranged at the fourth and last level of disaggregation. The GBD classification system is complementary to the WHO International Classification of Diseases revision 9 and 10, allowing for converting ICD coded data to the GBD disease classification system.

For the year 2004, a total of 1.52 billion DALYs were lost worldwide. Of these 1.52 billion DALYs about 730 (48% of the total burden) million DALYs were lost due to group II conditions, 187 (12.3% of the total burden) million DALYs due to group III conditions and 603 (39.7%) million DALYs due to group I conditions, respectively. Highlighting group I conditions, which include infectious and thus also zoonotic diseases about 301 million DALYs (19.8% of total burden) were attributable to infectious and parasitic diseases (WHO, 2008a). According to Coleman, who used WHO GBD data for 1999, 20 of the 27 infectious diseases listed in the 1999 GBD classification system by definition belong to the group of zoonotic infections (Coleman, 2002). 26 of the 27 diseases can also be found in the GBD classification of 2004. Hepatitis, caused by hepatitis E virus was not included in the 2004 GBD update. From the remaining 26 diseases there were then 19 conditions related to zoonotic origin. Thus, about 193 million DALYs (64.2% of the infectious burden) can be attributed to these 19 conditions. Figure 2 shows the percental distribution of the disease burden of those 19 disease entities sharing the definition of zoonotic diseases.

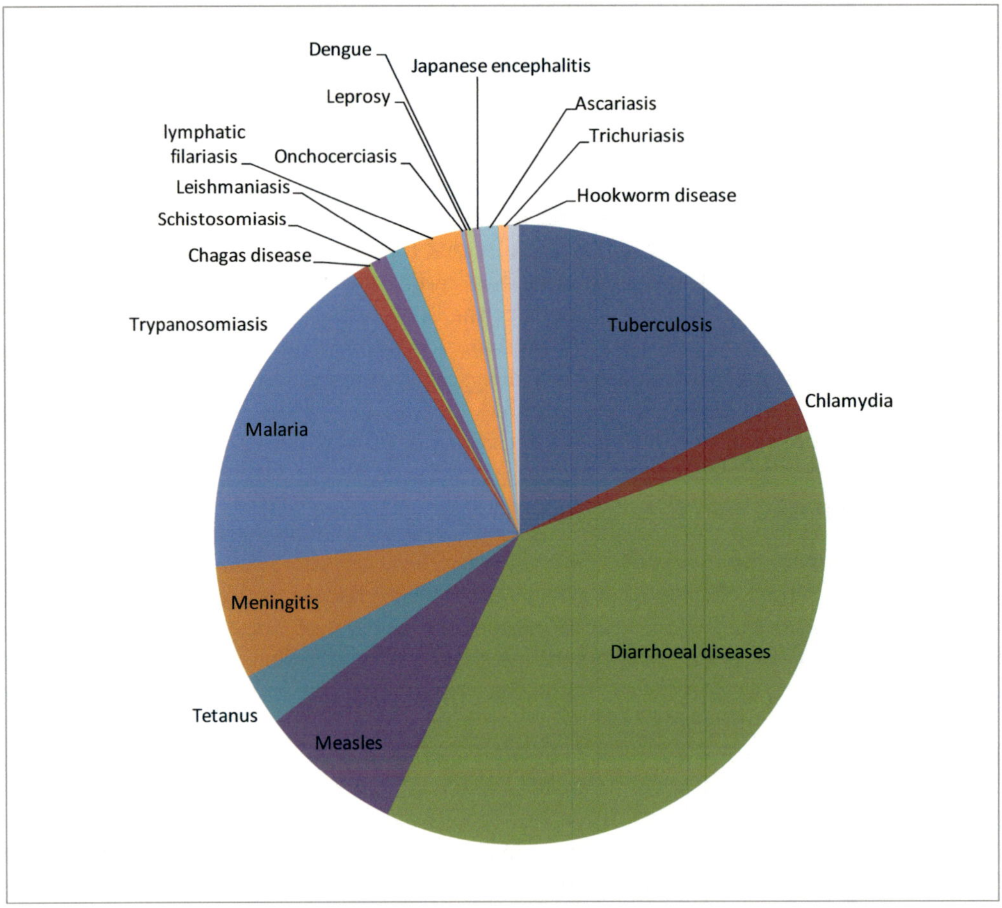

Fig. 2. Percental distribution of disease burden (120 Mio. DALY) due to zoonotic diseases

The figure indicates diarrheal diseases, tuberculosis, and malaria with 37.5, 17.7 and 17.5% as the major drivers of the zoonotic disease burden. Looking at the transmission cycle of the zoonotic disease described in figure one the entities can further be subdivided in two subgroups. 13 of the 19 zoonotic diseases can be attributed to the group with antrhoponotic (human-to-animal; human-to-human) transmission and for the remaining 6 diseases (trypanosomosis, schistosomiasis, leishmaniasis, chagas disease, Japanese B encephalitis, hookworm disease) increased evidence was provided for the high impact of animal-to-human transmissions indicating potential starting points for (veterinary) intervention measures to reduce the transmission and disease burden (Coleman, 2002).

The results of the Global Burden of Disease study indicate a high relevance of zoonoses for human health, including so-called food- and waterborne pathogens whereby some animals are often a reservoir for infections. The burden estimates for e.g. diarrheal disease also include cases that probably are not induced by a zoonotic agent. Therefore, it can be assumed that when focusing on the definition of Coleman and only using the GBD estimates one may overestimate the disease burden of Zoonoses. However, according to the different transmission cycles of the 19 disease entities, potential intervention measure should not only aim at reduction of human-to-human transmission but also take into account intervention measures, starting from the farm and moving to the table, to reduce the global zoonotic disease burden.

4. Using the DALY measure for assessing the disease burden of infectious diseases/zoonoses

In this section we will give a short overview of studies using DALY as an outcome-measure to present the disese burden of zoonotic agents and discuss the suitability and usefulness of the HALYs when used for estimating the burden of disease due to zoonotic pathgoens.

The heterogeneous characteristics and the dynamic nature of infectious diseases raise special requirements towards HALYs. In the GBD study the DALY is used for a set of very heterogeneous conditions such as non-communicable chronic diseases, injuries, or infectious diseases. Having the unique nature of infectious diseases in mind, it was argued that the DALY measure does not adequately capture the whole spectrum of infectious conditions and further seems to underestimate the true burden due to infectious diseases (Zou, 2001; Arnesen & Karpiriri, 2004; ECDC, 2010). As DALYs are based on epidemiological indicators (e.g. incidence, death cases) the quality of DALY estimates is highly dependent on data availability going further than notified data and mortality registration only.

For infectious diseases many countries have set up sophisticated surveillance measures whereby observed cases will have to be notified, but still high rates of under-estimation (under-reporting and under-ascertainment) are observed even in countries with high surveillance standards (Sethi et al. 1999; Wheeler et al. 1999; Food Standard Agency, 2000; Poggensee et al. 2009). Also there are high rates of asymptomatic cases (e.g. hepatitis B and C) not detected and therefore not reported to the health authorities and thus substantially mask the current true infectious disease burden. Having the example of hepatitis B, individuals with an infection who experience an asymptomatic disease course may later progress to severe disease states such as liver cirrhosis and hepatocellular carcinoma. These burdensome entities have a severe and sometime fatal course and thus would contribute to a high disease burden. However, GBD estimates usually take into account only acute symptomatic infectious cases and for most of the diseases neglected the disease burden caused by the sequelae associated with the initial infection. Further, the acute illness data e.g. from mandatory notification systems may be masked by under-estimation and thus only represent a small percentage of the real disease burden. Additionally to incomplete statistics, and inadequate attention towards long-term disease sequelae, coding practices of death cases also hamper the completeness of infectious disease burden as measured in the original GBD study. For example, an incidental death case has to be classified according to the ICD 10 classification system. The etiology of liver cirrhosis allows for multiple causes, such as alcohol use disorder, autoimmune disorders, viral hepatitis and many others. A certain number of deaths cases that result as a consequence from e.g. liver cirrhosis or hepatocellular carcinoma, though induced by a long lasting hepatitis B infection are incorrectly counted as e.g. neoplasms not related to an initial infection (Zou, 2001; Pinheiro et al. 2010). These misdiagnoses may lead to essential underestimation of infectious disease burden.

4.1 Incidence and pathogen-based approach

To better account for infectious disease characteristics several burden of infectious disease studies prefer the use of the so called pathogen-based approach rather than using the disease-specific one from the GBD study (e.g. Havelaar et al. 2004; Mangen et al 2005; Kemmeren et al., 2006; Cressey and Lake, 2007; ECDC, 2010). In the incidence and pathogen-based approach, the initial infection with a pathogen is used as the starting point for disease burden estimations. The pathogen-based approach is mainly based on so called outcome-trees that describe the natural course of a disease (figure 2). Starting with an initial infection the outcome-tree provides transition probabilities that inform about the percentage of people moving from one state to another after being infected by a certain pathogen. Using the outcome-trees allows for including all possible resulting short- and long-term sequelae and thus presenting the detailed pathways of an infection (see figure 2).

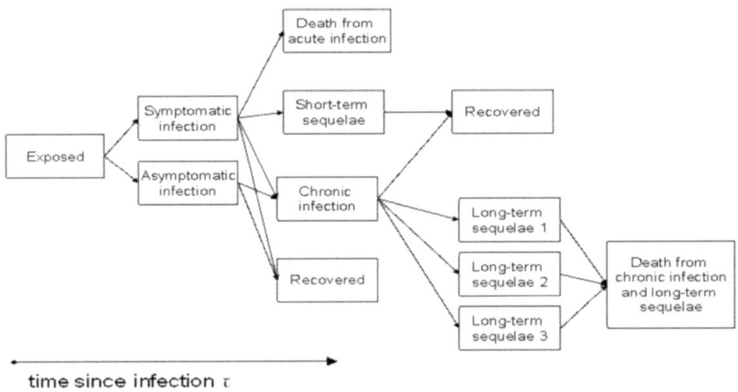

Fig. 3. The standard outcome-tree with possible sequelae (ECDC, 2010)

Using the information about the initial infection the pathogen-based and the included outcome-tree feature allow to comprehensively assess the disease burden due to infectious pathogens. The incidence and pathogen-based DALY approach is currently in use for a European study on infectious diseases (ECDC, 2010). In this study the disease burden of 32 infectious pathogens, including several zoonotic diseases is calculated for the European Union and EEA / EFTA countries (ECDC, 2010).

But next to this European study, there are also some national studies using the incidence and pathogen-approach, in particular for prioritization of foodborne pathogens (e.g. for the Netherlands (Kemmeren et al., 2006; Haagsma et al., 2009; and recently updated by Havelaar et al., 2012); for New Zealand (Cressey and Lake 2007)). In the recent update of Havelaar and colleagues, disease burden for a total of 14 foodborne pathogens was estimated. These were thermophilic Campylobacter spp.; Shiga-toxin producing Escherichia coli O157 (STEC O157); non-typhoidal Salmonella spp.; norovirus; rotavirus; Cryptosporidium spp.; Giardia spp.; C. aureus; Bacillus cereus; Clostridium perfringens; Staphylococcus aureus; hepatitis A virus; hepatitis E virus; Listeria monocytogenes and Toxoplasma gondii. The incidence of community-acquired non-consulting cases, patients consulting their general practitioner, those admitted to hospital, as well as the incidence of sequelae and fatal cases was estimated using surveillance data, cohort studies and published data. Data were combined with results from an expert survey to assess the fraction of cases attributable to food, and the main food groups contributing to transmission. The authors estimated that these fourteen pathogens would have in 2009 accounted for a total of 1.8 million cases of disease (approx. 10,600 per 100,000) and 233 deaths (1.4 per 100,000), resulting in 13,500 DALY (82 DALY per 100,000), or 11,300 DALY if discounted with 1.5% (according to Dutch guidelines) and 9,700 DALY if discounted with 3.5% (according to UK guidelines). Foodborne transmission was responsible for approximately 680,000 cases (approximately 4,100 per 100,000), 78 deaths (0.5 per 100,000) and 5,800 DALY (35 per 100,000) (Havelaar et al., 2012). In particular for pathogens like thermophilic Campylobacter spp.; Shiga-toxin producing Escherichia coli O157 (STEC O157); non-typhoidal Salmonella spp.; Listeria monocytogenes and Toxoplasma gondii did the associated sequelae result in far higher disease burden then if considering acute illness only (Havelaar et al, 2012). All studies that used the incidence and pathogen-based approach highlight the impact of short and long-term sequelae of infectious pathogens on the estimated disease burden. Therefore this approach allows for more comprehensive assessment of infectious disease burden.

4.2 Advantages, weaknesses and challenges of the DALY measure

The advantages of the DALY measure are in short:

- The biggest advantage is that morbidity (YLD) and mortality (YLL) effects are combined in one measure.
- DALY allow the comparison between different health hazards, why prioritization is possible.
- Also the DALY measure offers the ability to assess the impact of prevention strategies (as will be discussed in more detail in the following section)

The weakness of the DALY measure in short are:

- The used disability weights for YLD are based on subjective measures, whereby the applied technique and the used panel (e.g. experts, patients or lay-people) have a strong influence on the obtained disability weights.
- There is an on-going debate over their validity
- The DALY measure is not widely recognized outside the health sector.

The biggest challenges of the DALY measure consist in:

- Getting estimates of the total number of infections in the population due to a particular pathogen.
- When using the incidence and pathogen-based approach, defining the outcome tree with all relevant health outcomes for a particular pathogen.
- Getting appropriated transmission probabilities for the different health outcomes represented in the outcome tree.

5. Use of DALYs in economic analyses

This section will discuss the use of DALY in cost-effectiveness analysis. For a better understanding we will shortly highlight why to conduct an economic analysis; what economics is; list the potential perspectives that can be used in economic evaluations and shortly describe the different types of economic evaluations. Before then discussing the use of DALYs in cost-effectiveness analyses, illustrated by published studies of cost-effectiveness for controlling zoonotic diseases / foodborne pathogens. Foodborne pathogens will be included because they show some similarities with zoonotic diseases. Both have economic effects on all type of stakeholders from the stable to the table, and both affect also human health, though, foodborne pathogens do mostly not affect animal health. Consequently, monetary effects are obvious in several sectors of the society (e.g. farmers, food chain, consumers, health care sector).

5.1 Why conducting an economic analysis?

Once prioritization has taken place, interventions might be planned to tackle the problem. But given that most decision makers have to deal with limited budgets (e.g. the Minister of Health; Animal Health Authorities), the question is: "Which of the potential interventions will yield the best value for the money invested?". In order to answer this question, an economic analysis (e.g. cost-effectiveness analysis) is required (Drummond et al. 1997; Belli et al. 2001), in which either different potential interventions could be compared with each other (e.g. Is it more cost-effective to control Campylobacter at farm level, at slaughterhouse level or at consumer level? (Havelaar et al. 2007)), or a single intervention would be compared with no intervention (e.g. Is it cost-effective to introduce rotavirus vaccination in the National Immunization program? (Mangen et al. 2010a; Esposito et al. 2011)). In such an economic analysis, HALYs could be used to measure the intangible costs of bad health and premature mortality. HALYs and costs are estimated for each intervention separately and then compared. The incremental cost-effectiveness is then calculated in order to determine which intervention will offer the best value for money invested.

5.2 What is economics?

Economics, as a discipline, studies how people and societies make choices about scarce resources that could be used elsewhere or in another way (Belli et al, 2001). The main purpose of an economic analysis is hereby to provide a framework for analyzing the full implications of potential choices. Whereby an economic analysis is most useful if applied before the implementation of a new project, as supporting the decision-making process and identifying poor projects (Belli al. 2001). If conducted after the implementation of a project, economic analysis can only help in the decision of whether or not to continue with a project (Belli et al. 1998).

Opportunity-cost or the potential use of any scarce resource in alternative programs is an important factor in economic analyses. Opportunity-cost is what people give up, now and in the future, to accomplish a particular undertaking (Sassone and Schaffer 1978). The 'return' or 'opportunity' that could have been gained in other projects using the same resources is therefore the real cost of accomplishing an undertaking, not simply the money spend. Therefore opting to use resources for one particular purpose always means giving up the opportunity to use them in other desirable ways. The key question in economics is therefore: Are the benefits from what is 'chosen' greater than what is 'forgone? (Sassone and Schaffer 1978).

5.3 Economic evaluations

A full economic evaluation is characterized by two facts, namely:

- that there is a comparison with at least one alternative, even if this alternative is "do nothing" (or care-as-usual);
- and that both, costs and outcomes of the alternatives are analyzed.

If one of these two conditions is not fulfilled, because either the evaluation considers only costs, or only consequences, or there is no comparator, then it is only a partial evaluation that lacks the context to judge the relative performance of a program.

There are four techniques used to conduct full economic evaluations. These are: cost-minimization analysis (CMA); cost-effectiveness analysis (CEA); cost–utility analysis (CUA) and cost–benefit analysis (CBA). CMA requires equal effectiveness of all programs and is therefore only applied if two or more options have the same outcome (Drummond et al. 1997). Only monetary costs incurring in the alternative programs are considered and compared. Measuring consequences (outcomes) is not necessary. Interventions to control infectious diseases /zoonoses, however, usually have different effects, why CMA is seldom an adequate methodology to apply. Cost-effectiveness analysis is applied to interventions that have a single non-monetary effect, common to all of them but different in magnitude, and which is measured in physical units (Drummond et al. 1997; Belli et al. 1998; Belli et al. 2001). However, all other effects such as costs (inputs) and outcomes of the program under study are measured and evaluated in monetary terms. The ratio of interest in a CEA is then the net cost (monetary costs corrected for monetary benefits) per unit of effect (e.g. the net cost per averted Brucellosis infection; the net cost per averted Q-fever infection of goats, etc.). A big disadvantage of the CEA technique is that a comparison is only possible for program with the same outcome. However this non-monetary single effect is often more meaningful to specialist(s) than e.g. DALYs. Cost–utility analysis or weighted cost-effectiveness analysis is a variation on cost-effectiveness analysis (Belli et al. 2001). Although some authors prefer not to make a distinction between CEA and CUA (Drummond et al. 1997). CUA requires a valuation scheme that combines various effects into a single combined measurement, for which some weighting scheme is required (Belli et al. 2001). E.g. DALYs (disability-adjusted life years) and QALYs (quality-adjusted life years) are such metric units whereby effects on human morbidity and mortality are weighted and transferred into a single metric unit. The CUA methodology is then also widely used in public health economic evaluations (Gold et al. 1996; Drummond et al. 1997; Tan-Torres Edejer et al. 2003; WHO 2008b). All other consequences (costs and benefits), however, are measured and valued in monetary terms, as in a CEA. Also as in the CEA, the results of a cost–utility analysis are expressed in terms of net cost per unit of weighted combined effect (e.g. net costs per DALY averted). The most cost-effective program is the one with the lowest net cost per unit of weighted combined effect. By weighting and combining effects into a weighted unit, CUA allows the comparison of sometimes very different programs, such as vaccination programs and environmental programs. However, the terms (such as health outcome) have to be the same for all programs compared and, as with the CEA methodology, comparison with projects having different non-monetary effects is not possible. Theoretically cost-benefit analysis is the 'gold standard' in economic evaluation (Belli et al. 2001), whereby all effects, both monetary and intangible, direct and indirect, are measured and expressed in monetary terms. CBA results can be presented as net present value, internal rate of return (the remuneration against investment stated as a proportion or percentage) or as cost–benefit ratios. The main advantage of CBA is that all effects are valued in monetary terms, allowing the comparison of a given program with any other program, both in the same sector as well as in different sectors, and is therefore recommended by Belli et al. (2001) when health sector investments are compared with investments in other sectors. Unlike other economic evaluations, CBA allows you to consider allocated efficiency in its widest sense, by comparing the net economic impact of very different activities (Belli et al. 2001). For example, the societal gain from a newly introduced Brucellosis vaccination program of the cattle livestock might be compared with the gain to society from building a bridge. CBA is the most complete quantitative approach from an economic standpoint. However, assigning a monetary value to non-monetary benefits such as human health outcomes is much more complicated. Therefore one of the major problems, and also often the weakness in this type of evaluation, is the valuation of non-monetary factors.

There is no 'ideal' type of economic evaluation. All of them have their limitations. The analyst must therefore first identify the problem, define the boundaries, chose potential alternatives, define the target population (e.g. cattle livestock; children; inhabitants from country *x*; farmers; etc.); define the type of evalutions to evaluate; and choose the most appropriate perspective for answering the question, before then selecting the technique that best answers the question (Belli, Anderson et al. 2001). If the project objective is narrow, such as increasing the number of vaccinated livestock or increasing the number of vaccinated people, then the focus will be only at alternative ways of increasing the number of vaccinated livestock /persons and the success will be judged in terms of the number of vaccinated livestock /persons reached (Belli et al. 2001). Whereas if the program under study tries to achieve a broader objective, such as improvement of health status by e.g. vaccination of goats against Q-fever in order to reduce infections in humans, then in the evaluation we will not only look at alternative ways of reaching a maximum of goats, but also at alternative interventions that might reduce infections in humans, and as such reduce morbidity and mortality of the target human population. The judgment of success of the project is then the impact on human health status.

Therefore starting with a clear definition of the program reduces the number of alternatives to consider, and helps selecting the most appropriated type of evaluation and the performance indicators to look at (Belli, Anderson et al. 2001). The differences between the situation with and without the program are the basis for assessing the incremental costs and benefits of the project (Belli, Anderson et al. 2001), why it is important to clarify what happens if the program is carried out or not. Another important question is about the alternatives. Their choice has a fundamental impact on the type of evaluation, the data collected and the interpretation of the findings (WHO 2008). In the case of zoonoses, interventions might be targeted at the livestock and/or at human health. And might target either the whole human population and/or livestock in a country and geographic area, respectively, or at a specific group of persons/livestock within a country. In all cases does the target group strongly influence the choice of effects considered (monetary and non-monetary), as well as the results of an economic evaluation.

Economic evaluations can be applied at a number of levels. Potential perspectives that are used in public health economic evaluations are: individual perspective (e.g. patient); health care providers (e.g. hospital, doctor, etc.); third payer (i.e. often health insurance perspective); health authorities; manufacturers and society (a country, for example the Netherlands, or the international community, for example the EU; WHO; etc.). However, for zoonoses and foodborne pathogens the impact of these diseases does not only affect human health and as such the health care sector, but has also an impact on other sectors and stakeholders in the society. Therefore, other perspectives might be necessary. For example one of the following perspectives: another authority than health authorities (e.g. in the case of zoonosis it could be the animal health authority or ministry of agriculture, etc.); individual stakeholder affected (e.g. farmer; slaughterhouse; etc); another sector than health care (e.g. farmers' associations, slaughterhouses, or any other stakeholder in the chain or related industry); consumer. The chosen perspective determines which potential costs and consequences to be included in an economic evaluation.

Further should the time frame (the period over which the intervention is applied) and the analytic horizon (the period over which the costs and outcomes that occur as results of the intervention are considered) be long enough to capture all relevant positive and negative effects (WHO 2008b). Their respective durations are influenced by the type of intervention evaluated, the program itself, the target population and the model used (WHO 2008b).

The type of intervention to be analyzed determines what type of epidemiological model is required to capture key elements of the disease. Jit and Brisson (2011) conducted a literature review on infectious diseases and modeling, whereby looking at interventions such as vaccination, screening, social distancing, post-exposure treatment and culling (for animal and plant diseases only). Based on their findings they developed a flow diagram with seven key questions. Based on the answers to these seven key questions the analyst can evaluate which type of model would be the most appropriated choice.

5.4 Cost-effectiveness

After having assessed costs and effects of an intervention, and the comparator, the next step in an economic evaluation is to link these results in the form of a ratio, mostly in the form of an (incremental) cost-effectiveness ratio (ICER).

An ICER compares the differences between the costs and health outcomes of two alternative interventions that compete for the same resources. It is generally described as the additional cost per additional health outcome. The ICER numerator includes the differences in program costs and can include in addition the averted costs, depending on the choice of the perspective. Similarly, the ICER denominator is the difference in the measured effect e.g. DALY:

$$ICER = \left(\frac{C_{Intervention\ A} - C_{Intervention\ B}}{E_{Intervention\ A} - E_{Intervention\ B}}\right)$$

whereby C stays for costs and E for effects.

5.5 Cost-effectiveness studies using DALY in zoonoses and foodborne diseases

Most published cost-effectiveness studies in zoonoses and foodborne diseases are mostly only restricted to animal health and related industry. The impact on human health is seldom considered.

Nevertheless there are a few examples whereby also human health was considered, using DALY to measure the impact of the intervention on human health (e.g. Roth et al 2003; Budke et al 2005; Mangen et al 2007). A nice example of economic evaluations studying the impact of intervention on zoonoses and using DALY to express the intangible costs of bad health and premature mortality is the one by Roth et al. (2003). Using a dynamic model of livestock-to-human brucellosis transmission these authors simulate for Tibet the impact of vaccinating the livestock against brucellosis on the national animal health and national human health, and consequently expressed their results as costs per DALY averted. Another example of such an economic evaluation is the CARMA project (Havelaar et al. 2007; Mangen et al. 2007). These authors studied several interventions controlling campylobacter infections in the Dutch population. They looked at interventions at farm-level; in the slaughterhouse and at consumer level. For all these interventions the effect on human health was measured in averted infections, as well as in averted DALY. But also interventions costs were considered, as well as averted costs due to averted infections were considered in this study.

Both studies are nice demonstrations for the usefulness of the DALY approach in economic evaluations when aiming at measuring the impact of an intervention on human health.

6. Acknowledgment

Part of the work was done within the Burden of Communicable Diseases in Europe (BCoDE) project, a project funded by the European Centre for Disease Prevention and Control (Specific agreement No.1 to Framework Partnership Agreement GRANT/2008/03).
Further thanks go to Prof. Dr. Alexander Krämer as the supervisor of Dietrich Plass.

7. References

Anand S, Hanson K (1997) Disability-adjusted life years: a critical review. Journal of Health Economics; Vol. 16; pp 685–702

Anand S, Hanson K (1998) DALYs: efficiency versus equity. World Development Report; Vol. 26; pp 307–310

Arnesen T, Kapiriri L (2004). Can the value choices in DALYs influence global priority setting? Health policy (Amsterdam, Netherlands) Vol. 70; pp 137–149

Begg S, Voss T, Barker B, Stevenson C, Stanley L, Lopez AD (2007): Burden of Disease and Injury Australia 2003. Australian Institute of Health and Welfare

Belli P, Anderson J, et al. (1998) Handbook on economic analysis of investment operations. New York, Operational Core Services Network, Learning and Leadership Center

Belli P, Anderson JR, et al. (2001) Economic Analysis of Investment Operations Analytical Tools and Practical Applications. Washingtion, D.C., World Bank Institute

Boerma JT, Stansfield SK (2007) Health statistics now: are we making the right investments?" The Lancet; Vol. 369; pp 779-786

Bradshaw D, Groenewald P, Laubscher R, Nannan N, Nojilana B, Norman R, Pieterse D, Schneider M, Bourne DE, Timaeus IM, Dorrington R, Johnson L (2003) Initial burden of disease estimates for South Africa, 2000. South African Medical Journal. 38 Vol. 93; pp 682–688

Budke CM, Jiamin Q, et al. (2005) Economic effects of echinococcosis in a disease endemic region of the Tibetan Plateau. Am J Trop Med Hyg 73(1): 2-10

Coleman PG (2002) Zoonotic diseases and their impact on the poor. Appendix 9 In: Perry BD, McDermott JJ, Randolph TF, Sones KR, Thornton PK (2002). Investing in Animal Health Research to Alleviate Poverty. International 1 Livestock Research Institute (ILRI), Nairobi, Kenya.

Connecticut Department of Public Health (1999) Looking Toward 2000 - An Assessment of Health Status and Health Services; Hartford, Connecticut, page 368

Cressey PJ and Lake R (2008) Risk ranking: Estimates of the burden of foodborne disease for New Zealand. Institute of Environmental Science & Research Limited; Christchurch Science Center; http://www.foodsafety.govt.nz/elibrary/industry/risk-ranking-estimatesresearch-projects/FW07102_COI_estimates.pdf

Drummond MF (1997) Methods for the Economic Evaluation of Health Care Programmes. Oxford: Oxford University Press

Esposito DH, Tate JE, et al. (2011) Projected impact and cost-effectiveness of a rotavirus vaccination program in India, 2008. Clin Infect Dis 52(2); pp 171-177

European Centre for Disease Prevention and Control (2010) Methodology protocol for estimating burden of communicable diseases. Stockholm: European Centre for 19 Disease Prevention and Control (ECDC).
http://ecdc.europa.eu/en/publications/Publications/1106_TER_Burden_of_disea se.pdf

Field MJ, Gold MR (1998) Summarizing Population Health - Directions for the Development and Application of Population Metrics. Washington DC; National Academy Press

Food Standards Agency (2000) A Report of the Study of Infectious Intestinal Disease in England. Food Standards AgencyLondon: HMSO

Gold MR, Stevenson D, Fryback DG (2002). HALYS AND QALYS AND DALYS, OH MY: Similarities and Differences in Summary Measures of Population Health. Annual Review of Public Health; Vol. 23; pp 115–134

Gold MR, Siegel JE, et al. (1996) Cost-Effectiveness in Health and Medicine. New York, Oxford University Press, Inc

Greenberg AE, Ntumbanzondo M, Ntula N, Mawa L, Howell J, Davachi F (1989) Hospital based surveillance of malaria-related morbidity and mortality in Kinshasa, Zaire. Bulletin of the World Health Organisation; Vol. 67; pp 189–196

Havelaar AH, van Duynhoven YT, Nauta MJ, Bouwknegt M, Heuvelink AE, de Wit GA, Nieuwenhuizen MG, van de Kar N (2004) Disease burden in The Netherlands due to infections with Shiga toxin-producing Escherichia coli O157. Epidemiol Infect 132(3); pp 467-484

Havelaar AH, Mangen MJ, et al. (2007) Effectiveness and efficiency of controlling Campylobacter on broiler chicken meat. Risk Anal 27(4); pp 831-844

Havelaar AH, Haagsma JA, Mangen M-JJ, Kemmeren JM, Verhoef LP, Vijgen SM, Wilson M, Friesema IH, Kortbeek LM, Van Duynhoven YT, Van Pelt W (2012) Disease burden of foodborne pathogens in the Netherlands, 2009. International Journal of Food Microbiology (in press)

Jagger C, Gillies C, Moscone F, Cambois E, Van Oyen H, Nusselder W, Robine JM; EHLEIS team (2008) Inequalities in healthy life years in the 25 countries of the European Union in 2005: a cross-national meta-regression analysis. Lancet; Vol. 372; pp 2124–2 2131

Jit M and Brisson M (2011) Modelling the epidemiology of infectious diseases for decision analysis: a primer. Pharmacoeconomics 29(5); pp 371-86

Kemmeren JM, Mangen MJJ, van Duynhoven YTHP, HavelaarAH (2006) Priority setting of foodborne pathogens: disease burden and costs of selected enteric pathogens.

Bilthoven: National Institute of Public Health and Environment: RIVM rapport 330080001; Available online at: www.rivm.nl/bibliotheek/rapporten/330080001.pdf

Krauss H, Weber A, Enders B, Schiefer HG, Slenczka W, Zahner H (1997) Zoonosen. Von Tier zu Mensch übertragene Infektionskrankheiten. Deutscher Ärzte-Verlag

Krishnamoorthy K, Harichandrakumar KT, Krishna KA, Das LK (2009) Burden of chikungunya in India: estimates of disability adjusted life years (DALY) lost in 2006 epidemic. Indian Journal of Vector Bourne Diseases; Vol. 46; pp 26–35

Lopez AD, Mathers CD, Ezzati M, Jamison DT, Murray CJL (2006) Global and regional burden of disease and risk factors, 2001: systematic analysis of population health data. The Lancet Vol. 367; pp 1747–1757

Luz PM, Grinsztejn B, Galvani AP (2009) Disability adjusted life years lost to dengue in Brazil. Journal of Tropical Medicine and International Health Vol. 14; pp 237–246

Mangen M-JJ, Havelaar AH, Bernsen RAJAM, van Koningsveld R, de Wit GA (2005). The costs of human Campylobacter infections and sequelae in the Netherlands: A DALY and cost-of-illness approach. Acta Agriculturae Scandinavica Section C Food Economics 2(1); pp 35-51

Mangen MJ, Havelaar AH, et al. (2007) Cost-utility analysis to control Campylobacter on chicken meat: dealing with data limitations. Risk Anal 27(4); pp 815-30

Mangen MJM, van DuynhovenYTHP, et al. (2010a) Is it cost-effective to introduce rotavirus vaccination in the Dutch national immunization program? Vaccine 28(14); pp 2624-2635

Mangen MJM, Batz B, et al. (2010b) Integrated Approaches for the Public Health Prioritization of Foodborne and Zoonotic Pathogens. Risk Anal 30(5): 782-797.

Mathers CD (2002) Health expectancies: an overview and critical appraisal. In: Murray CJL, Salomon JA, Mathers CD, Lopez AD (2002) Summary Measures of Population Health; pp 177–204

Mathers CD, Bernard C, Iburg KM, Inoue M, Ma Fat D, Shibuya K, Stein C, Tomijima N, Xu H (2003) Global Burden of Disease in 2002: data sources, methods and results. World Health Organisation, Geneva

Mathers C (2006) Introduction to Burden of Disease. BoD Workshop Bielefeld, January 2006

Mathers CD, Ezzati M, Lopez AD (2007) Measuring the Burden of Neglected Tropical Diseases: The Global Burden of Disease Framework. PLoS Neglected Tropical Diseases; Vol. 1; e114

Mathers CD, Sadana R, Salomon JA, Murray CJL, Lopez AD (2001) Healthy life expectancy in 191 countries, 1999.The Lancet Vol. 357; pp 1685–1691

Melse JM, Essink-Bot ML, Kramers PG, Hoeymans NA (2000) National burden of disease calculation: Dutch disability-adjusted life-years. Dutch Burden of Disease Group; American Journal of Public Health. Vol. 90; pp 1241–1247

Michaud C, McKenna M, Begg S, Tomijima N, Majmudar M, Bulzacchelli 1 M, Ebrahim S, Ezzati M, Salomon J, Gaber Kreiser J, Hogan M, Murray CJL (2006): The burden of disease and injury in the United States; Population Health Metrics; Vol. 4:11

Murray CJL (1994) Quantifying the burden of disease: the technical basis for disability adjusted life years. Bulletin of the World Health Organisation. Vol.: 72; pp 429–445

Murray CJL (1996) Rethinking DALYs. In: Murray CJL, Lopez AD (eds.) The Global Burden of Disease: a comprehensive assessment of mortality and disability from diseases, injuries, and risk factors in 1990 and projected to 2020 (Global burden of disease and injuries series; I). Cambridge, Harvard School of Public Health on behalf of theWorld Health Organization and the World Bank

Murray CJL, Lopez AD (1996) The Global Burden of Disease: a comprehensive assessment of mortality and disability from diseases, injuries, and risk factors in 1990 and projected to 2020 (Global burden of disease and injuries series; I). Cambridge, Harvard School of Public Health on behalf of the World Health Organization and the World Bank

Murray CJL, Lopez AD (1997) The utility of DALYs for public health policy and research: a reply. Bulletin of the World Health Organisation; 1997; Vol. 75; pp 377-381

Murray CJL (2007) Towards good practice for health statistics: lessons from the Millennium Development Goal health indicators. The Lancet; Vol. 369; pp 862-73

Olshansky SJ, Ault AB (1986) The fourth stage of the epidemiologic transition: the age of delayed degenerative diseases. Milbank Quarterly Vol. 64; pp 355-391

Omran AR (1971) The Epidemiologic Transition: A Theory of the Epidemiology of Population Change. The Milbank Memorial Fund Quarterly. Vol. 49; pp 509–538

Organisation for Econcomic Co-operation and Development (2009) Health at a Glance 2009. OECD; Paris (France)

Palmer SR, Lord Soulsby, Simpson DIH (1998) Zoonoses: Biological, Clinical Practice and Public Health Control. Oxford University Press, Oxford, UK. 948 pp

Poggensee G, Reuss A, Reiter S, Siedler A (2009) Overview and assessment of available data sources to determine incidence of vaccine preventable diseases, vaccination coverage, and immune status in Germany. Bundesgesundheitsblatt; Vol. 52; pp 1019-1028

Roth F, Zinstag J, Orkhon D, Chimed-Ochir G, Hutton G, Cosivi O, Garrin G, Otte J (2003) Human Health benefits from livestock vaccination for brucellosis: case study. Bulletin of the World Health Organisation; Vol. 81; pp 867–876

Sassone PW and Schaffer WA (1978) Cost-benefit analysis: a handbook. New York, Academic Press

Sethi D, Wheeler JG, Cowden JM, Rodrigues LC, Socket PN, Roberts JA, Cumberland P, Tompkins DS, Wall PG, Hudson MJ, Roderick PJ (1999) A study on infectious intestinal disease in England: plan and methods of data collection. Communicable Disease and Public Health; Vol. 2; pp 101-107

Shi L (1993) Health care in China: a rural-urban comparison after socioeconomic reforms. Bulletin of the World Health Organisation; Vol. 71; pp 723-736 Smith KR (1988) The Risk Transition. East-West Center

Tan-Torres Edejer T, Baltussen R et al. (2003) Making choices in health: WHO guide to cost-effectiveness analysis. Geneva, World Health Organization

Tokarevich NK, Tronin AA, Blinova OV, Buzinov RV, Boltenkov VP, Yurasova ED, Nurse J (2011) The impact of climate change on the expansion of Ixodes persulcatus habitat and the incidence of tick-borne encephalitis in the north of European Russia. Global Health Action 2011, 4: 8448

van Lier EA, Havelaar AH (2007) Disease burden of infectious disease in Europe: a pilot study Bilthoven. National Institute for Public Health and the Environment. 86 pp. RIVM report 215011001
http://www.rivm.nl/bibliotheek/rapporten/215011001.html; Available online at:

http://www.rivm.nl/bibliotheek/rapporten/215011001.pdf

Wheeler JG, Sethi D, Cowden JM, Wall PC, Rodrigues LC, Tompkins DS, Hudson JM, Roderick JM on behalf of the Infectious Intestinal Disease Study Executive (1999) Study of infectious intestinal disease in England: rates in the community, presenting to general practice, and reported to national surveillance. BMJ; Vol. 318; pp 1046–1050

Voedsel en Waren Autoriteit (VWA) (2011) Eerdere uitbraken van Q-koorts. Ministerie van Economische Zaken, Landbouw en Economie; Voedsel en Waren Autorteit, Den Haag, Netherlands. www.vwa.nl/ondewerpen/dierziekten/dossier/q-koorts/eerdere-uitbraken-vanq-koorts Accessed on: 08-12-2011

World Health Organization (1959) Zoonoses. Second report of the Joint WHO/FAO Expert Committee. WHO, Geneva, Switzerland

World Health Organization (1980) International Classification of Impairments, Disabilities, Handicaps (ICIDH). A manual of classification relating to the consequences of disease. Published for trial purposes in accordance with resolution WHA29.35 of the Twenty- ninth World Health Assembly, May 1976, WHO, Geneva, 1980

World Health Organisation (2001) National Burden of Disease Studies: A practical guide. Edition 2.0. World Health Organisation, Geneva

World Health Organization (2008a) The global burden of disease: 2004 update. World Health Organisation, Geneva

World Health Organization (2008b) WHO guide for standardization of economic evaluations of immunization programmes. Geneva, World Health Organization; Department of Immunization, Vaccines and Biologicals

Zinstag J, Schelling E, Roth F, Bonfoh B, de Savigny D, Tanner M (2007) Human benefits of animal interventions for zoonosis control. Emerging Infectious Diseases; Vol. 13; pp 527–531

Zou S (2001) Applying DALYs to the burden of infectious diseases. Bulletin of the World Health Organisation. Vol. 79 No. 3

3

Sciences of Complexity and Chaos to Analyze Vectors and Zoonosis

Emilio Arch-Tirado and Alfonso Alfaro-Rodríguez
Instituto Nacional de Rehabilitación,
Laboratorio de Bioacústica, Mexico D.F.
Mexico

1. Introduction

In the late 1960s and early 1970s of the recently past century were consolidated the Sciences of complexity and chaos[1]. Complexity seems to follow a path through which the primary energy was transformed into particles, particles were amended and a force converted into atoms, molecules and atoms in molecules is polymerized into complex structures that are self-replication . There seems to also be a tangential force that includes information and knowledge [2].

On the other hand, chaos can be deterministic and non-deterministic. The first can predict their behavior although it can not be inferred, i.e., the number of external variables that infer it makes it almost impossible to manipulate, but you can know what will be the final behavior of the system. Likewise, we have the not deterministic, in that, as its name indicates it, the direction to take the system cannot be predicted, or the short life of human beings will not reach to analyse the final behavior of the system [3].

Dynamic systems are complex systems of elements which interact not only with the elements in the system, but also relations among them. It is known that some systems operate in a linear fashion that its action can be predicted by the information relating to its point of starting and its rules of operation. Many systems apparently deterministic can be regulated or extremely unpredictable. The chaos theory, to put it in some way, with two branches, the first emphasizes the hidden order that exists in a system called chaotic system; the second branch refers to the process of self-regulation and self-control spontaneous [4].

Lorenz contribution to knowledge of complex systems and the condition that can be chaotic is very important; Lorenz discovered, among other things, the fundamental characteristics of the systems that help us better understand what is known as chaos; Likewise, described the so-called Strange Attractors, which is popularly exemplify as "the butterfly effect", which refers to how a minimal variation in the initial conditions of a system can result in a totally unexpected effect, which would be equivalent to the idea of the "flutter of this insect in the Amazon could produce a storm a month later in Chicago". Lorenz contribution to knowledge of complex systems and the condition that can be chaotic is very important;

Lorenz discovered, among other things, the fundamental characteristics of the systems that help us better understand what is known as chaos; Likewise, described the so-called Strange Attractors, which is popularly exemplify as "the butterfly effect", which refers to how a minimal variation in the initial conditions of a system can result in a totally unexpected effect, which would be equivalent to the idea of the "flutter of this insect in the Amazon could produce a storm a month later in Chicago". This nomination is based on that there are many attractors in a given system, which increasingly are generating more changes in initial conditions, in this way each system is prone to certain attractors, such is the case of the large number of variables in the environment which in turn affect directly or indirectly in the system[5,6].

Bioterrorism is defined as the release or use of any microorganism, virus, infectious substance or biological product that may be modified as a result of biotechnology, natural or by components of bioengineering in any microorganism, virus, infectious substance, or biological product that can cause death, disease or disability in people, animals, plants or other living organisms 7,8,9 intentional. This paper aims to discuss and analyse the role of chaos in the proliferation of vectors and zoonosis induced and stochastic processes. The father of the linearity is Issac Newton; in its third Act set out that "every action has a reaction of the same magnitude but in the opposite direction", meaning a cause for effect. It is said that chaos theory breaks the paradigm of the linearity and Newtonian physics [10].

One of the basic foundations in the theory of chaos is that many independent variables affect a single dependent variable, i.e. many causes for a single effect [11, 12]. In chaotic systems the large number of independent variables present makes impossible their manipulation for what are complex processes. Given that all complex systems behave the same way, these concepts can be applied to health sciences. In this paper we propose the tools of the Sciences of complexity and chaos as a tool for the analysis of the proliferation of vectors and zoonosis in their potential use in bioterrorism.

There are about 400 type viral zoonoses in the world, in addition to numerous bacterial zoonoses. Likewise emerging diseases, approximately 75% are zoonotic 13. 1,415 Species of infectious organisms known as pathogens for humans, these were reported in 2001, 61% are zoonotic origin, similar to 75% of 175 considered pathogens as emerging.

Zoonoses can be introduced naturally or involuntarily (travel international, smuggling of goods, and animals) or by means of biological weapons. Zoonotic agents can be considered for their release or intentional introduction to cause damage and confusion that can run at the same time affect the health of animals and human having a serious socio-economic impact. On the other hand in a report published in the Journal of the American Medical Association concluded that 80% of common and likely to be used in biological warfare pathogens are zoonotic agents[7,14].

One of the important concepts in dynamical systems is "that small changes in initial conditions of the system can generate major changes in the final result", but in the surface forms of its evolution is likely to take different routes, such as self-organization, synchronization, no predictability of the effects of small changes in initial conditions and the existence of simplicity of some levels while chaos exists in other forms in the fundamental concepts of complexity [15].

Various properties spatiotemporal in complex systems emerge spontaneously from the interactions that occur in the system in question, which have an impact in a longitudinal manner over time, generating properties or unexpected effects in a given system; generating properties or unexpected effects in a given system; These properties has been called emergent processes. For example: it is known that when there is an overpopulation of a colony of lemmings, it enters into collective stress, then turns in droves to a cliff which precipitate. When the colony reaches a certain number you are calm and return to its territory. In this way, the colony regulates itself its population density. Complex systems can be critical systems characterized by the presence of spatiotemporals fluctuations in all possible scales existing in the system. It is important to mention that this phenomenon can be spontaneously and without the intervention of factors and forces external to the system, which is defined as self-organization. In many pathological processes in a particular community of animals, it is known that not all affected members will die; immunological properties of some is self-regulate and will compensate for the effects of the infectious agent[16].

Strange Attractors, not static or periodic, under the same conditions may diverge in a short period of time, making the system one chaotic and unpredictable [17], for example: the interaction between variables determines the transmission of infections in populations that are often complex and nonlinear, likewise involved individual life styles, which can only be understood in historical contextcultural and social in which occur. On zoonoses, daily living with pets or farm animals vary from family family 18,19 and 20 family economic status, so the flow of the spread can vary between each of these; Thus, with two equal systems at initial stage of a particular infectious disease will be different behaviors in its final phase. Strange Attractors, not static or periodic, under the same conditions may diverge in a short period of time, making the system one chaotic and unpredictable 17, for example: the interaction between variables determines the transmission of infections in populations that are often complex and nonlinear, likewise involved individual life styles, which can only be understood in historical contextcultural and social in which occur. On zoonoses, daily living with pets or farm animals can vary from family to family [18,19] and family economic status[20], so the flow of the spread can vary between each of these; Thus, with two equal systems at initial stage of a particular infectious disease will be different behaviors in its final phase.

There is ample evidence on the use of animals for early warning of a bioterrorist attack, has been observed that certain bioterrorism agents for, pets or livestock may prevent early, probably before manifested symptoms of the disease in humans to be detected in animals. Populations of animals such as wild birds, trade and shipping of livestock, as well as domestic animals involved in the local market or international trade could play a role in the maintenance and spread of an epidemic that is attributable to the deliberate release of a biological agent [7,14].

In the case of avian influenza virus H5N1 has been reported that direct contact with poultry is to be a major cause of infection in humans. Taking the initial changes in the same system, such as the time and the type of daily living with this species, the contagion will have different evolution. It is known that in many developing countries, as it is the case of Latin America, some families have animals in backyard; Thus customs in each household care and handling of the animals may differ, so a potential contagion and its dissemination will take different behaviors between different families[21].

The Center for prevention and Disease Control (CDC) classifies agents and bioterrorism in categories A, B and C diseases, placing with the letter A, to those with highest priority since they represent a national security risk already because, a) can be easily disseminated or transmitted from person to person, b) result in high mortality rates and have the potential to impact on public health, c) could cause panic among the population and social disorders and, d) require special public health measures. The main actors are anthrax, botulinum toxin, plague, smallpox, tularemia, and hemorrhagic fever viral. However, in addition to those already mentioned, there are other offensive players as it is the case of brucellosis, glanders, Hendra virus, avian flu, Nipah virus, avian psitacósis, Rift Valley fever melioidosis, cryptosporidiosis, Cryptococcosis, Q fever, fever of dengue, smallpox, equine viral encephalitis and viral hemorrhagic fevers which have been detected in animals other than smallpox and dengue fever[7,14, 22].

The majority of biological agents (especially of the type A) are effectively used spray; aerosols are the method most commonly used in a potential bioterrorism attack because they are the most effective means for wide dissemination[7].

Returning to the case of the H5N1 avian influenza, the modification of a variable, such as slight variations of the migratory routes, can generate completely different results, so that the follow-up to the transmission of avian influenza is complex[23]. We know that there are three clearly different States for the transmission of a zoonosis: excretion, presence in the environment and the entrance to the new host. Similarly there are two transmission mechanisms: caused by a vector and direct pollution from animal body fluids[24]. Another complex factor in the analysis and monitoring of a possible source of infection is the incubation period, as this can vary between the different subjects[25]. It is important to mention that many elements can contribute to emerge new zoonotic diseases of viral, or microbiological origin such as mutations, natural selection, progression would evolve, individual determinants of guests, acquisition of immunity, physiological determinants of the population of the host, behaviors, social characteristics of the guests, commercial transport, iatrogenic factors, ecological and climatic influences. Such is the case of the virus of swine influenza H1N1, cause of respiratory disease of pigs and that now their mutations have caused infection among humans[26, 27]. It is known that the H5N1 virus, which has been isolated in more than 90 bird species in wildlife, mainly ducks, geese and 49 species of shorebirds, has been able to cross the species barrier and has given rise to many human cases of influenza avian; some research studies report a fatality from 80%. Coupled with this is has isolated the virus in feces of cats that ate dead birds, so it is likely that these animals are also potential carriers[13,28,29,30,31,32]. The sum of these factors, in addition to migration routes and family customs, can give a chaotic model, making the analysis and follow-up of the epizootiology of influenza avian with conventional statistical tools[33]. It is important to mention that migratory birds may be reservoirs or mechanical vectors of numerous infectious agents with respect to a possible transmission of diseases from birds to humans[34]. Today it is known that many migratory birds have diverted their initial destinations and endings, as it has happened in the Lake of Guadalupe in Atizapan, State Mexico, where they currently live different kinds of migratory birds which have become the fauna of the place. New methods of study have been adapted to the increase in infectious diseases, using models of Bayesian analysis, theories of social, technical networks of systems posnormales, which generated an increase of the different variables affecting the study population, the biology of the multiple hosts in infectious complexes and social and ecological systems[35].

2. Usefulness of fractals in the theory of chaos

In nature there are countless formed whimsical figures to the length of time for the random sum of all its parts, so we could ask ourselves: when in nature is a completely spherical River stone or a hexagonal-shaped volcanic stone or a grotto with a cathedral-like vaults?[23]. It is obvious that man has simplified the capricious forms of nature in perfect geometric figures, starting from the basis for Euclidean geometry used today.

Based on the analysis of the figures of nature comes a new concept of these forms called "Fractals" by Mandelbrot[36]. Fractals have the characteristic that they may represent something more than a line and less than a plane can be larger than a one-dimensional form and lower than a two-dimensional[1]. The fractal depends on the scale of which is measured, so that the complexity of the forms and structures of nature are not accidental. Fractals can help to understand behaviors in different areas, from the distribution of galaxies in the universe until the spread of infectious diseases[23], to describe the formation of these random structures but with a certain pattern. For example, to observe the Gulf of Mexico from a satellite shown in the form of a semicircle, but approaching increasingly may distinguish forms that could not discriminate at the height of the satellite: large number of structures not symmetrical as bays, beaches, cliffs, stone, etc; When more detail will find more specific formations that break with the initial figure that would be the half circle. Another example would be the flower of broccoli; to the analyse in fragments increasingly smaller find structures similar to the original flower, which to the join form this, that, as mentioned, has a characteristic form, however, are not equal each other, share similar but not identical ways. A last example: the snow form irregular accumulations resulting in certain places be larger than others, in this way all clusters of snow are irregular and capriciously formed. Similarly, the grouping of cases in a particular epidemic could follow the trend groups in certain areas or regions. Based on this concept will be the utility of fractal geometry in epidemiology. Regarding social behavior in humans, we can say that some of them are still patterns of fractal formations, such as irregular settlements, where there is no defined order of the planning of streets and houses.

If he is a graph of dispersion of times and movements of the spread of a particular disease, we should possibly corresponding to fractal structures; in the graph, at each point you could see a new outbreak of the disease, for example: in a transmission of leptospirosis[37] by water contaminated in a given municipality, not concentrate the outbreaks of the disease near the source of the contaminated water, but in places where turned the carriers of the disease, either their homes or their sources of employment, which should be combined with the displacement of rats infected to places where the water stored for drinking contaminarían. Another example of spread of disease with this pattern would be that occurred at the beginning of the 20th century when the plague caused by *Yersinia pestis* killed millions of people to the Lake around the world[38], It is known that this bacteria infects small mammals, especially rodents and is transmitted to humans by fleas. It has identified more than 200 different mammals and about 80 different species of fleas in the prevalence of this disease; the flea in rat *Xenopsylla cheopis* is considered the most competent vector[39]. The chaotic spread was due to the displacement of the rats; If there will be a dispersion of times and movements of this spread chart we would possibly find a fractal formation. This type of graphics will give more information and understanding about the movement and spread of disease. The complexity of the swine influenza virus H1N1 is in their primary forms of infection, mainly people who have direct contact with these animals [27,40]; special cases like infection reported by a freshly dead animal viscera[41], the subtypes due to mutations of the virus[42], the first reports of infection between human[43], the resistance of the antiviral oseltamivir[44]. Uniting these factors, the threat of a pandemic is latent[45] because these factors are fundamental in viral diseases emerging, probably generating structures similar to fractals to analyse the cases that are registered to the length of the epidemic. This happened in Mexico during the recent outbreak by the subtype of the virus H1N1, appointed by the World Health Organization on April 30, 2009 as AH1N1 influenza virus human (to curb the indiscriminate slaughter of the pig), because this subtype spread from human to human. If he is a graph of regional States and municipalities, possibly it would be up to fractal structures, which could understand behavior following cases in its transmission.

Finally, we can mention the fractal geometry can be a useful tool for analyzing the chaotic systems [23].

3. Small world and social networks

Many times we have heard the phrase what little is the world!, mainly when two people are in a particular place and without knowing they have an acquaintance in common, resulting in the phrase "how small is the world". Societies, organizations and individuals are structured as a network of networks, interacting entities, who form "self-organized influence the quality and performance of their organizations"; self-organization is present in all of nature. The phenomenon of "small world" inherent in complex networks, shows that pooling is great but the distance from characteristic interconnection is very low. As a result, such networks are located in the complex area, between the total order and random. The "small world" phenomenon gives networks characteristics of optimization, such as computer and epidemiological flows: It is therefore essential to know in detail the social networks for phenomena that involve aspects of communication.

The usefulness of the small world on social networks implies that each of us are responsible for a given mode, where from, first, our relatives, friends and acquaintances, in turn each of them also has its node, so for them the primary node is for us our secondary node and so on. Using social networks in the analysis and monitoring of the spread of a disease, and its dissemination, displacements and the resulting direct contacts of relations that is daily with family, friends, coworkers and acquaintances may analyse more objectively. It is worth mentioning in addition to interpersonal relationships, long distances that are run on a daily basis make more complex this follow-up, for example: the inhabitants of big cities, as the case of the conurbados municipalities in the city of Mexico where people on average move approximately 20 Km or more to their places of work. Globalization implies that many people in the morning respondents in their hometown and eat or cenen in a city or country. According to airports and auxiliary services of Mexico, 2008 attended 28 million passengers in airports in Mexico[46], so the number of passengers who travel around the world by week is million; in this way, the infection of a disease can spread rapidly around the world; possibly a detailed analysis of aviation networks could be the cornerstone for the monitoring of the spread of disease [47]. For example: it is common that some businessmen in the morning are closing a business in any city of United States and in the afternoon are having dinner at his home in Mexico; determinant can occur with the migration with the theory of small world and the spread of diseases, we have as a result the complexity for the analysis and monitoring of a certain disease, mainly of the undocumented [48,49].

On the basis of the above examples by associating them; in the case of the zoonoses, little legislation in countries under development path, coupled with the little attachment is on the rules of transfer, the management of animal farm, which also affect the magnitude of the movements, and company result of commercial treaties between countries[50].

The existence of pet stores which allows children to interact with animals such as sheep, goats, cats, dogs and birds, without minimum hygiene conditions, both for animals and humans, with the potential risk of transmission of *Escherichia coli*[51], in addition to this, the almost non-existent participation of veterinary clinics in terms of education for the health of their clients [52,53], as well as the shortcomings of professional supervision of products of animal origin, can produce a complex spread of a particular zoonosis, in which disease appears at various points away from each other but with the same focus of origin. We know that *Brucella melitenesis* mainly affects goats, but can also affect cattle and pigs; on the other hand, the *Brucella abortus* is the primary responsibility for the bovine brucellosis. *Brucella* is excreted in the milk and vaginal excretions in high quantities, even in asymptomatic cases.

In humans, as well as direct contact with infected animals, you can purchase to consume dairy products, coupled with the variability of the trade routes that are complex, so it is almost impossible to know the source of original contamination[54,55] . Use the principles of "small world" and thorough analysis of the monitoring of relations between the different nodes (primary, secondary, tertiary, etc) of infected consumers, will be critical to understand the spread of this disease.

4. Usefulness of the analysis of processes of chaotic time series

The deterministic equations are structured to address a small number of variables, such form can ask few behaviors observed in nature describe deterministic equations with a small number of variables; on the contrary, the number of variables involved is high. To estimate the size of the strange attractors are useful time series, as they are generated by systems with many degrees of freedom [56]. There are many tools to analyze complex systems, in this article we will focus basically to time series for its ease of handling and understanding. A time series or chronological is a set of data recorded or observed in equal times; the purpose is to get a concise description of a series in particular, the construction of a model to explain the behavior of a series of time with respect to its history, or define a structure of behavior, i.e.

to establish a function of transfer and ultimately predict based on the results of the previous points[57]. In this way, time series are used to analyze the behavior of certain variable over time, so that its fundamental measurement are variables temporary, analyzing its influence on the trend, seasonality and cyclical fluctuations and irregular variations, the latter being the possible generators of chaotic models. It is worth noting that a chaotic process can not manipulate independent variables that affect the process but we know the effect generated by them; Thus the end of the system effect, is known to carry out a thorough analysis of the behavior of the different variables affecting the final outcome.

When you want to analyze the behavior of certain variable over time, usually we carry out analysis according to months, quarters or years, and on many occasions there are variables that to be averaged over the month, quarter or year are smoothed (when estimated an average between a lot of data there is a risk of that extreme values do not significantly alter the standard deviation) with respect to all data obtained during the period being analyzed.

Temporal analysis, the period to analyze is the smallest possible, i.e. in days, given that one of the characteristics of chaotic processes is that "small changes that can be generated in the initial conditions generate totally unexpected results". In this way, to analyse increasingly shorter periods daily behavior of the process, identified the modifier variables and changes that will generate these throughout the study period; may examine on many occasions when you have not expected natural events or the uncontrolled spread of a given pathology, or mutations in different pathogens adatando to various changes in the environment, it is difficult to predict their behaviour[58]. Investigate similar problems and describe the different scenarios where previous experiences known biases that occurred in the previous process, serves as background to generate campaigns of prevention or education for health in specific populations, for example: If in a certain area southeast of the Mexican Republic increases the amount of expected rain, may increase the population of *hemipteran insects,* sucking, as we know are responsible of transmitting *trypanosomiasis,* caused by the flagellate Protozoan *Trypanosoma cruzi*[59], Similarly, we know that the dog is the most important reservoir and found that it increases the risk of domestic transmission. If the increase in the population of dogs in the area add to the previous scheme, are not expected on the historical results. To use the analysis of time series include behavior that took the spread of Chagas disease in this area, is this way, certain actions will be taken. Another example would be the contamination of drinking water after a natural disaster: taking again as an example leptospirosis, where rodents dump large amount of Leptospira through urine, and transmission can occur through the skin and the mucous membranes to have direct contact with damp soil or vegetation contaminated, can be summarized that floods facilitated the proliferation of vectors, in association with the common proximity of rodents with humans[60]. Analysing the behaviour of the effects of this disease in a given population at the end of a month, the data that would would casuistry. Analysing shaped retrospective per day, the behavior of the spread of this disease correlating cases obtained by day by variable, such as dissemination, climate change, relocation of the population, and so on, the behavior of this zoonosis; will better understand Thus, predictability will only be possible when analysing short periods, mainly on models with dynamic and unpredictable behaviour[61,62].

5. Discussion

The variety of emerging diseases that are detected by the day make us reflect on the role of biological vectors as well as the transmission goes with coexistence with animals. Likewise, as mentioned in the text a percentage of emerging diseases are zoonotic origin. Diseases of high pathogenicity as the case of the H5N1 influenza avian in the reported a mortality rate above 65% coupled with cultural and social elements mainly in developing countries increases a potential direct transmission by the coexistence or possible bad cooking meat consumption, if we add this to the diversity of migratory routes as well as alternate routes derived from attractors a pandemic would be the result the sum of these factors. Genetic engineering has played a key role in what is the manipulation of the genetic engineering of several species, creating uncertainty and social dissatisfaction with regard to unexpected infections; If we add the elements you just mentioned with an intentional inoculation can generate incalculable catastrophes, which is why health teams should be prepared using tools such is the case of stochastic processes and chaos to analyse possible routes and modes of transmission of any zoonotic disease, medicine has tried to divorce of physicsWe must break the paradigm of the linearity and study, understand and analyze the role of complex systems in the transmission of diseases. The change or modification of the independent variables accelerates and slows the discontinuity thresholds, thus the thresholds indicated various endogenous processes or positive feedback, and these proportions you rulers of the change.

Two isolated chaotic systems can not be synchronized, because although they are particularly identical and begin to function at the same time, immediately their lower case differences will be amplified and this will increasingly be more divergent among themselves, similar to two outbreaks of a given disease in two different places. Hence the importance of the use of time series, that modifier effect on space and time variables may be known to decompose the system into smaller periods.

Human populations have a high degree of connectivity, addition to the increase in connections for ease of travel, hence the approach of the "small world", which makes us think about the increase in the likelihood of a pandemic[63,64].

The variables that should be considered in a complex dynamic model are susceptibility, exposure, infection, immunity, clinical manifestations, incubation period, in some cases healthy carriers and travel, among others[65].

It is important to emphasis that dynamic systems are independent, in particular the incidence of a particular disease, since this is a direct consequence of susceptibility. Thus, the incidence of certain zoonoses, starting simulators where deemed mobilizations, risk and possible susceptibility of individuals of the study population must analyze. Regardless of the understanding or not of a dynamic process, the use of time for analysis series serves to study the behavior of a particular infection in a subject, subgroup or a particular population, likewise gives the opportunity to use smaller periods of time[66].

We reiterate that there are many tools to analyze complex systems, such as the Scale-Free Model Barabasi-Albert, among others; in this work have exemplified time series for easy understanding and handling for the analysis of non-linear systems, because they are useful for interpreting and monitoring of a particular epidemic compared to linear models, for example: the trend of cases of a disease in particular is not linear over the yearsthey can identify cyclical fluctuations with respect to the seasons of the year, but this cyclical fluctuations will ever have identical behavior to analyze year by year, by which one may speak strictly of seasonality, that to ensure this, that you will need to have identical number of cases over the previous month year; so, irregular variations during the year of the cases of certain pathology will be the time series to analyze if it is possible to avoid the suavizamiento of data averaged over long periods of time in days. Finally, we believe that it is very important to know, disseminate and use the tools of the Sciences of complexity and chaos, as they represent a new paradigm that implies an advance to understand the dynamic processes of the biological and social phenomena.

The variety of emerging diseases that are detected by the day make us reflect on the role of biological vectors as well as the transmission goes with coexistence with animals. Likewise, as mentioned in the text a percentage of emerging diseases are zoonotic origin. Diseases of high pathogenicity as the case of the H5N1 influenza avian in the reported a mortality rate above 65% coupled with cultural and social elements mainly in developing countries increases a potential direct transmission by the coexistence or possible bad cooking meat consumption, if we add this to the diversity of migratory routes as well as alternate routes derived from attractors a pandemic would be the result the sum of these factors. Genetic engineering has played a key role in what is the manipulation of the genetic engineering of several species, creating uncertainty and social dissatisfaction with regard to unexpected infections; If we add the elements you just mentioned with an intentional inoculation can generate incalculable catastrophes, which is why health teams should be prepared using tools such is the case of stochastic processes and chaos to analyse possible routes and modes of transmission of any zoonotic disease, medicine has tried to divorce of physicsWe must break the paradigm of the linearity and study, understand and analyze the role of complex systems in the transmission of diseases.

The change or modification of the independent variables accelerates and slows the discontinuity thresholds, thus the thresholds indicated various endogenous processes or positive feedback, and these proportions you rulers of the change.

6. References

[1] Ruelas BE. Mansilla R. Las ciencias de la complejidad y la innovación médica. México: Plaza y Valdés; 2005.

[2] de Pomposo A. Las rupturas de simetría: principio y fin de las estructuras vitales. Conferencia Universidad La Salle. México, D.F., Septiembre de 2008.

[3] Batterman RW. Defining chaos. Philos Sci 1993;60:43-66.

[4] Ward M. Butterflies and bifurcation: can chaos theory contribute to the understanding of family systems? J Marriage Family 1995;57:629-638.

[5] Grenfell BT. Chance and chaos in measles dynamics. J R Static Soc B 1992;54:383-398.

[6] Nowak M. Sigmund K. Chaos and evolution cooperation. Proc Nat Acad Sci USA 1993;90:5091-5094.

[7] Patric R. Zoonoses likely to be used in bioterrorism. Public Health Reports 2008;123:276-281.

[8] Calisher CH. Let´s get something straight. Bioterrorism or Natural Disasters: What shall we worry about next?. Croat Med J 2007;48:574-578.

[9] Riedel S. Biologica warfare and bioterrorism: a historical review. BUMC PROCEEDINGS 2004;17:400-406.

[10] Sametband MJ. Entre el orden y el caos. La complejidad. México: Fondo de Cultura Económica/SEP/CONACyT/La Ciencia para Todos 167;1999.

[11] Philippe P. Chaos, population biology and epidemiology: some research implications. Hum Biol 1993;65:525-546.

[12] Thietart RA, Forgues B. Chaos theory and organization. Organiz Sci 1995;6:19-31.

[13] Ryan PC. Where do pets fit into human quarantines? J Public Health 2006;29:70-71.

[14] Gubemot DM, Boyer BL, Moses MS. Animals as early detectors of bioevents: veterinary tools and a framework for animal-human integrated zoonótico disease surveillance. Public Health Reports 2008;123:300-315.

[15] Pearce N. Merletti F. Complexity, simplicity and epidemiology. Int J Epidemiol 2006;35:515-519.

[16] Ramírez S. Los sistemas complejos como instrumentos de conocimiento y transfromación del mundo. México: Siglo XXI/CICH-UNAM; 1999.

[17] Prado VR, Ortiz MA, Ponce-de León CME. Evaluación del razonamiento clínico diagnóstico. Uso de atractores dinámicos como alternativa. Gac Med Mex 2002;138:411-420.

[18] Battelli G, Baldelli R. Ghinzelli M, Mantovani A. Occupational zoonoses in animal husbandry and related activities. Ann Ist Super Sanita 2006;42:391-396.

[19] Leighton FA. Veterinary medicine for world crisis. Can Vet J 2007;48:379-385.

[20] Stronks K. Van de Mhean HD, Casper WN, Mackenbach L, Mackenbach JP. Behavioural and structural factors in the explanation of socio-economic inequalities in health: an empirical analysis. Sociol Health Illness 1996;18:653-674.

[21] Norris JC. Van der Laan MJ. Lane S. Anderson JN. Block G. Nonlinearity in demographic and behavioral determinants of morbility. Health Serv Res 2003;38:1791-1818.

[22] Prakash N, Sharada P, Pradeep GL. Bioterrorism: challenges and considerations. J Forensic Dent Sci 2010;2:59-62.

[23] Talanquer V. Fractus, Fracta, Fractal. Fractales de laberintos y espejos. Tercera edición. México: Fondo de Cultura Económica; 2003. P. 79.

[24] Antonijevic B, Madle-Samardzija N, Turkulov V, Cana KG, Gavranic C, Petrovic-Milosevic I. Zoonoses a current issue in contemporary infectology. Med Pregl 2007;60:441-443.

[25] May R. Plagues and peoples. IUBMB Life 2006;58:119-121.

[26] Murphy FA. Emerging zoonoses. Emerg Infect Dis 1998;4:429-435.

[27] Damrongwatanapokn S, Parcheriyanon S, Pinochon W. Serological study of swine influenza virus H1N1infection in pigs of Thailand. 4th International Symposium on Emerging and Re-emerging Pig Diseases. Rome, June 29-July 2, 2003.
[28] Brown C. Commentary: Avian influenza. Am J Pathol 2006;168:176-178.
[29] Capua I, Maragon S. Control of avian influenza in poultry. Emerg Infect Dis 2006;12:1319-1324.
[30] Heeney JL. Zoonotic viral diseases and the frontier of early diagnosis, control and prevention. J Intern Med 2006;260:399-408.
[31] Sarikaya O, Erbaydar T. Avian Influenza outbreak in Turkey through Elath personnel´s views: a quantitative study. BMC Public Health 2007;7:330.
[32] Causey D. Edwards SV. Ecology of avian influenza virus in birds. J Infect Dis 2008; 197(suppl 1):S29-33.
[33] Ionides EL, Bretó C, King AA. Inference for nonlinear dynamics systems. PNAS 2006; 103:18438-18444.
[34] Tsiodras S, Kelesidis T, Kelesidis I, Bauchinger U, Falags ME. Human infections associated with wild birds. J Infect 2008;56:83-98. Epub 2007 Dec 21.
[35] Stephen C. Artsob H, Bowie WR, Drebot M, Fraser E, Leighton T, et al. Perspectives of emerging zoonótico disease research and capacity building in Canada. Can J Infect Dis Med Microbiol 2004;15:339-344.
[36] Mandelbrot B. The fractal geometry of nature. San Francisco: W.H. Freeman Company; 1982.
[37] De Igartúa LE, Coutiño RM, Velasco CO. Revisión breve de leptospirosis en México. Altepepaktli 2005;1:52-58.
[38] Keelin MJ, Gillian CA. Bubonic plague: a metapopulation model of a zoonoses. Proc R soc Lond B 2000;267:2219-2230.
[39] Bitam I, Baziz B, Rolain JM, Belkaid M, Raoult D. Zoonotic focus of plague, Algeria. Emerg Infect Dis 2006;12:1975-1977.
[40] Myers KP, Olsen CW, Gary GC. Cases of swine influenza in humans: a review of the literature. Clin infect Dis 2000;44:1084-1088.
[41] Newman AA, Reisdorf E, Beinemann J, Vyeki TM, Balish A, Shu B, et al. Human case of swine influenza A(H1N1) triple reassortant virus infection, Wisconsin. Emerg Infect Dis [serial of the Internet]. Available from http://www.cdc.gov/EID/content/14/9/1470.htm.
[42] Pekosz A, Glass GE. Emerging viral diseases. Md Med 2008;9:11-16.
[43] Dacso CC, Couch RB, Six HR, Young JF, Quarles JM, Kasel JA. Sporadic occurrence of zoonótico swine influenza virus infections. J Clin Microbiol 1984;20:833-835.
[44] Dharan NJ, Gubareva LV, Meyer JJ, Okomo-Adhiambo M, McClinton RC, Marshall SA, et al. Infections with oseltamivir-resistant influenza A(H1N1) VIRUS IN THE United States. JAMA 2009;301: 1034-1041.
[45] Gray GC, Trampel DW, Roth JA. Pandemic influenza planning: shouldn´t swine and poltry workers de included? Vaccine 2007;30:4376-4381.
[46] Secretaría de Comunicaciones y Transportes. Comunicado de Prensa No. 160. Incremente en 2008 el número de pasajeros atendidos en el AICM. Disponible en

http://www.set.gob.mx/nc/despliega-noticias/article/comunicado-de-prensa-no-160-incrementa-en-2008-el-numero-de-pasajeros-atendidos-en-el-aicm/

[47] Hufnagel L, Brockmann D, Geisel T. Forecast and control of epidemics in a globalized world. Proc Natl Acad Sci USA 2004;101:15124-15129. Epub 2004 Oct 11.

[48] Earn DJ, Rohani P, Grenfell BT. Persistence, chaos and synchrony in ecology and epidemiology. Proc Biol Sci 1998;265:7-10.

[49] Rohani P, Earn DJ, Grenfell BT. Opposite patterns of synchrony in sympatric desease metapopulations. Science 1999;286:968-971.

[50] Marano N, Arguin PM, Pappaioanou M. Impact of globalization and animal trade on infectious disease ecology. Emerg Infect Dis 2007;13:1807-1809.

[51] Stirling J, Griffith M, Dooley JS, Goldsmith CE, Loughrey A, Lowery CJ, et al. Zoonoses associated with petting farms and open zoos. Vector Borne Zoonotic Dis 2008;8:85-92.

[52] Stull JW, Carr AP, Chomel BB, Berghaus RD, Hird DW. Small animal deworming protocols, client education, and veterinarian perception of zoonótico parasites in western Canada. Can Vet J 2007;48:269-276.

[53] Palmarini M. A veterinary twist on pathogen biology. PloS Pathog 2007;3:e12.

[54] López MA, Migranas OR, Pérez MA, Magos C, Salvatierra-Izaba B, Tapia-Conyer R, et al. Seroepidemiología de la brucelosis en México, Salud Publica Mex 1992;34:230-240.

[55] Minas M, Minas A, Gourgulianis K, Stournara A. Epidemiological and clinical aspects of human brucellosis in central Greece. Jpn J Infect Dis 2007;60:362-366.

[56] Casdagli M. Chaos and deterministics versus stochastic non-linear modeling. J R Stat Soc B 1991;54:303-328.

[57] Martinez AG. Modelos y economía matemática. México: UAM-Iztapalapa; 1993. pp.73-95.

[58] Gupta S. Ferguson N, Anderson R. Chaos, persistence and evolution of strain structure in antigenically diverse infectious agents.

[59] Sosa JF, Zumaquero RJL, Reyes PA, Cruz-García A, Guzmán-Bracho C, Monteón VM. Factores bióticos y abióticos que determinan la seroprevalencia de anticuerpos contra Trypanosoma cruzi en el municipio de Palmar de Bravo, Puebla, México. Salud Publica Mex 2003;46:39-48.

[60] Watson JT, Gayen M, Connolly MA. Epidemics after natural disasters. Emerg Infect Dis 2007;13:1-5.

[61] Philippe P, Mansi O. Nonlinearity in the epidemiology of complex health and disease processes. Theor Med Bioethic 1998;19:591-607.

[62] Roth PA, Ryckman TA. Chaos, Clio, and scientific illusions of understanding. History Theory 1995;34:30-44.

[63] Peters DP, Pielke RA Sr, Bestelmeyer BT, Allen CD, Munson-McGee S, Havstad KM. Cross-scale interactions, nonlinearities and forecasting catastrophic events. Proc Natl Acad Sci USA 2004;101:15130-15135. Epub 2004 Oct 6.

[64] May R. Simple rules with complex dynamics. Science 2000;287:601-602.

[65] Korobeinikov A. Maini PK. Non-linear incidence and stability of infectious disease models. Math Med Biol 2005;22:113-128. Epub 2005 Mar 18.

[66] Belair J. Glass L, An Der Heiden U, Milton J. Dynamical disease identification, temporal aspects and treatment strategies of human illness. Chaos 1995;5:1-7.

4

Zoonotic Role of the Grasscutter

Maxwell N. Opara
Federal University of Technology, Owerri, Nigeria

1. Introduction

Zoonoses have affected human health throughout times, and wildlife has always played a role. Wildlife has long been recognized as potential sources for infectious diseases in humans and domestic animals. Diseases of wildlife have historically gained attention primarily when they were considered a threat to agricultural systems and the economic, social, or physical health of humans (Andrew et al, 2009). Today, zoonoses with wildlife reservoirs constitute a major public health problem, affecting all continents. The importance of such zoonoses is increasingly recognized, and the need for more attention in this area has to be addressed (Kruse et al., 2004). Wildlife can be defined as free-roaming animals such as mammals, birds, fish, reptiles, and amphibians living in a natural undomesticated state.

Zoonoses are infectious diseases which can be passed between vertebrate animals and humans. A high proportion of noticeable human diseases are zoonotic. They exclude diseases transmitted from human to human via an arthropod vector e.g. malaria (NR International managers of the Livestock Production Programme (LPP), 2006). Taylor et al, (2001) catalogued 1,415 known human pathogens and reported that 62% were of zoonotic origin. Wild animals seem to be involved in the epidemiology of most zoonoses and serve as major reservoirs for transmission of zoonotic agents to domestic animals and humans (Kruse et al., 2004). Zoonoses with wildlife reservoirs are typically caused by various bacteria, viruses, and parasites, whereas fungi are of negligible importance (WHO, 1999).

2. The grasscutter

The grasscutter (*Thryonomys swinderianus*), variously known as the marsh cane-rat , ground hog and in francophone West Africa, the aulacode or incorrectly, the agouti is a rodent but not a rat proper, since it belongs to the Hystricomorpha (porcupine family). This rodent subclass embraces similar species in both the old and new world, species which were originally classified according to the differentiation of the masticatory musculature (Simpson, 1974).

The grasscutter has thickset body, measuring up to 40cm to 60cm in addition to a 20cm - 25cm tail (Fitzinger, 1995), (See Plate 1). Its average weight fluctuates between 2kg to 4kg in the females and 3kg to 6kg in the males (Baptist and Mensah, 1986, Adjanahoun, 2002, Jori et al, 1995 and Merwe, 2000). Its furs comprise a mixture of brown reddish and gray hairs that vary depending on its habitat (Jori and Chardonnet, 2001). Some other authors reported that the skin and hair (fur) as well as limbs and tails are easily torn out (Rosevear, 1969; kingdom, 1974). This makes the animal very difficult to catch and even more difficult to handle after capture.

The grasscutter is a quick runner and a skilled swimmer, despite the blunt snout. Its visual powers are relatively poor, making communication to be based only on hearing and well developed sense of smell. This rodent can live up to four years in captivity (Jori and Chardonnet, 2001). It is a monogastric herbivore like the rabbit and other rodents; it is a good food converter and often practices coprophagy (Hemmer, 1992). They are considered delicacy, high prized source of protein and agricultural pest of cereals and other crops (Yeboah and Adamu, 1995).

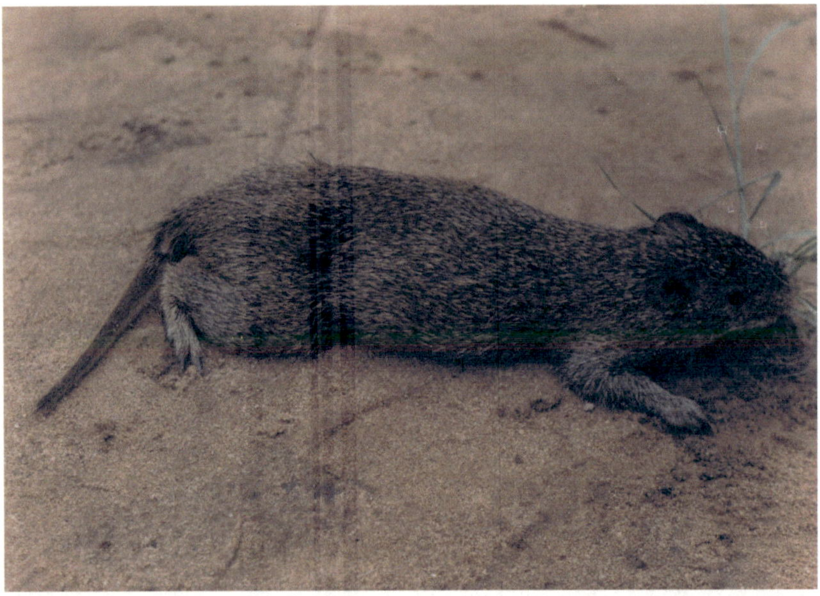

Plate 1. The grasscutter (*Thryonomys swinderianus*), matured adult measures 40-60cm long; weighs 2-6 kg; mixture of reddish brown and grey fur; monogastric herbivore; quick runner; skilled swimmer; poor vision; good sense of smell; lives up to 4 years in captivity; Induced ovulator; Gestation period 150-156 days; litter size up to 6.

3. Distribution and habitat of the grasscutter

The grasscutter is found only in Africa (Rosevear, 1969; Baptist and Mensah, 1986; Adoun, 1993). In West Africa where grass provides its main habitat and food, it is commonly known as the "grasscutter" or the "cutting grass", while in other parts of Africa particularly Southern Africa, where it is closely associated with cane fields, it is called the "Cane rat".

The grasscutter is found in grasslands and wooded savannah throughout the humid and sub-humid areas, south of the Sahara (National Research Council, 1991), specifically from Senegal to parts of the Cape Province in South Africa (Rosevear, 1969). The giant cane rat can also be found in any where there is dense grass, especially reedy grass growing in damp or wet places (Asibey, 1974a). They do not inhabit the rain forest, dry scrub or desert regions (National Research Council, 1991). Its distribution is determined basically by the availability of adequate or preferred grass species for food (National Research Council, 1991).

In West Africa, the grasscutter is not considered a threatened or disappearing species of wildlife (Baptist and Mensah, 1986). On the contrary, forest clearance in the Guinea zone has expanded its ecological habitat from the Savannah region into cropped areas and secondary forest, following agricultural encroachment on forests (Baptist and Mensah, 1986).

Similarly in Ghana, the grasscutter has penetrated the high forest where there is intensive maize, cassava, sugarcane, young cocoa, coconut, oil-palm, pineapple and egg plant cultivation (Asibey, 1974b). However, *Thryonomys swinderianus* has often been encountered in the vicinity of water courses just as both species have also been found in the same environment in East Africa (Kingdom 1974).

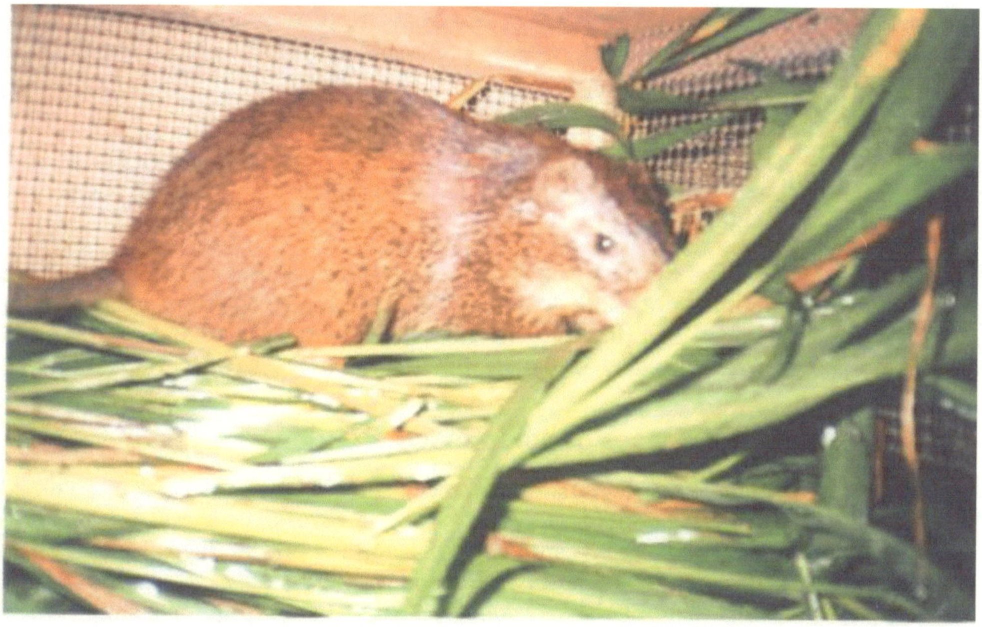

Plate 2. The grasscutter feeding on Guinea grass (*Panicum maximum*).

4. Characteristics of the grassutter

It has thickset body, measuring up to 40cm to 60cm, in addition to a 20cm -25cm tail (Fitzinger, 1995). Its average weight fluctuates between 2kg to 4kg in the females and 3kg to 6kg in the males (Baptist and Mensah, 1986, Adjanahoun, 1992, Jori et al, 1995 and Merwe, 2000). Its furs comprise a mixture of brown reddish and gray hairs that vary depending on its habitat (Jori and Chardonnet, 2001). Some other authors reported that the skin and hair (fur) as well as limbs and tails are easily torn out (Rosevear, 1969; kingdom, 1974). This makes the animal very difficult to catch and even more difficult to handle after capture. The grasscutter is a quick runner and a skilled swimmer, despite the blunt snout. Its visual powers are relatively poor, making communication to be based only on hearing and well developed sense of smell. It can live up to four years in captivity (Jori and Chardonnet, 2001). It is a monogastric herbivore like the rabbit and other rodents; a good food converter and often practices coprophagy (Hemmer, 1992). They are considered as high prized source of protein and agricultural pest of cereals and other crops (Yeboah and Adamu, 1995).

The grasscutter is found in grasslands and wooded savannah throughout the humid and sub-humid areas, south of the Sahara (National Research Council, 1991), specifically from

Senegal to parts of the Cape Province in South Africa (Rosevear, 1969). The giant cane rat can also be found any where there is dense grass, especially reedy grass growing in damp or wet places (Asibey, 1984). They do not inhabit the rain forest, dry scrub or desert regions (National Research Council, 1991). Its distribution is determined basically by the availability of adequate or preferred grass species for food (National Research Council, 1991).

The meat of the grasscutter is the most preferred among wild rodents (Asibey and Eyeson, 1973; Clottey 1981) and exploited in most areas as a source of animal protein (Vos, 1978; Asibey, 1974; National Research Council, 1991). Being the most preferred (Martin, 1985) and most expensive meat in West Africa (Baptist and Mensah, 1986; Asibey and Addo, 2000), it contributes to both local and export earnings of most of these countries (Asibey, 1969; National Research Council 1991; Baptist and Mensah, 1986; GEPC 1995; Ntiamoa-Baidu, 1998). For these reasons, the grasscutter is therefore hunted aggressively.

Unfortunately, its collection from the wild results in the destruction of the environment through setting of bush fires by hunters (National Research Council, 1991; Yeboah and Adamu, 1995; Ntiamoa-Baidu, 1998).

However, a great number of farmers in the sub-region have commenced the domestication of the grasscutter (National Research Council, 1991; Addo. 2002), thus making it more readily available. It is hoped that this venture will help the farmers to gain economic benefit and also reduce the environmental destruction that accompanies its collection from the wild.

5. Important zoonotic diseases in the grasscutter

Major diseases of economic and zoonotic importance in sub Sahara Africa are maintained by wildlife. The grasscutter serves as a reservoir host for several of these diseases, which includes human and animal trypanosomiasis, babesiosis, plasmodiasis, some zoonotic gastrointestinal helminths and protozoa (Opara and Fagbemi, 2008). Grasscutters harbor various types of parasites without showing obvious clinical manifestations, suggesting that they serve as reservoir hosts for parasitic agents that infect man and his animals. They are equally capable of transmitting some of the gastrointestinal parasites which are zoonotic in nature, especially if the meat is not properly cooked (Nwoke, 2001). For instance, some parasites responsible for zoonoses and communicable diseases to man and animals such as nematodes (*Ascaris, Bunostomum, Oesophagostomum, Strongyloides, Trichostrongylus Toxocara*); trematodes *(Fasciola, Schistosoma*); Cestodes (*Taenia*) and acanthocephalan (*Moniliformis*) occur in the grasscutter and their public health significance is worthy of note.

6. Blood protozoan parasites

There have been reports of few cases of naturally occurring blood parasites of the cane rats (Namso and Okaka, 1998), since they co-habit with other animal species. For example, Ntekim and Braide (1981) reported the occurrence of *Trypanosoma lewisi* in the blood of wild rats.

Much is not yet known about the blood parasites of the grasscutters.

Opara et al (2006) reported a natural infection of both the captive - reared and wild grasscutters with *Trypanosoma species.* The authors suggested that failure of establishment of clinical trypanosomiasis in these rodents could be attributed to the nature of food varieties the grasscutters consume.

They equally reported the occurrence of *Plasmodium* in the grasscutter. This is the causative organism of malaria in man and animals. It was commonly encountered in these rodents, suggesting that they serve as reservoirs of infection in the study areas. Malaria parasitaemia in humans is wide-spread in the study area and had been reported by Akpa and Iwuala, (1983) and Egwunyenga et al (1996).

Trypanosoma sp. recorded the highest prevalence of 25.0%, by the blood protozoan parasites. The organism causes African trypanosomiasis in animals and sleeping sickness in humans (Soulsby, 1982). Rodents are natural hosts of *Trypanosoma species* and the parasites are transmitted by fleas to these animals (Soulsby 1982). It is therefore likely that grasscutters may serve as reservoirs of infections for humans and their livestock, given the close proximity of these animals to human habitations and livestock houses. Perhaps, these rodents were equally infected during the course of their roaming around homes. For example, amplification of some genomic DNA for trypanosomes in his study (Opara, 2011), suggested that some of the grasscutters were infected with *Trypanosoma simiae*, which causes fulminating disease of pigs, trypanosomiasis in sheep, goats, and monkeys (Seifert, 1996). Human population expansion and encroachment, deforestation and other habitat changes have often driven wildlife close to human habitation.

Babesia sp. yielded a prevalence rate of 9.4%. This figure was close to that (5.4%) reported by Ajayi et al (2007) from rodents in Jos, Plateau State. Furthermore, Babesiosis caused by *Babesia bigemina* and *Babesia bovis* have been reported in Nigeria (Leeflang et al, 1976) and ticks have been incriminated in their transmission (Iwuala and Okpala, 1978, James-Rugu and Itse, 2001). Ticks were also observed on the bodies of the grasscutters examined.

7. Gastrointestinal helminth parasites

The examination of the GIT of wild grasscutters revealed endo-parasites comprising of 14 species of nematodes, 5 trematodes, 4 cestodes and 1 acanthocephalan (Opara and Fagbemi, 2008). The nematodes were identified as *Ascaris* sp., *Bunostonum* sp., *Cooperia* sp., *Gaigaria* sp., *Gongylonema* sp., *Haemonchus* sp., *Heterakis* sp., *Mammomonogamus* sp., *Metastrongylus* sp., *Oesophagostomum* sp., *Strongyloides* sp., *Toxocara* sp., *Trichostrongylus* sp. *and Trichuris* sp. The trematodes included *Cotylophoron* sp., *Dicrocoelium* sp., *Gastrodiscus* sp., *Paramphistomum* sp. *and Schistosoma* sp., while the cestodes were *Avitellina* sp., *Moniezia* sp., *Taenia* sp. *and Thysaniezia* sp. The acanthocephalan identified was *Moniliformis* sp. Other workers such as Mpoame (1995), Odumodu, (1999), Yeboah and Simpson (2001) and Ajayi et al (2007) had reported some of these parasites in Cameron, Anambra (Southeastern Nigeria), Ghana and Jos (North central Nigeria) respectively.

Some of the helminths encountered in the rodents in this study are of public health importance, because they cause zoonotic infections in both man and his livestock. For example, the prevalence of *Ascaris* in the grasscutters is enough to cause public health concern because of the closeness of the rodents to human habitation. Human ascariasis due to *Ascaris lumbricoides* is very common in Nigeria, with prevalence rates reaching 85.5% in primary school pupils (Holland et al, 1989). Judging by the relative ease with which *A. lumbricoides* establishes itself experimentally in pigs, a monogastric animal like man, it is not impossible that *Ascaris* transmission may be on-going between rodents and man with his livestock in the study area. *Bunostomum* sp. (a canine hookworm) is notable for its involvement in cutaneous larva migrans in man. Equally, some species of *Strongyloides* have also been incriminated in this phenomenon (Soulsby, 1982). It was a surprise to observe the infection of the grasscutters by *Mammomonogamus* sp., which is basically a nematode of mammals in Asia and South America. Although *M. loxodontus* occurs in the trachea of the African elephants and *M. nasicola* has also been observed in the nasal cavities of ruminants in Cameroon (Soulsby 1982 and Cox, 1982). The occurrence of *Oesophagostomum* sp. in these rodents suggests danger to man and his livestock because of the closeness of the grasscutters to human dwellings.

Furthermore, human oesophagostomiasis has been reported in Nigeria (Fabiyi, 2001). The prevalence of *Toxocara* sp. among grasscutters in this study shows that the rodents serve as reservoir hosts. The larvae of the helminth cause visceral larva migrans in children.

Trichuris sp. prevalence in the grasscutters was moderately high. This result has further confirmed that rodents transmit zoonotic parasites to man and animals. Trichuriasis is widespread in Nigeria and has been reported by Okpala (1961) and Holland et al (1989). The parasite causes rectal prolapse, anaemia, finger clubbing and retarded growth in man (Jung and Beaver 1951; Bowie et al, 1978 and Gilman et al 1983). Weight loss and formation of nodules in the caecal wall which leads to diarrhea and anorexia in pigs.

Trichostrongylosis is characterized by persistent diarrhea and wasting. In lambs and calves, heavy losses from lack of growth and death commonly occur.

Gastrodiscus sp., a trematode reported in this study causes gastrodiscoidiasis and has been reported in the caecum of man elsewhere (LaPage, 1963, Soulsby, 1982). It is not unlikely that human infections may exist in Nigeria because of the close proximity of these rodents to man and his habitation.

Dicrocoelium sp., although in a study carried out in our laboratory seemed to have lower prevalence rate (14.2%) than elsewhere (Manas et al, 1978) in cattle (34%), sheep (23%) and goats (45%), the rate is capable of infecting man and other livestock (Soulsby, 1982). Wild animals are commonly affected and serve as reservoir hosts for domestic stock, while rabbits maintain the infection for considerable periods (Soulsby, 1982).

Outbreaks of Paramphistomiasis generally occur in the drier months, when the snail population becomes concentrated around areas of natural water and these areas in the dry months also have the most palatable grazing and thus, there is concentration of animals including snails and metacercariae over a small area resulting in heavy infections.

Schistosomes of rodents and birds have often been proved to be the sources of human *Schistosoma* cercariae that cause "simmers Itch" when they penetrate human skin.

Tapeworm infection such as those from *Avitellina, Moniezia, Taenia* and *Thysaniezia species* have little or no effect on the health of adult farm animals, but infection in the young animals may cause failure to thrive. Tapeworms, when they increase in length, may coil and block the intestinal tract (small intestine), the result is that food passage becomes impossible and the animal develops emesis. Tapeworms feed on digested nutrients in the small intestine and hence the animal loses weight. The cestodes encountered in this study are very common in the tropics and subtropics. Heavy infection by these parasites may cause abdominal symptoms such as anorexia, vomiting, diarrhea and pains. Prevalence of these cestodes has been documented in Nigeria (Enyenihi, 1980) and rodents have been implicated in their transmission to man (Akinboade et al, 1981; Yunusa et al, 1998).

The occurrence of *Moniliformis* sp. among the grasscutters is of public health significance, especially in rural areas of tropical rainforest of southeastern Nigeria. *Moniliformis* is a rodent parasite of cosmopolitan distribution. It has been reported in man in different parts of the world (Moayedi et al, 1971), including Nigeria (Ikeh et al, 1992, Anosike et al, 2000). Of worry is the involvement of rodents and their allies in emergence or re-emergence of human and animal diseases.

8. Gastrointestinal protozoan parasites

Gastrointestinal protozoan parasites were also encountered among the wild grasscutters. Those found were *Eimeria, Entoamoeba* and *Gardia* species. This finding suggests that the grasscutters might have ingested the mature infective oocysts along with pastures contaminated with human and animal faeces. Some of these grasscutters were caught near human habitations, where faeces are indiscriminately passed in the bush. *Eimeria* is a major coccidia of importance in domestic animals, causing blood stained diarrhea, emaciation and constipation during the final stage of development (Soulsby, 1982). It also affects rats, mouse and guinea pigs.

Entoamoeba sp. causes dysentery in man and many species of monkey, dog, cat, rat and pig (Soulsby, 1982). The hosts acquire the infection orally with cysts or per rectum with the trophozoites leading to an acute amoebic dysentery.

Gardia sp. is always found in the duodenum, other parts of the small intestine and occasionally in the colon of man (Soulsby, 1982), causing acute, sub acute to chronic diarrhea and duodenal irritation with an excess mucous production.

9. Conclusion and recommendations

In recent years, domestication of the grasscutters is becoming popular as an alternative source of bush meat and animal protein which are seriously needed by Nigerians.

Grasscutters harbored various types of parasites without showing obvious clinical manifestations, suggesting that they may be serving as reservoir hosts for parasitic agents that infect man and his animals. They are equally capable of transmitting some of these parasites which are zoonotic in nature, if the grasscutter meat is improperly cooked. For instance, some parasites responsible for zoonoses and communicable diseases to man and animals such as nematodes (*Ascaris, Bunostomum, Oesophagostomum, Strongyloides, Trichostrongylus Toxocara*) ;trematodes (*Fasciola Dicrocoelium, Gastrodiscus, Schistosoma*); Cestodes (*Taenia*) and acanthocephalan (*Moniliformis*) and their public health significance especially in rural areas of tropical rainforest of southeastern Nigerian is worthy of note.

10. References

Addo, P.G. (2002): Detection of mating, pregnancy and imminent Parturition in the grasscutter (*Thryonomys swinderianus*). *Livestock Research for. Rural. Development,* 14 (4) 8-13.

Adjanahoun, E (2002): Gestation Diagnosis of the grasscutter (*Thryonomys swinderianus*): Field and Laboratory methods. *Proceedings of conference on grasscutter production. Cotonou, Benin,* pp 123-131.

Adoun, C. (1993): Place De L'aulacode ((*Thryonomys swinderianus)* Dan's Le Regne Animal ET SA Repartition Geographique. In: L "er conference Internationale, L' Aulacodiculture: Acquis ET Perspective" pp. 35-40.

Ajayi, O.O., Ogwurike, B.A., Ajayi, J.A., Ogo, N.I. and Oluwadare, A.T. (2007): Helminth parasites of rodents caught around human habitats in Jos, Plateau state, Nigeria. *Int.J.Nat.Appl.Sci.* 4(1):8-13

Akinboade,O.A..,Dipeolu,O.O.,Ogunji,F.O and Adegoke,G.O. (1981):The parasites obtained and bacteria isolated from house rat (*Rattus rattus*,Linnaeus 1758) caught in human habitations in Ibadan,Nigeria. *Int.J.Zoon.* 8:26-32.

Akpa, A.U.C. and Iwuala, M.O.E. (1983): Some aspects of the epidemiology of malaria in rural Owerri. *7th Annual Conference of the Nigeria Society for Parasitology* (Book of Abstracts) 7:11.

Andrew Thompson R.C., Susan J. Kutz, Andrew Smith (2009).Parasite Zoonoses and Wildlife: Emerging Issues. *Int. J. Environ. Res. Public Health.6*, 678-693; doi:10.3390/ijerph6020678.

Anosike, J.C., Njoku, A.J., Nwoke, B.E.B., Okoro, O.U., Okere,A.N., Ukaga,C.N. and Adimonye,R.N. (2000):Human infection with *Moniliformis moniliformis* (Bremger 1811) Travassus 1915 in southeastern Nigeria. .*Ann.Trop.Med.Parasitol.*94:837-838.

Asibey, E.O.A. (1969): Wild animals and Ghana's Economy (An Investigation into bush meat as a source of protein) Department of Game and Wild life, Ministry of Lands and Forestry Accra.

Asibey, E.O.A. (1974a): Wildlife as a source of protein in Africa South of the Sahara. *Biological Conservation*, 6:32-39.

Asibey, E.O.A (1974b): The Grasscutter (*Thryonomys swinderianus* Temminck*)* in Ghana. *Symposium, Zoological Society of London*, No. 34, 161-170.

Asibey, E.O.A and Addo, P.G. (2000): The Grasscutter, a promising animal for Meat Production. In: African Perspective Practices and Policies Supporting Sustainable Development (Turnham, D., ed.). Scandinavian Seminar College, Denmark, in association with weaver Press Harare. Zimbabwe. www.cdr.dk/sscafrica/as & ad-gh.htm.

Asibey, E.O.A. and Eyeson, K.K. (1973): Additional information on the importance of Wild Animals as Food Source in Africa South of the Sahara. *Bongo Journal of the Ghana Wildlife Society*. 1 (2): 13-17.

Baptist, R. and Mensah, G.A. (1986): Benin and West Africa: The cane Rat. Farm Animal of the Future? *World Animal Review*, 60:2-6.

Bowie, M.D., Morison, A. and Ireland, J.D. (1978): Clubbing and whipworm infestation. *Archives of Disease of Childhood*, 53:411-413.

Clottey St. John, A. (1981): Relation of Physical body composition to Meat yield in the grasscutter (*Thryonomys swinderianus* Temminck*)*. *Ghana Journal of Science*. 21:1-7.

Cox, F.E.G. (1982) :(ed).*Modern Parasitology: A textbook of Parasitology*.1st edition. Blackwell Scientific Publishers, Oxford, England.

Egwunyenga, O.A., Ajayi, J.A.and Duhlinska-Popova, D.D. (1996): Malaria in pregnancy in Nigerians: seasonality and relationship to splenomegaly and anaemia.Indian *Journal of Malariology*.34 (1):17-24.

Enyenihi, U.K. (1980): Zoonoses and public health planning in Nigeria in the 1980s'.*Nig.J.Parasitol.*1 (1):23-48.

Fabiyi, J.P. (2001): Parasitic Zoonoses in Nigeria. *African.Journal of.Natural.Sciences* .4:1-15.

Fitzinger, F. (1995): Cane rats. In: Nowak, R, (ed.) *Walker's Mammals of the World.* The John Hopkins University Press, pp 1650-1651.

Ghana Environmental Protection and Control (GEPC) (1995): In Addo, P.G (2002). Detection of mating, pregnancy and imminent parturition in the grasscutter (*Thryonomys swinderianus* Temminck*). Livestock Research for Rural Development,* 14 (4): 8-13.

Gilman,R.H.,Chong,Y.H.,Davis,C.,Greenberg,B,Virik,H.K.and Dixon,H.B. (1983):The adverse consequences of heavy *Trichuris* infestation. *Trans.R.Soc.Trop.Med.Hyg.* 70:313-316.

Hemmer, H. (1990): *Domestication, the decline of Environment Appreciation.* Cambridge University Press, Cambridge. Pp 24

Holland, C.V., Asaolu, S.O., Cromoton, D.W.T., Stoddart, R.C. Macdonald and Torimiro,S.E.A. (1989):The epidemiology of *Ascaris lumbricoides* and other soil transmitted helminthes in primary school children from Ile-Ife,Nigeria. *Parasitology,* 99:275-285.

Ikeh, E.I. Anosike, J.C. and Okon, E. (1992): Acanthocephalan infection in man in Northern Nigeria. *J.Helminth.*66:241-242.

Iwuala, M.O.E. and Okpala, J. (1978): Studies on the ectoparasites fauna of Nigerian livestock II: Season and infestation rates. *Bull.Anim.Hlth.Prod.Afr.* 16(4):360-372.

James-Rugu, N.N. and Itse, R. (2001): Ecological studies on tick infestation of domestic stocks in parts of Plateau state, Nigeria.*Int.J.Envir.Hlth.Hum.Dev.*2 (2):43-48.

Jori, F. and Chardonnet, P. (2001): Cane rat farming in Gabon. Status and Perspective. *Paper presented at the 5th International Wildlife Ranching Symposium, Pretoria, South Africa.* March, pp 33-51.

Jori, F; Mensah, G.A and Adjanohoun, E. (1995): Grasscutter Production. A model of rational exploitation of Wildlife. *Biodiversity and Conservation,* 4 (3): 257-265.

Jung, R.C. and Beaver, R.M. (1951): Clinical observation on *Trichocephalus trichuris* (whipworm) infestation in children. *Paediatrics,* 8:548-555

Kingdom, J. (1974): *East Africa Mammals* (Hares and Rodents) Academic Press London. Vol. 11 Part 3.

Kruse, H., Kirkemo, A and Handeland, K. (2004): Wild life as source of zoonotic infections. *Emerging Infectious Diseases* (EID).www.cdc.gov/eid, 10(12):2067-2072.

La Page, G. (1963): *Animal parasitic in man* (Rev.Edition). Dove Publications Inc.New York.320pp.

Leeflang, P., Oomen, J.M., Zwart, D. and Meuwissen, J.H.E.T. (1976): The prevalence of *Babesia* antibodies in Nigerians. *Int.J.Parasitol.*6:159-161.

Manas, A.I.,Gomez,G.V.,Lozano,M.J.,Rodriguez,O.M.and Campos,B.M. (1978):A study of the frequency of dicrocoeliasis in domestic animals in the province of Grenada. *Rev.Iberica Parasit.*38:751-773.

Martin, G.H.G. (1985): West Africa; Carcass Composition and Palatability of some Animal Commonly used As Food. *World Animal Review,* (53): 40-44.

Merwe, M (2000). Tooth Successions in the Greater Cane rat (*Thryonomys swinderianus*). *Journal of Zoology,* (251): 541-545

Moayedi, B., Izadi, M.and Maleki, B. (1971): Human infection with *Moniliformis moniliformis* Dublins). *Am.J.Trop.Med.Hyg.*20:445-448.

Mpoame, M. (1995): Gastro intestinal helminthes of the cane rat *Thryonomys swinderianus,* in Cameroon. *Tropical Animal Health and Production,* 26, 239-240.

National Research Council (NRC) (1991): *Micro-Livestock: Little Known small animals with a promising economic future.* National Academy Press, Washington D.C. Pp 192-282.

Namso, M.E. and Okaka, C.E. (1998): A Survey of Naturally occurring parasites of cane rats. *Nig J. Parasitol.*, Abstract 28:28-29.

NR International managers of the Livestock Production Programme (LPP) (2006). Zoonotic Diseases of Smallstock.

Ntekim, A. and Braide, E.I. (1981): A study of the parasites of wild Rats from the University of Calabar Poultry. *Nig J. Parasitol.*, 4:20-21.

Ntiamoa-Baidu, Y. (1998): Sustainable use of Bush meat. Wildlife development plan: 1998-2003. *Wildlife Department, Accra.* Vol. 6 VI Pp 78.

Nwoke, B.E.B. (2001): Urbanization and livestock handling and farming: The public health and parasitological implications.*Nig.J.Parasitol.*22:121-128.

Odumodu, I.O. (1999): A survey of the intestinal helminthes and blood parasites of rats in Ihiala LGA, Anambra state, Nigeria.M.Sc.Thesis, Imo state University, Owerri, Nigeria.

Okpala, J. (1961): A survey of the incidence of intestinal parasites among government workers in Lagos, Nigeria. *West Afr. Med.J.*, 10 (New series), 148-157.

Opara, M.N., Ike, K.A. and Okoli, I.C (2006): Haematology and Plasma Biochemistry of the Wild Adult African Grasscutter *(Thryonomys swinderianus,* Temminck). *The Journal of American Science* 2(2):17-22

Opara, M.N. (2011): Gastrointestinal and Blood parasitism in the Grasscutter (*Thryonomys swinderianus*, Temminck) under captive and wild conditions in Imo State Nigeria. PhD Thesis, University of Ibadan Nigeria

Opara, M.N. and Fagbemi, B.O. (2008a): Observations on the Gastrointestinal Helminth parasites of the wild Grasscutter (*Thryonomys swinderianus*, Temminck) in Imo State, Nigeria. Int. J. Trop. Agric. and Food Syst., 2(1): 105- 110.

Opara, M.N. and Fagbemi, B.O. (2008b): Haematological and Plasma Biochemistry of Adult Wild African Grasscutter (*Thryonomys swinderianus*): A Zoonosis Factor in the Tropical Humid Rainforest of Southeast Nigeria. Ann. N.Y. Acad. Sci.; 1149: 394 – 397.

Rosevear, D. R. (1969): *The Rodents of West Africa*, Trustees of the British Museum (National History) Publ. No. 677, London.

Seifert, H.S.H. (1996): *Tropical Animal Health.*Kluwer Academic Publishers, Boston/London.

Simpson, G.G (1974): Chairman's Introduction; Taxonomy Symposium. Zoological Society of London, 34, 1-5.

Soulsby, E.J.L. (1982): *Helminths, Arthropods and Protozoa of Domesticated Animals.* (Seventh Edition) Bailliere Tindall, London.Pp.359-589.

Taylor L.H., Latham S.M, Woolhouse M.E.(2001). Risk factors for human disease emergence. Philos Trans R Soc Lond B Biol Sci. 356:983–9.

Vos, A. De (1978): Game as Food. A report on its significance in Africa and Latin America. Unasylver, (4): 2-12.

World Health Organization Consultation on Public Health and Animal Transmissable Spongiform Encephalopathies (1999).Epidemiology, risk and research requirements. WHO/CDS/CSR/APH/2000.2. Geneva: The Organization.

Yeboah, S. and Adamu, E.K. (1995): The cane rat. *Biologist*, 42 (2):86-87.

Yunusa, Y.P., Audu, P.A. and Abdu, P.A. (1998): A survey of Helminth parasites of the gastro-intestinal tract of African giant rat (*Cricetomys gambianus*) in Zaria, Nigeria. *22nd Annual conference of the Nigerian Society for Parasitology.University of Benin, Benin City, Nigeria.*November,4-7 (Abstracts),7-11.

Part 2

Bacterial and Viral Zoonosis

5

Coxiella burnetii

Giorgia Borriello and Giorgio Galiero
Experimental Zooprophylactic Institute of Southern Italy, Italy

1. Introduction

Q fever is a zoonosis caused by *Coxiella burnetii*, a small obligate intracellular Gram-negative pathogen worldwide spread, except New Zealand (Maurin & Raoult, 1999).

Q fever has been described for the first time in 1935 as an outbreak of fever in workers of a slaughterhouse in Brisbane, Australia (Derrick, 1937). Derrick could not identify the aetiological agent therefore he defined the disease as "query fever". Afterwards, in 1937, Burnet and Freeman (Burnet & Freeman, 1937) isolated a troublesome intracellular pathogen from mice inoculated with blood or feces from Derrick's patients, and classified it as *Rickettia burnetii*. Only in 1948 Philip (Philip, 1948), according to cultural and biochemical characteristics, re-classified *R. burnetii* as a new genus, *Coxiella*, in honour of Herald R. Cox, who first isolated this microrganism in the USA.

Ruminants and pets represent the most important reservoirs of the infection, and transmission to man mainly occurs through inhalation of contaminated aerosols. The disease is characterized by a wide clinical spectrum, varying from asymptomatic seroconversion, self-limiting febrile episodes to hepatitis and pneumonia. The illness can also occur in a chronic form, mainly characterized by endocarditis, and sometimes can have a lethal outcome. In contrast in animals *C. burnetii* infection is generally asymptomatic, even if infected animals can shed intermittently this pathogen in feces, urine, milk and birth products. Clinical symptoms eventually occurring in ruminant herds are mainly represented by reproductive disorders, such as premature birth, dead or weak offspring and infertility.

2. Etiology

Philogenetic and molecular studies based on the 16S rRNA sequences locate *C. burnetii* in the order of Legionellales, in the gamma group of Proteobacteria, next to bacteria such as *Legionella* spp., *Francisella tularensis* and *Rickettsiella* spp. (Raoult et al., 2005). In eukaryotic cells *Coxiella* replicates inside vacuoles, in mammals prefers monocytes and macrophages. This pathogen exhibits a complex intracellular cycle, characterized by the formation of spore-like forms. In infected cells it can be found in two different forms, one metabolically inactive, denominated SCV ("Small-Cell Variant") and the other one metabolically active, LCV ("Large-Cell Variant"). The SCV form appears as a small and compact rod, and is highly resistant to physicochemical agents, such as desiccation and common disinfectants, therefore exhibiting high persistence in the environment. The LCV form is instead bigger and less dense if observed at the electronic microscope; it is metabolically active and can differentiate in the SCV form through a sporogenic differentiation. Following cell rupture, the spore-like forms are released in the external environment where they can survive for long periods.

When cultured on embrionated eggs or cell cultures, *C. burnetii* exhibits an antigenic variation associated with loss of virulence. Indeed this microrganism shows a pathogenic form denominated phase I, isolated from animal or human infected cells, and an avirulent form, denominated phase II, isolated after serial passages on embrionated eggs or cell cultures. The attenuated phase II is characterized by a deletion in the chromosome which causes the loss of some cell surface determinants (Maurin & Raoult, 1999).

The association between specific characteristics of *C. burnetii* and the virulence of the strain is still an open controversial question, and several theories have been proposed to address the ability of different isolates to induce the acute or the chronic form of the disease. Several researchers tried to correlate the virulence to specific phenotypic and genetic profiles of the microorganism. In particular, SDS-PAGE analysis of the LPS isolated from the phase I allowed to identify three phenotypic groups antigenically distinct, associated, the first one, with acute episodes of the infection in different sources (ticks, bovine milk and man), the second and the third one with chronic episodes in man (Hackstadt, 1986). Studies in literature show that *Coxiella* possesses four different plasmids, QpH1, QpRS, QpDV and QpDG7 (Valková & Kazár, 1995). According to the harboured plasmid and also to DNA restriction profiles, *C. burnetii* can be divided in six genetic groups, variably correlated to specific pathotypes (Hendrix et al., 1991). In particular, the groups from I to III, carrying the plasmid QpH1, have been isolated from ticks, human cases of acute Q fever, bovine milk and birth products of domestic ruminants; the groups IV and V, that respectively possess the plasmid QpRS or any plasmid (but, in the latter case, they possess plasmidic sequences integrated in the chromosomal DNA), have been associated with abortions of domestic ruminants and chronic human cases of endocarditis or hepatitis; the group VI, carrying the plasmid QpDG, isolated from rodents, results avirulent in experimental mouse models of the infection (Stoenner et al., 1959; Stoenner & Lackman, 1960). Subsequent studies classified 80 *C. burnetii* isolates in 20 different genetic profiles by RFLP analysis (analysis of the Restriction Fragments Length Polymorphisms). According to this characterization, four profiles correspond to the former genetic groups I, IV, V and VI, respectively. In general, the RFLPs profiles seem to be associated with the geographical origin of the analysed isolates (Jäger et al., 1998). More recent studies based on MST (Multispacer Sequence Typing) analysis have variedly confirmed the existence of the aforesaid genetic groups, and identified three great monophyletic groups, containing the groups I, II and III, the group IV and the group V, respectively. Moreover, these studies seem to confirm the association between the plasmid QpDV and acute infections, and between the plasmid QpRS and chronic infections, and between specific genotypes and specific courses of the disease (Glazunova et al., 2005). Subsequent studies (Beare et al., 2006) performed by microarray analysis, further confirm the RFLP genetic groups, and add to the previous groups from I to VI, other two big groups (VII and VIII). These studies, underline the importance of the polymorphisms of the genes involved in LPS biosynthesis for the virulence of *C. burnetii*. An opposite school of thought instead, considers the characteristics of the host as the main cause of the course of the infection in relation to the development of acute or chronic diseases. These theories follow on the fact that isolates carrying the plasmid QpH1 have been isolated in France from both acute and chronic human Q fever episodes, while isolates deprived of the plasmid QpH1 have been shown to be able to induce an acute syndrome as well (Stein & Raoult, 1993). Models of the disease have therefore been proposed in which the same isolate is able to cause either the chronic or the acute form of Q fever, exclusively according to the host immune response. Particularly, the establishment of the chronic syndrome has been associated with a compromised immune state of the host, as for instance in case of HIV infection, as well as with an increased production of IL-10, responsible of a diminution of the ability of the macrophages to eliminate *C. burnetii* due to an inhibitory effect on the phagosome maturation process (Raoult et al., 2005). Recent data (Russell-Lodrigue et al., 2009) on the behaviour of *C. burnetii* isolates belonging to the genetic groups I, IV, V and VI in mouse models of Q fever seem however to confirm the theory of the association genotype-pathotype. In this study, in fact, strains associated with mice acute episodes (group I) have been shown to cause a faster progression of the disease, to induce greater pathological changes and to exhibit a higher speed of proliferation *in vivo* if compared to isolates collected from chronic episodes (groups IV and V). Moreover, the isolates of the group I, if compared to the others, induce in mouse a stronger immune response, characterized by a greater production of inflammatory cytokines for a longer period of time.

3. Sources of infection and routes of transmission

Sources of infection of Q fever are diverse, and the principal for man is represented by the inhalation of infected particles (Fig. 1). Transmission of the bacterium through contaminated aerosol can occur following direct contact with infected animals, mostly, with birth products, such as amniotic fluid and placenta, which can in turn contaminate the new born or the skin of other animals. The extreme resistance of this pathogen to external agents makes it persistent in the environment, especially in areas where domestic ruminant farms are present. In fact *C. burnetii* can be easily transmissible through contaminated hay or contaminated dust, and spread in the surrounding environment by the wind. For this reason cases of Q fever can also be recovered in patients that have not had evident contacts with animals. Human-to-human transmission results extremely rare, although cases of transmission of Q fever occurred through contact with parturient, through the transplacental way (congenital infection), through sexual relations (shown in mouse models of the infection) (Kruszewska & Tylewska-Wierzbanowska, 1997), blood transfusions (van der Hoek et al., 2010) and intradermic inoculation. Ticks are considered as natural reservoirs of *C. burnetii*. They contribute to the maintenance of the infectious agent in the environment by transmitting the disease to animals (livestock, pets and wildlife) by bite or by expelling heavy loads of *C. burnetii* with their feces which can contaminate the skin of animals or be inhaled (Kazar, 1996). Cats, dogs, rabbits, foxes and rodents are thought to constitute a reservoir for maintenance of infection in the domestic cycle of Q fever (Aitken, 1989). The role of rats has not yet been clearly described, even if recent data suggest that they might be true reservoirs of the infection, capable of independent maintenance of *C. burnetii* infection cycles thereby contributing to spread and transmission of the pathogen (Reusken et al., 2011).

C. burnetii is secreted in the milk, therefore the ingestion of contaminated food such as raw milk and dairy products, represent a possible source of infection for humans (Maurin & Raoult, 1999). Hirai and colleagues analysed 147 cheese samples by PCR analysis and found

19% of positive results (Hirai et al., 2011). However, when inoculated in mice, none of the positive samples allowed the recover of viable *C. burnetii.* Also, the administration of contaminated milk to voluntaries provided contradictory results (Angelakis & Raoult, 2010). The notable transmissibility of *C. burnetii* makes this microorganism extremely dangerous, particularly for occupationally exposed workers (veterinarians, slaughterhouse workers and farmers) and for laboratory technicians in contact with potentially contaminated specimens which therefore require manipulation by experienced personnel in BL3 facilities (Angelakis & Raoult, 2010).

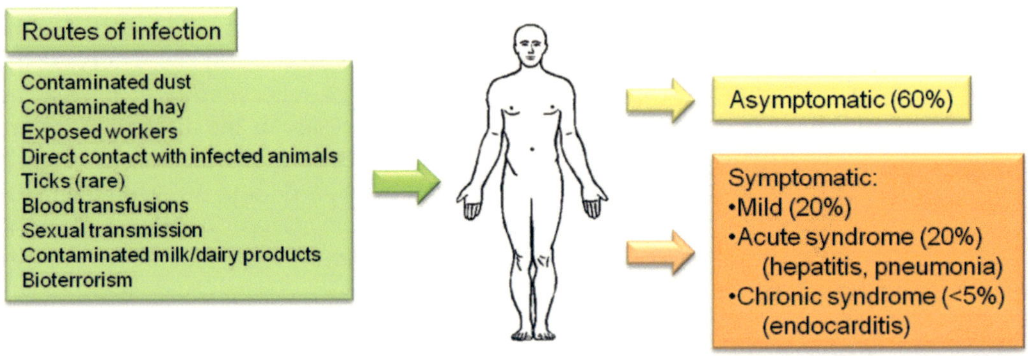

Fig. 1. Routes of transmission and pathophysiology of Q fever

C. burnetii is considered as a potential bioweapon, and is classified as class B agent (Madariaga et al., 2003). The high transmissibility of this pathogen, its extreme ability to persist in the environment and the aerial route of transmission make it a suitable bacterial agent for bioterrorism actions. In fact it has been evaluated that the inhalation of only one bacterial cell would be enough to induce the disease in man; moreover, the World Health Organization has esteemed that if 50 kg of *C. burnetii* were spread as an aerosol in an urban area of 500.000 inhabitants, 125.000 cases of acute illness, 9.000 cases of chronic Q fever and 150 dead people would be recorded (World Health Organization, 2004).

The aerial route of transmission of Q fever also represents the principal mode of infection for animals, for which however, unlike humans, an important role in the spread of the disease is also played by ticks. Other important ways of infection for animals are represented by direct contact with infected animals in the herd, by ingestion of contaminated placentas or milk, as well as possible ingestion of infected wild rodents (Angelakis & Raoult, 2010).

4. Pathogenesis

C. burnetii is a strictly intracellular bacterium capable of infecting different cellular types, mainly monocytes and macrophages. Its entry in the host cell is allowed by a mechanism of phagocytosis, much more efficient towards the phase II, avirulent, than to the phase I, virulent. This difference is due to the fact that the attachment to phase I bacteria is exclusively mediated by the integrin αvβ3, while attachment to phase II bacteria is mediated both by the integrin αvβ3 and by the complement receptor CR3. The most efficient internalization process determines a best intracellular replication and explains why bacteria in phase II grow faster than those in phase I, therefore justifying the conversion of the phase I to the phase II following growth in cell cultures. Both types can be recovered in the phagosomes, but only the phase I can survive in macrophages, while the phase II is quickly eliminated. The ability of *C. burnetii* to grow inside eukaryotic cells is due to the adaptation to the intracellular acidic pH. A pH value of 4.5, indeed, allows the entry of nutrients necessary for the metabolic functions of the bacterium, and, at the same time, confers protection from the action of numerous antibiotics, by altering their bactericidal activity. In macrophages this microorganism locates in vacuoles where its survival and proliferation are achieved by the control of phagocytosis and the prevention of phagosome lysosome fusion (Angelakis & Raoult, 2010; Raoult et al., 2005). The incomplete maturation of the phagosome is due both to the loss of the expression of the cellular marker cathepsin D, and to the exogenous production of IL-10, that also interferes with the microbicide activity of the macrophages. Interferon-γ restores the fusion between the phagosome and the lysosome, therefore allowing the elimination of *C. burnetii*. Moreover, it induces the alkalization of the vacuoles and controls the metabolism of the ions in the macrophages, inhibiting therefore the intracellular bacterial replication. Interferon-γ, finally contributes to the elimination of the infected macrophages through apoptosis, by inducing the expression of TNF on the cellular membrane. Following infection, the production of specific immunoglobulins is observed; in particular, while the phase I only stimulates the production of IgM, the phase II stimulates the production of both IgM and IgG1. The acute syndrome of Q fever determines a cell-mediated immune response and the formation of characteristic granulomatous lesions with a classical open space in the middle and a fibrin ring ("doughnut" granulomas). The control of the acute form includes the action of T cells, that however generally results insufficient for the complete elimination of the bacterium (Honstettre et al., 2004). When the infection assumes a chronic form, the level of inflammation becomes elevated, while cell-mediated immunity becomes defective. In fact, it has been observed that in patients affected by chronic endocarditis, the production of the inflammatory cytokines TNF and IL-6 is increased, while the ability of the lymphocytes to proliferate in response to the stimulation with *C. burnetii* antigen is decreased (Koster et al., 1985).

5. Epidemiology

Q fever is a worldwide zoonosis, prevalent in most countries in the world, with the exception of New Zealand. The reservoirs are large but partially known, and include many domestic and wild mammals, birds and arthropods like ticks (Fig. 2). The main sources of infection for man are domestic ruminants, mainly cattle, sheep and goats. Animals are often chronically infected, but mostly asymptomatic. In females *Coxiella* locates in the uterus and in the mammary glands and is shed in the environment through birth products, feces, urine and milk (Babudieri, 1959; Marrie & Raoult, 2002). Also pets, included dogs, cats and rabbits, can transmit the infection to man (Marrie & Raoult, 2002; Stein & Raoult, 1999). Animals can be infected by tick bites, ingestion of infected placentas or milk, and through the inhalation of contaminated particles. In ticks, as in mammals, *C. burnetii* is in phase I, and therefore highly contagious. Ticks, however, are not considered essential in the diffusion of the pathogen to domestic ruminants, but they play an important role in the transmission of *Coxiella* to the wild fauna, included vertebrates, lagomorphs and birds. Moreover they can spread high quantities of the microorganism through their feces, which in turn can be inhaled both by man and animals. Age and gender seem to have a role in the pathogenesis of Q fever; in particular, studies in man show that subjects less than 15 years old are less sensitive than older subjects (Angelakis & Raoult, 2010). Moreover, the number of cases in men is 2.5 times greater in comparison to that recorded in women (Gikas et al., 2010). During pregnancy, in animals, Q fever becomes chronic and *C. burnetii* remains in the uterus and in the mammary glands with the possibility to be reactivated by following pregnancies (Marrie et al., 1996).

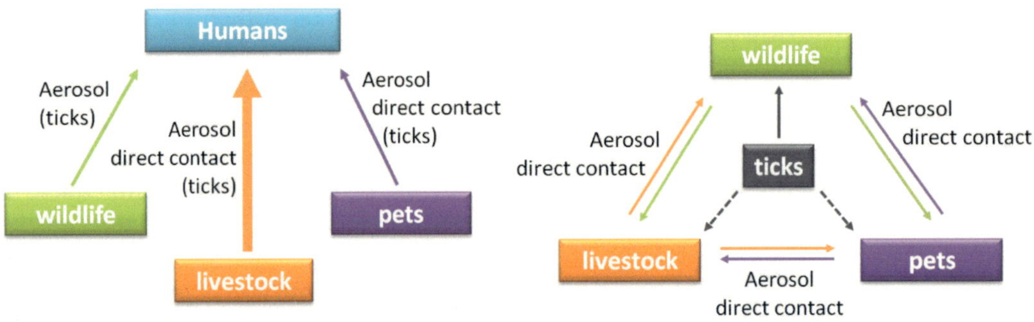

(a) Epidemiology of Q fever in humans (b) Epidemiology of Q fever in animals

Fig. 2. Epidemiology of Q fever

5.1 Occurrence of Q fever in man

Q fever can appear in the form of sporadic cases or outbreaks. It is a notifiable disease, but, as the infection is often asymptomatic, and its mild forms can be mistaken for other febrile episodes, sporadic forms of the disease are often undiagnosed and the true incidence of Q fever is still unknown. Moreover, the indiscriminate use of antibiotics in febrile patients hampers the clinical identification of Q fever as well as other rickettsioses and bacterioses. To the moment in the European states it is not clear yet the exact entity of Q fever in man, and in domestic ruminants. In Europe, preliminary data point out that during 2007, 585 human cases have been notified, while in 2008 they increased to 1594, with an increase of 172%. High risk groups include people working with possible infected material (slaughterhouse workers, veterinarians, meat-processing workers), persons living in or next to farms, and laboratory personnel processing eventually infected organs and tissues (Borriello et al., 2010; EFSA Panel on Animal Health and Welfare, 2010).

In abattoirs and wool-processing plants several epidemic outbreaks have occurred worldwide. Australia is considered an endemic area, with an outbreak characterized by 2000 cases in 1979-1980 (Hunt et al., 1983), while in Uruguay, in 1976, 310 of 360 workers and veterinary inspection personnel in a meat-packing plant contracted the disease in a month. The outbreak was attributed to the inhalation of contaminated aerosols, probably generated by the handling of infected material, as most cases were recorded among workers involved in bone-milling or collection of animal wastes. Three more outbreaks occurred in the same meat-packing plant in 1981 and 1984, mainly involving personnel working with slaughtering and animal wastes treatment (Somma-Moreira et al., 1987). Epidemics still occur in other slaughterhouse workers as well. Recent cases have been reported in New South Wales and in Scotland (Gilroy et al., 2001; Wilson et al., 2010).

Several Q fever epidemics have also been reported in farms and in geographic areas close to domestic ruminant herds (cattle, sheep and goats). Q fever cases have also been recorded in scientific institutes working with sheep as study models in different countries (Hall et al., 1982; Meiklejohn et al., 1981), or in human pathology institutes, as reported by Gerth and colleagues (1982) in Germany. Major outbreaks also occurred in the years following the World War II with estimated 20,000 cases in a two years period (Babudieri, 1959). In an urban school in central Israel a large Q fever outbreak has been reported in 2005, possibly transmitted by the air conditioning system (Amitai et al., 2005). This report highlights the importance to investigate the seroprevalence of Q fever in influenza-like outbreaks occurring outside the influenza season.

In addition to cattle, sheep and goats, parturient cats and newborn kittens can also represent a source of infection for man (Marrie et al, 1989). The role of cats in human Q fever epidemiology should not be underevaluated as it is the result of a combination of high prevalence of *C. burnetii* in rats and cats' predatory behavior towards these natural reservoirs (Reusken et al., 2011).

In the USA, 132 cases of Q fever with onset in 2008 have been reported; of these, 117 were acute Q fever and 15 were chronic Q fever (NASPHV & CDC, 2011). A serological survey in Japan reported prevalence values in healthy humans of 22.2% (Htwe et al., 1992). Moreover it has been observed that in Japanese children Q fever is often characterized by a clinical expression, mostly represented by atypical pneumonia (Hirai & To, 1998). A recent outbreak in the Netherlands started in 2007 and made the European Commission concerned about this zoonosis. The Dutch epidemic counted more than 2,200 confirmed human cases of the disease and more than 20 people died. In an effort to prevent the disease from spreading further, over 50,000 dairy goats were slaughtered and the government launched a mandatory animal vaccination campaign at the start of 2009. The main cause of infection has been attributed to infected goat and sheep farms located in the southern Brabant province (EFSA Panel on Animal Health and Welfare, 2010).

All the observed epidemics have common risk factors. Particularly, the greatest part of cases appear associated with a strict contact with domestic ruminant herds/flocks, mainly sheep and goats, both in relationship to the location and to the routes followed by the flocks. A great number of cases has often been recorded during or immediately after the period of the parturitions. Weather conditions characterized by dry and windy climate seem to play an important role in the transmission of the disease. Moreover, another risk factor is represented by living and/or working, sporting or performing social activities near agricultural zones covered with manure. Finally, also the presence of additional natural reservoir of infection (such as wild animals or ticks) near inhabited zones or herds further contributes to the maintenance of the pathogen in the environment (Borriello et al., 2010). The extreme persistence of *C. burnetii* in the environment and its diffusion in domestic ruminants and wild animals indicate therefore that good management practices play a critical role for the control of Q fever, not only in animals, but also in man (EFSA Panel on Animal Health and Welfare, 2010).

5.2 Occurrence of Q fever in animals

Q fever has been found in almost all species of domestic animals and many wild species. In India, the agent was isolated from amphibians (NASPHV & CDC, 2011) and a python. Q fever is endemic in domestic ruminants in the greatest part of the world. Serological surveys conducted in endemic areas have revealed a sizable proportion of reactors in the bovine, ovine and caprine populations. Although the infection is common, the disease is rare, and it has a limited impact on animal health.

Studies on the seroprevalence of the infection in cattle reported values of 67% in Ontario (Lang, 1989) and 40.4% in Sudan (Reinthaler et al., 1988). Similar prevalence values have also been reported in sheep and goats flocks in California (Ruppanner et al., 1982) and in Sudan (Reinthaler et al., 1988). In Japan, a survey on the presence of Q fever in domestic ruminants reported values of 25.4% in healthy cattle, 28.1% in sheep and 23.5% in goat. In Japanese bovine herds with reproductive disorders the seroprevalence of Q fever reached values of 84.3% (Htwe et al., 1992). In the European states to the moment it is not clear yet the exact entity of Q fever in domestic ruminants, since rules or recommendations are not harmonized for monitoring and report of the disease (EFSA Panel on Animal Health and Welfare, 2010). Epidemiological data on Q fever in animals point out that the general prevalence of the disease in domestic ruminants is increased from the 7.4% to the 10.0% within the period 2007 -2008. Particularly, the greatest increase has been recorded for goats, with values of 9.7% and 15.7% in 2007 and in 2008, respectively. Member States mostly affected are Bulgaria, France, Germany and, in particular way, the Netherlands (EFSA Panel on Animal Health and Welfare, 2010). In Italy *C. burnetii* is widely spread in domestic ruminants. Molecular analysis of milk in bovine farms has shown a prevalence of the infection of 40% (Magnino et al., 2009), and a significant association has been found between seropositive animals and abortion (Cabassi et al., 2006).

Reservoir species of *C. burnetii* can also be found among wildlife species and arthropods like ticks. A serological and molecular study in the Netherlands carried out on brown and black rats collected from both livestock farms and urban areas found the 15.8% of the brown rats seropositive, and detected *C. burnetii* DNA in the spleen of 4.9% of the brown rats and 3.0% of the black rats by PCR analysis (Reusken et al., 2011). A recent study in Northern Spain (Astobiza et al., 2011) identified as potential sources of the disease several wild species, such as roe deer, wild boar, European hares and birds, by PCR detection of *C. burnetii* DNA in spleen and liver (5.1%, 4.3%, 9.1% and 1.2%, respectively). Another study also carried out in Spain reported higher prevalence values in farmed red deer than in wild red deer (40% vs. 5.6%), probably indicating that in farmed animals direct contact may increase the risk of *C. burnetii* transmission (Ruiz-Fons et al., 2008). Moreover, several findings from different authors show an active role of ticks in maintaining *C. burnetii* in both wild and peridomestic cycles, therefore indirectly representing a risk factor for transmission of Q fever to humans (Mediannikov et al., 2010; Parola & Raoult, 2001; Toledo et al., 2009).

5.3 Occurrence of Q fever in domestic ruminants in Southern Italy

In Southern Italy the presence of *C. burnetii* in bovine and water buffalo herds, and in ovi-caprine flocks has been reported (Galiero et al., 1996; Parisi et al., 2006; Perugini et al., 2009), even if the exact prevalence of this pathogen is still largely unknown. The presence of *C. burnetii* in bovine and water buffalo herds of the Campania region was therefore investigated by molecular analysis carried out on aborted foetuses collected during the period 2009-2011.

For this purpose a total of 69 foetuses was analysed. The DNA from several organs (liver, lung, abomasum and placenta) was extracted by the DNA mini kit (QIAGEN) and was subsequently amplified by a single-tube nested PCR for the detection of *C. burnetii* (Parisi et al., 2006). The foetuses were considered positive when at least one of the sampled organs resulted positive.

The obtained results have shown that the 47% (8/17) of the analyzed bovine foetuses and the 29% (15/52) of the analyzed water buffalo foetuses resulted positive to *C. burnetii* PCR detection (Tab. 1).

Species	Examined Foetuses	Positive Foetuses
Bovine	17	8
Water buffalo	52	15
Total	69	23

Table 1. PCR detection of *C. burnetii* in bovine and water buffalo foetuses

Among the 8 positive bovine foetuses, 4 (50%) exhibited the presence of *C. burnetii* in the lungs, 1 (12%) in the liver and 5 (62%) in the abomasum. One foetus exhibited the presence of the pathogen both in lungs and liver.

Among the 15 positive water buffalo foetuses, 8 (53%) exhibited the presence of *C. burnetii* in the liver, 7 (47%) in the lungs, 3 (20%) in the abomasum and 4 (27%) in the placenta. Four foetuses exhibited the presence of *Coxiella* both in liver and lungs, one foetus in liver, lungs and placenta, and another foetus in liver, lungs and abomasum (Tab.2).

		Number of positive samples			
Species	Analysed foetuses	Lungs	Liver	Abomasum	Placenta
Bovine	8	4	1	5	0
Water buffalo	15	7	8	3	4
Total	23	11	9	8	4

Table 2. Detection of *C. burnetii* in organs

Abortions in bovine and water buffalo herds determine serious economic losses. In Southern Italy the incidence of abortions caused by infectious diseases is elevated and clear epidemiological data able to explain the possible causes of this phenomenon are still lacking (Capuano et al., 2004). Particularly, among the aetiological agents responsible of abortion, preliminary reports indicate that the presence of this pathogen is significant in Southern Italy. Indeed, Parisi and colleagues (2006) reported an incidence of *C. burnetii* in bovine herds and ovi-caprine flocks of 6% and 21.5%, respectively, while, in water buffalo herds, variable inter-herd prevalence values have been found, ranging from 17 to 23% (Galiero et al., 1996; Perugini et al., 2009).

The data reported in this study confirm the presence of *C. burnetii* both in bovine and water buffalo herds, and point out that this pathogen plays an important role as abortive agent for these animal species. Moreover, water buffalo seems to be more susceptible to this pathogen rather than cattle. Other studies will be therefore necessary to clarify the epidemiology and the pathogenesis of *C. burnetii* infection both in cattle and water buffalo. Particularly water buffalo needs careful investigation as the milk from this species can be used also crude for the production of the world famous "mozzarella di bufala" cheese.

The single-tube nested PCR proved to be an efficient diagnostic method to determine the presence of *C. burnetii* in organs from bovine and water buffalo foetuses. This technique, indeed, exhibited enhanced sensitivity, as it is based on the amplification of a secondary target sequence within the first run product. The use of a nested PCR therefore might increase the possibility to detect *C. burnetii* DNA in animal tissues, where DNA can easily be degraded due to autolysis phenomena, as it often happens in animal foetuses.

Moreover, these data underline the need of specific diagnostic methods to be carried out within proper monitoring plans aiming to provide a careful estimate of *C. burnetii* prevalence and its routes of transmission.

6. Description of the disease

Q fever is characterized by a polymorphic clinical spectrum, therefore the diagnosis of the disease can only be made if systematic laboratory tests are performed. Several factors are likely to influence the course of the infection by *C. burnetii*. Among these the route of infection, the infectious dose, age and gender play a major role (Angelakis & Raoult, 2010).

6.1 Q fever in man

In man the clinical demonstration of the disease can consist in an asymptomatic seroconversion, an acute form of the illness, varying from self-limiting fever episodes up to granulomatous hepatitis or severe pneumonia, or a chronic form, characterized by endocarditis. In the acute forms the incubation period has an average duration of 20 days, and the greatest part of cases presents no or mild symptoms. The combination of symptoms varies greatly from person to person, and it can include high fevers (up to 39-40°C), severe headache, general malaise, myalgia, chills and/or sweats, non-productive cough, nausea, vomiting, diarrhoea, abdominal pain and chest pain. Atypical pneumonia is among the most common acute manifestations of *C. burnetii* infection. In some patients serious respiratory stresses and diffusion of the bacterium in the pleura can occur. The duration of symptoms varies from 10 to 90 days, with a mortality of about 0.5-1.5%. Hepatitis is the most common clinical manifestation of Q fever, and it can be either asymptomatic, or associated with hepatomegaly or with characteristic granulomas and prolonged fever (Angelakis & Raoult, 2010). Rarely (2% of the cases) other symptoms can occur, such as perycarditis, myocarditis, neurological symptoms (varying from the most common headaches to meningitis, meningoencephalitis or peripheral neuropathies). Dermatological lesions are more common than generally thought and they include transient punctiform rashes, maculopapular eruptions and, more rarely, erythema nodosum (Raoult et al., 2005). Post-Q fever fatigue syndrome can be observed in some (10-25%) acute patients, characterized by constant or recurring fatigue, night sweats, severe headaches, photophobia, pain in muscles and joints, mood changes and difficulty sleeping. In pregnant women *Coxiella* settles in the uterus and mammary glands, often resulting in pre-term delivery or miscarriage.

Chronic Q fever is a severe disease occurring in <5% of acutely infected patients. It may present soon (within 6 weeks) after an acute infection, or may manifest years later. The chronic forms are mostly characterized by endocarditis and vascular infections, less frequently by aortic aneurysms and infections of the bone, liver or reproductive organs, such as the testes in males. They almost exclusively affect individuals with predisposing conditions, such as lesions of cardiac valves, vascular problems or immunodeficiency, and symptoms can also occur months or years after the infection. The endocarditis and the vascular infections from chronic Q fever generally have a lethal outcome if they are not treated with an appropriate antibiotic for a period of at least 18 months up to a life treatment (Maurin & Raoult, 1999).

6.2 Q fever in animals

In domestic ruminants *C. burnetii* infection is mostly asymptomatic. During the acute phase *C. burnetii* can be found in blood, lungs, spleen and liver, whereas during chronic Q fever it is persistently shed in urine and feces.

In cattle the main pathological demonstrations of Q fever associated with chronic infections are represented by ipofertility, metritis and low birth weight calves, more rarely by abortions and stillbirths. In asymptomatic but seropositive herds, *Coxiella* is almost exclusively shed in milk. The excretion can last several months (up to 32) and can be continuous or intermittent, and, in some cases, can be associated with chronic subclinical mastitis (Rodolakis et al., 2007). In bovine herds with reproductive disorders, infected females primarily shed *Coxiella* through birth products, but also through feces, urine and milk (Arricau Bouvery et al., 2003). Elimination of the microorganism through these ways can persist for several months, also for subjects that have not exhibited problems during the parturition (Berri et al., 2005b). None of these shedding patterns however appears to have a predominant role in the eliminatory subjects, often exhibiting one excretion route only.

Sheep and goats, like cattle, are considered as the main reservoirs of infection for man. They almost always result asymptomatic and the most common pathological manifestations of chronic Q fever are abortions and stillbirths. In sheep and goats flocks with reproductive disorders, animals contemporarily shed the bacterium through vaginal mucus, feces and milk. Particularly, in a recent work, goats have been shown to eliminate *C. burnetii* mostly through milk, sheep mainly through vaginal mucus or feces (Rodolakis, 2009).

Asymptomatic but seropositive ovine flocks, instead, always resulted negative to *C. burnetii* detection by PCR analysis in bulk tank milk.

Differences in shedding patterns can explain why sheep and goats are identified more frequently than cattle as the main source of infection for man (Rodolakis, 2009).

7. Diagnostic techniques

The extreme virulence of *C. burnetii* requires the use of bio-containment level 3 facilities for contaminated specimens processing, and isolation and cultivation of the pathogen should be performed by experienced laboratory personnel only (OIE, 2010). *Coxiella burnetii* can be demonstrated in various ways, depending on the type of sample and the purpose of investigations (Samuel & Hendrix, 2009; Sidi-Boumedine et al., 2010).

For human diagnosis of Q fever the most appropriate tests are PCR analysis of whole blood samples (most sensitive if blood is collected during the first week of illness; rapidly decreasing in sensitivity when antibodies reach a high level) and PCR or immunohistochemistry of biopsy specimens. Negative PCR results should not rule out the diagnosis, and treatment should not be withheld. Culture isolation of *C. burnetii* is possible in specialized laboratories only, as routine hospital blood cultures cannot detect the microorganism. The gold standard serologic test for diagnosis of Q fever is the indirect immunofluorescence assay (IFA), performed on paired serum samples collected the first as early in the disease as possible (preferably in the first week of symptoms), and the second 2 to 4 weeks later. The first IgG IFA titer should therefore be typically low or negative, and the second should instead exhibit a significant (four-fold) increase. Analysis of two samples is necessary as antibodies to *C. burnetii* may remain elevated for months or longer after the disease has resolved, or may be detected in persons previously exposed to antigenically related organisms, therefore, interpretation of one sample may be difficult. Humans can develop antibody response against both *C. burnetii* phase I and phase II. In particular, in acute infection, an antibody response to *C. burnetii* phase II antigen is predominant and is higher than phase I antibody response; the reverse is true in chronic infection which is associated with a rising phase I IgG titer (according to current U.S. case definitions >1:800) that is often much higher than phase II IgG (NASPHV & CDC, 2011).

For animal diagnosis in the context of serial abortions and stillbirths, samples should be collected from aborted foetuses, placenta and vaginal discharges soon after abortion or parturition. The diagnosis should always include a differential investigation of major abortive agents. Early detection of a Q fever outbreak of abortions in a herd or flock and correct biocontainment measures are essential to prevent and limit both environmental and farm-based routes of infection. A positive case is a herd or flock with clinical signs (abortion and/or stillbirth) for which the presence of the agent has been confirmed. As a rule, in the veterinary practice, a breeding or a flock can be considered clinically affected by Q fever if three circumstances occur: abortions or stillbirths, presence of *C. burnetii* in samples from affected animals (evaluated by Quantitative PCR analysis) and presence of seropositive animals (evaluated by ELISA test). EFSA criteria (Sidi-Boumedine et al., 2010) suggested for a correct diagnosis of *C. burnetii* as abortive agent in bovine herds and ovi-caprine flocks are summarized in the figures 3 and 4, respectively.

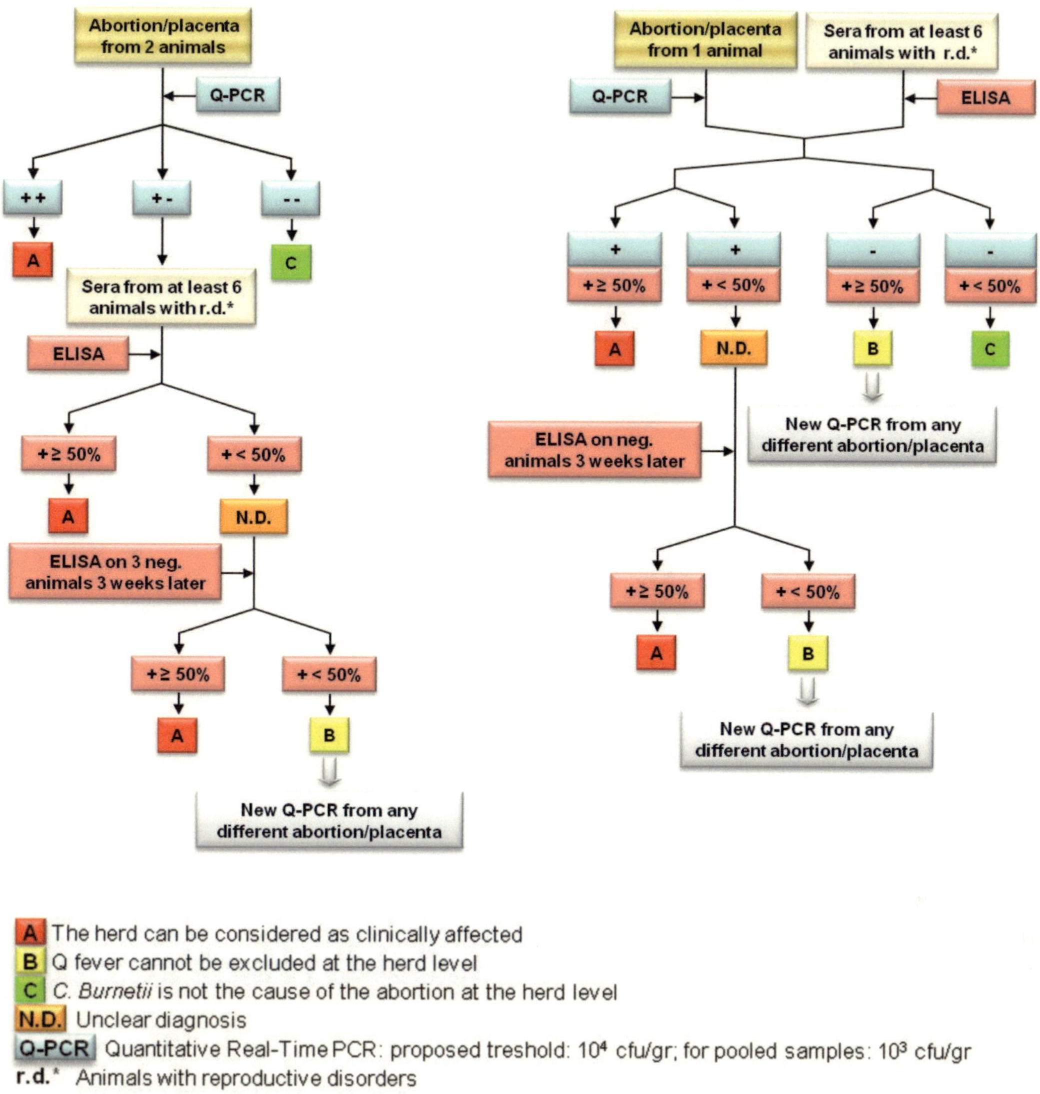

Fig. 3. EFSA criteria for a correct diagnosis of Q fever in bovine herds

7.1 Direct techniques

For specific laboratory investigations, it may be necessary to isolate the agent. The direct methods for the isolation and the identification of the infectious agent require proper samples, mainly represented by placenta, vaginal mucus, milk, colostrum, feces and tissues of the aborted foetus, such as liver, lung and content of the stomach, collected immediately after the abortion.

Several techniques are available for *C. burnetii* identification (OIE, 2010), even if they are often characterized by low specificity.

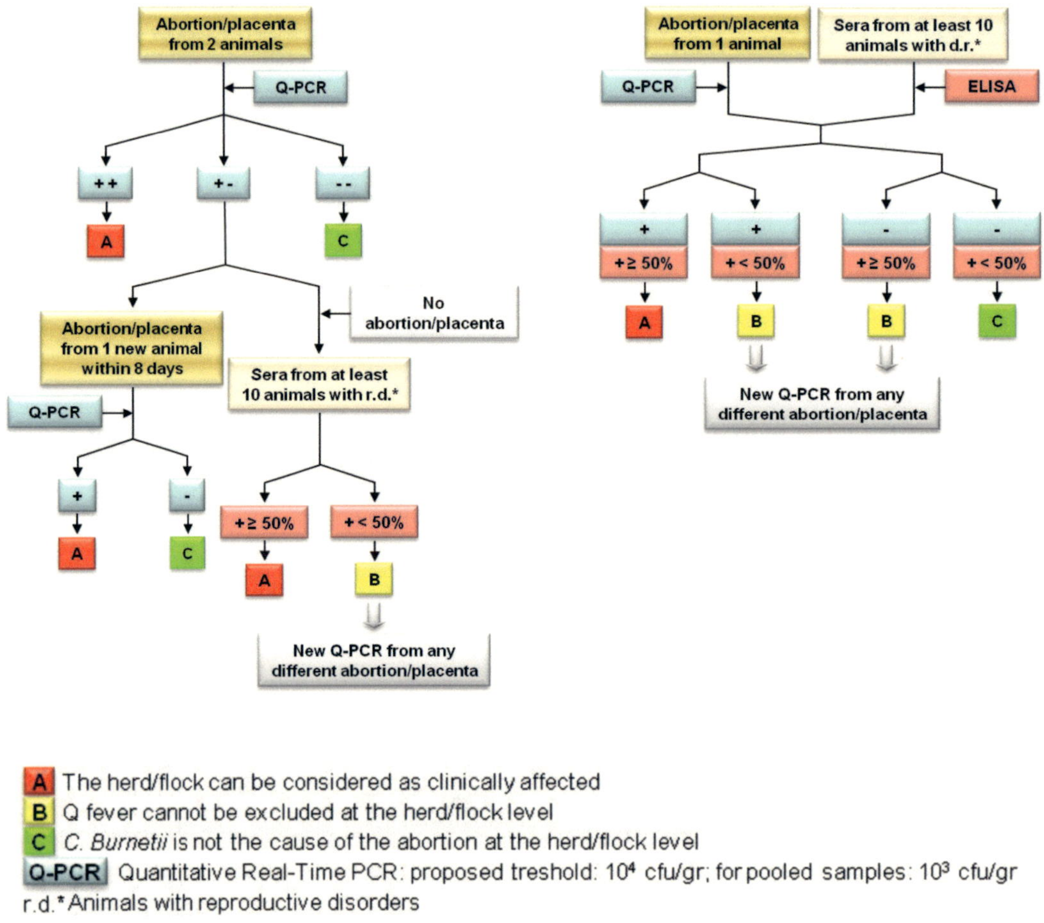

Fig. 4. EFSA criteria for a correct diagnosis of Q fever in ovi-caprine flocks

7.1.1 Staining techniques

These techniques can be carried out in case of abortions suspected to have an infectious origin. Best results can be obtained by smears of placental cotyledon prepared on microscope slides, but lung, liver and abomasum contents of the aborted foetus or vaginal discharges may be used as well. Several methods are suitable for *Coxiella* identification: Stamp, Gimenez, Macchiavello, Giemsa and modified Koster (Gimenez, 1964; Quinn et al., 1994; Samuel & Hendrix, 2009). The first three techniques give the best results (OIE, 2010). These methods are close to the modified Ziehl-Neelsen method involving basic fuchsin to stain bacteria. The Stamp method is preferred in veterinary laboratories whereas the Gimenez method is very fast for monitoring infected cultural cells in research laboratories. Attention must be taken in the interpretation of the results as, microscopically, *C. burnetii* can be confused with *Chlamydophila abortus* or *Brucella* spp. When biological staining is inconclusive, one of the other methods may be used as a confirmatory test.

7.1.2 Isolation of the agent

These techniques have been abandoned because of their high risk level, even if they can be necessary when isolation of *Coxiella* is required from samples contaminated with more than a bacterial species (OIE, 2010). When *C. burnetii* is present in large numbers and is combined with a low contamination rate with other bacteria, direct isolation by inoculation of embryonated chicken eggs or cell culture is possible (Maurin & Raoult, 1999; Samuel & Hendrix, 2009). A cell microculture system from a commercially available method used for virus culture, the shell vial cell culture, has been adapted for isolating strict or facultative intracellular bacteria, including *C. burnetii*. Such a method was described for *C. burnetii* in 1990 (Raoult et al., 1990). Suspensions of samples are inoculated into a cell line to observe the characteristic vacuoles of *C. burnetii* multiplication. This method was developed for humans but could be adapted for animals. With heavily multi-contaminated samples, such as placentas, vaginal discharges, feces, or milk, the inoculation of laboratory animals may be necessary as a filtration system. Mice and guinea-pigs are the most appropriate animals for this purpose (Scott et al., 1987).

7.2 Indirect techniques

Indirect techniques include the indirect immunofluorescence assay (IFA), the ELISA test and the complement fixation test (FDC) to be performed on serum samples, or, in the case of the ELISA, also on milk samples. Such methods result useful for the screening of high numbers of samples, as in the case of entire herds/flocks, but do not provide clear results for single animal investigations. In fact some animals can remain seropositive for quite several years following acute infection, other animals can shed *C. burnetii* before seroconversion and therefore represent a risk factor for infection, while other animals never seroconvert (Maurin & Raoult, 1999). To the moment tests able to discriminate between infected and vaccinated animals do not exist yet.

7.2.1 Indirect Immunofluorescence Assay (IFA)

In human medicine, the IFA adapted as a micro-immunofluorescence technique is the current method for the serodiagnosis of Q fever (Tissot-Dupont et al., 1994). Both phase I and phase II *C. burnetii* antigens are used. The two forms of the infection, acute and chronic, have different serological profiles: during acute Q fever, IgG antibodies are elevated against phase II only whereas during chronic Q fever, high levels of IgG antibodies to both phase I and II of the bacteria are observed (Tissot-Dupont et al., 1994).

7.2.2 Complement Fixation Test (CFT)

The test detects complement-fixing antibodies present in the serum. The CFT is specific but less sensitive than the ELISA or IFA (Kittelberger et al., 2009; Rousset et al., 2007; 2009). The CFT is still used by laboratories in many countries. This method often uses antigen in phase II prepared from a mixture of two strains (Nine Mile and Henzerling) or a mixture of antigens in phase I and II prepared from Nine Mile strain.

7.2.3 Enzyme-Linked Immunosorbent Assay (ELISA)

This technique has a high sensitivity and a good specificity (Kittelberger et al., 2009; Rousset et al., 2007; 2009). It is easy to perform. The ELISA is preferred to IFA and CFT, particularly for veterinary diagnosis, because it is convenient for large-scale screening and, is a reliable technique for demonstrating *C. burnetii* antibody in various animal species (Jaspers et al., 1994; Soliman et al., 1992). Ready-to-use kits are commercially available and can detect anti-phase II antibodies or both anti-phase I and II antibodies.

7.3 Specific detection methods

Detection of *C. burnetii* in samples can also be achieved by specific immunodetection (capture ELISA, immunohistochemistry), in-situ hybridisation or DNA amplification (Jensen et al., 2007; Samuel & Hendrix, 2009; Thiele et al., 1992). Immunohistology may be used with paraffin-embedded tissues or on acetone-fixed smears (Raoult et al., 1994). The method is an indirect immunofluorescence or immunoperoxidase assay using polyclonal *C. burnetii* specific antibodies. Fluorescent in-situ hybridisation using specific oligonucleotide probes targeting 16s rRNA may be used on paraffin-embedded tissues, especially placenta samples (Jensen et al., 2007).

C. burnetii detection is today mainly performed by PCR. This method has many advantages because it is highly specific and sensitive, it allows the inactivation of the microorganism by heating to 90°C for 30-60 min, it allows working on different kinds of samples without the need to isolate the bacterium. Unfortunately this method does not allow the isolation of the agent. Target sequences for PCR are numerous, and the most used is the IS1111 (accession number M80806), which renders the technique even more sensitive as this insertion sequence is broadly repeated in the genome of *Coxiella*. PCR is therefore an effective method for the identification of shedding animals. Recently a Real-Time PCR protocol has been set up for the identification and the quantification of the number of bacteria present in a biological matrix. The quantification of *C. burnetii* in the abortion products is an extremely important information as it is the core part of a correct diagnosis of this pathogen as the real cause of the abortion (Sidi-Boumedine et al., 2010).

7.4 Genotyping methods

Detection, isolation and identification of *C. burnetii* can be completed with a molecular characterization, useful for epidemiological studies. Several typing methods have been used for the characterisation of *C. burnetii* strains, such as restriction endonuclease of genomic DNA (Hendrix et al., 1991), PFGE (Pulsed-Field Gel Electrophoresis) (Jäger et al., 1998), and sequence and/or PCR-RFLP (Restriction Fragment Length Polymorphism) analysis of *icd, com1* and *mucZ* genes. More recently, the two PCR-based typing methods MLVA (Multi-Locus Variable number of tandem repeats Analysis) (Arricau-Bouvery et al., 2006; Svraka et al., 2006) and multispacer sequence typing (MST) (Glazunova et al., 2005) are gaining importance for several reasons. Indeed they permit the typing of *C. burnetii* without the need for isolation of the organism. Moreover they exhibit high discriminating power with relatively low costs. MLVA analysis is currently the reference method for the genetic characterization of important pathogens such as *M. tuberculosis, B. anthracis* and *Y. pestis*. Recent studies have shown that the application of this technique to *C. burnetii* isolates both of animal and human origin allowed the identification of 36 different genetic profiles on a total of 42 isolates (Arricau-Bouvery et al., 2006). Moreover, databases have been established, http: //minisatellites.u-psud.fr/MLVAnet/ and http://ifr48.timone.univ-mrs.fr for MLVA and MST, respectively. The availability of such databases allows easy inter-laboratory comparisons which might lead to a better understanding of the propagation of *C. burnetii* isolates.

These tools are very useful for epidemiological investigation, particularly to clarify links regarding sources of infection, for better understanding of the epidemiological emerging factors, and to a lesser extent, for evaluating control measures.

8. Therapy and prophylaxis

In man doxycycline is the first line treatment for all adults, and for children with severe illness. Doxycycline is most effective at preventing severe complications if it is started early in the course of disease. Failure to respond to this antibiotic indicates that *C. burnetii* is not the aetiological agent of the illness, as resistance to doxycycline has never been documented. The recommended dosage for acute Q fever in adults is 100 mg every 12 hours, while for children under 45 kg is 2.2 mg/kg of body weight given twice a day. Standard duration of treatment is 2-3 weeks, or for at least three days after the fever subsides, or until there is evidence of clinical improvement. The recommended treatment for adults affected by chronic Q fever includes 100 mg of doxycycline every 12 hours and 200 mg of hydroxychloroquine every 8 hours. Standard duration of treatment is 18 months (NASPHV & CDC, 2011).

In animals little information is available on the effectiveness of antibiotic treatments, which are often used for reducing the number of abortions and the level of elimination of *C. burnetii* during parturition. Antimicrobial treatment is in fact used mainly to minimize shedding of the organism in the placenta and birth fluids rather to eliminate it. This treatment doesn't prevent entirely neither the abortion (Berri et al., 2005a), nor the elimination of *Coxiella* during parturition (Arricau-Bouvery & Rodolakis, 2005). The prophylaxis based on antibiotic treatment provides therefore the advantage to reduce the risk of abortion, but it doesn't determine the eradication of the disease. In fact, following antibiotic treatment, the animals can still shed *Coxiella* even if they result clinically recovered from the disease.

During Q fever outbreaks the spreading of *Coxiella* in the herd can be prevented or at least reduced by applying control measures including severe hygiene protocols, aiming to prevent environmental contamination (manure composting, fight against natural reservoirs, separation of the areas used for parturition and new born, ready elimination of vaginal discharges and abortion products) and possible culling of seropositive and/or shedding animals.

Vaccination seems to be the only efficient strategy for the control of the disease. Currently two typologies of vaccines exist, one developed against the phase I (virulent), and one against the phase II (avirulent). The commercial available products are Q-VAX ® (for human use), Coxevac ® (for veterinary use) and Chlamivax FQ ® (for veterinary use, developed also against *Chlamydophila abortus*). The use of vaccine does not avoid the risk of shedding of the microorganism from infected animals. Vaccination is therefore suitable only for seronegative herds/flocks. The use of the anti-phase I vaccine in the veterinary practice results useful not only for the control of the disease inside the herd/flock, but also effective against the spreading of the infection in the neighbouring herds as well as in man.

9. Conclusion

The numerous cases of Q fever in animals and in man recently occurred in the Netherlands renewed the interest of the sanitary authorities and of the scientific community on a disease for too long neglected. The presence of this pathology worldwide and the underestimation of this disease highlight the need of specific serological and molecular investigations including careful examination of all the ipofertility and abortion cases recorded in domestic ruminant herds/flocks. Epidemiological data should be used to set up effective monitoring and prophylaxis strategies for the control of Q fever. Particular attention should be posed on the control of this pathology in domestic and wildlife animals, aiming to contain the economic and sanitary impact that the uncontrolled spread of Q fever would have on human health.

10. References

Aitken, I.D. (1989). Clinical aspects and prevention of Q fever in animals. *European Journal of Epidemiology*, Vol.5, No.4, (December), pp.420-424, ISSN

Amitai, Z., Bromberg, M., Bernstein, M., Raveh, D., Keysary, A., David, D., Pitlik, S., Swerdlow, D., Massung, R., Rzotkiewicz, S., Halutz, O. & Shohat, T. (2005). A large Q fever outbreak in an urban school in central Israel. *Clinical Infectious Diseases*, Vol.50, No.11, (June 1), pp. 1433-1438, ISSN 1537-6591

Angelakis, E. & Raoult, D. (2010). Q Fever. *Veterinary Microbiology*, Vol.140, No.3-4, (January 27), pp. 297-309, ISSN 0378-1135

Arricau Bouvery, N., Souriau, A., Lechopier, P. & Rodolakis, A. (2003). Experimental *Coxiella burnetii* infection in pregnant goats: excretion routes. *Veterinary Research*, Vol.34, No.4, (July-August), pp. 423-433, ISSN 0378-1135

Arricau-Bouvery, N. & Rodolakis, A. (2005). Is Q fever an emerging or reemerging zoonosis? *Veterinary Research*, Vol.36, No.3, (May-June), pp. 327-349, ISSN 0378-1135

Arricau-Bouvery, N., Hauck, Y., Bejaoui, A., Frangoulidis, D., Bodier, C.C., Souriau, A., Meyer, H., Neubauer, H., Rodolakis, A. & Vergnaud, G. (2006). Molecular characterization of *Coxiella burnetii* isolates by infrequent restriction site-PCR and MLVA typing. *BMC Microbiology*, Vol.6, (April 26), pp. 38, ISSN 1471-2180

Astobiza, I., Barral, M., Ruiz-Fons, F., Barandika, J.F., Gerrikagoitia, X., Hurtado, A. & García-Pérez, A.L. (2011). Molecular investigation of the occurrence of *Coxiella burnetii* in wildlife and ticks in an endemic area. *Veterinary Microbiology*, Vol.147, No.1-2, (January 10), pp. 190-194, ISSN 0378-1135

Babudieri, B. (1959). Q fever. A zoonosis. *Advances in Veterinary Science*, Vol.5, pp. 82-182, ISSN 0096-7653

Beare, P.A., Samuel, J.E., Howe, D., Virtaneva, K., Porcella, S.F. & Heinzen, R.A. (2006). Genetic diversity of the Q fever agent, *Coxiella burnetii*, assessed by microarray-based whole-genome comparisons. *Journal of Bacteriology*, Vol.188, No.7, (April), pp. 2309-2324, ISSN 1098-5530

Berri, M., Crochet, D., Santiago, S. & Rodolakis, A. (2005a). Spread of *Coxiella burnetii* infection in a flock of sheep after an episode of Q fever. *The Veterinary Record*, Vol.157, No.23, (December 3), pp. 737-740, ISSN 0042-4900

Berri, M., Rousset, E., Hechard, C., Champion, J.L., Dufour, P., Russo, P. & Rodolakis, A. (2005b). Progression of Q fever and Coxiella *burnetii* shedding in milk after an outbreak of enzootic abortion in a goat herd. *The Veterinary Record*, Vol.156, No.17, (April 23), pp. 548-549, ISSN 0042-4900

Borriello, G., Iovane, G. & Galiero, G. (2010). La febbre Q negli animali domestici. *Large Animal Review*, Vol.16, pp. 273-283, ISSN 1124-4593

Burnet, F.M. & Freeman, M. (1937). Experimental studies on the virus of "Q" fever. *Reviews of Infectious Diseases*, Vol.5, No.4, (July August), PP. 299-305, ISSN 0162-0886

Cabassi, C.S., Taddei, S., Donofrio, G., Ghidini, F., Piancastelli, C., Flammini, C.F. & Cavirani, S. (2006). Association between *Coxiella burnetii* seropositivity and abortion in dairy cattle of Northern Italy. *New Microbiologica*, Vol.29, No.3, (July), pp. 211-214, ISSN 1121-7138

Capuano, F., Parisi, A., Cafiero, M., Picaro, L. & Fenizia, D. (2004). *Coxiella burnetii*: what is the reality?. *Parassitologia* Vol.46, No.1-2, (June), pp. 131–134, ISSN: 0048-2951

Derrick, E.H. (1937). Q fever, a new fever entity clinical features, diagnosis and laboratory investigation. *The Medical Journal of Australia*, Vol.2, pp. 281-299, ISSN 1326- 5377

EFSA Panel on Animal Health and Welfare (AHAW), (2010) Scientific opinion on Q fever. *EFSA Journal* Vol.8, No.5, (May 12), pp. 1595-1708, ISSN 1831-4732

Galiero, G., Goffredi, C.G. & D'Orazi, A. (1996). Epidemiology of Q fever: seroprevalence in buffalo dairies of Salerno province. *Selezione Veteterinaria*, Vol.6, pp. 407-412, ISSN 0037-1521

Gerth, H.J., Leidig, U. & Riemenschneider, T. (1982). Q-fever epidemic in an institute of human pathology. *Deutsche medizinische Wochenschrift*, Vol.107, No.37, (September 17), pp. 1391-5, ISSN 1439-4413

Gikas, A., Kokkini, S. & Tsioutis, C. (2010). Q fever: clinical manifestations and treatment. *Expert Review of Anti-Infective Therapy*, Vol.8, No.5, (May), pp. 529-539, ISSN: 1478-7210

Gilroy, N., Formica, N., Beers, M., Egan, A., Conaty, S. & Marmion, B. (2001). Abattoir-associated Q fever: a Q fever outbreak during a Q fever vaccination program. *The Australian and New Zealand Journal of Public Health*, Vol.25, No.4, (August), pp. 362-367, ISSN 1753-6405

Gimenez, D.F. (1964). Staining rickettsiae in yolk-sack cultures. *Stain technology*, Vol.39, (May), pp. 135–140, ISSN 0038-9153

Glazunova, O., Roux, V., Freylikman, O., Sekeyova, Z., Fournous, G., Tyczka, J., Tokarevich, N., Kovacava, E., Marrie, T.J. & Raoult, D. (2005). *Coxiella burnetii* genotyping. *Emerging Infectious Disease*, Vol.11, No.8, (August), pp. 1211-1217, ISSN 1080-6059

Hackstadt, T. (1986). Antigenic variation in the phase I lipopolysaccharide of *Coxiella burnetii* isolates. *Infection and Immunity*, Vol.52, No.1, (April), pp. 337-340, ISSN 1098-5522

Hall, C.J., Richmond, S.J., Caul, E.O., Pearce, N.H. & Silver, I.A. (1982). Laboratory outbreak of Q fever acquired from sheep. *The Lancet*, Vol.1, No.8279, (May 1), pp. 1004-1006, ISSN 0140-6736

Hendrix, L.R., Samuel, J.E. & Mallavia, L.P. (1991). Differentiation of *Coxiella burnetii* isolates by analysis of restriction-endonuclease-digested DNA separated by SDS-PAGE. *Journal of General Microbiology*, Vol.137, No.2, (February), pp. 269-276, ISSN 0022-1287

Hirai, K. & To, H. (1998). Advances in the understanding of *Coxiella burnetii* infection in Japan. *Journal of Veterinary Medical Science*, Vol.60, No.7, (July), pp. 781-790, ISSN 0916-7250

Hirai, A., Nakama, A., Chiba, T. & Kai, A. (2011). Development of a Method for Detecting *Coxiella burnetii* in Cheese Samples. *Journal of Veterinary Medical Science*, (October 7), Epub ahead of print, ISSN 0916-7250

Honstettre, A., Ghigo, E., Moynault, A., Capo, C., Toman, R., Akira, S., Takeuchi, O., Lepidi, H., Raoult, D. & Mege, J.L. (2004). Lipopolysaccharide from *Coxiella burnetii* is involved in bacterial phagocytosis, filamentous actin reorganization, and inflammatory responses through Tolllike receptor 4. *Journal of Immunology*, Vol.172, No.6, (March 15), pp. 3695-3703, ISSN 1550- 6606

Htwe, K.K., Amano, K., Sugiyama, Y., Yagami, K., Minamoto, N., Hashimoto, A., Yamaguchi, T., Fukushi, H. & Hirai, K. (1992). Seroepidemiology of *Coxiella burnetii* in domestic and companion animals in Japan. *The Veterinary Record*, Vol.131, No.21, (November 21), pp. 490, ISSN 0042-4900

Hunt, J.G., Field, P.R. & Murphy, A.M. (1983). Immunoglobulin responses to *Coxiella burnetii* (Q fever): single-serum diagnosis of acute infection, using an immunofluorescence technique. *Infection and Immunity*, Vol.39, No.2, (February), pp. 977-981, ISSN 1098-5522

Jäger, C., Willems, H., Thiele, D. & Baljer G. (1998). Molecular characterization of *Coxiella burnetii* isolates. *Epidemiology and Infection*, Vol.120, No.2, (March), pp. 157-164, ISSN 1469-4409

Jaspers, U., Thiele, D. & Krauss, H. (1994). Monoclonal antibody based competitive ELISA for the detection of specific antibodies against *Coxiella burnetii* in sera from different animal species. *Zentralblatt für Bakteriologie*, Vol.281, No.1, (June), pp. 61–66, ISSN 0934-8840

Kazar, J. (1996). Q fever. In: *Rickettsiae and Rickettsial Diseases*, Kazar, J., Toman, R. (Eds.), 353-362, Slovak Academy of Sciences, ISBN 978-052-1821-49-0, Bratislava, Slovakia

Jensen, T.K., Montgomery, D.L., Jaeger, P.T., Lindhardt, T., Agerholm, J.S., Bille-Hansen, V. & Boye M. (2007). Application of fluorescent in situ hybridisation for demonstration of *Coxiella burnetii* in placentas from ruminant abortions. *Acta Pathologica, Microbiologica et Immunologica Scandinavica*, Vol.115, No., pp. 347–353, ISSN 1600-0463.

Kittelberger, R., Mars, J.,Wibberley, G., Sting, R., Henning, K., Horner, G.W., Garnett, K.M., Hannah, M.J., Jenner, J.A., Pigott, C.J. & O'keefe, J.S. (2009). Comparison of the Q fever complement fixation test and two commercial enzyme-linked immunosorbent assays for the detection of serum anibodies against *Coxiella burnetii* (Q-fever) in ruminants: Recommandations for use of serological tests on imported animals in New Zealand. *New Zealand Veterinary Journal*, Vol.57, No.5, (October), pp. 262–268, ISSN 1176-0710

Koster, F.T., Williams, J.C. & Goodwin, J.S. (1985). Cellular immunity in Q fever: specific lymphocyte unresponsiveness in Q fever endocarditis. *Journal of Infectious Diseases*, Vol.152, No.6, (December), pp. 1283-1289, ISSN 1537-6613

Kruszewska, D. & Tylewska-Wierzbanowska, S. (1997). Isolation of *Coxiella burnetii* from bull semen. *Research in Veterinary Science*, Vol.62, No.3, (May June), pp. 299-300, ISSN 0034-5288

Lang, G.H. (1989). Q fever: an emerging public health concern in Canada. *Canadian Journal of Veterinary Research*, Vol.53, No.1, (January), pp.1-6, ISSN 0830-9000

Madariaga, M.G., Rezai, K., Trenholme, G.M. & Weinstein, R.A. (2003). Q fever: a biological weapon in your backyard. *The Lancet infectious diseases*, Vol.3, No.11, (November), pp. 709-721, ISSN 1474-4457

Magnino, S., Vicari, N., Boldini, M., Rosignoli, C., Nigrelli, A., Andreoli, G., Pajoro, M. & Fabbi, M. (2009). Rilevamento di *Coxiella burnetii* nel latte di massa di alcune aziende bovine lombarde. *Large Animal Review*, Vol.15, pp. 3-6, ISSN 1124-4593

Marrie, T.J., Langille, D., Papukna, V. & Yates, L. (1989). Truckin' pneumonia--an outbreak of Q fever in a truck repair plant probably due to aerosols from clothing contaminated by contact with newborn kittens. *Epidemiology and Infection*, Vol.102, No.1, (February), pp. 119-127, ISSN 1469-4409

Marrie, T.J., Stein, A., Janigan, D. & Raoult, D. (1996). Route of infection determines the clinical manifestations of acute Q fever. *Journal of Infectious Diseases*, Vol.173, No.2, (February), pp. 484-487, ISSN 1537-6613

Marrie, T.J. & Raoult, D. (2002). Update on Q fever, including Q fever endocarditis. *Current Clinical Topics in Infectious Diseases*, Vol.22, pp. 97-124, ISSN 0195-3842

Maurin, M. & Raoult, D. (1999). Q fever. *Clinical Microbiology Reviews*, Vol.12, No.4, (October), pp. 518-553, ISSN 0893-8512

Mediannikov, O., Fenollar, F., Socolovschi, C., Diatta, G., Bassene, H., Molez, J.F., Sokhna, C., Trape, J.F. & Raoult, D. (2010). *Coxiella burnetii* in humans and ticks in rural Senegal. *PLoS Neglected Tropical Diseases*, Vol.4, No.4, (Apr 6), e654, ISSN 1935-2735

Meiklejohn, G., Reimer, L.G., Graves, P.S. & Helmick, C. (1981). Cryptic epidemic of Q fever in a medical school. *Journal of Infectious Diseases*, Vol.144, No.2, (August), pp. 107-113, ISSN 1537-6613

NASPHV (National Association of State Public Health Veterinarians, Inc.) & CDC (Centers for Disease Control and Prevention), (2011). Compendium of measures to prevent disease associated with animals in public settings, 2011: National Association of State Public Health Veterinarians, Inc. *MMWR Recommendations and reports*, Vol.60, No.RR-4, (May 6), pp. 1-24, ISSN 1545-8601

OIE, Manual of Diagnostic Tests and Vaccines for Terrestrial Animals, (2010). Q fever, World Organisation for Animal Health, Chapter 2.1.12, (May), pp.1-13, ISBN 978-92-9044-718-4

Parisi, A., Fraccalvieri, R., Cafiero, M., Miccolupo ,A., Padalino, I., Montagn,a C., Capuano, F. & Sottili, R. (2006). Diagnosis of *Coxiella burnetii*-related abortion in Italian domestic ruminants using single-tube nested PCR. *Veterinary Microbiology*, Vol.118, No.1-2, (November 26), pp. 101-106, ISSN 0378-1135

Parola, P. & Raoult, D. (2001). Ticks and tickborne bacterial diseases in humans: an emerging infectious threat. Clinical Infectious *Diseases*, Vol.32, No.6, (March 15), pp. 897-928, ISSN 1537-6591

Perugini, A.G., Capuano, F., Esposito, A., Marianelli, C., Martucciello, A., Iovane, G. & Galiero, G. (2009). Detection of *Coxiella burnetii* in buffaloes aborted foetuses by

IS111 DNA amplification: a preliminary report. *Research in Veterinary Science*, Vol.87, No.2, (October), pp. 189-191, ISSN 0034-5288

Philip, C.B. (1948). Comments on the name of the Q fever organism. *Public Health Reports*, Vol.63, pp. 58-59, ISSN 0033-3549

Quinn, P.J., Carter, M.E., Markey, B. & Carter, G.R. (1994). Bacterial pathogens: microscopy, culture and identification. In: *Clinical Veterinary Microbiology*. Wolfe Publishing, Mosby-Year Book Europe Limited, 21–30, ISBN 978-072-3417-11-8, London

Raoult, D., Vestris, G. & Enea, M. (1990). Isolation of 16 strains of *Coxiella burnetii* from patients by using a sensitive centrifugation cell culture system and establishment of the strains in HEL cells. *Journal of Clinical Microbiology*, Vol.28, pp. 2482-2484, ISSN 0095-1137

Raoult, D., Laurent, J.C. & Mutillod, M. (1994). Monoclonal antibodies to *Coxiella burnetii* for antigenic detection in cell cultures and in paraffin-embedded tissues. *American Journal of Clinical Pathology*, Vol.101, No.3, (March), pp. 318–320, ISSN 1943-7722

Raoult, D., Marrie, T. & Mege, J. (2005). Natural history and pathophysiology of Q fever. *The Lancet infectious diseases*, Vol.5, No.4, (April), pp. 219-226, ISSN 1474-4457

Reinthaler, F.F., Mascher, F., Sixl, W. & Arbesser, C.H. (1988). Incidence of Q fever among cattle, sheep and goats in the Upper Nile province in southern Sudan. *The Veterinary Record*, Vol.122, No.6, (February 6), pp. 137, ISSN 0042-4900

Reusken, C., van der Plaats, R., Opsteegh, M., de Bruin, A. & Swart, A. (2011). *Coxiella burnetii* (Q fever) in *Rattus norvegicus* and *Rattus rattus* at livestock farms and urban locations in the Netherlands; could *Rattus* spp. represent reservoirs for (re)introduction? *Preventive Veterinary Medicine*, Vol.101, No.1-2, (august 1), pp.124-130, ISSN 0167-5877

Rodolakis, A., Berri, M., Héchard, C., Caudron, C., Souriau, A., Bodier, C.C., Blanchard, B., Camuset, P., Devillechaise, P., Natorp, J.C., Vadet, J.P. & Arricau-Bouvery, N. (2007). Comparison of *Coxiella burnetii* shedding in milk of dairy bovine, caprine, and ovine herds. *Journal of Dairy Science*, Vol.90, No.12, (December), pp. 5352- 5360, ISSN 0022-0302

Rodolakis, A. (2009). Q Fever in dairy animals. *Annals of the New York Academy of Sciences*, Vol.1166, (May), pp. 90-93, ISSN 1749-6632

Rousset, E., Durand, B., Berri, M., Dufour, P., Prigent, M., Russo, P., Delcroix, T., Touratier, A., Rodolakis, A. & Aubert, M.F. (2007). Comparative diagnostic potential of three serological tests for abortive Q fever in goat herds. *Veterinary Microbiology*, Vol.124, No.3-4, (October 6), pp. 286–297, ISSN 0378-1135

Rousset, E., Berri, M., Durand, B., Dufour, P., Prigent, M., Delcroix, T., Touratier, A. & Rodolakis, A. (2009). *Coxiella burnetii* shedding routes and antibody response after outbreaks of Q fever-induced abortion in dairy goat herds. *Applied and Environmental Microbiology*, Vol.75, No.2, (January), pp. 428–433, ISSN

Ruppanner, R., Brooks, D., Franti, C.E., Behymer, D.E., Morrish, D. & Spinelli, J. (1982). Q fever hazards from sheep and goats used in research. *Archives of Environmental Health*, Vol.37, No.2, (March - April), pp. 103-110, ISSN 0003-9896

Ruiz-Fons, F., Rodríguez, O., Torina, A., Naranjo, V., Gortázar, C. & de la Fuente, J. (2008). Prevalence of *Coxiella burnetti* infection in wild and farmed ungulates. *Veterinary Microbiology*, Vol.126, No.1-3, (January 1), pp. 282-286, ISSN 0378-1135

Russell-Lodrigue, K.E., Andoh, M., Poels, M.W., Shive, H.R., Weeks, B.R., Zhang, G.Q., Tersteeg, C., Masegi, T., Hotta, A., Yamaguchi, T., Fukushi, H., Hirai, K., McMurray, D.N. & Samuel, J.E. (2009). *Coxiella burnetii* isolates cause genogroup-specific virulence in mouse and guinea pig models of acute Q fever. *Infection and Immunity*, Vol.77, No.12, (December), pp. 5640-5650, ISSN 1098-5522

Samuel, J.E. & Hendrix, L.R. (2009). Laboratory maintenance of *Coxiella burnetii*. *Current Protocols in Microbiology*, Vol.6C, No.suppl.15, pp. 1–16, ISSN 1934-8533

Scott, G.H., Williams, J.C. & Stephenson, E.H. (1987). Animal models in Q fever: pathological responses of inbred mice to phase I *Coxiella burnetii*. *Journal of General Microbiology*, Vol.133, No. 3, (March), pp. 691–700, ISSN 0022-1287

Sidi-Boumedine, K., Rousset, E., Henning, K., Ziller, M., Niemczuck, K., Roest, H.I.J. & Thiéry, R. (2010). Development of harmonised schemes for the monitoring and reporting of Q-fever in animals in the European Union. EFSA Scientific Report on Question No EFSA-Q-2009-00511., (May 5), pp. 1-48. Available from: http://www.efsa.europa.eu

Soliman A.K., Botros B.A. & Watts D.M. (1992). Evaluation of a competitive immunoassay for detection of *Coxiella burnetii* antibody in animal sera. *Journal of Clinical Microbiology*, Vol.30, No.6, (June), pp.1595–1597, ISSN 0095-1137

Somma-Moreira, R.E., Caffarena, R.M., Somma, S., Pérez, G. & Monteiro, M. (1987). Analysis of Q fever in Uruguay. *Reviews of Infectious Diseases*, Vol.9, No.2, (March - April), pp. 386-387, ISSN 0162-0886

Stein, A. & Raoult, D. (1993). Lack of pathotype specific gene in human *Coxiella burnetii* isolates. *Microbial Pathogenesis*, Vol.15, No.3, (September), pp. 177-185, ISSN 0882-4010

Stein, A. & Raoult, D. (1999). Pigeon pneumonia in Provence. A bird borne Q fever outbreak. *Clinical Infectious Diseases*, Vol.29, No.3, (September), pp. 617-620, ISSN 1537-6591

Stoenner, H.G., Holdenried, R., Lackman, D. & Orsborn, J.S. Jr. (1959). The occurrence of *Coxiella burnetii*, *Brucella*, and other pathogens among fauna of the Great Salt Lake Desert in Utah. *The American Journal of Tropical Medicine and Hygiene*, Vol.8, (September), pp. 590-596, ISSN 0002-9637

Stoenner, H.G. & Lackman, D.B. (1960). The biologic properties of *Coxiella burnetii* isolated from rodents collected in Utah. *American journal of hygiene*, Vol.71, (January), pp. 45-51, ISSN 0096-5294

Svraka, S., Toman, R., Skultety, L., Slaba, K. & Homan, W.L. (2006). Establishment of a genotyping scheme for *Coxiella burnetii*. *FEMS Microbiology Letters*, Vol.254, No.2, (January), pp. 268–274, ISSN 1574-6968

Thiele, D., Karo, M. & Krauss, H. (1992). Monoclonal antibody based capture ELISA/ELIFA for detection of *Coxiella burnetii* in clinical specimens. *European Journal of Epidemiology*, Vol.8, No.4, (July), pp. 568–574, ISSN 1573-7284

Tissot-Dupont, H., Thirion, X. & Raoult, D. (1994). Q fever serology: cutoff determination for microimmunofluorescence. *Clinical and Diagnostic Laboratory Immunology*, Vol.1, No.2, (March), pp. 189–196. ISSN 1098-6588

Toledo, A., Jado, I., Olmeda, A.S., Casado-Nistal, M.A., Gil, H., Escudero, R. & Anda, P. (2009). Detection of *Coxiella burnetii* in ticks collected from Central Spain. *Vector-Borne and Zoonotic Diseases*, Vol.9, No.5, (October), pp. 465-468, ISSN 1530-3667

Valková, D. & Kazár, J. (1995). A new plasmid (QpDV) common to *Coxiella burnetii* isolates associated with acute and chronic Q fever. *FEMS Microbiology Letters*, Vol.125, No.2-3, (January 15), pp. 275-280, ISSN 1574-6968

van der Hoek, W., Dijkstra, F., Schimmer, B., Schneeberger, P.M., Vellema, P., Wijkmans, C., ter Schegget, R., Hackert, V. & van Duynhoven, Y. (2010). Q fever in the Netherlands: an update on the epidemiology and control measures. *Euro Surveillance*, Vol.25, No.12, (March 25), pp. 15-26, ISSN 1560-7917

Wilson, L.E., Couper, S., Prempeh, H., Young, D., Pollock, K.G., Stewart, W.C., Browning, L.M. & Donaghy, M. (2010). Investigation of a Q fever outbreak in a Scottish co-located slaughterhouse and cutting plant. *Zoonoses and Public Health*, Vol.57, No.7-8, (December), pp. 493-498, ISSN 1863-2378

World Health Organization, (2004). Public health response to biological and chemical weapons: In. *WHO guidance*, 2nd ed., ISBN 978-924-1546-15-7, Geneva

6

Helicobacter – An Emerging New Zoonotic Pathogen

Okjin Kim
Center for Animal Resources Development, Wonkwang University, Republic of Korea

1. Introduction

The genus *Helicobacter* contains 35 named species and numerous provisionally named species. It is likely that several novel *Helicobacter* species await discovery. Members of this genus are microaerobic, have a fusiform or curved to spiral rod morphology and are motile by flagella that vary in number and location among different species (Vandamme et al., 1990). All known *Helicobacters* live in human and animal hosts, where colonization occurs primarily in the gastrointestinal tract. The type species, *Helicobacter pylori (H. pylori)*, was isolated from the stomach of humans and has been associated with a variety of gastric anomalies including gastritis, peptic ulcer disease, gastric carcinoma, and gastric mucosa-associated lymphoma (Parsonnet, 1998). Like *H. pylori*, other species of *Helicobacter* have also been shown to colonize the stomach and cause disease in animals. Gastric colonizers include *H. felis, H. mustelae, H. acinonychis, H. bizzozeronii, H. heilmannii, H. salomonis*, and a recently isolated novel *Helicobacter* sp. of dolphins (Hodzic et al., 2001). Several species of *Helicobacter* have been identified in rodents, including the species *H. hepaticus, H. bilis, H. muridarum, H. aurati, H. cinaedi, H. cholecystus, H. trogontum, H. rodentium*, and a bacterium morphologically resembling *H. Flexispira* taxon 8 (formerly *Flexispira rappini*) (Hodzic et al., 2001). Evidence is accumulating that especially pigs, dogs, and cats constitute reservoir hosts for gastric *Helicobacter* species with zoonotic potential.

2. History of *Helicobacter* research

The first well-known report of gastric *Helicobacters* was by Bizzozero in Turin in 1893 (Bizzozero, 1893). Bizzozero was a well-known anatomist, famous already for his proof that all dividing cells required cell nuclei (Castiglioni, 1947). In his anatomical observations of the gastric mucosa of dogs, Bizzozero reported "spirochetes" inhabiting the gastric glands (Figura & Orderda, 1996) and even the canaliculi of the parietal cells. In hand-drawn color illustrations, Bizzozero showed gram-negative organisms with approximately 10 wavelengths within the parietal cells and gastric glands. We now know these organisms variously identified as *H. canis, H. felis* (Lee et al., 1988), and/or *H. heilmannii* (Heilmann & Borchard, 1991). Bizzozero's work was extended by Salomon, who was able to propagate these spiral organisms in mouse stomachs after feeding ground-up gastric mucosa from cats and dogs to his mouse colony (Salomon, 1896). Salomon's work was a precursor to current studies where the *H. felis*-infected mouse is an important model in vaccine and therapeutic studies of *Helicobacter* eradication (Chen et al., 1995). Warren had observed patients with spiral organisms on their gastric mucosa since 1979 and had documented the inflammation associated with the bacteria by the time he and Marshall began a concerted attempt to study the organisms in patients with various upper gastrointestinal symptoms. After August 1981, the team studied patients attending for endoscopy and was able to demonstrate the gram-negative bacteria on Gram stains but could not culture them at that time. They tentatively treated one patient with tetracycline and were able to observe a decrease in the number of neutrophils in the gastric mucosa as well as apparent disappearance of the bacteria. They recognized, however, that anecdotal evidence of the bacteria's role in gastric inflammation was of little value and therefore commenced a study in 100 consecutive endoscopy patients to try to culture the bacteria, as well as determine their association with gastritis and/or other clinical syndromes. Initially, they did not focus specifically on the etiology of peptic ulcer disease, although they were aware that gastritis was strongly associated with duodenal and gastric ulcers, as well as with gastric cancer (Warren & Marshall, 1983).

3. Classification of *Helicobacter* species

The genus *Helicobacter* contains 35 named species and numerous provisionally named species. It is likely that several novel *Helicobacter* species await discovery. Members of this genus are microaerobic, have a fusiform or curved to spiral rod morphology and are motile by flagella that vary in number and location among different species (Vandamme et al., 1990). All known *Helicobacters* live in human and animal hosts, where colonization occurs primarily in the gastrointestinal tract. The type species, *H. pylori*, was isolated from the stomach of humans and has been associated with a variety of gastric anomalies including gastritis, peptic ulcer disease, gastric carcinoma, and gastric mucosa-associated lymphoma (Parsonnet, 1998). Like *H. pylori*, other species of *Helicobacter* have also been shown to colonize the stomach and cause disease in animals. Gastric colonizers include *H. felis*, *H. mustelae*, *H. acinonychis*, *H. bizzozeronii*, *H. heilmannii*, *H. salomonis*, and a recently isolated novel *Helicobacter* sp. of dolphins (Hodzic et al., 2001). Several species of *Helicobacter* have been identified in rodents, including the species *H. hepaticus*, *H. bilis*, *H. muridarum*, *H. aurati*, *H. cinaedi*, *H. cholecystus*, *H. trogontum*, *H. rodentium*, and a bacterium morphologically resembling *Helicobacter Flexispira* taxon 8 (formerly *Flexispira rappini*) (Hodzic et al., 2001). A number of *Helicobacter* species may confound experimental data because of their association with disease progressing in various kinds of animals (Chin et al., 2000, Ward et al., 1994, Eaton et al., 1996). *H. hepaticus and H. bilis* were initially reported as pathogens associated with hepatitis and inflammatory bowel diseases (Shomer et al., 1997, Ward et al., 1996), and *H. typhlonicus* caused proliferative typhlocolitis in SCID mice (Franklin 1999). *H. suncus* was isolated from house musk shrews as a pathogenic agent (Goto et al., 2000).

Most routine laboratories apply the same basic biochemical tests for the identification and differentiation of all *Campylobacter*-like organisms and would fail to identify many *Helicobacter* species. Although the number of *Helicobacter* species encountered in human clinical samples is fairly small, the lack of application of highly standardized procedures and the well-known biochemical inertness of *Campylobacter*-like organisms render biochemical identification of all of these bacteria very difficult. Whereas *Arcobacter* strains can be differentiated from *Campylobacter* and *Helicobacter* strains by their ability to grow in air and at low temperature (Vandamme et al., 1991), there are no clear biochemical characteristics to separate the genus *Helicobacter* from the genus *Campylobacter*. Theoretically, one has to differentiate over 35 validly named species and subspecies, as well as various unnamed taxa. An overview of biochemical and other methods to differentiate *Campylobacter* and *Arcobacter* species was described earlier (Vandamme, 2000). A summary of the characteristics of cultivated *Helicobacter* species shows that discrimination between some species may rely on only one differential feature. Moreover, some species, notably *H. pylori* and *H. acinonychis*, and *H. felis* and *H. bizzozeronii*, cannot be differentiated with conventional phenotypic tests.

4. Clinical sequels of *Helicobacter* infection

Helicobacter pylori (*H. pylori*) is a Gram-negative, spiral-shaped, microaerophilic bacterium that infects the human gastric mucosa (Warren and Marshall, 1983). Chronic infection is thought to be associated with chronic active gastritis, peptic ulcer and gastric malignancies, such as mucosa-associated B cell lymphoma and adenocarcinoma (NIH, 1994). In particular, this organism has been categorized as a class I carcinogen by the World Health Organization (International Agency for Research on Cancer, 1994) and previous studies have confirmed that long-term infection with *H. pylori* induces adenocarcinoma in Mongolian gerbils (Honda et al., 1998; Watanabe et al., 1998). The association between *H. pylori* and gastric cancer has been explained by two possible mechanisms.

Gastric mucosal infection with *H. pylori* is accompanied by infiltration of neutrophils, and activated inflammatory cells are known to produce oxygen radicals (Evans et al., 1995; Ramarao et al., 2000). Oxygen radicals are known as inducers and initiators because they cause direct DNA damage (Clemens, 1991), but the relationship of these radicals with the onset of gastric cancer has not been sufficiently explored. Ammonia/ammonium concentrations increase in the gastric mucosa due to infection with *H. pylori*, and Tsujii et al. have found that ammonia acts as a promoter in a rat model of gastric cancer induced by N-methyl-N-nitro-N-nitrosoguanidine (MNNG) (Tsujii et al., 1992). To consider the association between *H. pylori* infection and the onset of diffuse type of gastric cancer, unlike intestinal type gastric cancer, the process from infection with *H. pylori* through gastric mucosal atrophy, intestinal metaplasia, and development of cancer must be excluded (Correa et al., 1994; Fay et al., 1994). Direct evidence must therefore be found to indicate progression from infection with *H. pylori* through persistent inflammatory cell infiltration resulting in DNA damage by oxygen radicals, point mutations of genes, and finally carcinogenesis.

5. Host ranges of *Helicobacters*

Since *H. muridarum* was first reported in the intestinal mucosal of mice and rats (Lee 1992), additional *Helicobacter* species have been isolated from laboratory animals. Several *Helicobacter* species such as *H. hepaticus* (Fox 1994), *H. muridarum, H. bilis* (Fox et al., 1995), *H. rodentium* (Shen et al., 1997), *Flexispira rappini* (Schauer et al., 1993), *H. typhlonicus* (Franklin et al., 1999) have been identified in rodents. The genus *Helicobacter* contains 24 named species and numerous provisionally named species. It is likely that several novel *Helicobacter* species await discovery. Members of this genus are microaerobic, have a fusiform or curved to spiral rod morphology and are motile by flagella that vary in number and location among different species (Vandamme et al., 1990). All known *Helicobacters* live in human and animal hosts, where colonization occurs primarily in the gastrointestinal tract. The type species, *H. pylori*, was isolated from the stomach of humans and has been associated with a variety of gastric anomalies including gastritis, peptic ulcer disease, gastric carcinoma, and gastric mucosa-associated lymphoma (Parsonnet, 1998). Like *H. pylori*, other species of *Helicobacter* have also been shown to colonize the stomach and cause disease in animals. Gastric colonizers include *H. felis, H. mustelae, H. acinonychis, H. bizzozeronii, H. heilmannii, H. salomonis*, and a recently isolated novel *Helicobacter* sp. of dolphins (Hodzic et al., 2001). Several species of *Helicobacter* have been identified in rodents, including the species *H. hepaticus, H. bilis, H. muridarum, H. aurati, H. cinaedi, H. cholecystus, H. trogontum, H. rodentium*, and a bacterium morphologically resembling *H. Flexispira* taxon 8 (formerly *Flexispira rappini*) (Hodzic et al., 2001).

6. Transmission of *Helicobacters*

In-depth knowledge of the transmission patterns may constitute important information for future intervention strategies. In the absence of consistent and verified environmental reservoirs, a predominantly person-to-person transmission has been postulated. *H. pylori* infection is associated with poor living conditions, and possible transmission routes are fecal-oral, oral-oral, or gastro-oral, but firm evidence is lacking (Torres et al., 2000). Young children are particularly vulnerable to infection by transmission of *H. pylori* from their infected parents, especially infected mothers (Rothenbacher et al., 1999), and it is generally believed that such transmission is influenced by socio-economic status. However, little is known about how and when maternal transmission occurs during perinatal period, especially whether this occurs before or after parturition. In the present study, we examined these issues in an experimental murine model, Mongolian gerbil model that have been reported as a most optimal laboratory animal model to study *H. pylori in vivo* (Hirayama et al., 1996).

In the previous study, Lee & Kim (2006) examined these issues in an experimental murine model, Mongolian gerbil model that have been reported as a most optimal laboratory animal model to study *H. pylori*. Pregnant Mongolian gerbils, infected experimentally with *H. pylori*, were divided as four groups. Following the experimental design, the stomachs of the mother and litters were isolated and assessed for transmission of *H. pylori* at prenatal period, parturition day, 1-week old age and 3-week old age respectively. Bacterial culture and polymerase chain reaction (PCR) was used to examine the presence of transmitted *H. pylori*. All litters showed no transmission of *H. pylori* during pregnancy and at parturition day. However, they reveled 33.3% and 69.6 % at 1-week old age and 3-week old age respectively by PCR. These results suggested that vertical infection during prenatal period or delivery procedure is unlikely as a route of mother-to-child *H. pylori* infection. It might be acquired *H. pylori* through breast-feeding, contaminating saliva and fecal-oral during co-habitat (Lee & Kim, 2006).

Half of the world's population is estimated to be infected with *H. pylori* and the infection is mainly acquired in early childhood but the exact routes of transmission remain elusive. Infected mothers are generally considered to be the main source of the pathogen (Weyermann et al., 2006; Escobar & Kawakami, 2004; Rothenbacher et al., 2002). The epidemiology of *H. pylori* infection is variable, with prevalence being significantly higher and incident infection occurring earlier in developing countries compared with developed countries (Frenck & Clemens 2003; Ahuja & Sharma, 2002; Graham et al., 1991). There is an obvious public health impact of *H. pylori* infection and thus, to design targeted and cost-effective prevention strategies, elucidation of the mode of transmission for this bacteria is crucial (Fendrick et al., 1999). It is known that *H. pylori* infection is typically acquired in early childhood and usually persists throughout life unless specific treatment is applied (Crone & Gold 2004). Definitive modes of transmission have not yet been characterized and the principal reservoir appears to be humans. Person-to-person transmission via fecal-oral, oral-oral and gastro-oral routes have been proposed (Mladenova et al., 2006). Numerous studies also indicate low socioeconomic status, including domestic overcrowding in childhood, as major risk factors for higher infection prevalence rates (Frenck & Clemens 2003). Little is known about when and how often maternal transmission of *H. pylori* occurs during perinatal stage. In the previous study, Lee & Kim (2006) examined these issues in an experimental murine model.

The results of the vertical-transmission experiment indicated that vertical transmission of *H. pylori* was not occurred at pregnant and delivery staged. However, they reveled 33.3% and 69.6 % at lactating and weaning stage respectively. Recent epidemiological studies in humans suggest that the acquisition of *H. pylori* occur during childhood. For example, Rothenbacher et al (2000) reported that *H. pylori* acquisition seems to occur mainly between the first and second year of life: that is, after the age of weaning. Our results are in agreement with this report. Also, Rothenbacher et al (2000) reported that infected parents, especially infected mothers, play a key role in the transmission of *H. pylori* within families. Maternal contact behaviour during the breastfeeding period may be responsible for the high frequency of maternal transmission (Kurosawa et al., 2000). Our results also showed that the maternal-transmission of *H. pylori* was not observed during pregnancy and delivery stage, but detected at lactating and weaning stage. On the basis of these findings, vertical infection during pregnancy or at delivery is unlikely as a route of mother-to-child *H. pylori* infection. Lee & Kim (2006) suggested that *H. pylori* infection of transplacental route during pregnancy might not be occurred and that *H. pylori* transmission by discharges of uterine or vagina, obstetric delivery tract, during parturition might not be occurred. It might be acquired *H. pylori* through breast-feeding, contaminating saliva and fecal-oral during co-habitat.

7. Diagnostic methods of *Helicobacters*

To detect *Helicobacter* species, serologic tests (Livingston et al., 1997), the culture method (Russel et al., 1995), and the PCR (Engstrand et al., 1992) have been used. Serologic test may be not available for animal screening because of absence of available species-specific antibodies against *Helicobacter* species. Also, culture assay is labor-intensive. It has been reported that PCR assays is easy and useful method and can be performed even on feces as a noninvasive means of rapidly screening large numbers of animals for *Helicobacter* species (Beckwith et al., 1997). However, those kinds of PCR assays requires multiple assays because of a lot of *Helicobacter* species (Grehan et al., 2002). There is no doubt that a bacteriological culture is the best method for diagnosing a bacterial infection. However, it is not easy to cultivate *Helicobacters* because the specimens are usually obtained from several different locations by biopsy or necropsy. In addition, the sensitivity of the culture-isolation method is low (Hammar et al., 1992). Therefore, a culture is not considered to be the most practical diagnostic method. As a result, the CLO test and staining methods are preferred in many clinical laboratories. Nonetheless, they also have problems such as accuracy of species-specific identification (Megraud, 1997). PCR which is a specific and sensitive molecular method for detecting *Helicobacter* DNA, can supplement the above methods. However, PCR methods using species-specific primers require multiple assays because of a lot of *Helicobacter* species (Grehan et al., 2002). In this study, the RNA polymerase ß-subunit-coding gene (*rpo*B) was used for the detection of novel *Helicobacter* species by a simple PCR analysis. *rpo*B is an important transcription apparatus in all microorganisms. Because this region is highly conserved, this *rpo*B DNA PCR could be used as a consensus PCR analysis method to detect *Helicobacter* species. Therefore, it is clear that PCR methods targeting a stable gene such as *rpo*B would give more reliable results. Mutiple PCR assays using *Helicobacter* species-specific primers may be considered an expensive, laborious, and thus impractical procedure for many samples in clinical laboratory settings. On the other hand, this consensus PCR can be used alone without multiple assays. Therfore, the cost, which is higher than those of other methods, including culture, will be reduced. *Helicobacter* species may be identified in this single PCR and the presence of a novel species may be detected. Fecal samples may be stored at room temperature for up to a week without affecting the outcome of PCR for *Helicobacter* species (Beckwith et al., 1997). Therefore, monitoring of *Helicobacter* infection could be conducted very easily by this consensus PCR with feces. In the previous study, the consensus PCR using *rpo*B primers was able to detect successfully *Helicobacter* species (Kim & Kim, 2004). A set of primers (HF, 5'-ACTTTAAACGCA TGAAGATAT-3'; and HR, 5'-ATATTTTGACCTTCTGGGGT-3') was used to amplify *rpo*B DNA (458 bp) encompassing the Rif^r region. Amplification of *rpoB* DNAs (458 bp) from *Helicobacter* species PCR products was electrophoresed on a 1.2% agarose gel. The PCR products (458 bp) were observed from the *Helicobacter* species such as *H. felis, H. cinaedi, H. mustelae, H. hepaticus, H. pylori* ATCC43504, *H. pylori* ATCC 43579, *H. pylori* ATCC 43619, *H. pylori* ss1, *H. pylori* isolate. There was no amplification from other bacteria such as *E. coli, Bacilus subtilis, Corynebacterium diphtheriae, Haemophilus influenzae, Moraxella catarrhalis, Enterococcus faecalis,* suggesting that the primers (HF and HR) are *Helicobacter* specific. This consensus PCR will be useful and effective for monitoring *Helicobacter* species including human and animals and could be used for detection of a new *Helicobacter* species by combination with partial sequencing (Kim & Kim, 2004).

8. Preventive and therapeutic methods of *Helicobacters*

Various pharmacological regimens have been studied in the treatment of *H. pylori* infection. Antibiotics (Fera et al., 2001), proton–pump inhibitors (Park et al., 1996), H_2-blockers (Sorba et al., 2001), and bismuth salts (Midolo et al., 1997) are suggested standard treatment modalities, which are typically combined in dual, triple and quadruple therapy regimens in order to eradicate *H. pylori* infection (Worrel et al., 1998). Some problems may arise upon administration of these eradication regimens, i.e. the cost (Worrel et al., 1998), the efficacy of antibiotics regarding the pH (for instance, amoxicillin is most active at a neutral pH and tetracycline has greater activity at a low pH) (Worrel et al., 1998) and resistance to the antibiotics (Ferrero et al., 2000). However, above 15% of the patients undergoing such drug regimens experienced therapeutic failure (Worrel et al., 1998).

Hence, numerous studies have concentrated on the eradication of *H. pylori* infection using traditional herbal medicines. Garlic and Pteleopsis extracts exhibited weak and modest, respectively, anti-*H. pylori* activity (Germano et al., 1998). Fifty-four Chinese herbs were screened for anti-*H. pylori* activity, exhibiting *Rheum palmatum, Rhus javanica, Coptis japonica* and *Eugenia caryophyllata* strong anti-*H. pylori* activity (Bae et al., 1998). Cranberry juice possesses modest anti-*H. pylori* activity (Burger et al., 2000). The anti-*H. pylori* activities of *Aristolochia paucinervis,* black myrobalan and cinnamon were also examined (Gadhi et al., 2001). Anti-*H. pylori* compounds from the Brazilian medicinal plant *Myroxylon peruiferum* have successfully isolated (Ohsaki 1999). Extracts and fractions from seven Turkish plants were also demonstrated to elicit anti-*H. pylori* activity (Yesilada et al., 1999). The leaves, roots and stems of Korean and Japanese wasabi exhibited bactericidal activities against *H. pylori,* having the leaves the highest bactericidal activity (Shin et al., 2004). In addition, some flavonoids and isoflavonoids isolated from licorice such as licochalcone A, licoisoflavone B, and gancaonols have been reported to exhibit inhibitory activities against *H. pylori* (Fukai et al., 2002).

Lee et al (2010) conducted the study of anti-*H. pylori* efficacy with 81 folk medicinal plants. They confirmed that 3 herbal compounds, *Melia azedarach, Cinnamomum cassia* and *Magnolia officinalis* showed an antibiotic effect on *H. pylori* infection. It could be a promising native herb treatment for patients with gastric complaints including gastric ulcer caused by *H. pylori.* These results will be able to develop the therapeutics against *H. pylori* infection. *Melia azedarach, Cinnamomum cassia* and *Magnolia officinalis* will be useful to treat *H. pylori* infected patients with high therapeutic efficacy and safety (Lee et al., 2010).

9. *Helicobacters* as an emerging new zoonotic pathogen

The genus *Helicobacter* contains at least 24 named species and an additional 35 or more novel *Helicobacters* wait formal naming (Fox, 2002). Members of this genus are microaerobic, have a fusiform or curved to spiral rod morphology and are motile by flagella that vary in number and location among different species (Vandamme et al., 1990). All known *Helicobacters* live in human and animal hosts, where colonization occurs primarily in the gastrointestinal tract. The type species, *H. pylori,* was isolated from the stomach of humans and has been associated with a variety of gastric anomalies including gastritis, peptic ulcer disease, gastric carcinoma, and gastric mucosa-associated lymphoma (Parsonnet, 1998). Like *H. pylori,* other species of *Helicobacter* have also been shown to colonize the stomach and cause disease in animals. Gastric colonizers include *H. felis, H. mustelae, H. acinonychis, H. bizzozeronii, H. heilmannii, H. salomonis,* and a recently isolated novel *Helicobacter* sp. of dolphins (Hodzic et al., 2001). The initial interest in animal *Helicobacters* arose from the need for a suitable animal model for studying *H. pylori* infection, and subsequently from an ecological perspective (Fox et al., 1997; Lee et al., 1988). However, there have been recent concerns regarding the potential of animals, notably domestic pets, to be a source of zoonotic *Helicobacter* infection. Dogs and cats used for biomedical research have been occasionally found to harbor *H. pylori* strains (Handt et al., 1995), while *H. felis* has been implicated as a potential human pathogen in a few cases (Wegmann et al., 1991). *H. pylori* has also been found in pet animals, and it can promote gastritis when introduced into specific-pathogen-free cats. The significance of this infection as a cause of gastritis in pet dogs and cats is nevertheless unclear. The main gastric *Helicobacter* species in dogs and cats are primarily *H. heilmannii* (formerly "*Gastrospirillum hominis*") and *H. felis.* These two species are collectively referred to as gastric *Helicobacter*-like organisms (GHLO) because they cannot be distinguished by light microscopy. So far, *H. heilmannii* has not been reliably cultured *in vitro.*

10. Conclusions

Clinical symptoms associated with non-*H. pylori Helicobacters* in humans can be characterized by atypical complaints such as acute or chronic epigastric pain and nausea. Other aspecific symptoms include hematemesis, recurrent dyspepsia, irregular defecation frequency and consistency, vomiting, heartburn, and dysphagia, often accompanied by a decreased appetite. Evidence is accumulating that especially pigs, dogs, and cats constitute reservoir hosts for gastric *Helicobacter* species with zoonotic potential. The recent successes with in vitro isolation of these fastidious microorganisms from domestic animals open new perspectives for developing typing techniques that can be directly applied on gastric biopsies from humans. These techniques should make it possible to determine whether animal and human strains belonging to the same *Helicobacter* species are clonally related.

11. Acknowledgment

This research was supported by the Basic Science Research Program through the National Research Foundation of Korea (NRF) funded by the Ministry of Education, Science, and Technology (2010-0021940).

12. References

[1] Ahuja V, Sharma MP. High recurrence rate of *Helicobacter pylori* infection in developing countries. *Gastroenterology* 2002;123:653-654.

[2] Bae EA, Han MJ, Kim NJ, Kim DH. Anti-*Helicobacter pylori* activity of herbal medicines. *Biol. Pharm. Bull.* 1998;21:990–992.

[3] Beckwith CS, Franklin CL, Hook RR Jr, Besch-Williford CL, Riley LK. Fecal PCR assay for diagnosis of helicobacter infection in laboratory rodents. *J. Clin. Microbiol.* 1997;35:1620-1623.

[4] Bizzozero G. Ueber die schlauchformigen drusen des magendarmkanals und die bezienhungen ihres epithels zu dem oberflachenepithel der schleimhaut. *Arch. Mikr Anat.* 1893;42:82.

[5] Burger O, Ofek I, Tabak M, Weiss EI, Sharon N, Neeman I. A high molecular mass constituent of cranberry juice inhibits *Helicobacter pylori* adhesion to human gastric mucus. *FEMS Immunol. Med. Microb* .2000; 29:295–301.

[6] Castiglioni A. *A History of Medicine*, 2nd ed. Alfred A. *Knopf, New York, N.Y.* 1947

[7] Chen M, Lee A, Hazell S. Immunisation against gastric helicobacter infection in a mouse/*Helicobacter felis* model. *Lancet* 1995;339:1120–1121.

[8] Chin EY, Dangler CA, Fox JG, Schauer DB. *Helicobacter hepaticus* infection triggers inflammatory bowel disease in T cell receptor alpha beta mutant mice. *Comp. Med.* 2000;50:586-594.

[9] Clemens MR. Free radicals in chemical carcinogenesis. *Klin. Wochenschr.* 1991;69:1123–1134.

[10] Correa P, Chen VW. Gastric cancer. *Cancer Surv.* 1994;19–20:55–76.

[11] Crone J, Gold BD. *Helicobacter pylori* infection in pediatrics. *Helicobacter* 2004;9 Suppl 1:49-56.

[12] Eaton KA, Dewhirst FE, Paster BJ, Tzellas N, Coleman BE, Paola J, Sherding R. Prevalence and varieties of *Helicobacter* species in dogs from random sources and

pet dogs: animal and public health implications. *J. Clin. Microbiol.* 1996;34:3165–3170.

[13] Engstrand L, Nguyen AH, Graham DY, El-Zaatari FAK. Reverse transcription and polymerase chain reaction amplification of rRNA for detection of helicobacter species. *J. Clin. Microbiol.* 1992;30:2295-2301.

[14] Escobar ML, Kawakami E. Evidence of mother-child transmission of *Helicobacter pylori* infection. *Arq. Gastroenterol.* 2004;41:239-244.

[15] Evans DJ Jr, Evans DG, Takemura T, Nakano H, Lampert HC, Graham DY, Granger DN, Kvietys PR. Characterization of a *Helicobacter pylori* neutrophil-activating protein. *Infect. Immun.* 1995;63:2213–2220.

[16] Fay M, Fennerty MB, Emerson J, Larez M. Dietary habits and the risk of stomach cancer: a comparison study of patients with and without intestinal metaplasia. *Gastroenterol. Nurs.* 1994;16:158–162.

[17] Fendrick AM, Chernew ME, Hirth RA, Bloom BS, Bandekar RR, Scheiman JM. Clinical and economic effects of population-based *Helicobacter pylori* screening to prevent gastric cancer. *Arch. Intern. Med.* 1999;159:142-148.

[18] Fera MT, Carbone M, Pallio S, Tortora A, Blandino G, Carbone M. Antimicrobial activity and postantibiotic effect of flurithromycin against *Helicobacter pylori* strains. *Int. J. Antimicrob. Ag.* 2001;17:151–154.

[19] Ferrero M, Ducons JA, Sicilia B, Santolaria S, Sierra E, Gomollon F. Factors affecting the variation in antibiotic resistance of *Helicobacter pylori* over a 3-year period. *Int. J. Antimicrob. Agents* 2000;16:245–248.

[20] Figura N, Orderda G. Reflections on the first description of the presence of *Helicobacter* species in the stomach of mammals. *Helicobacter.* 1996;1:4–5.

[21] Fox JG, Yan LL, Dewhirst FE, Paster BJ, Shames B, Murphy JC, Hayward A, Belcher JC, Menders En . *Helicobacter bilis* sp. Nov., a novel *Helicobacter* species isolated from bile, liver, and intestines of aged, inbred mice. *J. Clin. Microbiol.* 1995;33:445-454.

[22] Fox JG, Dangler CA, Sager W, Borkowski R, Gliatto JM. *Helicobacter mustelae*-associated gastric adenocarcinoma in ferrets (*Mustela putorius furo*). *Vet. Pathol.* 1997;34:225–229.

[23] Franklin Cl, Riley LK, Livingston RS, Beckwith CS, Hook RR Jr, Besch-Wiliford CL, Hunziker R, Gorelick PL . Enteric lesions in SCID mice infected with "*Helicobacter typhlonicus*" a novel urease-negative *Helicobacte*r species. *Lab. Anim. Sci.* 1999;48:496-505.

[24] Frenck RW Jr, Clemens J. Helicobacter in the developing world. *Microbes Infect.* 2003;5:705-713.

[25] Fukai T, Marumo A, Kaitou K, Kanda T, Terada S, Nomura T. Anti-*Helicobacter pylori* flavonoids from licorice extract. *Life Sci.* 2002;71:1449–1463.

[26] Gadhi CA, Benharref A, Jana M, Lozniewski A. Anti-*Helicobacter pylori* of *Aristolochia paucinervis* pomel extract. *J. Enthnopharm.* 2001;75:203–205.

[27] Germano MP, Sanogo R, Guglielmo M, Pasquale RD, Crisafi G. Effects of *Pteleopsis suberosa* extracts on experimental gastric ulcers and *Helicobacter pylori* growth. *J. Enthnopharm.* 1998;59:167–172.

[28] Goto K, Ohashi H, Ebukuro S, Itoh T .Pathogenicity of *Helicobacter* species isolated from the stomach of the house musk shrew (*Sncus murinusu*). *Comp. Med.* 2000;50: 73-77.

[29] Graham DY, Adam E, Reddy GT. Seroepidemiology of *Helicobacter pylori* infection in India. Comparison of developing and developed countries. *Dig. Dis. Sci.* 1991;36:1084-1088.

[30] Grehan M, Tamotia G, Robertson B, Mitchell H . Detection of Helicobacter Colonization of the Murine Lower Bowel by Genus-Specific PCR-Denaturing Gradient Gel Electrophoresis. *Appl. Environ. Microbiol.* 2002;68:5164–5166.

[31] Hammar M, Tyszkiewicz T, Wadstrom T, O'Toole PW . Rapid detection of *Helicobacter pylori* in gastric biopsy material by polymerase chain reaction. *J. Clin. Microbiol.* 1992;30: 54-58.

[32] Handt LK, Fox JG, Stalis IH, Rufo R, Lee G, Linn J, Li X, Kleanthous H. Characterization of feline *Helicobacter pylori* strains and associated gastritis in a colony of domestic cats. *J. Clin. Microbiol.* 1995;33:2280–2289.

[33] Heilmann K L, Borchard F. Gastritis due to spiral shaped bacteria other than *Helicobacter pylori*: clinical, histological, and ultrastructural findings. *Gut* 1991;32:137–140.

[34] Hirayama F, Takagi S, Yokiyama Y. Establishment of gastric *Helicobacter pylori* infection in Mongolian gerbils. *J. Gastroenterol.* 1996;31:24-28.

[35] Hodzic E, McKisic M, Feng S, Barthold SW . Evaluation of diagnostic methods for *Helicobacter bilis* infection in laboratory mice. *Comp. Med.* 2001;51:406-412.

[36] Honda S, Fujioka T, Tokieda M. Development of *Helicobacter pylori*-induced gastric carcinoma in mongolian gerbils. *Cancer Res.* 1998; 58:4255-4259.

[37] International Agency for Research on Cancer. Schistosomes, liver flukes and *Helicobacter pylori*. *IARC Monogr. Eval. Carcinog. Risks Hum.* 1994; 61:1-241.

[38] Kim SH, Kim O. Application of Consensus Polymerase Chain Reaction for Monitoring of Helicobacter Species. *Kor. J. Lab. Anim. Sci.* 2004; 20:316-320.

[39] Kurosawa M, Kikuchi S, Inaba Y, Ishibashi T, Kobayashi F. *Helicobacter pylori* infection among Japanese children *J. Gastroenterol. Hepatol.* 2000;15:1382-1385.

[40] Lee A, Hazell SL, O'Rourke J, Kouprach S. Isolation of a spiral-shaped bacterium from the cat stomach. *Infect. Immun.* 1988;56:2843–2850.

[41] Lee H, Hong S, Oh H, Park S, Kim Y, Jeong G, Kim O. *In vitro* and *in vivo* Antibacterial Activities of *Cinnamomum cassia* Extracts against *Helicobacter pylori*. *Laboratory Animal Research* 2010;26:21-29.

[42] Lee JU, Kim O. Natural maternal transmission of Helicobacter pylori in Mongolian gerbils. *J. World Gastroenterol.* 2006;12:5663-5667.

[43] Lee A, Hazell SL, O'Rourke J, Kouprach S. Isolation of a spiral-shaped bacterium from the cat stomach. *Infect. Immun.* 1988;56:2843–2850.

[44] Livingston RS, Riley LK, Steffen EK, Besh-Williford CL, Hook RR Jr, Franklin CL. Serodiagnosis of Helicobacter hepaticus infection in mice by an enzyme-linked immunosorbent assay. *J. Clin. Microbiol.* 1997;35:1236-1238.

[45] Megraud F. How should *Helicobacter pylori* infection be diagnosed? *Gastroenterology* 1997;113:S93-S98.

[46] Midolo PD, Norton A, Itzstein MV, Lambert JR. Novel bismuth compounds have in vitro activity against *Helicobacter pylori*. *FEMS Microb. Lett.* 1997;157: 229–232.

[47] Mladenova I, Durazzo M, Pellicano R. Transmission of *Helicobacter pylori*: are there evidences for a fecal-oral route? *Minerva Med.* 2006;97:15-18.

[48] NIH Consensus Conference. *Helicobacter pylori* in peptic ulcer disease. *J.A.M.A.* 1994; 272:265-269.

[49] Ohsaki A, Takashima J, Chiba N, Kawamura M. Microanalysis of a selective potent anti-*Helicobacter pylori* compound in a Brazillian medicinal plant, *Myroxylon peruiferum* and the activity of analogues. *Bioorg. Med. Chem. Lett.* 1999;9:1109–1112.

[50] Park JB, Imamur LL, Kobashi K. Kinetic studies of *Helicobacter pylori* urease inhibition by a novel proton pump inhibitor, rabeprazole. *Biol. Pharm. Bull.* 1996;19:182–187.

[51] Parsonnet J. *Helicobacter pylori. Infect. Dis. Clin. N. Am.*1998;12:185-197.

[52] Ramarao N, Gray-Owen S. D., Meyer T. F. *Helicobacter pylori* induces but survives the extracellular release of oxygen radicals from professional phagocytes using its catalase activity. *Mol. Microbiol.* 2000;38:103–113.

[53] Rothenbacher D, Inceoglu J, Bode G. Acquisition of *Helicobacter pylori* infection in a high-risk population occurs within the first 2 years of life. *J. Pediatr.* 2000;136:744-748.

[54] Rothenbacher D, Winkler M, Gonser T. Role of infected parents in transmission of *Helicobacter pylori* to their children. *Pediatr. Infect. Dis. J.* 2002;21:674-679.

[55] Rothenbacher D, Winkler M, Gonser T. Role of infected parents in transmission of Helicobacter pylori to their children. *Pediatr. Infect. Dis. J.* 2002;21: 674-679.

[56] Russel RJ, Haines DC, Anver MR, Battles JK, Gorelick PL, Blumenauer LL, Gonda MA, Ward JM . Use of antibiotics to prevent hepatitis and typhlitis in male scid mice spontaneously infected with *Helicobacter hepaticus. Lab. Anim. Sci.* 1995;45:373-378.

[57] Salomon H. Ueber das spirillum saugetiermagens und sien verhalten zu den belegzellen (abstract 1). *Zentralbl. Bakteriol.* 1896;19:433–442.

[58] Schauer DB, Ghori N, Falkow S. Isolation and characterization of *Flexispira rappini* from laboratory mice. *J. Clin. Microb.* 1993;31:2709-2714.

[59] Shen Z, Fox JG, Dewhirst FE, Paster BJ, Foltz CJ, Yan L, Shames B, Perry L. *Helicobacter rodentium* sp. Nov., a urease-negative Helicobacter species isolated from laboratory mice. *Int. J. Syst. Bacteriol.* 1997;47:627-634.

[60] Shin IS, Masuda H, Naohide K. Bactericidal activity of wasabi (*Wasbia japonica*) against *Helicobacter pylori. Int. J. Food Microbiol.* 2004;94:255–261.

[61] Shomer NH, Dangler CA, Schrenzel MD, Fox JG. *Helicobacter bilis*-induced inflammatory bowel disease in scid mice with defined flora. *Infect. Immun.* 1997;65: 4858-4864.

[62] Sorba G, Bertinaria M, Stilo AD, Gasco A, Scaltrito MM, Brenciaglia, M.I., Dubini, F. Anti-*Helicobacter pylori* agents endowed with H_2-antagonist properties. *Bioorg. Med. Chem. Lett.* 2001;11:403–406.

[63] Torres J, Perez-Perez G, Goodman KJ. A comprehensive review of the natural history of *Helicobacter pylori* infection in children. *Arch. Med. Res.* 2000;31:431-469.

[64] Tsujii M, Kawano S, Tsuji S, Nagano K, Ito T, Hayashi N, Fusamoto H, Kamada T, Tamura K. Ammonia: a possible promotor in *Helicobacter pylori*-related gastric carcinogenesis. *Cancer Lett.* 1992;65:15–18.

[65] Vandamme P, Falsen E, Pot B, Kersters K, De Ley J. Identification of *Campylobacter cinaedi* isolated from blood and feces of children and adult females. *J. Clin. Microbiol.* 1990;28:1016-1020.

[66] Vandamme P, Pot B, Kersters K. Differentiation of campylobacters and *Campylobacter*-like organisms by numerical analysis of one-dimensional electrophoretic protein patterns. *Syst. Appl. Microbiol.* 1991;14:57–66.

[67] Vandamme P. Taxonomy of the family *Campylobacteriaceae. In* M. Blaser (ed.), *Campylobacter. American Society for Microbiology, Washington, D.C.* 2000;3–26

[68] Ward JM, Anver MR, Haines DC, Melhorn JM, Gorelick P, Yan L, Fox JG . Inflammatory large bowel disease in immunodeficient mice naturally infected with Helicobacter hepaticus. *Lab. Anim. Sci.* 1996;46: 15-20.

[69] Warren JR, Marshall B. Unidentified curved bacilli on gastric epithelium in active chronic gastritis. *Lancet* 1983;1:1273–1275.

[70] Watanabe T, Tada M, Nagi H. *Helicobacter pylori* infection induces gastric cancer in Mongolian gerbils. *Gastroenterology* 1998;115:642-648.

[71] Wegmann W, Aschwanden M, Schaub N, Aenishanslin W, Gyr K. Gastritis associated with *Gastrospirillum hominis*—a zoonosis? *Schweiz Med. Wochenschr.* 1991;121:245–254.

[72] Weyermann M, Adler G, Brenner H, Rothenbacher D. The Mother as Source of *Helicobacter pylori* Infection. *Epidemiology* 2006;17:332-334.

[73] Worrel JA, Stoner SC. Eradication of *Helicobacter pylori. Med. Update Psychiat.* 1998;4:99–104.

[74] Yesilada E, Gurbuz I, Shibata H. Screening of Turkish anti-ulcerogenic folk remedies for anti-*Helicobacter pylori* activity. *J. Enthnopharm.* 1999;66: 289–293.

Bovine Tuberculosis in European Bison as Possible Zoonotic Impact in Poland

Kita Jerzy[2*], Anusz Krzysztof[1*], Salwa Andrzej[3], Welz Mirosław[4], Orłowska Blanka[1] and Zaleska Magdalena[5]
[1]*Department of Food Hygiene and Public Health Protection, Faculty of Veterinary Medicine, Warsaw University of Life Sciences - SGGW*
[2]*Faculty of Veterinary Medicine, Warsaw University of Life Sciences - SGGW*
[3]*Veterinary Hygiene Institute, Gdańsk*
[4]*Voivodeship Veterinary Inspectorate, Krosno*
[5]*Department of Pathology and Veterinary Diagnostics, Faculty of Veterinary Medicine, Warsaw University of Life Sciences - SGGW, Nowoursynowska, Warsaw, Poland*

1. Introduction

Tuberculosis remains the most prevailing disease worldwide. This infectious disease is caused by various strains of mycobacteria - *Mycobacterium tuberculosis, M. bovis, M. bovis BCG, M. microti* and *M. africanum* all known under one name *Mycobacterium tuberculosis* complex. Each of the aforementioned agents is recognized as dangerous both to humans and animals. Bovine tuberculosis (bTB) results from infection by *M. bovis.*

Suspicions of tuberculosis incidents in wildlife of Bieszczady Mountains (Poland, Podkarpackie Province) have a long history, however, first records on the confirmed bTB cases date back 1996 and concern European bison found dead within Brzegi Dolne Forest Inspectorate (Fig. 1, 3, 4) (Żurawski et al.1997). Culling of the European bison for diagnostic purposes, carried out in the period 1997-2001, revealed 13 bTB cases of 18 individuals tested (Welz et al.2006).

2. Molecular epidemiology of *M. bovis* isolates

In 2005-2008 in Bieszczady Mountains the next study was conducted. 5 strains of *M. bovis* were isolated - from 2 European bison (of 3 investigated), 2 cows and badger (of 2 investigated).

The whole study covered 215 free - ranging animals: red deer, wild boar, roe deer, a few examples of European bison, badger, wolf and lynx (Fig. 2). All of the animals were examined for mycobacterial infections. The studied material also involved 4 domestic cows. The examination of the collected material resulted in isolation of 14 strains of acid-resistant mycobacteria. The strains were distinguished as follows: 4 strains of *M. tuberculosis* (3 wolfs

---

* Corresponding Authors

and a cow), 5 strains of *M. bovis* (2 European bison, 2 cows and badger), 4 strains of *M.avium* (4 red deer), and a strain of *M. species* (1 red deer) (Salwa et al. in prep.).

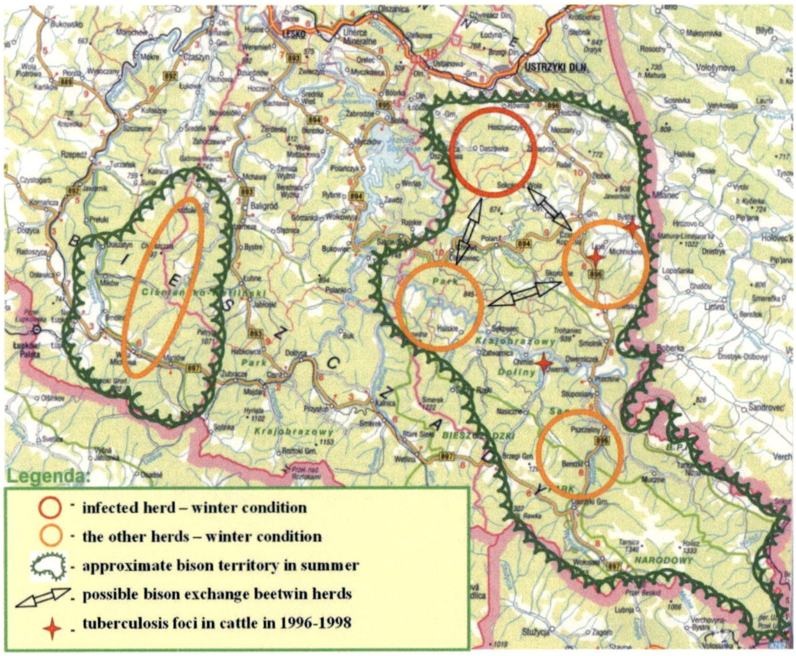

Fig. 1. European bison herds localization in the Bieszczady area in 1996-1998.

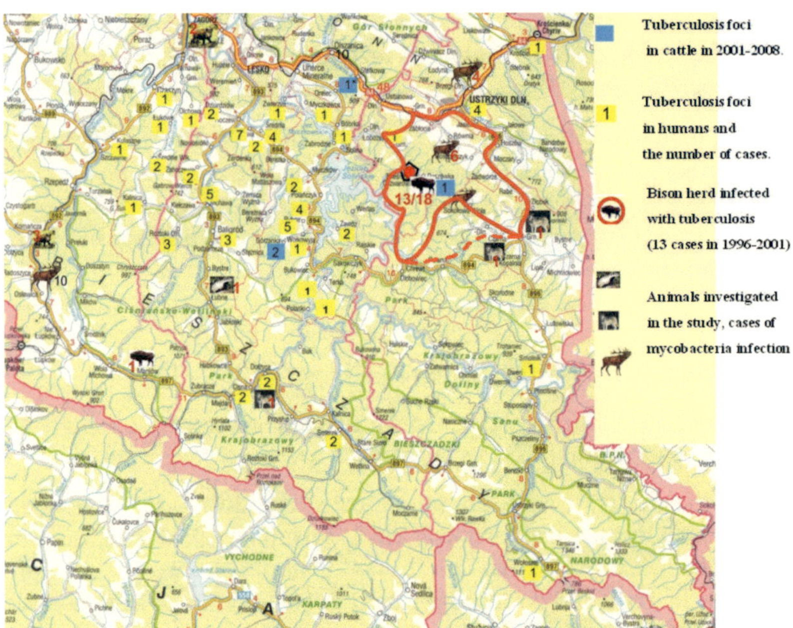

Fig. 2. The localization of tuberculosis foci in animals and humans in the Bieszczady in 2001 - 2008.

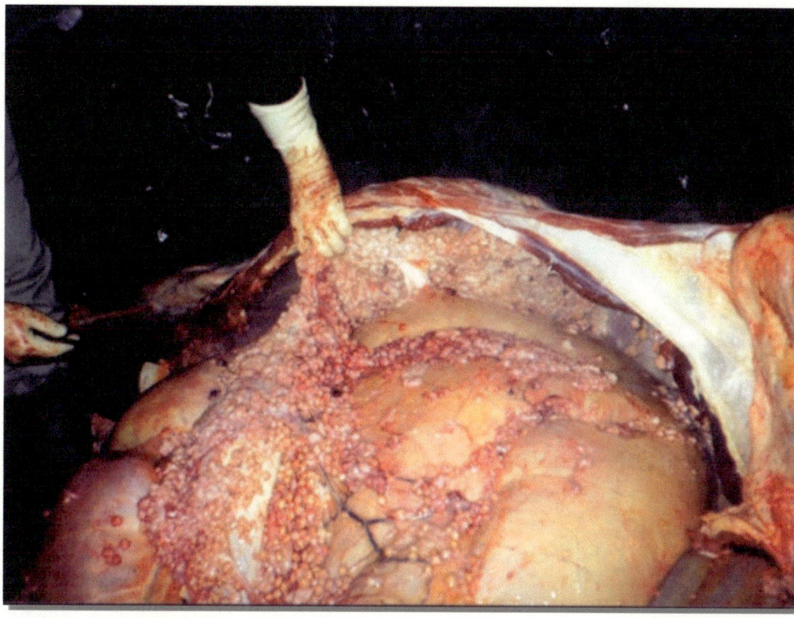

Fig. 3. Lesions characteristic for *M. bovis* infection - European bison, diagnostic cull; February, 1997 (fot. J. Polityński - Brzegi Dolne).

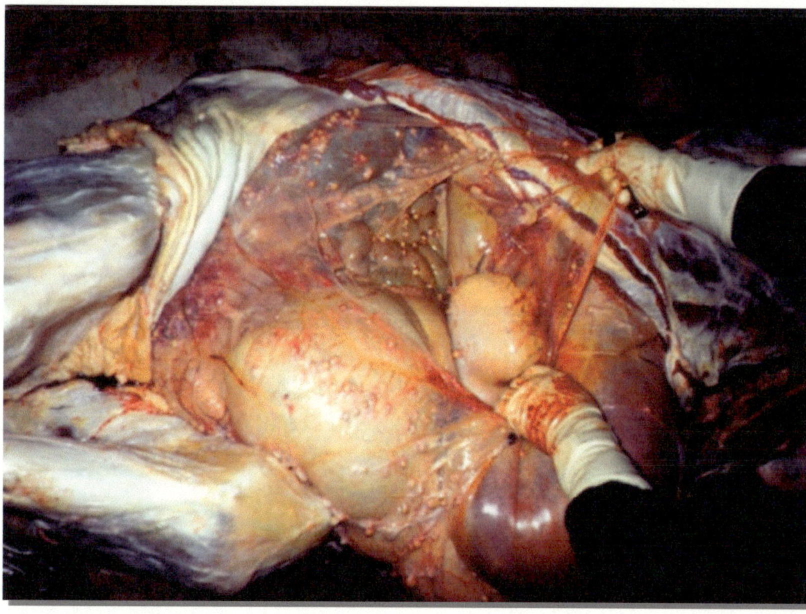

Fig. 4. Lesions characteristic for *M. bovis* infection - European bison, diagnostic cull; February, 1997 (fot. J. Polityński - Brzegi Dolne).

The examination toward the isolation and identification of tuberculosis mycobacteria was carried out by culture technique with the use of biological tests recommended by the Microbiology Unit of State Veterinary Institute in Pulawy. Lymph nodes were microsectioned and chosen tissue fragments were homogenized. The inoculation was carried out in solid medium according to Lowenstein-Jansen and Stonebrink. Identification of isolated bacteria was carried out by the culture and biochemical methods.

Parallel to bacteriological identification of isolated Mycobacterium strains, a confirmation via PCR methods was performed. DNA isolation from examined strains was carried out by the column method using Genomic Mini AX Tissue set (A&A Biotechnology, Gdynia), according to the producer's instructions. The amplification of the selected fragment of region 16S-23 rRNA ITS was carried out utilizing 2 starters complementary to 5′ and 3′ with the following sequences:

ITS-F1-1 5′- TTG ATC CGA CGA AGT CGT AAC AAG g-3′

Mycom-3 5′- ATG CTC GCA ACC ACT ATC CA-3′

Oligonucleotides were synthesized by using a DNA Synthesizer (Genmed Synthesis, Inc.-USA). After finished reaction, the amplification products were analysed electrophoretically in 2% agarose gel (Sigma, Chemical Co.) with addition of ethydine bromide. After electrophoresis the gel was photographed wit an UV transiluminator (Fotodyne Inc.).

Restriction analysis based on the enzyme Sau 961 (Fermentas, Lithuania) to digest bacterial DNA, identifying and cutting the DNA chain in the region of a specific nucleotide sequence. The electrophoresis was carried out in polyacrylamide gel electrophoresis apparatus filled with TAE buffer. The electrophoresis was carried out at voltage 100V/3 hours.

Sequencing was carried out using an automatic sequencer ABI PRISM 3100 Avant Genetic Analyzer, Applied Biosystem. The analysis involved a chosen area of the 16S-23 ITS region of all strains included in the examination. The obtained DNA sequences were then subjected to comparative analysis and subsequently a phylogenetic tree image was created by the Tree View program (version: 1.6.6).

The following strains were used for comparative examination: *M. tuberculosis* isolated from humans (strain PBG/28) and *M. bovis* isolated from a cow (strain DG/358-9). The strains were supplied by the Tuberculosis Diagnostic Pomeranian Center of Infectious Diseases and Tuberculosis in Gdansk, Poland and from the Tuberculosis Diagnostic Laboratory Veterinary Hygiene Institute in Bydgoszcz, Poland.

Among the compared *M. bovis* strains, the highest affinity was displayed by strain derived from two European bisons. Sequence comparision of the analyzed fragment 16S-23S rDNA revealed that it was homologous except for only two nucleotides. What is important, the animals came from two herds living in different regions of Bieszczady. A high genetic differentiation was demonstrated comparing nucleotide sequences od *M. bovis* strains isolated from the badger and cattle. These evidence indicate that *M. bovis* spread within the Bieszczady region is represented by different variants (Salwa et al. in prep.). Consistent with this observation, studies of others authors have shown DNA diversity of *M. bovis*. (Skuce et al. 1996, Sechi et al.1999)

The result of the aforementioned study suggest that tuberculosis had been transmitted to European bison from the cattle when grazing the same pastures. The role of badgers in the spreading of *M. bovis* in Bieszczady Mountains is not yet fully recognized. It is necessary to underline that *M. bovis* was not isolated from deer and boars in Bieszczady Mountains.

3. Discussion

According to the report listing the local zoonotic disease in Bieszczady found during 1960-2008, in the sixties tuberculosis was common in cattle of Bieszczady. Although in the seventies the disease was believed to be eradicated, some isolated cases of tuberculosis positive cows were being found regularly every year thereafter. The report pointed at Daszówka as the location with the highest density of tuberculosis loci (Fig. 2).

A natural reservoir of *M. bovis* can be both a livestock, cattle in particular, and wildlife. Mutual contacts of animals from these two groups, taking place at pastures and meadows, facilitate an interspecies transmission of mycobacteria. Long term observations point at farm animals and humans as a primary source for Mycobacterium infections (Pavlik et al.2005, Tessaro et al.1990). Free-ranging animals might in term become a reservoir of bTB and a secondary source of infection for other free-ranging animals or livestock. Infections may have a direct or indirect character. There are also many routes of *M. bovis* spreading (via air, with feces, urine, etc.). In England Courtenay et al. (2006) studied the route of *M. bovis* transmission and found out that infections of cattle had an indirect character and took place on the pastures via water and soil contaminated with urine of infected badger. A further support for this finding came from DNA comparative analysis of *M. bovis* strains isolated from cattle and badger that revealed a genetic similarity (Cheeseman et al. 1981, Costello et al. 2006). What is important, in Great Britain badgers are the main wildlife reservoir for bTB and there are different badger control strategies for reducing bTB in cattle (ex. culling, vaccination)(defra.gov.uk). During 1992-2001 cases of tuberculosis were reported in buffaloes of the Kruger National Park, South Africa (De Vos et al.2001, Miller et al. 1997). Further epidemiological and molecular studies pointed at wild felids to play an important role in spreading the bacilli (De Vos et al.2001).

Tuberculosis can have a chronic or rapidly progressive course. In free-ranging animals it is very often diagnosed after the onset of the typical clinical signs. This fact favours a prolonged period of the disease transmission.

The implementation of numerous cattle tuberculosis control programs have efficiently decreased the number of mycobacteria - infected animals to the level below 0.5%. Hence there are now countries, including Poland, regarded as free from bTB (WHO Report 2006). The presence of the disease in free-ranging wildlife in the Bieszczady region is a considerable threat to cattle and can lead to the loss of officially bTB free status of the region.

Epidemiological situation of Great Britain and New Zealand clearly demonstrates that the natural reservoir of *M. bovis* circulating in wildlife impedes the efficient eradication of tuberculosis in farm animals, especially in cattle. Numerous studies have concluded that the prevalence of tuberculosis in free-ranging animals is related to cases of tuberculosis in cattle (Bengis et al.2002, De Lisle et al. 2001, Gallagher et al. 2000, Mathews 2006, Nishi et al.2006).

According to the study bTB is endemic in the herds of free-ranging European bison of Bieszczady Mountains. The transmission of *M. bovis* probably originated from the infected cattle. Despite the actions taken in order to eliminate infections, new cases of bTB in European bison are still being reported. Last two cases are quite recent (2011) and they legitimate further studies on the spread of tuberculosis also in many wildlife species, also from the orders Carnivora (wolf - *Canis lupus*, red fox - *Vulpes vulpes*, badger – *Meles meles*) and Rodentia.

M. bovis has been isolated from many free-ranging animals worldwide (Aranaz et al. 2004, Delahay et al. 2007). First world reports on tuberculosis in wildlife related to the kudu antelope in South Africa (Griffith 1929). Since then the disease have been observed in other species inhabiting different countries for example: the red deer, elks and coyotes from Texas (Perumaalla et al. 1996), red deer, elks, lynxes and hares from Spain (Aranaz et al. 2004), the African buffalo from Southern Africa (De Vos et al. 2001, Michel et al. 2006) and the bison from Canada (Schmit et al. 2002). Tuberculosis was also found in the baboon, lion, panther and cheetah (Michel et al. 2006). In Poland tuberculosis in wildlife was described for the first time in roe deer in the Gdańsk district (Czarnowski 1956). Later research showed quite frequent occurrence of Mycobacterium infection in the zoo animals (Dąbrowski 1974, Żurawski et al. 1980)

Tuberculosis, one of the oldest recognized disease in humans and animals, still remains a serious health hazard. It is estimated that one third of the human world population is infected with TB. The number of the strains showing a multi-drug resistance is still increasing (Augustynowicz-Kopeć et al. 2009). Human tuberculosis due to *M. bovis* has become very rare in countries with pasteurized milk and bovine tuberculosis eradication programs. In the region of Bieszczady Mountains there had been over 100 outbreaks of tuberculosis noted in humans over last 20 years. *Mycobacterium tuberculosis* complex was described as a causative agent of infections. Further procedures of mycobacteria identification were not performed. Cases of infections with *M. bovis* in cattle are also more numerous here as compared to any other regions of Poland. For this reason, there was a time when the bovine tuberculin tests were performed on some area every year (normally when the area is considered a tuberculosis free, the law stipulates a three-year interval between obligatory tuberculin tests). The analysis of epidemiological background of tuberculosis in the region revealed that the role of *M. bovis* in spreading the disease among people is underestimated.

Bovine tuberculosis can only be eradicated by controlling *M. bovis* infection in both wildlife and domestic animals. Otherwise cattle herds can be continually re-infected. The persistence of bovine tuberculosis in wildlife and the subsequent spread to farmed animals has stimulated research into new methods for controlling the disease in wildlife as well as cattle. A promising option for control of *M. bovis* infection in wildlife in the longer term is the development of a tuberculosis vaccine for wildlife and oral bait vaccines are the most practical means of delivering vaccines to wildlife. *M. bovis* bacilli Calmette-Guerin (BCG) is the world's most widely used human vaccine (intradermal vaccination). BCG is a live attenuated strain of *M. bovis* and was originally derived from a cow with tuberculous mastitis (Aldwell et al. 2003). Oral BCG vaccination of wildlife reservoirs of bTB is being extensively researched for application in many countries, including New Zealand (brushtail possum), Great Britain, Ireland (badger), United States (white-tailed deer) and South Africa (African buffalo) (Nol et al. 2008). Nol and all 2008. indicate that oral BCG Danish 1331 is effective in protecting white-tailed deer against disease caused by experimental *M. bovis* infection. Orally vaccinated deer had fewer tuberculosis lesion. The results of the present experiment indicate that white-tailed deer can be vaccinated orally using BCG incorporated in a lipid-formulated bait. This oral bait has successfully induced protection against *M. bovis* and *M. tuberculosis* infection in a number of species, including laboratory mice (Aldwell et al., 2003), brushtail possum (*Trichosurus vulpecula;* Aldwell et al., 2003a) and domestic cattle (Buddle et al., 2005). White-tailed deer are a good candidate for oral vaccination programs to control bovine tuberculosis in the field (Nol et al. 2008). Trial with oral BCG vaccination in

European bison in Bieszczady Mountains should also be undertaken (evaluation of vaccine efficacy by microbiological and molecular examination - samples from characteristic pathological lesions; gamma interferon and lymphocyte proliferation tests, ELISA - blood samples). Oral administration of vaccines has a number of advantages including ease of administration, low cost, and the avoidance of needles. Furthermore, oral immunization more effectively targets the mucosal immune response. Oral bait vaccines have been successfully used to prevent rabies in foxes and other wildlife carriers (Schneider 1995).

It is necessary to remind that the European bison (*Bison bison*) is the largest terrestrial mammal in Europe (Fig. 5.). Long since being exterminated, it has been eventually returned to the wild. Considering health threats to European bison, the fact that those alive today descent from just 12 individuals (5 males and 7 females) survived in zoos and animal parks should be taken into account. Limited genetic variability characterizes all the European bison living now. That may lead to the appearance of genetic defects, less-flexibility and tolerance to unfavorable environmental changes, or a lowering of resistance and consequent vulnerability to disease. The threats to the European bison not only concern infectious disease, but also genetically derived problems such as testicular anomalies and environmental limitation like lack of opportunity for migration between isolated populations, limitations on food resources, competition with other ungulates (Krasińska et al. 2007). There are 5 free-ranging population of European bison in Poland, four in the east of the country and one in the north-west. The total number of bison present in the wild is about 750 individuals. The largest population is in Białowieża Forest, about 370 individuals. Bieszczady Mountains are the only place in Poland where bison of the Białowieża-Caucasian Line are present, about 300 individuals. Unfortunately, a serious threat to this population is posed by the tuberculosis.

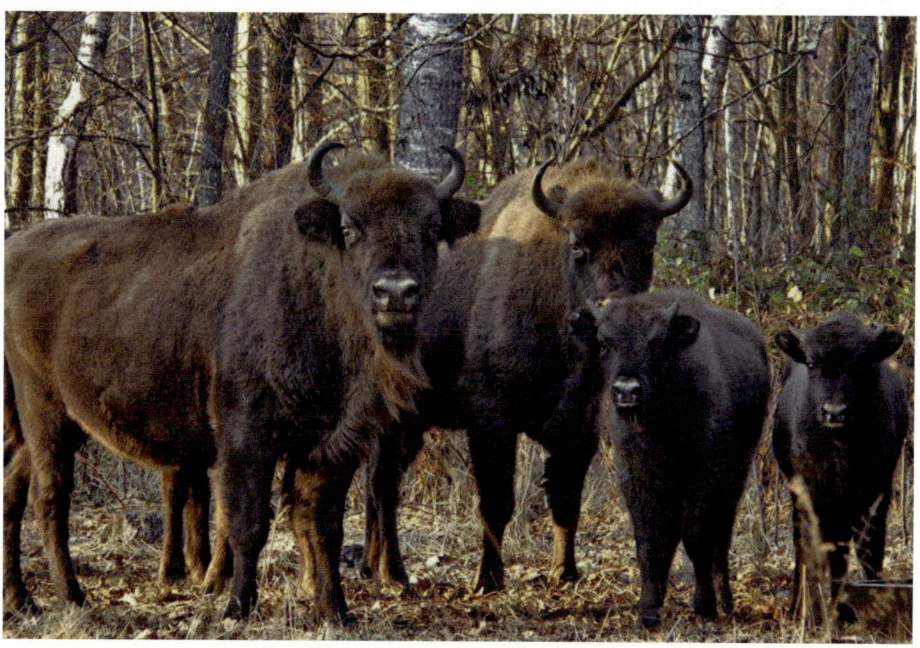

Fig. 5. European bison (*Bison bison*) is the largest terrestrial mammal in Europe.

Bieszczady Mountains is one of the most valuable Polish mainstays for many species. It houses about 230 species of vertebrates, including protected animals as European bison, the wolf, brown bear, lynx and badger.

4. References

[1] Aldwell F. E., Keen D. L., Parlane N. A., Skinner M. A., Lisle G. W., Buddle B. M.: Oral vaccination with *Mycobacterium bovis* BCG in a lipid formulation induces resistance to pulmonary tuberculosis in brushtail possums. Vaccine 2003, 22, 70–76.

[2] Aranaz A., Juan L., de Montero N., Sánchez C., Galka M., Delso C., Alvarez J., Romero J., Bezos J., Vela A.I., Briones V., Mateos A., Domínquez L.: Bovine tuberculosis (*Mycobacterium bovis*) in wildlife in Spain. J. Clin. Microbiol. 2004, 42, 2602-2608.

[3] Augustynowicz-Kopeć E., Zwolska Z.: Drug resistant tuberculosis in Poland. Nowa Medycyna 2009, 1, 50-55.

[4] Bengis R.G., Kock R.A., Fischer J.: Infectious animal diseases: the wildlife/ livestock interface. Rev. Sci. Tech. Int. Epiz. 2002, 21, 53 – 65.

[5] Buddle B. M., Aldwell F. E., Skinner M. A., De Lisle G. W., Denis M., Vordermeier H. M., Hewinson R. G., and Wedlock D. N.: Effect of oral vaccination of cattle with lipid-formulated BCG on immune responses and protection against bovine tuberculosis. Vaccine 2005, 23, 3581–3589.

[6] Cheeseman C.L., Jones G.W., Gallagher J., Mallinson P.J.: The Population Structure, Density and Prevalence of Tuberculosis (*Mycobacterium bovis*) in Badgers (Meles meles) from Four Areas in South-West England. J. Appl. Ecol. 1981, 18, 795 - 804.

[7] Costello E., Flynn O., Phil M., Quigley F., O'Grady D., Griffin J., Clegg T., McGrath G.: Genotyping of *Mycobacterium bovis* isolates from badgers in four areas of the Republic of Ireland by restriction fragment length polymorphism analysis. Vet. Rec. 2006, 159, 619 - 623.

[8] Courtenay O., Reilly L., Sweeney F., Hibberd V., Bryan S., Ul-Hassan A., Newmann C., Macdonald D., Delahey R., Wilson G., Wellington E.: Is *Mycobacterium bovis* in the environment for the persistence of bovine tuberculosis. Biol Lett. 2006, 2, 460-462.

[9] Czarnowski A.: Tuberculosis in deer due to human *Mycobacterium* bacilli. Medycyna Wet. 1956, 12, 348.

[10] Dąbrowski J.: Tuberculosis in animals of Łódź Zoological Garden. Medycyna Wet. 1974, 30, 596 - 597.

[11] Delahay R.J., Smith G.C., Barlow A.M., Walker N., Harris A., Clifton-Hadley R.S., Cheeseman C.L.: Bovine tuberculosis infection in wild mammals in the South-West region of England: a survey of prevalence and a semi-quantitative assessment of the relative risks to cattle. Vet J. 2007, 173, 287-301.

[12] De Lisle G.W., Mackintosh C.G., Bengis R.G.: *Mycobacterium bovis* in free-living and captive wildlife, including farmed deer. Rev. Sci. Tech. Int. Epiz. 2001, 20, 86 – 111.

[13] De Vos V., Bengins R.G., Kriek N.P., Michel A.A., Keet D.F., Raath J.P., Huchzermeyer H.F.: The epidemiology of tuberculosis In free-ranging African Buffalo (*Syncerus caffer*) In the Kruger Natinal Park, South Africa. J.Vet.Res. 2001, 68, 119 - 130.

[14] Gallagher J., Clifton-Hadley R. S.: Tuberculosis in badgers; a review of the disease and its significance for other animals. Res. Vet. Sci. 2000, 69, 203 - 217.

[15] Griffith A.S.: Infections of wild animals with tubercle and other acid-fast bacilli. Proc. R. Soc. Med. 1939, 32, 1405 - 1412.

[16] Krasińska M., Krasiński Z.A.: European Bison, The Nature Monograph, Mammal Research Institute Polish Academy of Science, Białowieża, 2007, 221-234; 258-262.
[17] Mathews F., Macdonald D.W., Taylor G.M., Gelling M., Norman R.A., Honess P.E., Foster R., Gower C.M., Varley S., Harris A., Palmer S., Hewinson G., Webster J.P.: Bovine tuberculosis (*Mycobacterium bovis*) in British farmland wildlife: the importance to agriculture. Proc. R. Soc. B. 2006, 273, 357-365.
[18] Michel A.L., Bengins R.G., Keet D.F., Hofmeyer M., Klerk L.M., Cross P C., Jalles A.E., Cooper D., Whyte I.J., Buss P., Godfroid J.: Wildlife tuberculosis in South African conservation areas: implications and challenges. Vet. Microbiol. 2006, 112, 91 - 100.
[19] Miller J., Jenny A., Rhyan J., Saari D., Suarez D.: Detection of *Mycobacterium bovis* in formalin-fixed, paraffin-embedded tissues of cattle and elk by PCR amplification of an IS6110 sequence specifc for *Mycobacterium tuberculosis* complex organisms. J.Vet.Diagn. Invest. 1997, 9, 244-249.
[20] Nishi J.S., Shury T., Elkin B. T.: Wildlife reservoirs for bovine tuberculosis (*Mycobacterium bovis*) in Canada: strategies for management and research. Vet Microbiol. 2006, 112, 325 - 338.
[21] Nol P., Palmer M.V., Waters W.R., Aldwell F.E., Buddle B.M., Triantis J.M., Linke L.M., Philips G.E., Thacker T.C., Rhyan J.C., Dunbar M.R., Salman M.D.: Efficacy of oral and parenteral routes of *Mycobacterium bovis* bacille calmette-guerin vaccination against experimental bovine tuberculosis in white-tailed deer (*Odocoileus virginianus*): a feasibility study. Journal of Wildlife Diseases. 2008, 44, 247-259.
[22] Pavlik, I., Machackova M., Ayele W.Y., Lamka J., Parmova I. , Melicharek I., Hanzlikova M., Körmendy B., Nagy G., Cvetnic Z., Ocepek M., Lipiec M.: Incidence of bovine tuberculosis in wild and domestic animals other than cattle in six Central European countries during 1990–1999. Vet. Med. - Czech, 2002, 47, 122–131.
[23] Perumaalla V.S., Adams L.G., Payeur J.B., Jarnagin J. L., Baca D.R., Guemes F. S., Ficht T. A.: Molecular Epidemiology of *Mycobacterium bovis* in Texas and Mexico. J. Clin. Microbiol. 1996, 34, 2066 - 2071.
[24] Schmit S.M., O'Brien D.J., Bruning-Fann C.S.: Bovine tuberculosis in Michigan wildlife and livestock. Ann N. Y. Academy Scie. 2002, 969, 262-268.
[25] Salwa A., Anusz K., Śmigielska M., Welz M., Wozikowski R., Burkiewicz A., Zaleska M., Kita J.: An assessment of genetic variability of mycobacteria isolated from free-ranging and farm animals in the Bieszczady area.- publication in preparation.
[26] Schneider LG.: Rabies virus vaccines. Dev Biol Stand. 1995, 84, 49–54.
[27] Sechi LA, Leori G, Lollai SA, Duprè I, Molicotti P, Fadda G, Zanetti S.: Different strategies for molecular differentiation of *Mycobacterium bovis* strains isolated in Sardinia, Italy. Appl Environ Microbiol. 1999, 65, 1781-1785.
[28] Skuce R.A., Brittain D., Hughes M.S., Neill S.D.: Differentation of *Mycobacterium bovis* isolates from animals by DNA typing. J. Clin.Microbiol. 1996, 34, 24- 27.
[29] Tessaro S.V., Forbes L.B., Turcotte C.: A survey of brucellosis and tuberculosis in bison in and Wood Buffalo National Park. Canada. Can. Vet. J. 1990, 31, 174 - 180.
[30] Welz M., Anusz K., Salwa A., Zaleska M., Bielecki W., Osińska B., Kaczor S., Kita J.: Bovine tuberculosis in European bison in the Bieszczady Region. Health threats for the European bison particulary in the free-roaming population in Poland. Monograph, The SGGW Publishers, 2006, 70-77.
[31] WHO Raport.: Tuberculosis. Global and regional incidence. Geneva, 2006.
[32] www.defra.gov.uk

[33] Żurawski C., Lipiec M.: Generalized tuberculosis in European bison. Medycyna Wet. 1997, 53, 90 - 92.

[34] Żurawski C., Stankiewicz M., Skwarek P.: Enzootic of tuberculosis in monkeys caused by a niacin positive strain of *Mycobacterium bovis*. Medycyna Wet. 1980, 36, 328 - 330.

8

Anthrax

Antonio Fasanella
Istituto Zooprofilattico Sperimentale della Puglia e della Basilicata, Foggia, Italy

1. Introduction

1.1 Definition

Anthrax is a non-contagious infectious disease hitting a high range of animal species including humans, although the animals that are most susceptible are domestic and wild ruminants. The bacterial agent is *Bacillus anthracis* whose main characteristic is to form spores that can survive outdoors for several decades. Anthrax in susceptible animals generally has a fatal evolution characterised by sudden deadly bleeding from natural openings. In humans, the disease develops in three forms depending on the route of penetration of the bacterium: cutaneous (non-fatal), pulmonary and gastrointestinal. Recently a fatal form was reported characterised by a subacute evolution in drug users as a result of injection of drugs contaminated with anthrax spores. Due to its high capacity to maintain its viability and pathogenicity and for low cost production, B. *anthracis* is considered one of the pathogen agents of greatest interest for use as a bacteriological weapon in bioterroristic attack.

1.2 History

Anthrax is a disease known since ancient times. Probably the first record of the disease can be found in the Bible in the Book of Exodus Chapter 7-9. It is thought that the V plague that struck Egyptian people is a disease that has clinical features very similar to anthrax. Another allusion to a disease very similar to anthrax is made by Homer in the Iliad when he speaks of a "burning wind of plague". Then Hippocrates (5th century B.C.), using the Greek word for "coal", defined a disease characterised by skin dark lesions and fluid blood.

But it is the Roman poet Virgil in his Georgics who described anthrax in detail and for the first time hypothesized on the transmission from animals to humans, suggesting attention to the ongoing slaughter of animals with the disease.

Anthrax has been for a long time the main and most feared disease among animals and the epizootics of anthrax have been responsible for real massacres of animals up to the 19th century. A serious outbreak in the mid-18th century seems to have destroyed half of the entire population of sheep in Europe. Chaber in 1780 described in detail the disease in animals and over the same period Barthelemy showed the transmission in healthy animals by the inoculation of infected blood. The appearance of zoonotic anthrax had been widely highlighted by the fact that human cases of this disease increased during the epidemic among animals. Maret and Fournier in 1769 studied this aspect of the disease due to the fact that people who came into contact with sick animals often developed skin ulcers, which if not properly treated could lead to a fatal septicaemia. Pulmonary anthrax had long been known, especially as the "wool-sorter disease". If untreated, it rapidly leads to death. As for gastro-intestinal anthrax, due to consumption of meat from diseased animals, it caused considerable human fatalities simultaneous with anthrax epidemics in animals. Thus, for instance, in 1613, the disease caused 60,000 human fatalities in Southern Europe (Schwartz, 2009). In 1958, the WHO estimated the annual incidence of human cases of anthrax worldwide to be between 20,000 and 100,000.

Anthrax is not only a disease of the past. It is still with us today, not only as a potential weapon for bioterrorists.

In developed countries, due to the application of adequate prophylactic measures, it is sporadic. In contrast, in developing countries, anthrax may still represents a major problem, for animals as well as for human (Hugh-Jones, 1999; Hugh-Jones & Blackburn, 2009). A massive outbreak occurred in Zimbabwe during the period 1978–1980, which caused 9,711 human cases with 151 deaths (WHO, quoted by Turnbull). More recent examples are the epidemics in Kyrgyzstan and Zimbabwe. In the former, large but unknown numbers of animal cases were accompanied by at least 50 human cases in 2008. In Zimbabwe, in 2008, anthrax added its toll to the severe epidemic of cholera in a totally disorganised country where actual numbers of disease victims are difficult to ascertain; WHO reported some 200 human cases with eight confirmed deaths. In Bangladesh in 2010 there were 104 animal cases of anthrax and 607 associated human cases from contact with contaminated meat from sick livestock (Fasanella et al., 2011).

2. Characteristic of *Bacillus anthracis*

2.1 Aspect

B. anthracis belongs to the family of Bacillaceae and has a rod-shape (long 3 - 6 μ and wide 1 - 1.5 μ). It is motionless and aerobic. Often there are different elements assembled in a chain. In preparations fixed and stained the extremities appear at right angles or enlarged and the surface of contact between the individual elements is concave, similar to the epiphysis of a bone, and that gives them a particular look similar to "bamboo canes" (fig. 1). Bacilli in the animal organism are surrounded by a clear capsule that is usually lacking in culture media and is considered as a defence by the forces of the germ-bacterial organism. Sometimes the *B. anthracis* undergoes lysis phenomena: the capsules are intact while the inside contains only remains of the bacillary body, some are completely empty capsules (shadows). This is especially true in the material in the process of putrefaction. Outside the body and with temperatures between 14°C and 42°C (optimum between 21°C and 37°C) *B. anthracis* will sporulate. The spores are oval and are released after lysis of the bacterium. Sporulation is completed within 48 hours, but it does not happen in the presence of high concentrations of CO_2, a condition that occurs in infected putrefacting carcasses.

2.2 Staining

B. anthracis is coloured with all the aniline dyes. It is Gram-positive. In blood or organ smears stained with methylene blue Löffer, the bacillary body is coloured in blue and purple capsule (sometimes only purple spots are observed, probably due to the material of the capsule: reaction of Mc. Fadyean).

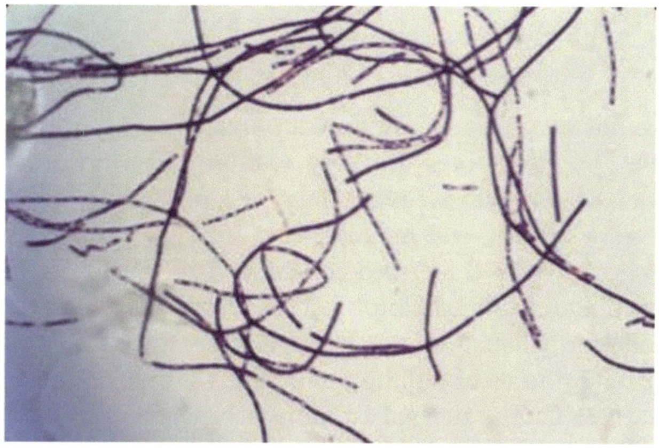

Fig. 1. Gram stain of *Bacillus anthracis* vegetative form from a colony growth on agar TSP 5% sheep blood. It is evident the typical bamboo-shaped filaments

2.3 Cultivation

B. anthracis grows well on ordinary culture media under aerobic or microaerofilia, at temperatures between 12°C and 44°C, but optimal growth occurs around 37°C and at a pH of 7.0 to 7.4. In tryptose broth there is a flocculation and then it forms a silky deposit. Colonies on plates form a magnificent plot called caput medusae (phase R or rough) (fig. 2). For this reason is generally believed that the R phase of B. *anthracis* is the normal and virulent one, while the attenuated (vaccine germs) grow mostly in S phase. This would be an exception, as with other microbial species S phase is the normal and virulent phase. But it seems that the physiological condition for the growth of anthrax bacilli, including the presence of carbon dioxide concentration of at least 5% (which occurs in the alveoli), permits

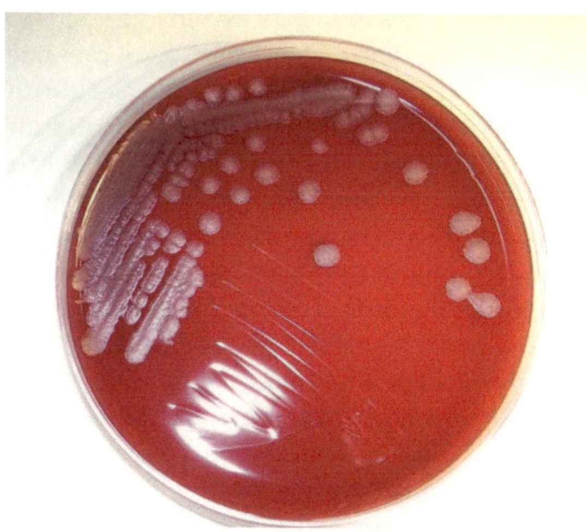

Fig. 2. Colony of *Bacillus anthracis* growth on TSP agar 5% sheep blood

the germs to grow in an S virulent phase (mucosal aspect of colonies). Probably the growth in the R phase, which occurs in an ordinary atmosphere, would be a temporary phenomenon of adaptation.

2.4 Resistance

Vegetative forms are not very robust and they are inactivated within 30 minutes at 60°C - 65°C (Turnbull, 1998), but its spores are very resistant. The action of direct sunlight is significant as ultraviolet rays will inactivate them in a few hours, however the spores that live a few inches deep in the soil will remain active for years. In fertiliser prepared so that the temperature reaches over 60°C (aerated compost, rich in horse faeces) spores are killed in a few days. In the cold and salting samples spores resist for a long time: frozen meat and skins remain virulent for years and the same is true for dried skins. The spores are destroyed only after ten minutes of boiling temperatures, they are destroyed in 20 minutes in an autoclave set at 121°C. The normal fixation techniques do not kill the spores, which can successfully germinate even after many years, so it is necessary to flame slides several times before assuming the spores are dead. The spores are sensitive to 2%-3% formaldehyde solutions at 40°C for 20 minutes or 0.25% at 60°C for six hours or at 4% after a contact of at least two hours. The spores are destroyed by 5% phenol and mercury chloride, and 1% solutions of caustic soda and potash.

3. Ecology of anthrax

Anthrax spores survive best in soils rich in organic matter and calcium. In the Kruger National Park (Africa) *B. anthracis* spores have been isolated from animal bones estimated to be about 200 years old (Smith et al., 2000). Saile and Koehler (2006) have demonstrated that spores will germinate and establish stable populations of vegetative cells in the rhizosphere of fescue (*Festuca arundinacea*) grass in the laboratory in an otherwise sterile environment. In natural circumstances the vegetative cells are fragile and die even in simple environments, such as water or milk (Turnbull et al., 1989). In conclusion it seems that soil encourages sporulation, not germination, and this would explain why vegetative bacilli are not found in nature. Van Ness (1971) defined the "incubator areas" as depressions which collect water, dead vegetation, calcium and other salts washed in from the surrounding slightly higher ground and thus provide a medium suitable for germination and multiplication. However, this hypothesis was never confirmed by scientific study. It has been proposed that rainy water may collect and concentrate spores in 'storage areas' (Dragon & Renie, 1995). Spores have a high surface hydrophobicity and so could be carried during a rain runoff in clumps of humus and organic matter to collect and concentrate in standing pools or puddles. As they have a high buoyant density, this would result in them and their organic matter clumps remaining suspended in the standing water to be further concentrated as the water evaporated. Thus theoretically 'storage areas' may collect more spores from extended areas to reach increasing spore concentrations over time and be lethally available to potential incidental grazing hosts. Most *B. anthracis* is held in the ground as spores until the ideal conditions are created for its reproductive cycle that occurs in a different habitat, primarily domestic and wild ruminants. Nature provides few opportunities to the bacterium for its replicative cycle and the development of an exceptional pathogenicity is the effective strategy aimed to significantly increase the probability of success against the host's immune mechanisms. Rapid intense multiplication by the vegetative cells quickly takes the host to death. Although many of the new generations of bacteria will be neutralised by putrefactive processes, a good part survives and spreads into the surrounding soil as spores, ensuring the standard of environmental density of the bacteria that is an essential condition for the continuation of the species. In summary, the few cases of anthrax that occur each year are merely the result of a natural ecological balance that seeks through these extraordinary events simply to promote the maintenance of a bacterial species that otherwise would have been extinguished some time ago. It is widely believed that the vegetative forms of *B. anthracis* tend to sporulate when exposed to oxygen. Under these assumptions it is assumed that in an intact carcass putrefactive processes should destroy almost all bacteria in a period of time ranging from 48 to 72 hours (Stein, 1947a). But rarely in nature are carcasses of dead animals left undisturbed by scavengers. Spores will survive passage through the scavenger's intestinal tract, but vegetative cells will not. Anthrax spores were recovered from approximately half of the faeces from jackals (*Canis mesomelas*), vultures (*Gyps africanus, Torgos tracheliotus, Trigonoceps occipitalis*) and hyaenas (*Crocuta crocuta*) collected in the vicinity of carcasses in the Etosha National Park, but not at a distance; the faecal spore density was extremely variable (Lindeque and Turnbull, 1994). Insects, primarily necrophilic and haemophagic flies, have been associated in the spreading of anthrax spores. Fasanella et al. (2010) demonstrated that, under experimental condition, *Musca domestica* can spread the bacterium and additionally that *B. anthracis* is able to germinate within their intestines.

4. Toxic factors of *B. anthracis*

The pathogenic action of *B. anthracis* is closely linked to the following two plasmids:

- pXO1, 182 Kb, which contains the genes encoding the three anthrax protein factors: the oedema factor (EF), the lethal factor (LF) and the protective antigen (PA);
- pXO2, 96 Kb, which contains the genes encoding the biosynthesis of the capsule (Uchida et al., 1997).

The results of a study demonstrated that *B. anthracis* virulence is related to clonality (as indicated by MLVA genotype cluster) and pXO1 and pXO2 copy number (Cocker et al., 2003).

The capsule is a linear polymer of D-glutamic acid which plays an important role in the ability of anthrax to resist phagocytosis by macrophages. The exact mechanism by which this occurs, however, is still unknown. In contrast, the three protein factors have been, and still are, the object of much attention. Interestingly, the idea that the bacterium could secrete a molecule involved in pathogenesis was mentioned by Pasteur as early as 1877. Pasteur noted that filtrates prepared from the blood of diseased animals induced the agglutination of red cells in blood from healthy animals. Smith and his associates showed the complex to be composed of the three protein factors mentioned above: PA (83 kDa), EF (89 kDa) and LF (90 kDa). Independently, these three factors are innocuous. Intravenous injection of PA + LF, however, provokes death, whereas intradermal injection of PA + EF produces oedema in the skin. In the early 1990s, Singh et al. discovered that PA was the component involved in the specific binding of LF and EF to the target cell, as well as in the transport of these virulence factors into the cell (Singh et al., 1991).

Contrary to earlier studies suggesting that the toxins were responsible for death (Keppie et al., 1955; Smith et al., 1955), recent research indicates that their primary targets are cells of innate immunity that would otherwise impair anthrax multiplication (Tournier et al., 2009) . They do so by altering the cyclic adenosine monophosphate (c-AMP) and mitogen-activated protein kinase (MAPK) signalling pathways essential for the activation of immune cells. In brief, the two anthrax toxins derive from the combination of three different proteins: PA, EF and LF. PA binds to two cell surface receptors, the tumour endothelium marker 8 (TEM8) and the capillary morphogenesis protein 2 (CMG2), both of which are widely expressed on many cell types, including immune cells (Collier & Young, 2003; Scobie & Young, 2005). The proteolytic release of the C-terminal domain (20 kDa) of PA results in spontaneous oligomerisation of truncated PA (PA63) into heptamers, which bind EF and LF. The (PA63)7–EF and the (PA63)7–LF complexes enter rafts and - after endocytotic uptake - are transported to late endosomes, whose low pH induces a conformational change of the complex, with the insertion of a part of PA into the membrane and the translocation of EF and LF into the cytosol. EF is a calmodulin-dependent adenylate cyclase (Leppla, 1982) which creates a gradient of cAMP with a high concentration in the perinuclear area, whilst LF is a metalloprotease which cleaves most isoforms of MAPKKs (MEKs) throughout the cytosol (Vitale et al., 2000). This does not exclude the possibility that it may act on other cytosolic proteins as well, a possibility raised in recent reports suggesting that LF acts on the inflammasome (Boyden & Dietrich, 2006; Muehlbauer et al., 2007). MEKs are part of a major signalling pathway linking the activation of membrane receptors to the transcription of several genes, including those encoding pro-inflammatory cytokines and other proteins involved in the immune response.

5. Epidemiology

Knowledge of the disease, the agent, the transmission, the development of a vaccine and especially understanding that a relevant rule in the control of anthrax is the removing of infected carcasses from the environment to reduce the process of spore production, has contributed to the almost complete disappearance of anthrax.

In agricultural areas of industrialised and rich countries, the sporadic outbreaks of anthrax still tend to occur where in the past infected animals were buried or leather industry waste was collected. More frequently, outbreaks are reported that develop as a consequence of the introduction of contaminated feed. Probably the most serious incident occurred in 1923 in South Africa where in one year it killed between 30,000 and 60,000 animals (Sterne, 1967). Though worldwide it is now an uncommon disease in much of Western Europe, Northern America and Australia, with exceptions in endemic foci in wild fauna in the African national parks (Hugh-Jones, 1999). In Canada it is enzootic in specific locations in the North-West Territories (Slave River Flats) and Alberta (Wood Bison National Park) (Nischi et al., 2002), and has the potential if control is relaxed to form epidemics in the Canadian Prairie provinces, while in the US. the disease is a persistent threat in Eastern North and South Dakota and North-West Minnesota, is enzootic in South-West Texas (Hugh-Jones, 1999) and suddenly 'appeared' in 2008 in South-West Montana where it had not been recorded . In Australia, anthrax is sporadic, although a sudden and severe epidemic occurred in Northern Victoria in 1997 (Turner et al., 1999). In Europe, the major enzootic areas are Greece, Spain, Turkey, Albania, France and Southern Italy (Fouet et al., 2002; Fasanella et al., 2005), but essentially absent from Northern Europe.

While the incidence is generally falling worldwide, it persists in certain countries; for example it is hyper-enzootic in Haiti and still enzootic in Bolivia, Mexico and Peru. This follows from ineffective control programmes. In contrast, vaccination programmes in Belize, Nicaragua and Chile have resulted in good control. It is still absent from the Guianas. In Russia and in countries of the former Soviet Union, lack of effective control programmes is evidenced by the high percentage of human cases, reflecting the inadequacies of both the public health systems and the veterinary services (Hugh-Jones, 1999). In Asia, anthrax is widespread in the Philippines, South Korea, Eastern India and in mountainous zones of Western China and Mongolia; porcine anthrax is frequently reported in the highlands of Papua New Guinea. Africa remains severely afflicted, with major epidemic areas in wildlife areas such as Queen Elizabeth National Park (Uganda), Mago National Park Omo (Ethiopia), Selous National Reserve (Tanzania), Luangwa Valley (Zambia), Etosha National Park (Namibia), Kgalagadi Transfrontier Park (Botswana and South Africa) and Vaalbos and Kruger National Parks (South Africa) (Ebedes, 1976; Turnbull et al., 1991; Hugh-Jones and de Vos, 2002). An anthrax-like disease has been found in wild primates living in tropical rainforests, a habitat not previously known to harbour *B. anthracis* (Leendertz et al., 2004) and characterised by an unusually high number of sudden deaths observed over nine months in three communities of wild chimpanzees *(Pan troglodytes resus)* in the Tai National Park, Ivory Coast. However, *Bacillus* strains associated with this outbreak were toxigenic *B. cereus* and not typical *B. anthracis*.

6. Receptive animals

Under natural conditions the animals that are more susceptible to anthrax are ruminants, both domestic (cattle, buffalo, sheep, goats, camels, etc.) and wild (deer, roe deer, elephant, etc.). Horses are also receptive and pigs to a lesser extent.

Horses in natural conditions are less receptive to anthrax than cattle when the infection is transmitted via food, probably because they are monogastric and the spores ingested with food are quickly neutralised by the acid chloride present in the stomach. In cattle, however, before arriving in the stomach the spores make a long trip and this favours their implantation. On the contrary in anthrax infection transmitted through the skin, horses seem to be more sensitive because in the past, when the Pasteur vaccines were used, vaccination accidents were more frequent in the horse compared to ruminants. In anthrax outbreaks, because of the activity of biting flies, the value of horses affected/horse population is higher than the value of ruminants affected/ruminant population.

Carnivores are sick only exceptionally while birds are refractory.

Humans contract the infection almost always from infected products of animal origin.

7. Transmission

Anthrax ordinarily is a disease characterised by indirect transmission by means of materials (feed, straw, water, etc.) that have been polluted with spores.

As for the great resistance of the spores, polluting materials retain their infectivity for several years. It follows that in the pastures where dead animals or their residues have been abandoned the spores are durable and new infections happen when other animals graze or eat forages coming from these fields (telluric origin).

However, if the carcass was buried at shallow depth, the spores of anthrax can easily be brought to the surface of the ground thanks to an elevation of the waterbed and by movement of the earth due to the activity of earthworms and snails.

Another danger of infection is given to waste waters of tanneries where skins of infected animals are worked. This water often ends up in the irrigation canals and when the water flows out very slowly (e.g. stagnant) it leaves anthrax spores and other material on the vegetation. The import of food, wool, bristles, etc. from high risk anthrax areas are frequently the cause of the spread of infection. The infection can also be spread by animals, being naturally resistant to infection, that distribute anthrax spores in the faeces ingested with the food. Additionally, in cases of carnivores (dogs, foxes, vultures) that eat infected meat, outbreaks of anthrax have spread to distant points.

Laboratory studies have shown, using mouse and guinea pig models, that stable flies *Stomoxys calcitrans* and *Aedes aegypti and Aedes taeniorhyncus* mosquitoes are able to transmit the infection. The percentage of transmission is very low (about 17% in the flies and 12% in the mosquitoes), but it is suspected that when the insect population density is high, they could be an important vehicle in the spread of the disease (Turell and Knudson, 1987). The role of tabanid *Haematobia irritans* in the spread of the disease was confirmed in two old scientific papers (Mitzmain, 1914; Morris, 1918). Recently Blackburn et al. (2010) isolated *B. anthracis* from flesh-eating flies and demonstrated the importance of these kinds of insects with a wildlife anthrax outbreak in North America and the potential role in anthrax epizootics. Moreover, the hypothesis that blood-sucking insects such as tabanids (gadflies or horse-flies) can play an important role in spreading diseases among livestock and other animals is widely accepted (Krinsky, 1976) (fig. 3).

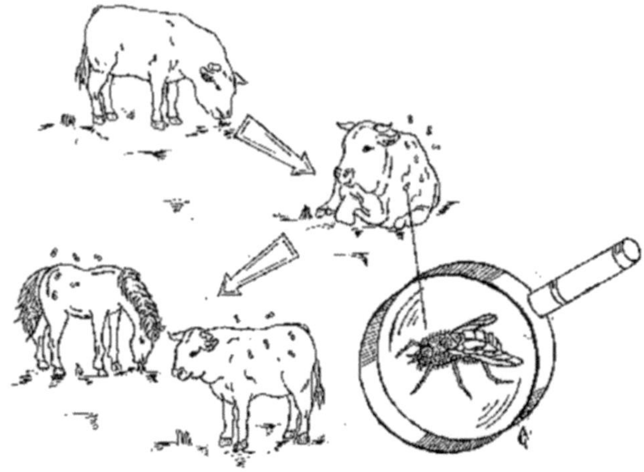

Fig. 3. Circulation of anthrax by means of horseflies (drawing by Gabriella Abbatangelo)

Anthrax human infection is rare in developed countries. However, recent outbreaks in the US and Europe, and potential use of the bacteria for bioterrorism have focused interest on it. Furthermore, while anthrax was known to typically occur as one of three syndromes related to the site of entry (i.e. cutaneous, gastrointestinal or inhalational), a fourth syndrome including severe soft tissue infection in injectional drug users is emerging. However, the 2010 anthrax epidemic in Bangladesh, where 607 associated human cases were registered from contact with contaminated meat from sick livestock, underlined that anthrax has the potential to be a serious zoonotic disease in low income countries where there are few resources for an optimal infectious diseases control system in humans or livestock. It underscored the high risk to humans when exposed to infected animals through slaughtering and butchering.

8. Pathogenesis

The most common way of penetration by spores is via the digestive system after the ingestion of spore contaminated feed, forages and water. The ports of entry are micro-wounds that can be found in the mucous membranes of the mouth, pharynx and along the entire gastrointestinal tract. The infection can also occur through skin abrasions or skin lesions that may be caused by haematophagous insects (e.g. biting flies) acting as passive carriers or biological vectors. Although less frequent, spread is possible through the inhalation of dust containing spores. The severity of the disease depends on the sensitivity of the host, on the infectious dose and on the route of penetration. Regardless of the route of penetration, it is considered that the spores of *B. anthracis* are carried by macrophages from the initial site of entry to the draining lymph nodes. The spores germinate, giving rise to vegetative forms that are capable of producing the main virulence factors: toxins and capsule.

Whatever the route of infection, it is believed that *B. anthracis* spores are transported by macrophages from the original site of introduction to draining lymph nodes and then enter the blood stream where they continue to rapidly multiply. The pathogenicity of *B. anthracis* depends on the quality of the capsular coat and the amounts of toxins produced (Coker et al., 2003; Shoop et al., 2005) and on the sensitivity of the host species (Smith, 1973). In Fischer 344 rats, the injection of the toxin causes death in about 30 minutes and a severe pulmonary oedema can be seen. Rabbits experimentally infected with *B. anthracis* show respiratory symptomatology due to the intense action of the oedematous toxin on the lung. The leakage of blood from the nose is always just before or just after the death of the animal (personal observations).

9. Anthrax in animals

The incubation period of the disease under natural conditions varies from one to 14 days, but usually three to five days.

9.1 Ruminants

In cattle, the symptom picture is quite variable. Some animals suddenly fall down and die in few minutes, without having presented any symptoms (fig. 4). Other times the death occurs after one to two days (rarely three to five) and the disease is characterised by the following symptoms: rapid pulse and respirations, anorexia, decrease or cessation of milk secretion, cyanotic mucous membranes, colic, outflow bleeding from the body's natural openings and oedematous swelling under the skin (especially in the neck, chest and belly).

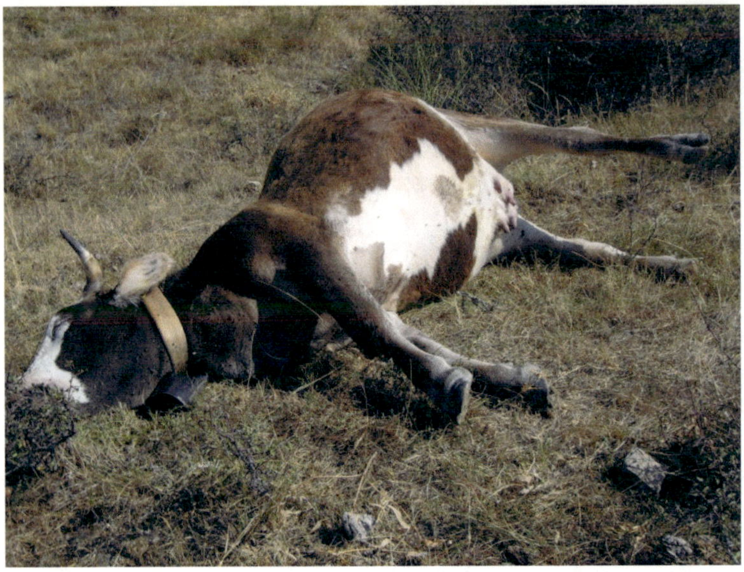

Fig. 4. Hyperacute form of anthrax in cattle

These events are always accompanied by high fever (41°C and beyond) that tends to settle very early. In farms with active outbreaks it is possible detect the sick animals by measuring body temperature before clinical symptoms appear. In sheep and goats most of the time evolution is hyperacute. The animals are suddenly struck by dizziness, staggering, falling to the ground and die in a few minutes with leakage of blood from the body's natural openings.

In ruminants the disease is characterised by splenomegaly, bleeding and diffuse oedema predominantly in the connective tissues (Marcato, 1981). The carcass rapidly decomposes and swells (de Vos, 1994); *rigor mortis* is incomplete and blood is dark red, uncoagulable and sometimes extravasates via natural openings (nostrils, mouth, anus, vulva). The blood clots are gelatinous because the normal blood coagulation processes are altered. This is accompanied by cyanosis and apparent mucosal bleeding, a gelatinous infiltration of the subcutaneous connective tissue and congestion of the serosa, often with haemorrhagic petechiae (Contini, 1995), which collect a blood coloured liquid, particularly in the peritoneum, pleura and pericardium. But haemorrhages can be found throughout the internal organs. Sometimes small quantities of serum sweat from tissues of the neck and inguinal regions (Marcato, 1981). There may also be blood mixed with urine in the bladder (Contini, 1995). The organ with the greatest changes is the spleen (de Vos, 1994), which has congestive-haemorrhagic tumefactions in the red pulp as a result of septicaemia. There is a significant increase in the volume of this organ and the capsule tense; on dissection, the pulp is red and black, and the white pulp hard to see (Marcato, 1981). Splenomegaly, however, is inconstant. The lesions may also affect the intestine; the internal mucosa is hyperaemic and full of punctiform haemorrhages. There are round tumefactions in the lymphoid tissue of the Peyer plaques that are haemorrhagic-necrotic and ulcerative. The lesions can extend to the mesentery. Haemorrhage and oedema may be found in relation to the pharynx, larynx and lungs (Contini, 1995). Sometimes there are cases of cutaneous oedema because of local infections (Marcato, 1981). Sheep are less resistant than cattle and therefore for them the disease develops faster.

9.2 Equines

The clinical manifestations and the course of the disease are almost always of an acute form with death occurring in two to three days. The disease develops with colic syndrome and septicaemia associated with muscle tremors, sensory depression, a very high fever, cyanosis, tachypnoea and tachycardia. In horses, anthrax involves oedematous subcutaneous swelling of the neck, shoulders, chest, abdomen and perineum (Sterne, 1959). The cutaneous oedema suggests a cutaneous reaction to bites from contaminated horseflies. When there is an infection of the pharynx or intestine from contaminated feed or forage there is often a diffuse haemorrhagic ulcerative enteritis. The regional lymph nodes are red and swollen with yellowish areas of necrosis. Splenic lesions will be absent if the animal dies as a result of local reaction, without septicaemia.

9.3 Pigs

This species is more resistant and the disease is usually subclinical (Smith, 1973). It manifests as a localised swelling in the pharynx - the so-called "anthrax angina" - or in the intestine. There may be a profuse diarrhoea after an intestinal infection. When the lesions are severe, death occurs within three to seven days. It seems that the nature of the contaminated feed can play an important role since a fibrous abrasive feed can kill while the same spore dose in a soft feed will pass through the pig without apparent harm (Ferguson, 1981). With pigs, the primary lesions are located in the pharynx and intestine as a result of the ingestion of infected meat leading to the formation of the "anthrax angina". There is a haemorrhagic oedematous swelling of the mucosa and sub-mucosa of the pharynx and glottis, of peripharyngial tissues, and of the subcutaneous connective tissue of the throat and neck (Henning, 1956). It is characterised by diphtheric membranes on the surface and deep, haemorrhagic, necrotic, grey-yellowish grey-brownish processes (Marcato, 1981). The regional lymph nodes - sublingual, retropharyngeal, sub-parotid - increase to several times their normal size. They are coloured dark red because of the adenopathy from the oedema, the iperemia, the haemorrhage and secondary necrosis (Ferguson, 1981). Anthrax pustules may form in the intestines and be localised or diffuse, with haemorrhagic areas of inflammation affecting the wall of the intestine and corresponding mesentery. Only the mesenteric lymph nodes may be affected (Henning, 1956).

9.4 Carnivores

These animals are fairly resistant, but if affected, they show signs of acute gastroenteritis and oro-pharyngitis due to ingestion of large volumes of infected meat. Usually it heals spontaneously.

10. Anthrax in humans

10.1 Cutaneous form

More than 95% of all naturally occurring *B. anthracis* infections worldwide are cutaneous. This form of anthrax is associated with the handling of infected animals or contaminated items such as meat, wool, hides, leather or hair products from infected animals (Lucey, 2005). The majority of cutaneous anthrax lesions develop in exposed areas such as the face, neck, arms and hands. The lesion begins as a small, often pruritic papule that quickly enlarges and develops a central vesicle or bulla, which ruptures or erodes, leaving an underlying necrotic ulcer. Another characteristic that is firmly adherent is black eschar developing over the surface of the ulcer, however, the risk for person-to-person transmission of cutaneous anthrax is very low (Heyworth et al., 1975). The incubation period for cutaneous disease is reported to be five to seven days (range: one to 12 days) (Carucci, 2002). However, during the 1979 Sverdlovsk outbreak, cutaneous cases reportedly developed over up to 13 days after the aerosol release of spores (Meselsen et al., 1994) and an outbreak in Algeria was reported with a median incubation period of 19 days (Abdenour et al., 1987).

10.2 Gastrointestinal form

Gastrointestinal anthrax typically occurs after eating raw or undercooked contaminated meat, although spores consumed through any route, including spores that are inhaled and subsequently swallowed, can result in gastrointestinal anthrax. The intestinal form develops when spores infect the gastrointestinal tract epithelium after consumption of undercooked, contaminated meat. Signs and symptoms range from subclinical gastrointestinal disturbances to clinical illness with nausea and vomiting, fever, anorexia and abdominal pain and tenderness, and can progress to haematemesis and bloody diarrhoea. Abdominal distension with voluminous, haemorrhagic ascites might be present. The disease might progress to septicaemia and toxaemia, cyanosis, shock and death (the incubation period for gastrointestinal disease is estimated to be one to six days; the case-fatality ratio is unknown, but is estimated to range from 25% to 60% (Sirisanthana & Brown, 2002; Kanafani et al., 2003; Ndybahinduka et al., 1984; Beatty et al., 2003).

10.3 Pulmonary form

Inhalation anthrax is a systemic infection caused by inhalation of *B. anthracis* spores. This form of the disease results from the inhalation of aerosolised *B. anthracis* spore-containing particles that are ≤5 microns (Druett et al., 1953). Spore-containing aerosols can be generated through industrial processing or work with spore-contaminated animal products such as wool, hair or hides; by laboratory procedures such as vortexing of cultures or as a result of the intentional release of aerosolised spores. Early studies of inhalation anthrax demonstrated that inhaled spores are phagocytosed by macrophages in the lungs and transported to the pulmonary-associated lymph nodes where germination and vegetative growth occur, followed by bacteraemia and dissemination to the rest of the body (Lyncoln et al., 1964; Henderson et al., 1956; Ross, 1957). Initial signs and symptoms of inhalation anthrax are non-specific and might include sore throat, mild fever and muscle aches; these symptoms might initially be mistaken for an upper respiratory infection (Temte & Zinkel, 2004; Lucey, 2005). Approximately two to three days later, infected patients generally become progressively ill as respiratory symptoms develop, including severe dyspnoea and hypoxaemia and the disease progresses with development of hypotension, diaphoresis, worsening dyspnoea, shock, cyanosis and stridor (Holty et al., 2006). Chest radiography often reveals the characteristic widened mediastinum (Jernigan et al., 2001; Lucey, 2005).

Case-fatality ratios of 86% and 89% were reported after the 1979 Sverdlosk outbreak in the former Soviet Union and in the United States during in the 20th century, respectively (Meselsen et al., 1994; Brachman, 1980; Brachman & Fridlander, 1994). During the bioterrorism events of 2001, the case-fatality ratio for patients with inhalation anthrax treated in intensive care units was 45% (five of 11 cases) (Jernigan et al., 2002).

10.4 Bacteraemic dissemination and meningitis

After infection at the primary cutaneous, gastrointestinal or inhalation site, lymphatic and haematogenous proliferation of anthrax bacilli can result in dissemination to other organs and organ systems (i.e. systemic anthrax). Massive septicaemia with 107 to 108 bacteria per millilitre of blood and toxaemia can develop, systemic effects, including high fever and shock, develop quickly and death usually follows rapidly (Dixon et al., 1999). Anthrax meningitis has been reported with all three clinical forms of anthrax and likely results from haematogenous spread across the blood-brain barrier, generally presenting as haemorrhagic meningitis. Anthrax meningitis is characterised by a fulminant, rapidly progressive clinical course; even with aggressive therapy, cases are usually fatal (Lanska, 2002; Sejvar et al., 2005). The likelihood of the development of clinical or subclinical meningitis in patients with severe systemic *B. anthracis* infections is high. In rare cases, anthrax meningitis has been reported without any other associated primary (i.e. cutaneous, gastrointestinal or inhalation) manifestation of anthrax (Lanska, 2002; Sejvar et al., 2005). A review of 82 cases of inhalation anthrax that occurred during 1900--2005 included 70 fatal cases. Among the 70 patients who died, 11 of 61 patients for whom data were available, had signs of meningeal involvement, compared with none of 12 patients who survived; 44 of the 70 patients who died developed meningoencephalitis during the course of their disease, compared with none of the 12 patients who survived. Development of meningoencephalitis during the course of the disease was found to be significantly associated with death ($p = 0.003$) (Holty et al., 2006). Studies in non-human primates have demonstrated meningeal involvement in 33%--77% of experimental inhalation anthrax cases (Friedlander et al., 1993; Gleiser et al., 1963; Fritz et al., 1995; Vasconcelos et al., 2003).

10.5 Anthrax in drug users

A new form of anthrax was observed in drug users in Scotland in December 2009 and similar cases were seen in England during 2010. Drug users may become infected with anthrax when heroin has become contaminated with anthrax spores. This could be a source of infection if injected, smoked or snorted. Patients have not presented with classic anthrax (cutaneous, inhalational or gastrointestinal) but represented a new pattern. The clinical presentation may vary.

The patients that developed intracranial or subarachnoid haemorrhage with anthrax bacilli in their blood died rapidly—i.e. in the late stages of disseminated anthrax. Gastrointestinal symptoms occasionally predominated, probably reflecting disseminated disease. Most have presented as atypical, but severe, soft tissue infections, with significant soft-tissue oedema (one inducing compartment syndrome). Findings differ from classic necrotising fasciitis or classic cutaneous anthrax and can present as variants of cellulitis or abscess. Patients can present with vague prodromal symptoms or excessive bruising at the index injection site, which may be difficult to identify. Despite appearing very unwell, with tachycardic and peripherally shut down, they maintain an almost normal blood pressure, respiratory function, oxygenation and acid-base, and are lucid. Systemic features might otherwise be non-specific. Haematology and biochemistry are also non-specific; typically the white-cell count, C-reactive protein and lactate are not grossly abnormal. A decline in platelet count may predict clinical deterioration, even if remaining within the normal range. Coagulopathy may develop, with significant bleeding. In cases of severe soft tissue infection, fluid requirements may exceed 10 L per 24 h. Surgical debridement removes the nidus of infection and provides diagnostic material (Gram stain, culture and PCR). Characteristic surgical features include profound capillary bleeding, necrosis of predominantly the superficial rather than deep fat, oedema not fasciolysis and the finding of needle tracks containing necrotic material (Booth, et al., 2010).

11. Diagnosis

Suspicion of anthrax arises from the observation of clinical symptoms, the anatomic-pathological findings and epidemiological data. The ecology of the bacterium limits the distribution of the disease that is almost always confined to well-defined territories. Less frequent and certainly more dangerous are introductive events that affect animals living in fixed stalling and which contract anthrax by eating contaminated food (usually forages) coming from high risk areas. This can, and does, happen in areas normally deemed free of anthrax and commonly in winter when livestock need extra feed which will have been purchased and may be contaminated. Thus, despite a careful epidemiological analysis, this can lead health professionals to misdiagnose suspect cases and, consequently, the subsequent inappropriate management of infected carcasses that leads to an inevitable increase in the risk of infection in humans and other livestock (Kreidl et al., 2006).

11.1 Differential diagnosis

In cattle, anthrax should be differentiated from the following diseases:

- lightning strike and accidental electrocutions,
- pasteurellosis,
- piroplasmosis ,
- blackleg, malignant oedema and other clostridial diseases,
- food intoxications.

However, we should consider any disease causing sudden death or haemorrhagic septicaemia. In horses, we should consider colic syndromes, because of their symptomatology and infectious anaemia and dourine, because of the oedemas. However, in infectious anaemia, sublingual haemorrhages can be found.

11.2 Laboratory diagnosis

When there is suspicion that an animal has died of anthrax it is important to take precautions to avoid both infection and the shedding of blood that could pollute the surrounding environment. Live animals' blood can be collected from main superficial veins; while with dead animals it can be taken from the peripheral veins, such as in the ear after removal of the auricle with a hot knife; in this way the wound is cauterised and we prevent the spilling of blood and ground contamination with spores. The blood can be either on a cotton swab or in a vacutainer; the former is better. When using a cotton swab the blood should be allowed to dry, killing the contaminants and encouraging any *B. anthracis* to sporulate. Putrefaction quickly destroys vegetative *B. anthracis* and in this case it is much better to make a swab from nasal turbinates which are well vasculated and therefore should, and do, have plenty of spores, but with minimal tissue are little affected by putrefaction. If the carcass is too dehydrated, which can present diagnostic problems, one can collect soil from the ground under the animal that may have been contaminated by the leakage of blood and other body fluids from the natural openings and seepage. It should be noted that the longer an animal has been dead the smaller is the probability of getting a positive diagnosis, even with an experienced diagnostic laboratory.

11.3 Microscopic test

A preliminary examination with an unstained fresh blood smear will highlight the presence of stick forms or typical "*bamboo canes*". The organisms are immobile and well capsulated. The slide may be fixed and stained with Gram stain when *B. anthracis* is coloured in violet. Preferably one can use Giemsa which colours the bacilli purple and the capsule a characteristic red mauve or with MacFadyean stain, which is blue methyl polychromatic and stains the capsule pink. Löffler uses methylene blue to which K_2CO_3 to 1% has been added (Turnbull, 1998). This with *Bacillus anthracis* leads to the metachromatic phenomenon with the bacterial bodies stained blue, while the capsule takes on a reddish colour. In the preparation of the slide one must take care to pass the slide several times over the flame because the usual methods of fixing colours do not inactivate the spores, which can represent a significant danger to the staff who will handle these microscopic preparations (personal observation). Anecdotally there are stories of students getting cutaneous lesions from handling sharp-edged broken blood smear slides that were decades old.

11.4 Cultural test

Bacillus anthracis grows easily on normal agars, whether liquid or solid media. Using a sterile loop the plates can be sown with material from samples of blood, exudates, oedematous infiltrations, organs or parts of them taken from infected or suspect animals. When one suspects the presence of spores in the material used in the sample (wool, hair, leather, environmental samples) it is necessary to first incubate the material 72°C for 30 minutes to destroy contaminating bacteria, yeasts and moulds. It is always better to use a semi-selective medium to isolate the bacterium. Moreover, blood-containing media are preferable in comparison to the often-used PLET or a Knisly agar, such as TSPB Agar, which is made highly selective against Gram-negative bacteria by supplementation with trimethoprim (13.1 mg/L), sulfamethoxazole (20 mg/L) and polymyxin B (30000 IU/L) (Tomaso et al., 2006). The plates are then incubated at 37°C for 24 hours. If the bacterium is present in the materials collected, white colonies will develop, 2-5 mm in diameter, of a pasty consistency and non-haemolytic. At a small magnification one can see long filaments folded several times on their own that seem to have the appearance of the foliage of a jellyfish, the so-called Medusa's Head.

11.5 Biological test

It is usual with this kind of test to use particularly sensitive laboratory animals such as guinea pigs. The inoculation of suspect material subcutaneously or intramuscularly is not recommended, especially when the inoculate is full of secondary putrefactive bacteria. It is better to set up a test infection by coating the material on an area of abdominal skin which has been previously shaved and scarified. This technique takes advantage of the ability of *B. anthracis* to penetrate scarified skin, selecting it from the mixed microbial flora. Rabbits die within 72 to 166 hours (Fasanella et al., 2009) and this depends on the virulence of the different strains of anthrax and the number of organisms. However, after a few hours a gelatinous, haemorrhagic oedema forms at the point of inoculation, which is then followed by all the other characteristics of an anthrax lesion.

11.6 Polymerase Chain Reaction (PCR)

To confirm suspicious colonies specific PCR represent the best method to identify *Bacillus anthracis*. To identify virulent *B. anthracis* strains, and for the differentiation of non-virulent strains, the presence of both of the plasmids pXO1 (toxins) and pXO2 (capsule formation) must be confirmed. However, some chromosomal targets of rpoB, S-layer protein genes and Ba813 very often lead to false-positive results from environmental samples (Papaparaskevas et al., 2004), while *plcR* is able to differentiate *Bacillus anthracis* from *Bacillus cereus* and *Bacillus thuringiensis* (Easterday et al., 2005).

11.7 Molecular characterisation

The genomic diversity is the result mainly of events in the evolution of the bacterium and the genomic analysis must rely on molecular markers as polymorphic as possible with a high rate of mutation. The anthrax genotyping methods currently in use test different types of markers in relation to the utility of the analysis.

The genotyping method, considered to be at low resolution, is the analysis of SNPs (Single Nucleotide Polymorfisms) and identifies point mutations of the genome. These markers have a good stability with a genomic mutation rate of 10^{-10}. While there is a low rate of mutation some 35,000 SNPs comprise the entire genome of anthrax (Pearson et al., 2004; Read et al., 2002). At present the opportunity to test all the identified SNPs in any isolate is technically hard and financially expensive. However, some studies have helped identify 12 canonical SNPs that are the most stable and homoplastic which can be used for phylogenetic investigations. Polymorphism analyses may be carried out using Snapshot or with real time PCR assays with TaqMan MGB probes (Van Ert et al., 2007).

The high resolution typing assay par excellence is that of Multiple Locus VNTR Analysis (MLVA) as it seeks to identify specific genomic regions known as Variable Number Tandem Repeat (VNTR). These regions of repeated DNA in tandem by their nature have a higher rate of mutation. The frequency of mutation of these markers in *B. anthracis* is comparable to 10^{-5} with a high variability depending on the locus (Keim et al., 2004). This technique initially with eight VNTR was able to identify 89 genotypes from 400 isolates from around the world (Keim et al., 2000), while the 15 VNTR assay increased this to 221 genotypes with 1033 isolates. This method has now been increased up to 25 loci (Lista et al., 2006), which allows an excellent organism discrimination with this high genetic homology. Technically, the VNTR are searched for using capillary sequencers to analyse DNA fragments.

Latterly, high resolution assays were discovered that examine markers called SNRs (Single Nucleotide Repeats), a sort of VNTR consisting of repeated sequences of poliA. Stratilo et al. (2006), through a bioinformatics analysis, identified specific regions with a mutation rate of 10^{-4}. Utilisation of these regions allows discrimination between organisms with the same MLVA pattern and thus allows sub-genotyping. The instability of these loci does not make them homoplastic because back-mutations often occur. Their use can differentiate strains within the same outbreak or epidemic. A recent study has suggested the use of a panel of four SNR markers that may be discriminated with an advanced method of analysis of DNA fragments (Kenefic et al., 2008).

These briefly described genotyping methods can be understood in a hierarchical way. The SNPs being at low-power of discrimination can be used for phylogenetic investigations. On the other hand, VNTRs and SNRs have high discriminatory powers. The first for their high diversity and homoplasia are able to correctly define genotype, while the latter, searching for any signs of redundancy, are considered suitable for identifying sub-genotypes. All the methods described are best run by specialised laboratories experienced in molecular biology (Keim et al., 2004).

12. Anthrax vaccines and their mechanism of protection

Toxin formation is known to occur when PA binds to receptors on cells (Little et al., 2004; Bradley et al., 2001), undergoes proteolysis which exposes a binding site for LF or EF and forms heptamers (Milne et al., 1994). The shared cell-binding component, PA, when combined with LF, forms a lethal toxin, which kills laboratory animals (Beall & Dallford, 1966; Stanley & Smith, 1961) and is cytotoxic to certain macrophage cell lines (Friedlander, 1986). When combined with EF, on the other hand, PA forms an oedema toxin, which causes oedema and inhibits neutrophil functions (O'Brien et al., 1985) due to the calmodulin-dependent adenylate cyclase activity of EF. Clearly, then, blocking PA leads to the neutralisation of the toxic activity of anthrax. Indeed, protection of certain animal models (guinea pig, rabbit, non-human primate) against infection with *B. anthracis* can be achieved by inoculation with a variety of vaccine preparations that contain PA as their main immunogen (Ivins et al., 1990; Ivins et al., 1992; Ivins et al., 1998). Moreover, a strong correlation has been found between the level of PA-specific toxin-neutralising antibodies (TNA) and protection.

Toxin neutralisation is probably not the only antibody-mediated mechanism of protection. The kinetics of PA production during *B. anthracis* growth and the role of anti-PA antibody in host immunity are not clearly defined, however. Recently, anti-PA antibodies (Abs) have also been shown to exhibit anti-spore activities. Rabbit anti-rPA polyclonal Abs (pAbs) were shown to enhance the phagocytosis and subsequent killing of spores by macrophages, and to partially inhibit spore germination in vitro. Further, PA was found to be associated with spores and to induce anti-PA Abs which retard germination in vitro, and enhance the phagocytic and sporicidal activities of macrophages (Cote et al., 2005; Welkos et al., 2001; Stepanov et al., 1996; Welkos et al., 2002).

An important aspect of the protective ability of the immune system is the persistence of PA-specific IgG memory B cells allowing animals to remain resistant to infection even after their serum Ab response has waned. In a study on mice, for example, half of the animals immunised with CpG-adjuvanted AVA (Synthetic Oligodeoxynucleotides containing Unmethylated CpG motifs to AVA) with anti-PA titers 10-fold below the protective baseline, survived a 100 LD_{50} Sterne strain spore challenge. This contrasted with only 1/35 mice with the same Ab titer that had been immunised with AVA alone. These findings suggest that an important goal of anthrax vaccine development should be that of attaining a vaccine able to generate a durable pool of high-affinity memory B cells (Tross & Klinman, 2008; Ivins et al., 1994).

Another important aspect of immunity is with regard to T cells which may play a role beyond simply enhancing adaptive humoral response. Immunisation with formaldehyde-inactivated *B. anthracis* spores resulted in the generation of CD4 T lymphocytes, which responded in an MHC-restricted manner by producing interferon γ (IFNγ) (Glomski et al., 2007). This suggested that the production of IFNγ leads to the activation of phagocytes and consequently increases sporicidal and bactericidal activity. IFN was shown to protect up to 60% of mice against lethal inhalational anthrax (Walberg et al., 2008). Finally, nasal (i.n.) immunisation of deeply anesthetised rabbits with rPA+IL-1α consistently induced rPA-specific serum IgG ELISA titers that were not significantly different than those induced by intramuscular (IM) immunisation with rPA+alum, although lethal toxin-neutralising titers induced by nasal immunisation were lower than those induced by IM immunisation (Gwinn et al., 2010).

12.1 First generation of anthrax vaccine for human use

The observation that the injection of sterilised oedema fluid from anthrax lesions in laboratory animals protected against challenge with a fully virulent strain, suggested that the acellular vaccine can protect against anthrax. Investigations followed on the protective role of artificially cultivated *B. anthracis* filtrates as vaccines for human use. The first US product was developed in 1954. It was a cell-free filtrate from an aerobic culture of the Vollum strain of *Bacillus anthracis*, precipitated with aluminium potassium sulphate. In the 1960s, the strain used was changed from Vollum to V770-NP1-R, a toxigenic, non-capsulated and non-proteolytic mutant (Puzzis et al., 1963) and the microaerophilic culture method adopted. A significant increase in the stability and immunogenicity of the vaccine was obtained as a result. This vaccine, named Anthrax Vaccine Adsorbed (AVA), was licensed by the NIH in 1970 and reapproved by the FDA in 1985. In December 2008, the FDA approved a biologics licence application supplement for AVA, submitted by Emergent BioSolutions. The current licensed schedule consists of five of 0,5 ml intramuscular injections (at zero and four weeks, and at six, 12 and 18 months) followed by yearly 0,5-ml booster doses. Intramuscular injection causes fewer local reactions, but it entails a reduction in anti-PA antibody response from week eight to six months after vaccination, during which protection may also be reduced (Wright et al., 2009).

The Anthrax Vaccine Precipitated (AVP) was licensed in Great Britain in 1979. It was developed by the Centre for Applied Microbiology and Research at Porton Down, Salisbury, using an avirulent toxigenic, non-capsulated 34F2 strain of *B. anthracis* originally isolated by Sterne in 1937. It contains PA, LF and EF. The main indication for using the vaccine is risk of infection by inhalation of *B. anthracis* spores.

The AVP vaccine is administered in a three-dose primary regimen three weeks apart, followed by the fourth dose after six months and annual booster doses. The main active component of the vaccine is a sterile filtrate of alum-precipitated *B. anthracis* antigens in solution for injection. Other ingredients are aluminium potassium sulphate, sodium chloride and purified water. The preservative is thimerosal (0.005%). Immunisation by the vaccine induces production of IgG antibodies, which guarantees good immunogenicity. No serious side effects have been reported. Reactions are uncommon, but occasionally a mild rash or swelling at the site of injection, or even at the site of an earlier injection, may occur and last for a couple of days. More rarely, swollen glands, mild fever, flu-like symptoms, a rash, itching or other allergic reactions may occur (Baillie, 2009; Friedlander & Little, 2009; Splino et al., 2005).

Compared to AVA, the British AVP contains lower levels of PA and higher concentrations of additional *B. anthracis* antigens, such as LF and EF, and certain bacillus surface proteins (Turnbull, 1991; Baillie et al., 2003). These differences, owing to the strain used and/or to vaccine preparation techniques, may be the cause of the slightly enhanced protection conferred by AVP (Baillie et al., 2004) and of the increased transient reactogenicity seen in comparison to AVA (Turnbull, 2000). First-generation vaccines are, thus, relatively safe and efficacious, but they do present a number of important limitations, making them less than ideal for urgent mass vaccinations or for use in non-industrialised or remote regions.

12.2 Second generation of anthrax vaccine for human use

12.2.1 PA vaccines

Several high-level PA expression systems have been developed based on a variety of microbial and eukaryotic organisms such as attenuated strains of *B. anthracis, B.subtilis, B. brevis, Baculovirus, Escherichia coli* (Baillie, 2006).

rPA102 (formerly produced by Vaxgen Inc., South San Francisco, California, later acquired by Emergent BioSolutions, Maryland) is a purified protein obtained from culture supernatant of *B. anthracis* ΔSterne-1, an asporogenic, avirulent, non-toxigenic strain, which contains a recombinant plasmid encoding PA. PA is adsorbed in aluminium hydroxide adjuvant with a final aluminium concentration of approximately 82.5 μg per dose. This vaccine protected rabbits and non-human primates from inhalational challenge and was found to be safe and immunogenic in a randomised trial performed on healthy volunteers (Gorse et al., 2006). SparVax, an rPA vaccine obtained from *E. coli* (Baillie, 2009) and manufactured by Pharmathene in the US, is undergoing US National Institute of Health-sponsored human safety and immunogenicity trials. SparVax was developed by researchers at the Defence Science and Technology Laboratory, Porton Down, Wiltshire UK.

In preclinical studies, SparVax has demonstrated the capability to protect rabbits and non-human primates against a lethal aerosol spore challenge of the anthrax Ames strain.

A recently published report described a phase I clinical trial testing the safety and immunogenicity of an anthrax vaccine using *Escherichia coli*-derived, *B. anthracis* rPA. Sixty seven healthy adults received two injections, four weeks apart, of either rPA in increasing doses (5, 25, 50, 100 μg), formulated with or without 704 μg/ml Alhydrogel adjuvant, or buffered saline placebo. Participants were followed for one year. No serious adverse events were recorded. The most robust humoral immune responses were observed in subjects receiving 50 µg of rPA formulated with Alhydrogel, while the strongest cellular response was observed in the group receiving 25 µg Alhydrogel-formulated rPA. The vaccine was safe, well tolerated and stimulated a robust humoral and cellular response after two doses (Brown et al., 2010).

12.3 Third generation of anthrax vaccine for human use

12.3.1 Epitope–specific vaccines

The efficacy of PA domain was demonstrated in mice: all animals immunised with PA proteins containing domain 4 were fully protected against anthrax spore challenge while a decrease in protection was seen in mice immunised with a mutated strain of *B. anthracis* that expressed PA without domain 4 (Flick-Smith et al., 2002; Brossier et al., 2000).

12.3.2 Oral vaccines

Aloni-Grinstein et al. showed the efficacy of an attenuated non-toxigenic non-capsulated *B. anthracis* spore vaccine as an oral vaccine in guinea pigs (Aloni - Grinstein et al., 2005).

Another orally delivered vaccine for human use is that derived from *Salmonella enterica* serovar *Typhimurium*. Vaccines based on either full-length PA, PA domains 1 and 4 or PA domain 4 were tested on A/J mice. The study compared oral vaccines with rPA vaccines showing, for the first time, the efficacy of an oral *S. enterica*-based vaccine against an aerosolised *B. anthracis* challenge (Stokes et al., 2007; Baillie et al., 2008).

Orally administered *Lactobacillus gasseri* engineered to express the PA-DCpep fusion proteins was proven effective against anthrax Sterne challenge. This vaccine showed efficacious adjuvanticity and a safe delivery to mucosal immune cells, including dendritic cells. Both mucosal and systemic immune responses were elicited, resulting in complete animal survival (Mohamadzadeh et al., 2010).

12.3.3 Nasal vaccines

Rapid protective immunity has been achieved in mice through a combination of a nasal prime with a *S. Typhi* vaccine strain expressing PA, followed by a parenteral rPA boost. The same immunising strategy using a *S. enterica* serovar *Typhi*-derived PA83 fused with the export protein ClyA (ClyA-PA83) was also tested in rhesus and cynomolgus macaques. Monkeys developed high levels of serum TNA. Having been successful in non-human primates, this anthrax vaccine strategy based on heterologous mucosal immunisation followed by a parenteral vaccine booster is considered very interesting for human application (Mikszta et al., 2005).

12.3.4 DNA vaccines

A human serotype 5 adenovirus (ad5) expressing PA (AdsechPA) was tested and compared with the new US military rPA/Alhydrogel vaccine in a mouse model. AdsechPA afforded approximately 2.7-fold more protection than the rPA vaccine against *B. anthracis* lethal toxin challenge four weeks after a single intramuscular administration, suggesting the potential of this vaccine to protect the civilian population against *B. anthracis* in response to a bioterrorism attack (Tan et al., 2003). Chimeric virus-like particles (VLPs), which are very effective at eliciting humoral as well as cellular immunity, were also tested. VLPs complexed with PA elicited a powerful TNA response that protected rats from anthrax lethal toxin challenge after a single dose without adjuvant. This highly effective, dually-acting reagent can be used both for protection against anthrax and as post-infection treatment (Manayani et al., 2007).

12.4 Vaccine for veterinary use

The history and theory of anthrax vaccines for veterinary use are closely linked to the first developments of modern vaccinology science. Louis Pasteur, a pioneer in this field, developed the first anthrax vaccine in 1881 (Shlyakhy et al., 1996). His method was widely used for livestock immunisation until the 1930s. Pasteur's schedule consisted of a first inoculation of *B. anthracis* cells from cultures incubated at 42°- 43°C for 15-20 days (Pasteur type I) followed by an inoculation, after 14 days, of less attenuated *B. anthracis* cells from cultures incubated at 42°- 43°C for 10-12 days (Pasteur type II) (Turnbull, 1991).

The live attenuated vaccines for veterinary use can be divided into three main categories: Pasteur vaccines, Carbozoo vaccines and Sterne vaccines. The division is not merely historical, but based on different attenuation mechanisms (Hambleton et al., 1984) . The Pasteur method of attenuation results in the loss of the pXO1 plasmid that encodes the major virulence factors (PA, LF, EF), thus producing a non-toxigenic and capsulated (pXO1-,pXO2+) vaccine. The Sterne type is a *B. anthracis* strain lacking the pXO2 plasmid encoding the capsule. It is, therefore, toxigenic and non-capsulated (pXO1+,pXO2-), resulting in a non-virulent stable phenotype which still conserves the main antigen, anthrax toxins. The Carbozoo attenuation mechanism is still unknown, but studies on Carbosap demonstrated the presence of both plasmids (pXO1+ pXO2+) placing this strain in the category of toxigenic and capsulated, and suggesting different mechanisms of attenuation (Fasanella et al., 2001). At present, most veterinary vaccines are live attenuated vaccines, produced worldwide according to the requirements for anthrax spore vaccine (live- for veterinary use), the requirements for biological substances No. 13 (WHO, 1967), the manual for the production of anthrax and blackleg vaccines (FAO, 1991), the manual of diagnostic tests and vaccines for terrestrial animals (OIE, 2008) and the updated European Pharmacopoeia. The Sterne 34F2 strain is used worldwide, with the exception of Russia, China and Romania, where other, analogous toxigenic and non-capsulated strains are used. The formulation consists of about 10^7 spores suspended either in glycerin with saponin or in physiological solution with saponin. The effectiveness of this vaccine soon emerged, with a sharp reduction in outbreaks observed in South Africa during the period 1925-1941. Moreover, epidemiological data suggest that, in the past 50 years, vaccination has drastically reduced anthrax in industrialised countries where it is now considered rare.

New animal vaccines are sorely needed. First studies reporting the use of recombinant or edible vaccines for veterinary use have been conducted. These proved the efficacy of two experimental vaccines against *B. anthracis* for veterinary use: an rPA mutant vaccine and a trivalent vaccine (TV) composed of rPA, an inactive LF mutant (mLF-Y728A; E735A) and an inactive EF mutant (mEF-K346R), both emulsified with mineral oils. Although this was only a preliminary study on a rabbit model, the possibility of administering these vaccines with antibiotics to halt incubating infections or during an anthrax epidemic was underlined (Fasanella et al., 2008).

Preliminary attempts to generate transgenic PA-producing plants successfully explored the possibility of creating a safe and protective vaccine. The use of an edible vaccine would be useful for the vaccination of herbivores - both domesticated and feral. Anthrax control programmes would be improved above all in non-industrialised countries, where syringes and needles are normally in short supply.

For example, in the search for an alternative, less expensive method to produce PA, a transgenic tobacco chloroplast was developed, that expressed the 83 kDa immunogenic *B. anthracis* PA. Crude plant extracts contained up to 2.5 mg full length PA/g of fresh leaf tissue and this showed exceptional stability for several months in stored leaves or crude extracts . The recently demonstrated efficacy of plant-expressed domain 4 of *B. anthracis* PA opens new horizons for the mass vaccination of animals in areas where the risk of anthrax is high (Watson et al., 2004; Brodzik et al., 2005; Gorantala et al., 2011).

13. Conclusions

Anthrax is an infectious disease which is still widespread in many areas of the planet and its presence is recorded mainly in poor or developing countries where the lack of an efficient health system able to prevent or counteract health emergencies favours the spread of infections, which often tend to result in an epidemic form. The source of anthrax infection is animals and the controlling of the disease in animals reduces the risk of human infection. The vaccine is still the most effective means of control, but mass vaccinations are not always possible in underdeveloped areas, where in addition to the lack of infrastructure such as roads or passable roads, an information system on the real animal population to submit to the vaccine treatment is often absent. Programmes to combat zoonoses, and anthrax in particular, need to have a fruitful collaboration between health authorities and farmers who need to be active players in the programme and not passive spectators. The process of training and information of those active in agriculture on the real dangers of the infection is fundamental, envisaging the adoption of restrictive measures in the case of outbreaks and not penalising the fragile economy of the livestock sector. The recent epidemic in Bangladesh owes its spread to the fact that farmers, fearing economic losses linked to the deaths of their animals, slaughtered them during the illness or even in that pre-agonising phase to sell the meat at a reduced price to limit losses.

With regard to developed countries, except for the anthrax threat represented by its use as a bacteriological weapon or potential bioterrorist attacks and episodes in drug users, anthrax is a sporadic disease characterised by few outbreaks that tend to occur where infected animals were buried in the past or where collected waste from the leather industries was placed. More frequently are reported outbreaks that develop consequent to the introduction of contaminated feed.

In wild areas like natural parks or natural reservations, human control is not always efficacious and often the carcasses of dead animals are left undisturbed by scavengers. Since the carnivores are less susceptible to the disease compared to herbivores, they can ingest larger quantities of infected viscera and meat, but the vegetative cells do not survive passage through their acid stomachs; but if they have been eating older carcasses with spores they may spread spores in their faeces (Turnbull et al., 1989). In wild areas scavenger birds such as ravens (*Corpus corax*) and vultures (*various spp*), can contaminate pastures or small bodies of water far from the original outbreak. These events permit generation of a relevant amount of spores that spread in the environment. It seems that *B. anthracis* has found in wild areas its natural habitat that permits the completion of its cycle and the production of a sufficient amount of spores ensuring its survival.

The area located between agricultural and wild areas where generally human activity is limited to the exploitation of pastures represents the contact point between the wild and the agricultural world, the habitat where domestic and wild animals divide the same space and where the ecology systems tend to influence each other. The proximity to the sources of production of anthrax spores, that are located in the wild area, guarantees the standard level of contamination of soil, favouring the realisation of the events that cause the disease in the domestic animals that pasture on this area, in conclusion, the area where anthrax crosses the border of its habitat and shows its presence. Animals from areas free of anthrax placed in areas at risk would be much more receptive to the disease. The project for the reintroduction of deer in some nature reserves of Basilicata (South Italy) is facing major obstacles just because of the receptivity of this particular animal species to anthrax infection (Fasanella et al, 2007). We do not know if this is a form of sensibility related to animal species or related to a lack of natural antibodies, but it is certain they are subjects who come from ecosystems in which anthrax is not present. In nature there are no behaviours which are an end in themselves and every living being has evolved its own strategies, not only in terms of preservation of their species, but also in that of its ecosystem. So why not hypothesise that *Bacillus anthracis* returned to its protective role of the delicate balance of its ecosystem, protecting the animal species that are an integral part of that particular area from a possible risk of extinction, due to infectious diseases introduced by unknown animals from different environments.

In developed countries, where the disease is sporadic, anthrax can cause serious health problems when it develops outbreaks in areas considered free of the disease, because the real risk is that health authorities can intervene in a misdiagnosis and not take the necessary precautionary measures. In conclusion, we must begin to consider anthrax as a neglected disease and undertake all activities that tend to reduce the risk for humans related to the underestimation of the disease. It is necessary to continue in the research activity on new and more sensitive and rapid diagnostic tests, on the development of more effective vaccines for human and veterinary use, and also on the improvement of the information and training of health personnel responsible for the control of zoonoses.

14. Acknowledgements

Thanks to Gabriella Abbatangelo collaborating author in the drawing on anthrax cycle

15. References

[1] Abdenour, D.; Larouze, B.; Dalichaouche, M.; Aouati, M. (1987) Familial occurrence of anthrax in Eastern Algeria. *J Infect Dis*; 155:1083-4.

[2] Aloni-Grinstein, R.; Gat, O.; Altboum, Z.; Velan, B.; Cohen, S.; Shafferman, A. (2005) Oral spore vaccine based on live attenuated nontoxinogenic Bacillus anthracis expressing recombinant mutant protective antigen. *Infect Immun*; 73(7):4043-53.

[3] Baillie, L.; Hebdon, R.; Flick-Smith, H. Williamson D. (2003) Characterisation of the immune response to the UK human anthrax vaccine. *FEMS Immunol Med Microbiol;* 36(1-2):83-6.

[4] Baillie, L.; Townend, T.; Walker, N.; Eriksson, U.; Williamson, D. (2004) Characterization of the human immune response to the UK anthrax vaccine. *FEMS Immunol Med Microbiol;* 42(2):267-70.

[5] Baillie, LW. (2006) Past, imminent and future human medical countermeasures for anthrax. *J Appl Microbiol;* 101(3):594-606.

[6] Baillie, LW. (2009) Is new always better than old?: The development of human vaccines for anthrax. *Hum Vaccin;* 5(12):806-16.

[7] Baillie, LW.; Rodriguez, AL.; Moore, S.; Atkins, HS.; Feng, C.; Nataro, JP.; Pasetti, MF. (2008) Towards a human oral vaccine for anthrax: the utility of a Salmonella Typhi Ty21a-based prime-boost immunization strategy. *Vaccine;* 26(48):6083-91

[8] Beall, FA.; Dalldorf, FG. (1966) The pathogenesis of the lethal effect of anthrax toxin in the rat. *J Infect Dis;* 116(3):377-89.

[9] Beatty, ME.; Ashford, DA.; Griffin, PM.; Tauxe, RV.; Sobel, J. (2003) Gastrointestinal Anthrax: Review of the Literature. *Arch Intern Med;* 163:2527-2531.

[10] Blackburn, JK.; Curtis, A.; Hadfield, TL.; O'Shea, B.; Mitchell, MA.; Hugh-Jones, ME. (2010) Confirmation of Bacillus anthracis from flesh-eating flies collected during a West Texas anthrax season. *J Wildl Dis;* 46(3):918-22.

[11] Booth, MG.; Hood, J.; Brooks, TJ.; Hart, A. (2010) Anthrax infection in drug users. *Lancet;* 375(9723):1345-6.

[12] Boyden, ED.; Dietrich, WF. (2006) Nalp1b controls mouse macrophage susceptibility to anthrax lethal toxin. *Nat Genet;* 38:240-244.

[13] Brachman, P.; Friedlander, A. Anthrax. In: Plotkin S, Mortimer E, eds. Vaccines. Philadelphia, PA: WB Saunders; 1994:729--39.

[14] Brachman, PS. (1980) Inhalation anthrax. *Ann N Y Acad Sci;* 353:83-93.

[15] Bradley, KA.; Mogridge, J.; Mourez, M.; Collier, RJ.; Young, JA. (2001) Identification of the cellular receptor for anthrax toxin. *Nature;* 414(6860):225-9.

[16] Brodzik, R.; Bandurska, K.; Deka, D.; Golovkin, M.; Koprowski, H. (2005) Advances in alfalfa mosaic virus-mediated expression of anthrax antigen in planta. *Biochem Biophys Res Commun;* 338:717-22.

[17] Brossier, F.; Weber-Levy, M.; Mock, M.; Sirard, JC. (2000) Role of toxin functional domains in anthrax pathogenesis. *Infect Immun;* 68(4):1781-6.

[18] Brown, BK.; Cox, J.; Gillis, A.; VanCott, TC.; Marovich, M.; Milazzo, M.; Antonille, TS.; Wieczorek, L.; McKee, KT, Jr.; Metcalfe, K.; Mallory, RM.; Birx, D.; Polonis, VR.; Robb, ML. (2010) Phase I study of safety and immunogenicity of an Escherichia coli-derived recombinant protective antigen (rPA) vaccine to prevent anthrax in adults PLoS One; 5(11): e13849.

[19] Carucci, JA.; McGovern, TW.; Norton, SA.; Daniel, CR.; Elewski, BE.; Fallon-Friedlander, S., Lushniak, BD.; Taylor, JS.; Warschaw, K.; Wheeland, RG. (2002) Cutaneous anthrax management algorithm. *J Am Acad Dermatol;* 47:766--9.

[20] Coker, PR.; Smith, KL.; Fellows, PF.; Rybachuck, G.; Kousoulas, KG.; Hugh-Jones, ME. (2003) Bacillus anthracis virulence in guinea pigs vaccinated with anthrax vaccine

adsorbed is linked to plasmid quantities and clonality. *Journal of Clinical Microbiology;* 41(3):1212-1218.

[21] Collier, RJ.; Young, JA. (2003) Anthrax toxins. *Annu Rev Cell Dev Biol;* 19:45-70.

[22] Contini, A. (1995) *Bacillus.* In: Andreani, E., Buonavoglia, C., Compagnucci, M., Contini, A., Farina, R., Flammini, C., Gentile, G., Gualandi, G., Mandelli, G., Panina, G., Papparella, V., Pascucci, S., Poli, G., Redaelli, G., Ruffo, G., Scatozza, F., Sidoli, L., Malattie infettive degli animali, UTET, Torino, 20, 290-295.

[23] Cote, CK.; Rossi, CA.; Kang, AS.; Morrow, PR.; Lee, JS.; Welkos, SL. (2005) The detection of protective antigen (PA) associated with spores of Bacillus anthracis and the effects of anti-PA antibodies on spore germination and macrophage interactions. *Microb Pathog;* 38(5-6):209-25.

[24] de Vos, V. (1994) Antrax. In: Coetzer J., Thomson G.R., Tustin R., Kriek N., (eds.) Infectious diseases of livestock, volume II, Oxford University Press. 153:1262-1289.

[25] Dixon, TC.; Meselson, M.; Guillemin, J.; Hanna, PC. (1999) Anthrax. *N Engl J Med;* 341:815-26.

[26] Dragon, DC.; Rennie, RP. (1995) The ecology of anthrax spores: tough but not invincible. *Can Vet J;* 36(5):295-301.

[27] Druett, HA.; Henderson, DW.; Packman, L.; Peacock, S. (1953) Studies on respiratory infection. I. The influence of particle size on respiratory infection with anthrax spores. *J Hyg (Lond);* 51:359--71.

[28] Easterday, WR.; Van Ert, MN.; Simonson, TS., Wagner, DM.; Kenefic, LJ.; Allender, CJ.; Keim, P. (2005) Use of Single Nucleotide Polymorphisms in the *plcR* Gene for Specific Identification of *Bacillus anthracis. J Clin Microbiol;* 43(4):1995–1997.

[29] Ebedes, H. (1976) Anthrax epizootics in Etosha National Park. *Modoqua;* 10:99-118.

[30] Fasanella, A.; Losito, S.; Trotta, T.; Adone, R.; Massa, S.; Ciuchini, F.; Chiocco, D.; (2001) Detection of anthrax vaccine virulence factors by polymerase chain reaction. *Vaccine;* 19:4214–4218.

[31] Fasanella, A.; Van Ert, M.; Altamura, SA.; Garofolo, G.; Buonavoglia, C.; Leori, G.; Huynh, L.; Zanecki, S.; Keim, P. (2005) Molecular diversity of *Bacillus anthracis* in Italy. J *Clin Microbiol;* 43:3398-3401.

[32] Fasanella, A.; Palazzo, L.; Petrella, A.; Quaranta, V.; Romanelli, B.; Garofolo, G. Anthrax in red deer (Cervus elaphus), Italy. Emerg Infect Dis. 2007 Jul;13(7):1118-9

[33] Fasanella, A.; Tonello, F.; Garofolo, G.; Muraro, L.; Carattoli, A.; Adone, R., Montecucco, C. (2008) Protective activity and immunogenicity of two recombinant anthrax vaccines for veterinary use. *Vaccine;* 26(45):5684-8

[34] Fasanella, A.; Scasciamacchia, S.; Garofolo, G. (2009) The behaviour of virulent *Bacillus anthracis* strain AO843 in rabbits. *Vet Microbiol;* 133(1-2):208-9.

[35] Fasanella, A.; Scasciamacchia, S.; Garofolo, G.; Giangaspero, A.; Tarsitano, E.; Adone, R. Evaluation of the house fly Musca domestica as a mechanical vector for an anthrax. PLoS One. 2010 Aug 17;5(8):e12219.

[36] Fasanella, A.; Garofolo, G.; Hossain, MJ.; Shamsuddin, M.; Blackburn, JK.; Hugh-Jones, M. A 2010 anthrax field investigation in Bangladesh. *Epidemiology & Infection,* 2011 *in submission*

[37] Ferguson, LC. (1981) Anthrax. In: Leman A. D., Glock R. D., Mengeling W. L., Penny R. C. H., Scholl E. & Straw B.(eds). Diseases of Swine. 5th edn. Ames, Iowa: Iowa State University Press

[38] Flick-Smith, HC.; Walker, NJ.; Gibson, P.; Bullifent, H.; Hayward, S.; Miller, J.; Titball, RW.; Williamson, ED. (2002) A Recombinant Carboxy-Terminal Domain of the Protective Antigen of Bacillus anthracis Protects Mice against Anthrax Infection. *Infect and Immu;* 70(3):1653-1656.

[39] Fouet, A.; Smith, KL.; Keys, C.; Vaissaire, J.; Le Doujet, C.; Lévy, M.; Mock, M.; Keim, P. (2002) Diversity Among French *Bacillus anthracis* Isolates. *J Clin Microbiol;* 40:4732–4734.

[40] Friedlander, AM. (1986) Macrophages are sensitive to anthrax lethal toxin through an acid-dependent process. *J Biol Chem;* 261(16):7123-6.

[41] Friedlander, AM.; Little, SF. (2009) Advances in the development of next-generation anthrax vaccines. *Vaccine;* 27 Suppl 4:D28-32.

[42] Friedlander, AM.; Welkos, SL.; Pitt, ML.; Ezzell, JW.; Worsham, PL.; Rose, KJ.; Ivins, BE.; Lowe, JR.; Howe, GB.; Mikesell, P.; Lawrence, WB. (1993) Postexposure prophylaxis against experimental inhalation anthrax. *J Infect Di;* 167:1239-43.

[43] Fritz, DL.; Jaax, NK.; Lawrence, WB.; Davis, KJ.; Pitt, ML.; Ezzell, JW.; Friedlander, AM. (1995) Pathology of experimental inhalation anthrax in the rhesus monkey. *Lab Invest;* 73:691-702.

[44] Gleiser, CA.; Berdjis, CC.; Hartman, HA.; Gochenour, WS. (1963) Pathology of experimental respiratory anthrax in *Macaca mulatta. Br J Exp Pathol;* 44:416-26.

[45] Glomski, IJ.; Corre, JP.; Mock, M.; Goossens, PL. (2007) Cutting Edge: IFN-gamma-producing CD4 T lymphocytes mediate spore-induced immunity to capsulated Bacillus anthracis. *J Immunol;* 178(5):2646-50

[46] Gorantala, J.; Grover, S.; Goel, D.; Rahi, A.; Jayadev Magani, SK.; Chandra, S.; Bhatnagar, R. (2011) A plant based protective antigen [PA(dIV)] vaccine expressed in chloroplasts demonstrates protective immunity in mice against anthrax. *Vaccine;* 29(27):4521-33.

[47] Gorse, GJ.; Keitel, W.; Keyserling, H.; Taylor, DN.; Lock, M.; Alves, K.; Kenner, J.; Lynne Deans, L.; Gurwith, M. (2006) Immunogenicity and tolerance of ascending doses of a recombinant protective antigen (rPA102) anthrax vaccine: A randomized, double-blinded, controlled, multicenter trial. *Vaccine;* 24(33-34):5950-5959

[48] Gwinn, WM.; Kirwan, SM.; Wang, SH.; Ashcraft, KA.; Sparks, NL.; Doil, CR.; Tlusty, TG.; Casey, LS.; Hollingshead, SK.; Briles, DE.; Dondero, RS.; Hickey, AJ.; Foster, WM.; Staats, HF. (2010) Effective induction of protective systemic immunity with nasally administered vaccines adjuvanted with IL-1. *Vaccine;* 28(42):6901-14.

[49] Hambleton P; Carman JA; Melling J. Anthrax: the disease in relation to vaccines Vaccine 1984; 2: 125-32)

[50] Henderson, DW.; Peacock, S.; Belton, FC. (1956) Observations on the prophylaxis of experimental pulmonary anthrax in the monkey. *J Hyg (Lond);* 54:28-36.

[51] Henning, MW. (1956) Anthrax. In: Animal diseases in South Africa. 3rd ed. South Africa: Central News Agency Ltd.

[52] Heyworth, B.; Ropp, ME.; Voos, UG.; Meinel, HI.; Darlow, HM. (1975) Anthrax in The Gambia: an epidemiological study. *Br Med J;* 4:79-82.

[53] Holty, JE.; Bravata, DM.; Liu, H.; Olshen, RA.; McDonald, KM.; Owens, DK. (2006) Systematic review: a century of inhalational anthrax cases from 1900 to 2005. *Ann Intern Med;* 144:270-80.

[54] Hugh-Jones, ME. (1999) 1996-97 Global Anthrax report. *J Appl Microbiol;* 87:189-191.

[55] Hugh-Jones, ME.; Blackburn, J. (2009) The ecology of *Bacillus anthracis. Molecular Aspects of Medicine. in press*

[56] Hugh-Jones, ME.; de Vos, V. (2002) Anthrax and wildlife. *Rev Sci Tech;* 2:359-389.

[57] Ivins, BE.; Fellows, PF.; Nelson, GO. (1994) Efficacy of a standard human anthrax vaccine against Bacillus anthracis spore challenge in guinea-pigs. *Vaccine;* 12(10):872-4.

[58] Ivins, BE.; Pitt, ML.; Fellows, PF.; Farchaus, JW.; Benner, GE.; Waag, DM.; Little, SF.; Anderson, GW Jr.; Gibbs, PH.; Friedlander, AM. (1998) Comparative efficacy of experimental anthrax vaccine candidates against inhalation anthrax in rhesus macaques. *Vaccine;* 16(11-12):1141-8.

[59] Ivins, BE.; Welkos, SL.; Knudson, GB.; Little, SF. (1990) Immunization against anthrax with aromatic compound-dependent (Aro-) mutants of Bacillus anthracis and with recombinant strains of Bacillus subtilis that produce anthrax protective antigen. *Infect Immun;* 58(2):303-8.

[60] Ivins, BE.; Welkos, SL.; Little, SF.; Crumrine, MH.; Nelson, GO. (1992) Immunization against anthrax with Bacillus anthracis protective antigen combined with adjuvants. *Infect Immun;* 60(2):662-8.

[61] Jernigan, DB.; Raghunathan PL.; Bell, BP.; Brechner, R.; Bresnitz, EA.; Butler, JC. (2002) Investigation of bioterrorism-related anthrax, United States, 2001: epidemiologic findings. *Emerg Infect Dis;* 8:1019–1028.

[62] Kanafani, ZA.; Ghossain, A.; Sharara, AI.; Hatem, JM.; Kanj, SS. (2003) Endemic gastrointestinal anthrax in 1960s Lebanon: clinical manifestations and surgical findings. *Emerg Infect Dis;* 9:520-5.

[63] Keim, P.; Price, LB.; Klevytska, AM.; Smith, KL.; Schupp, JM.; Okinaka, R.; Jackson, PJ.; Hugh-Jones, ME. 2000. Multiple-Locus Variable-Number Tandem Repeat Analysis Reveals Genetic Relationships within Bacillus anthracis. *J. Bacteriology.* 182, 2928-2936.

[64] Keim, P.; Van Ert, MN.; Pearson, T.; Vogler, AJ.; Huynh, LY.; Wagner, DM. (2004) Anthrax molecular epidemiology and forensics: using the appropriate marker for different evolutionary scales. *Infect Genet Evol;* 4:205-213.

[65] Kenefic, LJ.; Beaudry, J.; Trim, C.; Huynh, L.; Zanecki, S.; Matthews, M.; Schupp, J., Van Ert, M.; Keim, P. (2008) A high resolution four-locus multiplex single nucleotide repeat (SNR) genotyping system in Bacillus anthracis. *J Microbiol Methods;* 73(3):269-72.

[66] Keppie, J.; Smith, H.; Harris-Smith, PW. (1955) The chemical basis of the virulence of Bacillus anthracis. III. The role of the terminal bacteraemia in death of guinea-pigs from anthrax. *Br J Exp Pathol;* 36(3):315-22.

[67] Kreidl, P.; Stifter, E.; Richter, A.; Aschbachert, R.; Nienstedt, F.; Unterhuber, H.; Barone, S.; Huemer, HP.; Carattoli, A.; Moroder, L.; Ciofi Degli Atti, ML.; Rota, MC.; Morosetti, G.; Larcher, C. (2006) Anthrax in animals and a farmer in Alto Adige, Italy. *Euro Surveill;* 11(7).

[68] Krinsky, WL. (1976) Animal disease agents transmitted by horse flies and deer flies (Diptera: Tabanidae). *J Med Entomol;* 13(3):225-75.

[69] Lanska, DJ. (2002) Anthrax meningoencephalitis. *Neurology;* 59:327-34.

[70] Leendertz, FH.; Ellerbrok, H.; Boesch, C.; Couacy-Hymann, E.; Matz-Rensing, K.; Hakenbeck, R., Bergmann, C.; Abaza, P.; Junglen, S.; Moebius, Y.; Vigilant, L.; Formenty, P.; Pauli, G. (2004) Anthrax kills wild chimpanzees in a tropical rainforest. *Nature;* 430:451-452.

[71] Leppla, SH. (1982) Anthrax toxin edema factor: a bacterial adenylate cyclase that increases cyclic AMP concentrations of eukaryotic cells. *Proc Natl Acad Sci USA;* 79:3162-3166.

[72] Lincoln, RE.; Walker, JS.; Klein, F.; Haines, BW. (1964) Anthrax. Advan *Vet Sci;* 9:327-68.

[73] Lindeque, PM.; Turnbull, PC. (1994) Ecology and epidemiology of anthrax in the Etosha National Park, Namibia. Onderstepoort. *J Vet Res;* 61(1):71-83.

[74] Lista, F.; Faggioni, G.; Valjevac S.; Ciammaruconi, A.; Vaissaire, J.; le Doujet, C.; Gorge, O.; de Santis, R.; Carattoli, A.; Ciervo, A.; Fasanella, A.; Orsini, F.; D'Amelio, R., Pourcel, C.; Cassone, A.; Vergnaud, G. (2006) Genotyping of *Bacillus anthracis* strains based on automated capillary 25-loci multiple locus variable-number tandem repeats analysis. *BMC Microbiology;* 6-33.

[75] Little, SF.; Ivins, BE.; Fellows, PF.; Pitt, ML.; Norris, SL.; Andrews, GP. (2004) Defining a serological correlate of protection in rabbits for a recombinant anthrax vaccine. *Vaccine;* 22(3-4):422-30.

[76] Lucey, D. *Bacillus anthracis* (anthrax). In Mandell G, Bennett J, Dolin R, eds. Mandell, Douglas, and Bennett's principles and practice of infectious diseases. Philadelphia, PA: Churchill Livingstone; 2005:2485--91.

[77] Manayani, DJ.; Thomas, D.; Dryden, KA.; Reddy, V.; Siladi, ME.; Marlett, JM.; Rainey, GJ.; Pique, ME.; Scobie, HM.; Yeager, M.; Young, JA.; Manchester, M.; Schneemann, A. (2007) A viral nanoparticle with dual function as an anthrax antitoxin and vaccine. *PLoS Pathog;* 3(10):1422-31.

[78] Marcato, PS. (1981) Anatomia e istologia patologica speciale dei mammiferi domestici, *Edagricole,* Bologna

[79] Meselson, M.; Guillemin, J.; Hugh-Jones, ME.; Langmuir, A.; Popova, I.; Shelokov, A.; Yampolskaya, O.; (1994) The Sverdlovsk anthrax outbreak of 1979. *Science;* 266(5188):1202-8.

[80] Mikszta, JA.; Sullivan, VJ.; Dean, C.; Waterston, AM.; Alarcon, JB.; Dekker, JP.; Brittingham, JM.; Huang, J.; Hwang, CR.; Ferriter, M.; Jiang, G.; Mar, K.; Saikh, KU.; Stiles, BJ.; Roy, CJ.; Ulrich, RG.; Harvey, NG. (2005) Protective immunization against inhalational anthrax: A comparison of minimally-invasive delivery platforms. *J Infect Dis;* 191:278–288.

[81] Milne, JC.; Furlong, D.; Hanna, PC.; Wall, JS.; Collier, RJ. (1994) Anthrax protective antigen forms oligomers during intoxication of mammalian cells. *J Biol Chem;* 269(32):20607-12.

[82] Mitzmain, MB. (1914) Experimental insect transmission of anthrax. *Public Health Reports;* 29:75-7716.

[83] Mohamadzadeh, M.; Durmaz, E.; Zadeh, M.; Pakanati, KC.; Gramarossa, M.; Cohran, V.; Klaenhammer, TR. (2010) Targeted expression of anthrax protective antigen by Lactobacillus gasseri as an anthrax vaccine. *Future Microbiol;* 5(8):1289-96.

[84] Morris, H. (1918) Blood-sucking insects as transmitters of Anthrax or Charbon, *Louisiana Bulletin No;* 163:pp15.

[85] Muehlbauer, SM.; Evering, TH.; Bonuccelli, G.; Squires, RC.; Ashton, AW.; Porcelli, SA.; Lisanti, MP.; Brojatsch, J. (2007) Anthrax lethal toxin kills macrophages in a strain-specific manner by apoptosis or caspase-1-mediated necrosis. *Cell Cycle;* 6(6):758-66.

[86] Nishi, JS.; Dragon, DC.; Elkin, BT.; Mitchell, J.; Ellsworth, TR.; Hugh-Jones, ME. (2002) Emergency response planning for anthrax outbreaks in bison herds of northern Canada: A balance between policy and science. *Ann NY Acad Sci;* 969:245-50.

[87] O'Brien, J.; Friedlander, A.; Dreier, T.; Ezzell, J.; Leppla, S. (1985) Effects of anthrax toxin components on human neutrophils. *Infect Immun;* 47(1):306-10.

[88] Papaparaskevas, J.; Houhoula, DP.; Papadimitriou, M.; Saroglou, G.; Legakis, NJ.; Zerva, L. (2004) Ruling out *Bacillus anthracis*. *Emerg Infect Dis;* 10:732-735.

[89] Pearson, T.; Busch, JD.; Ravel, J.; Read, TD.; Rhoton. SD.; U'Ren, JM.; Simonson, TS.; Kachur, SM.; Leadem, RR.; Cardon, ML.; Van Ert, MN.; Huynh, LY.; Fraser, CM.; Keim, P. (2004) Phylogenetic discovery bias in *Bacillus anthracis* using single-nucleotide polymorphisms from whole-genome sequencing. *Procl Nat Acad Sci USA;* 101(37):13536-13541.

[90] Puziss, M.; Manning, Lc.; Lynch, Jw.; Barclaye Abelow, I.; Wright, Gg. (1963) Large-scale production of protective antigen of Bacillus anthracis in anaerobic cultures. *App Microbiol;* 11:330-4.

[91] Read, TD.; Salzberg, SL.; Pop, M.; Shumway, M.; Umayam, L.; Jiang, L.; Holtzapple, E.; Busch, JD.; Smith, KL.; Schupp, JM.; Solomon, D.; Keim, P.; Fraser, CM. (2002) Comparative genome sequencing for discovery of novel polymorphisms in Bacillus anthracis. *Science;* 296(5575):2028-2033.

[92] Ross, J. (1957) The pathogenesis of anthrax following the administration of spores by the respiratory route. *J Path Bact;* 73:485-94.

[93] Saile, E.; Koehler, TM. (2006) *Bacillus anthracis* multiplication, persistence, and genetic exchange in the rhizosphere of grass plants. *Appl Environ Microbiol;* 72(5):3168-3174.

[94] Schwartz, M. (2009) Dr. Jekyll and Mr. Hyde: a short history of anthrax. *Molecular Aspect of Medicine;* 30:347-355

[95] Scobie, HM.; Young, JA. (2005) Interactions between anthrax toxin receptors and protective antigen. *Curr Opin Microbiol;* 8(1):106-112.

[96] Sejvar, JJ.; Tenover, FC.; Stephens, DS. (2005) Management of anthrax meningitis. *Lancet Infect Dis;* 5:28795.

[97] Shlyakhov, E.; Blancou, J.; Rubinstein, E. (1996) Vaccines against anthrax in animals, from Louis Pasteur to our day. *Rev Sci Tech;* 15:853-62.

[98] Shoop, WL.; Xiong, Y.; Wiltsie, J.; Woods, A.; Guo, J.; Pivnichny, JV.; Felcetto, T.; Michael, BF.; Bansal, A.; Cummings, RT.; Cunningham, BR.; Friedlander, AM.; Douglas, CM.; Patel, SB.; Wisniewski, D.; Scapin, G.; Salowe, SP.; Zaller, DM.; Chapman, KT.; Scolnick, EM.; Schmatz, DM.; Bartizal, K.; MacCoss, M.; Hermes, JD. (2005) Anthrax lethal factor inhibition. *Proc Natl Acad Sci USA;* 102(22):7958-7963.

[99] Singh, Y.; Klimpel, KR.; Quinn, CP.; Chaudhary, VK.; Leppla, SH. (1991) The carboxyl-terminal and of protective antigen is required for receptor binding and anthrax toxin activity. *J Biol Chem;* 266:15493-15497.

[100] Sirisanthana, T.; Brown, AE. (2002) Anthrax of the gastrointestinal tract. *Emerg Infect Dis;* 8:649-51.

[101] Smith, H.; Keppie, J.; Stanley, Jl. (1955) The chemical basis of the virulence of Bacillus anthracis. V. The specific toxin produced by B. Anthracis in vivo. *Br J Exp Pathol;* 36(5):460-72.

[102] Smith, IM. (1973) A brief review of Anthrax in domestic animals. *Postgrad Med J;* 49(574):571-572. Review.

[103] Smith, KL.; De Vos, V.; Bryden, H.; Price, LB.; Hugh-Jones, M.; Kleuytska, A.; Price, LB.; Keim, P. (2000) *Bacillus anthracis* diversity in Kruger National Park. *J Clin Micro;* 38(10):3780-3784.

[104] Splino, M.; Patocka, J.; Prymula, R.; Chlibek, R. (2005) Anthrax vaccines. *Ann Saudi Med;* 25(2):143-149.

[105] Stanley, Jl.; Smith, H. (1961) Purification of factor I and recognition of a third factor of the anthrax toxin. *J Gen Microbiol;* 26:49-63.

[106] Stein, CD. (1947) 1947a. Some observations on the tenacy of Bacillus anthracis. *Vet Med;* 13-22.

[107] Stepanov, AV.; Marinin, LI.; Pomerantsev, AP.; Staritsin, NA. (1996) Development of novel vaccines against anthrax in man. *J Biotechnol;* 44(1-3):155-60.

[108] Sterne, M. (1959) Anthrax. In: Stableforth A. W. & Galloway I. A., (eds). *Infectious Diseases of Animal Diseases due to Bacteria.* Vol I. London: Butterworths Scientific Pubblication.

[109] Sterne, M. (1967) Distribution and economic importance of Anthrax. *Fed Proc;* 26(5),1493.

[110] Stokes, MG.; Titball, RW.; Neeson, BN.; Galen, JE.; Walker, NJ.; Stagg, AJ.; Jenner, DC.; Thwaite, JE.; Nataro, JP.; Baillie, LW.; Atkins, HS. (2007) Oral administration of a Salmonella enterica-based vaccine expressing Bacillus anthracis protective antigen confers protection against aerosolized B. anthracis. *Infect Immun;* 75(4):1827-34.

[111] Stratilo, CW.; Lewis, CT.; Bryden, L.; Mulvey, MR.; Bader, D. (2006). Single-nucleotide repeat analysis for subtyping Bacillus anthracis isolates. *J Clin Microbiol;* 44(3):777-778.

[112] Tan, Y.; Hackett, NR.; Boyer, JL.; Crystal, RG. (2003) Protective immunity evoked against anthrax lethal toxin after a single intramuscular administration of an adenovirus-based vaccine encoding humanized protective antigen. *Hum Gene Ther;* 14(17):1673-82.

[113] Temte, JL.; Zinkel, AR. (2004) The primary care differential diagnosis of inhalational anthrax. *Ann Fam Med;* 2:438-44.

[114] Tournier, JN.; Rossi Paccani, S.; Quesnel-Hellmann, A.; Baldari, CT. (2009) Anthrax toxins: a weapon to systematically dismantle the host immune defenses. *Mol Aspects Med;* 30(6):456-66.

[115] Tross, D.; Klinman, DM. (2008) Effect of CpG oligonucleotides on vaccine-induced B cell memory. *J Immunol;* 181(8):5785-90.

[116] Turell, MJ.; Knudson, GB. (1987) Mechanical transmission of *Bacillus anthracis* by stable flies *(Stomoxys calcitrans*) and mosquitoes (*Aedes aegypti and Aedes taeniorhynchus). Infect Immun;* 55:1859-1961.

[117] Turnbull, PC. (1991) Anthrax vaccines: past, present and future. *Vaccine;* 9(8):533-539.

[118] Turnbull, PC. (2000) Current status of immunization against anthrax: old vaccines may be here to stay for a while. *Curr Opin Infect Dis;* 13(2):113-120.

[119] Turnbull, PC.; (1998) Guidelines for the surveillance and control of Anthrax in human and animals.3rd edition.

[120] Turnbull, PC.; Bell, RH.; Saigawa, K.; Munyenyembe, FE.; Mulenga, CK.; Makala, LH. (1991b) Anthrax in wildlife in the Luangwa Valley, Zambia. *Vet Rec;* 17:399-403.

[121] Turnbull, PCB.; Barman, JA.; Lindeque, DM.; Joubert, F.; Hubschle, OJB.; Snoeyenbos, GS. (1989) Further progress in understanding anthrax in Etosha National Park. *Mdoqua;* 16:93-104.

[122] Turner, AJ.; Galvin, JW.; Rubira, RJ.; Condron, RJ.; Bradley, T. (1999) Experiences with vaccination and epidemiological investigations on anthrax outbreak in Australia in 1997. *J Appl Microbiol;* 87:294-297.

[123] Uchida, I.; Sou-ichi, M.; Tsutomu, S.; Nobuyuki, T. (1997) Cross-talk to the genes for Bacillus anthracis capsule synthesis by atxA, the gene encoding the frans-activator of anthrax toxin synthesis. *Molecular Microbiol;* 23(6):1229–1240.

[124] Van Ert, M.; Easterday, WR.; Huynh, LY.; Okinaka, RT.; Hugh-Jones, ME.; Ravel, J.; Zanecki, SR. Pearson, T.; Simonson,TS.; U'Ren, JM.; Kachur, SM.; Leadem-Dougherty, RR.; Rhoton, SD.; Zinser, G.; Farlow, J.; Coker, PR.; Smith, KL.; Wang, B.; Kenefic, LJ.; Fraser-Liggett, CM.; Wagner, DM.; Keim, P. (2007) Global Genetic Population Structure of *Bacillus anthracis. PlosOne;* 5:461-471.

[125] Van Ness, GB. (1971) Ecology of anthrax. *Science;* 172(990):1303-1307.

[126] Vasconcelos, D.; Barnewall, R.; Babin, M.; Hunt, R.; Estep, J.; Nielsen, C.; Carnes, R.; Carney, J. (2003) Pathology of inhalation anthrax in cynomolgus monkeys (*Macaca fascicularis*). *Lab Invest;* 83:1201-9.

[127] Vitale, G.; Bernardi, L.; Napolitani, G.; Mock, M.; Montecucco, C. (2000) Susceptibility of mitogen-activated protein kinase family members to proteolysis by anthrax lethal factor. *Biochem. J;* 352:739-745.

[128] Walberg, K.; Baron, S.; Poast, J.; Schwartz, B.; Izotova, L.; Pestka, S.; Peterson, JW. (2008) Interferon protects mice against inhalation anthrax. *J Interferon Cytokine Res;* 28(10):597-601.

[129] Watson, J.; Koya, V.; Leppla, SH.; Daniell, H. (2004) Expression of Bacillus anthracis protective antigen in transgenic chloroplasts of tobacco, a non-food/feed crop. *Vaccine;* 22: 4374-84.

[130] Welkos, S.; Friedlander, A.; Weeks, S.; Little, S.; Mendelson, I. (2002) In-vitro characterisation of the phagocytosis and fate of anthrax spores in macrophages and the effects of anti-PA antibody. *J Med Microbiol;* 51(10):821-31.)

[131] Welkos, S.; Little, S.; Friedlander, A.; Fritz, D.; Fellows, P. (2001) The role of antibodies to Bacillus anthracis and anthrax toxin components in inhibiting the early stages of infection by anthrax spores. *Microbiology;* 147(Pt 6):1677-85.

[132] Wright, JG.; Quinn, CP.; Shadomy, S.; Messonnier, N. (2010) Centers for Disease Control and Prevention (CDC) Use of anthrax vaccine in the United States: recommendations of the Advisory Committee on Immunization Practices (ACIP), 2009. *MMWR Recomm Rep;* 59(RR-6):1-30.

9

Brucellosis Vaccines: An Overview

Seyed Davar Siadat, Ali Sharifat Salmani and
Mohammad Reza Aghasadeghi
Pasteur Institute of Iran
Iran

1. Introduction

Brucella is α-*Proteobacteria* causing an infectious disease in mammals that could be transmitted to humans. Ruminant and swine are prone to be infected by such microorganism all over the world, thus acting as a potential reservoir for domestic livestock and therefore, affecting humans. *Brucella* species differ in their hosts' preference, physiological abilities and cell surface structural characteristics. Those affecting domestic livestock are *B. melitensis* (sheep and goats), *B. abortus* (cattle), *B. suis* (swine), and *B. ovis* (sheep). Because domestic ruminants and swine are essential to the economy of millions of people, particularly in low income countries, brucellosis is a major cause of direct economical losses and a major impediment for trade. Moreover, human brucellosis is a severe and debilitating disease requiring a prolonged antibiotic treatment and often leaving permanent and disabling sequel. Thus, its control and if it possible its eradication are major goals of public health programs in affected countries (1,2).

2. The bacterium

Brucella belongs to the α- 2 subdivision of the *proteobacteria*, along with *ochrobactrum*, *rhizobium*, *rhodobacter*, *agrobacterium*, *bartonella*, and *rickettsia*. The traditional classification of *Brucella* species is largely based on its preferred hosts. There are six classic pathogens, of which four are recognized human zoonoses. The presence of rough or smooth lipopolysaccharide is correlated to the virulence of the disease in humans. Two new *Brucella* species, provisionally called *Brucella pinnipediae* and *B. cetaceae*, have been isolated from marine hosts within the past few years (3,4,).

Brucella is a monospecific genus that should be termed *B. melitensis*, and all other species are subtypes, with an interspecies homology above 87 percent. The phenotypic differences and host preferences can be attributed to various proteomes, as exemplified by specific outer-membrane protein markers. All *Brucella* species seem to have arisen from a common ancestor to which *B. suis* biotype 3 shares particular similarity. Although the scientific accuracy of this classification cannot be disputed, its practicality has been under scrutiny (5).

3. Nomenclature and classification

The Manchester report assumed the paper by Verger et al. on DNA hybridization studies and the proposition that all *Brucella* are just one species, with biovars; it was necessary to reclassify *Brucella* abortus biovar 9 as *Brucella melitensis* biovar abortus 7, following deletion of biovars 7 and 8. It is remarkable that, according to the Manchester nomenclature, all 'biovars' Melitensis 1-3, Abortus 1-7 and Suis 1-5 were assigned to the same level of differentiation, irrespective of previous nomenspecies; this is undoubtedly correct and is based on genome studies, but misleading for brucellosis epidemiology considering the relatedness of nomenspecies with host animals and geographical spreading. Moreover, McGillivery et al. (1988) found that the restriction endonuclease profiles produced by *BamHI* from DNA of five *Brucella abortus* isolates and the reference strain *B. abortus* biovar 2 were very similar. These results reinforced the existence of significant genetic homogeneity in *Brucella* genus. The report also emphasizes the relatedness of genus *Brucella* with the genera *Agrobacterium*, *Phyllobacterium* and *Rhizobium*. De Ley et al. identified *B. abortus* as a member in the α-2 subgroup of Proteobacteria on the basis of 16S rRNA gene sequence comparison and Moreno et al. suggested a close phylogenetic relation within the same group as a result of studying the composition of *Brucella* lipid A; later, Corbel published dendrogram considered it as serologically related (*Yersinia enterocolitica* O: 9, *Yersinia pseudotuberculosis*, *Salmonella typhimurium*, *Vibrio cholerae*, *Francisella tularensis*, *Escherichia coli* O: 157, *Pseudomonas putida*, *Rickettsia prowazekii*) (6,7).

4. Genetics of the *Brucella*

Classic genetic studies of *Brucella* was begun by spontaneous mutants in the early 20th century .The most widely studied spontaneous mutants are vaccine strains, such as *B. melitensis* Rev 1, *B. abortus* strain 19 and recently *B. abortus* strain RB51. The classic genetic studies are focused on phenotypic appearance, stability, metabolism and virulence of mutant colonies. Smoothness and roughness of the colonies usually attribute to high and low virulence of *B. abortus*, *B. suis*, and *B. melitensis*. Mutation causing changes in appearance of the colonies (smoothness → roughness) usually decreases the virulence of these species and decreases or eliminates the stimulation of antibodies to the O antigen in animal hosts. *B. abortus* strain RB51 illustrates this well, it is a rough strain which is highly attenuated and does not induce anti-O antibodies. The *Brucella* genome has a GC content of approximately 58%. *B. melitensis*, *B. abortus*, *B. ovis*, *B. neotomae, and B. suis* biovar 1, each has two chromosomes of 2,100 kb and 1,150 kb. However, *B. suis* biovar 2 and 4 have two chromosomes of 1.85 Mb and 1.35 Mb, and *B. suis* biovar 3 has only one chromosome with a size of 3.1 Mb. These differences in size and number of chromosomes can be explained by rearrangements resulting from homologous recombination at chromosome regions containing the three *rrn* genes. The DNA sequences amongst different *Brucella* species share more than 90% homology. According to the present taxonomy and phylogeny based on 16S RNA, the classic 6 species belong to a single species. This fact has been used to propose that the genus *Brucella* contains only a single species *B. melitensis*, and that the remaining classic species be considered biovars .Insertion sequences (IS) are discrete segments of DNA that can transpose from one genomic site to another and promote genetic rearrangements. Insertion sequences are found on both chromosomes of *Brucella*. All *Brucella* species contain approximately 8-35 copies of an insertion sequence denominated IS711 (also known as IS6501). The position and copy number of this insertion sequence seems to vary in different species, a characteristic which can be used to differentiate them. For example, the *wboA* gene in *B. abortus* RB51 is disrupted by an IS711-like element. Based on this, a PCR assay has been developed to distinguish strain RB51 from other *Brucella* spp. and strains including its parent strain 2308. Many PCR assays based on gene differences have been developed to detect or differentiate various *Brucella* strains. There are more than 50 *Brucella* genes with a variety of functions listed in GenBank. For example, GenBank includes genes that encode the chaperones such as dnaK, groEL, and groES. Both 16S RNA and 23S RNA DNA sequences of *Brucella* are found in GenBank. No resident plasmids have been found in *Brucella*. However, several plasmids have been shown to be able to replicate in the *Brucella* (8,9).

5. Antigenic composition

A substantial number of antigenic components of *Brucella* have been characterized. However, the lipopolysaccharide constituents of the cell wall in *Brucella* species cause the antibody to response to such species. *Brucella* devoid of the o-polysaccharide (O-PS) are termed rough or "R" because their colonial surface contrasts with the glistening, smooth aspect of those carrying S-LPS. They can naturally be members of the R *Brucella* species (*B. canis* and *B. ovis*) or mutants derived from the S *Brucella* species (*B. melitensis, B. abortus* and *B. suis*)(18,19,20). Cultures of S *Brucella* spontaneously dissociate to generate mixtures of S and R colonies, the latter is formed by R mutants. Owing to their lack of antigenic O-PS, true R mutants neither induce anti O-PS antibodies nor react with antibodies of this specificity. They also show other outer membrane topology and physiological changes due to lack of O-PS. Manifestations of these changes are the uptake of crystal violet, the auto agglutination in acryflavin solutions and the sensitivity to *Brucella* phages specific for the R species. Since the S → R dissociation occurs spontaneously with a frequency that depends on the strain and growth conditions, repeated *in vivo* or *in vitro* passage has been used to obtain R- mutant strain for vaccines production. The *B. abortus* 45/20 and RB51 strains were developed in this way. Alternatively, R mutants can be generated by new molecular genetics techniques such as transposon mutagenesis or deletion of genes involved in S-LPS biosynthesis. It has been known for a long time that *Brucella* R mutants are attenuated spontaneously. This attenuation has been ascribed to the increase in both the antibody independent complement activation and the sensitivity to polycationic bactericidal peptides. In addition, R mutants display altered attachment to cells. Moreover, since the S *Brucella* are intracellular parasites able to alter constitutively intracellular trafficking (i.e. the one followed by inert particles or non-virulent *Brucella*), other factors related to the interplay of R mutant is the importance of the host cell, an aspect that has not been investigated so far. The outer membrane topology of rough mutants is altered LPS acylation patterns and could be relevant in this regard (4,21,22). The structure of S-LPS content of *Brucella* is known in part. According to nuclear magnetic resonance studies, the O-PS is a homopolymer of N-formyl-perosamine either exclusively in α-(1-2) linkages (for example in *B. abortus* biotype 1) or in α- (1-2) plus α- (1-3) in a ≥ 4:1 proportion (4:1 in *B. melitensis* biotype 1). These O-PSs carry three basic types of overlapping epitopes: C (common to all chemical types of *Brucella* O-PS), M (present in those O-PS with α (1-3) linkages) and A (present in those O-PS with no α (1-3) linkages or with a proportion of α- (1-2) to α- (1-3) linkages higher than 4:1). Nuclear magnetic resonance studies also show that the S-LPS of *Yersinia enterocolitica* O:9 carries a homopolymer of N-formyl-perosamine in α- (1-2) linkages and, accordingly, it should be identical to O-PS such as those of the *B. abortus* biotype 1. It might be, however, that some aspect of these structures has escaped the nuclear magnetic resonance analyses because, whereas some monoclonal antibodies of O-PS specificity react equally with *S Brucella* and *Y. enterocolitica* O:9 (Cyb epitopes), others recognize epitopes common to all S *Brucella* but not to *Y. enterocolitica* O:9 (Cb epitopes), strongly suggests subtle structural differences (4,23,24,25). The structure of the LPS core in *Brucella* is largely unknown and qualitative studies show 3-deoxy-D-manno-2- octulosonic acid, mannose, glucose, glucosamine and quinovosamine as the main sugars. The synthesis of LPS in *Brucella* is largely unknown but the genetic evidence available is fully consistent with a mechanism similar to that existing in some of the best studied gram-negative bacteria. First, lipid A is synthesized on the inner face of the cytoplasmic membrane. Second, through the sequential action of glycosyltransferases, sugars are added to lipid A until the core oligosaccharide is completed. These two pathways are intermingled since two 3-deoxy-D-manno- 2-octulosonate residues are added before lipid A synthesis is finished. On the contrary, the O-PS is synthesized in an independent pathway and, once its biosynthesis is carried through, it is linked to the acceptor sugar of the completed lipid A-core (19,24,25). Depending on the particular O-PS, there are three known types of mechanisms of synthesis, and that of *Brucella* belongs to the so-called ABC transporter-dependent (or *wzy*-independent) type. In this pathway, a lipid carrier (undecaprenol pyrophosphate) on the cytoplasmic side of the membrane is first primed with an amino sugar by the *WecA* protein. Then, O-PS sugar units are inserted successively at the non-reducing end (i.e. the "tip" of the growing polysaccharide) by glycosyltransferases .Finally, the ABC proteins translocate the amino sugar-O-PS (possibly still linked to the undecaprenol) to the periplasmic side of the membrane where a ligase (*WaaL)* binds the amino sugar-O-PS to the completed lipid A-core. Thus, when the synthesis of the core is blocked, the O-PS is generally not incorporated to the LPS (25). In addition to the lipid A, core, and O-PS pathways, there are subsidiary pathways that provide the necessary nucleotide-sugar precursors. Some of them are exclusive to LPS biosynthesis whereas others are housekeeping pathways. The more recent nomenclature for the genes coding for the enzymes of LPS synthesis uses four letters:1 (i), *lpx** for those involved in the early steps of lipid A synthesis; (ii), *wa*** for those involved in the late steps of lipid A synthesis, in core synthesis and in the ligation of the amino sugar-O-PS to the lipid A-core (*waaL*); (iii), *wb*** for those involved in the OP-S synthesis; and (iv), *wz*** for those involved in OP-S processing (for example, *wzm/wzt* are the genes coding for the ABC transporters such as those acting on *Brucella* OP-S). The genes coding for the enzymes belonging to the precursor pathways follow a conventional nomenclature (for example man* for mannose biosynthesis, per for perosamine synthetase, etc.) even though they functionally belong to LPS pathways. Sometimes there are two different genes for the same enzymatic function as there can be two pathways for the same sugar when it is present in both the core or the O-PS and, in this case, sub-indexes are used (for example, *manBcore* and *manBOAg* for the phosphomannomutases of core and O-PS [O Antigen] mannose synthesis). At least sixteen genes have been proven to be involved in *Brucella* LPS synthesis by analysis of the corresponding mutants and, as in many bacteria, most of the O-PS ones are clustered in a region *(wbk)* region. Although mutations in some genes outside *wbk* also bring about an R phenotype, their assignation to the core or O-PS pathways is less clear. As judged by the analyses derived from the complete sequence of the *B. melitensis* and *B. suis* genomes, genes encoding for LPS in *Brucella* are scattered in chromosomes with the exception of the *wbk* region (26). R strains of *B. melitensis, B. abortus* and *B. suis* should result from mutations in some *wa*** genes (including *WaaL*), in all *wb*** genes, in the *wzm/wzt* genes, and in genes of the pathways that lead to precursors of core and O-PS sugars (for example *manBcore* and *per,* respectively). But for the absence of an O-PS linked to the remaining LPS molecule, it can be predicted that not all these mutants are equivalent and they can be hypothetically grouped as follows: (i), R mutants have a complete lipid A-core plus a cytoplasmic O-PS, the incorporation of which to the LPS is blocked (at least the *wzm/wzt* and possibly the *WaaL* mutants); (ii), R mutants have a complete lipid A-core but no O-PS (mutants in *wb*** glycosyltransferases, in *wecA,* and in genes coding for enzymes necessary to synthesise some precursors, such as *manBOAg, gmd* and *per*) and (iii), R mutants have progressive deficiencies in the core and that may or may not accumulate cytoplasmic O-PS (mutants in some *wa*** genes and in some precursor genes such as *manBcore*). Mutants of each of these three groups have in fact been described, and the question then arises as to what extent they are equivalent in attenuation and immunizing abilities (27,28,29,30). Numerous outer and inner membranes, cytoplasmic, and periplasmic antigenic proteins have also been characterized. Some are recognized by the immune system during infection and are potentially useful in diagnostic tests. Hitherto, tests based on such antigens have suffered from low sensitivity as infected persons tend to develop a much less consistent response to individual protein antigens than to LPS. Thus, tests such as immuno-blotting against whole-cell extracts may have some advantages over more quantitative tests that employ purified individual antigens. Recently, ribosomal proteins have reemerged as immunologically important components. Interest in these, first arose more than 20 years ago when crude ribosomal preparations were demonstrated to stimulate both antibody and cell-mediated responses and to confer protection against challenge with *Brucella.* However, the individual components responsible for such activity were not identified until recently. It has been established that the L7/L12 ribosomal proteins are important in stimulating cell-mediated responses. They elicit delayed hypersensivity responses as components of brucellins, and as fusion proteins, they have been shown to stimulate protective responses to *Brucella.* They appear to have potential as candidate vaccine components (31,32).

Bacterial pathogens that maintain long-term residence within host phagocytes probably express a variety of genes to help them adapt to the harsh environmental conditions of pH, nutrition deprivation, ROIs, and reactive nitrogen intermediates (RNIs) as well as lysosomal enzymes encountered within the phagosome .Prominent among these responses is the induction of heat shock proteins, suggesting that considerable protein misfolding and damage occurs within this compartment. However, the role of these proteins in *Brucella* pathogenesis was uncertain. B. abortus Lon transposon mutants were attenuated in BALB/c resident peritoneal macrophages but persistent in BALB/c mice except for a minor attenuation at 1 week postinfection, suggesting that Lon protease is important for *Brucella* survival during early infection. *B. suis dnaK* insertional mutants, defective in a member of the Hsp70 family, were attenuated in the human macrophagic cell line, U937. *B. abortus htrA* deletion mutants, deficient in a serine protease called high temperature- requirement A protein, have been considered to be attenuated in vitro and in vivo, but a recent report suggests that *htrA* mutants were in fact *htrA cycL* double deletion mutants. An additional report suggests that a B.melitensis authentic htrA deletion mutant was not attenuated in goats, suggesting that *HtrA* is not involved in *Brucella* pathogenesis. Also, the B. suis *clpA* deletion mutant was not attenuated in vitro or in vivo. Taken together, these reports suggest that not all heat shock proteins are critical to *Brucella* pathogenesis or that redundant function of heat shock proteins will compromise the functional deficiency caused by the loss of one heat shock protein (33,34,35,36).

6. Virulence

The basis for the virulence of *Brucella* can be attributed to the ability of these bacteria to escape the host defense mechanisms and to survive and replicate within the host cells.

Attempts to identify *Brucella* virulence factors have been made. The first studies reported that intracellular multiplication of *Brucella* was attributable to erythritol .Virulent *Brucellae* are capable of invading and residing in professional phagocytes, such as macrophages, as well as non-phagocytic cells. The mechanism of attachment and entry into these cells by *Brucella* has yet to be clearly elucidated. Virulence mechanisms identified so far is associated with the ability to reside within phagocytic and/or non-phagocytic cells are as follows: the ability to inhibit phagolysosome fusion, degranulation and activation of the myelo-peroxidase-halide system, and the production of tumor necrosis factor (37,38).

In both phagocytic and non-phagocytic cells, *Brucella* has the ability to replicate within membrane-bound compartments. In non-phagocytic cells, such as *HeLa* cells, virulent *B .abortus* 2308 has been documented to replicate in the endoplasmic reticulum by utilizing the auto phagic machinery of the *HeLa* cell. In professional phagocytes, the membrane-bound compartment within which virulent *Brucella* organisms can replicate is the phagosome. By some unknown mechanism, *Brucella* is able to block phagolysosome fusion. It is now thought that the production of adenine and guanine monophosphate can inhibit phagolysosome fusion. The ability to produce these compounds is therefore considered as virulence factor of *Brucella*. In contrast, attenuated strains of *Brucella* are unable to prevent such fusion and are thereby destroyed by the lysosomal contents. Research on intracellular survival and replication of *Brucella* within professional phagocytes has mainly focused on macrophages (39,40). Survival within macrophages is apparently associated with the production of many different proteins. These proteins tend to be stress induced proteins such as heat shock or acid-induced proteins. They include 17, 24, 28, 60, and 62 KD proteins . Two of these proteins, the 17 and 28 KD proteins, seem to be induced only during intracellular cohabitation of *Brucella* with macrophages (41,42). *HtrA*, another stress-induced protein, has been examined for its possible role in virulence and intracellular survival. Using deletion mutants, *HtrA* has been shown to be involved in inducing a granulomatous reaction and thus reduces the levels of infection during the early phase of infection (murine model). However, this does not result in reduced levels in the later phases of infection. In fact, overall, *htrA*-deficient mutants produce spleenic bacterial loads comparable to their 11 wild-type counterparts. *RecA* mutants produce similar results as *htrA* mutants in early- and late-phase spleenic load (43).Two other types of proteins that have been put forth as possible virulence factors are siderophores and Cu-Zn superoxide dismutase (Cu-Zn SOD). Iron-sequestration by siderophores may be an integral virulence factor in intracellular survival of *Brucella* species. Low levels of iron *in vivo* aid the host's ability to restrict microbial growth. *Brucella* species do carry iron-sequestering proteins and other siderophores, but their role in pathogenesis has not been clearly elucidated. Cu-Zn SOD may play a significant role in the early phase of intracellular infection, but contradictory results have been reported. Further studies are needed before the role of Cu-Zn SOD as a virulence factor of intracellular survival of *Brucella* can be accurately assessed (33,44). An auxotrophic mutation encoding for an essential enzyme (5′-phosphoribosyl-5-amino-4-imidazole carboxylase) necessary for the *de novo* synthesis of purines has been demonstrated to be essential for the intracellular survival of *B. melitensis*. Deletion of the gene, *purE*, encoding this enzyme in virulent *B. melitensis* drastically reduced its ability to survive within macrophages and demonstrated attenuated behavior in mice and goats. Recently, a two-component regulatory system has been discovered in *B. abortus*. The *Brucella* virulence related proteins *(Bvr)* system consists of a regulatory *(BvrR)* and a sensory protein *(BvrS)*. This regulatory system, *BvrR-BvrS*, may play a critical role in the ability of *B.abortus* to invade and multiply within cells. BvrR-deficient mutants were obtained by transposon mutagenesis. Morphologically, these mutants produced smooth-type LPS (45). They were found to be increasingly sensitive to polycations surfactants and showed decreased *in vivo* replication and persistence in mouse spleens. This occurred even though no obvious 12 growth defects could be detected in the mutants *in vivo*. Complementation with the *bvrR* gene restores resistance to polycations and partially restored the ability of these mutants to multiply intracellularly. The results further suggest that restoration of full virulence requires both components of the regulatory system to be intact. Interestingly, LPS core and lipid A are known to be involved in polycationic resistance. Therefore, it is possible that these LPS features involved in polycationic resistance are under the *BvrR-BvrS* regulatory system. Analysis at the DNA level of *bvrR* and *bvrS* genes revealed that they are highly homologous to other regulatory systems being found within symbiotic plant pathogens such as *Rhizobium meliloti* (*ChvI-ExoS* system) and *Agrobacterium tumefaciens* (*ChvI-ChvG* system). It has been established that *B. abortus, R. meliloti*, and *A. tumefaciens* are phylogenetically related. Therefore, this suggests that the *BvrR-BvrS* system co-evolved with the other two systems listed above to aid in the ability of *Brucella* to survive intracellularly (22,46). Recently in *B .suis*, genes encoding a type IV secretion system homologous to the *Agrobacterium tumefaciens VirB* and *Bordatella perutussis* Pt1 systems have been identified to be essential for the intracellular survival in *HeLa* cells and human macrophages. Further research is needed to clearly understand the actual role of this secretion system in the virulence of *Brucella* species (47). At present, there is no evidence to support a secretion system within *Brucella*. If *Brucella* is capable of secreting, it is probably in very small amounts. Non-protein components of *Brucella* may also contribute to its ability to survive within cells. One such cellular component, lipopolysaccharide (LPS) will be discussed in the section below (46,47).

The LPS of smooth strains of *Brucella* are comprised of a lipid A molecule, fatty acids, a core region, and a polysaccharide O-side chain. This O-side chain is made from a homopolymer of perosamine and is found on the surface of smooth strains, while rough organisms lack this chain on their LPS. Smooth *Brucellae* are able to survive intracellularly as compared to their rough counterparts. Therefore, smooth lipopolysaccharide (S-LPS) probably plays a significant role in pathogenesis. The simple explanation of rough versus smooth morphology and virulence, however, does not explain how naturally occurring rough species *B. ovis* and *B. canis* retain their virulence. Using *Tn5* transposon mutagenesis, several genes necessary for the synthesis of S-LPS have recently been identified. Both *in vitro* and *in vivo* studies with the rough mutants derived from the deletion of these genes clearly established that S-LPS is necessary for efficient intracellular survival and virulence of *B. melitensis, B. abortus*, and *B. suis*. *B. abortus* S-LPS is 100 times less potent than that of *E. coli* and *Salmonella* in inducing TNF from macrophages as well as oxidative metabolism and lysozyme release by human neutrophils. This feature of S-LPS has been proposed to contribute to the survival of *B. abortus* within phagocytic cells. In addition, *Brucella* S-LPS is not susceptible to the actions of polycationic molecules, suggesting that smooth *Brucella* can resist the cationic bactericidal peptides of the phagocytes. S-LPS has also been found to confer anti-phagocytic properties to *Brucella* and does not activate the alternate pathway of the complement cascade (37,48,49).

7. *Brucella* vaccines

7.1 Live, attenuated vaccines

Both killed and live, attenuated vaccines have been examined for their potential role in the control and eradication of brucellosis in cattle, goats, and swine. Live, attenuated vaccines carry several advantages over their killed counterparts. First, immunity derived from their use tends to be cell-mediated and long lasting. Also, as they are administered live, the organism is allowed to replicate within the host, thus making them less expensive. However, some live, attenuated vaccines may cause abortion in pregnant females and therefore their use is often relegated to males and non-gravid females.

The two main live, attenuated vaccines used in the control of *B. abortus* infection in cattle are *B. abortus* strain 19 and *B. abortus* strain RB51. A brief discussion of each, plus the use of B. melitensis strain Rev. 1 in goats, follows (48,50).

7.2 Killed vaccines

Killed vaccines can offer protection to a disease while still retaining safety for those animals that are young, immuno-suppressed, or pregnant. Over the years, a variety of killed vaccines have been developed for protection against brucellosis. They have had limited success. None have approached the protection status afforded by the live, attenuated vaccines. Examples of vaccines in this category are *B. abortus* strain 45/20 and *B. melitensis* H38. In addition to the lack of sufficient protection in the face of challenge, killed vaccines such as 45/20 and H38 can induce persistent antibody titers that can interfere with common serological tests used (51,52,53).

7.3 *Brucella abortus* vaccines

7.3.1 *B. abortus* strain 19

Brucella abortus strain 19 (S19) is a smooth but attenuated strain. The molecular basis for the attenuation is not known. The strain S19 has been shown to contain a deletion in the erythritol catabolic genes rendering it sensitive to erythritol. However, such a deletion in virulent strains has been shown not to result in attenuation. Prior to the introduction of vaccine strain RB51 in 1996, *B. abortus* S19 was known to be the official vaccine strain. The strain S19 was quite effective in protecting cattle against subsequent infection with virulent strains of *B. abortus* (54). However, S19 did have several problems that restricted its use within the cattle. During protection studies, it was discovered that S19, when given to adult cattle (>1yr), often caused persistent titers which could not be distinguished from titers resulting from a natural infection using standard serological tests. The tests like a plate agglutination test, complement fixation (CFT), and tube agglutination tests can only detect the presence of antibodies against O-antigens. This directly undermined the brucellosis eradication program that was dependent on a test and slaughter strategy to reduce numbers of infected cattle within the United States. Persistent antibodies could be detected for up to 10-11 months post vaccination when vaccinating adult cattle with the standard dose (3×10^{10} CFU). Although a rare finding, even some calves vaccinated S19 produced persistent antibodies (55,56). Use of S19 in pregnant cattle also resulted in abortions. Even when a reduced dose of S19 (1/20-1/100 of the standard dose) was used to vaccinate pregnant cattle, abortions in post-inoculation were still observed, although this reduced dose appeared to be less abortigenic (57,58). The use of the reduced dose vaccine did not eliminate the problem of persistent titers (51,59,60). In fact, these titers lasted about the same amount of time as the full dose (60). For this reason, Erasmus and Erasmus recommended that vaccination of adults with the reduced dose of S19 be relegated to herds heavily infected with *B. abortus*. As a result of the overwhelming experimental evidence, S19 was designated for use as a calf hood vaccine (4 to 12 month of age) (60). Calf hood vaccination with S19 is not completely without side effects. As with all other brucellosis vaccines, S19 cannot be administered to bulls or bull calves due to the resulting persistent orchitis (61). There have also been reports of an arthropathy (gonitis) linked to vaccination of female calves with S19. Immunological studies by *Wyn-Jones* and colleagues indicated the presence of *B. abortus* strain S19 antigenic material within the cells of the stifle, synovial membrane and the drainage lymph nodes (54). With the discovery of *B. abortus* strain RB51, the benefits of S19 vaccination diminished and RB51 replaced S19 as the official vaccine for the brucellosis eradication program. The use of S19 has also raised concerns about human exposure to brucellosis vaccines.

There have been several reports of illness following accidental self-inoculation with the S19 vaccine (54,62). This stresses the importance of safe-handling practices when vaccinating herds for brucellosis using the S19 vaccine. It also led investigators to try and develop a more efficacious cattle vaccine that would also be safer in terms of potential human exposure (62,63,64).

7.3.2 *B. abortus* strain RB51

The use of *B. abortus* strain RB51 was approved to be the official strain employed to manufacture calf hood vaccine for protection against brucellosis in 1996. Vaccine strain RB51 is a stable, rifampin-resistant, and derived from rough mutant of *B. abortus* 2308. It was derived by serial passage of parental strain 2308 on trypticase soy agar supplemented with varying concentrations of rifampin and penicillin. Colonies of RB51 are rough in morphology as indicated by their ability to absorb crystal violet as well as auto-agglutinate when in suspension. The LPS of RB51 is deficient in O-side chain, unlike its parental strain 2308. Metabolically, RB51 shares the ability to use erythritol with strain 2308 and RB51 has proven to be an extremely stable rough mutant of *B. abortus*. Its stability and efficacy have been shown in vitro and in vivo (65,66). Like the strain S19 vaccine, calves must be vaccinated with strain RB51 between the ages of 4-12 months of age with the calf dose (1.0-3.4×10^{10} CFU) and in high risk area animals receive the vaccine after 12 month of age (67). Advantages of RB51 over other vaccines for protection against bovine brucellosis are numerous. It does not produce any clinical signs post-vaccination, nor does it produce a local reaction at the site of injection (65). It is rapidly cleared from the bloodstream, as early as 2 weeks after post-inoculation. It is not shed in the nasal secretions, saliva, or urine. Therefore, the organism appears to be unable to spread from vaccinated to non-vaccinated animals through these routes. In immuno-suppressed animals, no recrudescence of infection has been documented. In addition, vaccination with RB51 affords a high level of protection, characterized by good cell mediated immunity. In one study, vaccination of cattle at least one year prior to mating induced 100% protection against abortion caused by exposure to field conditions of high and low brucellosis levels .The use of RB51 has also helped clear up the issue of *Brucella*-positive/"reactor" animals. Since RB51 lacks O-side chain, vaccination with the strain (unlike strain 19) produces no antibodies to O-side chain. This is particularly advantageous because all of the diagnostic tests used to screen for brucellosis in herds are directed toward the detection of O-antibodies in the serum or milk. Cattle vaccinated with RB51 are negative on all subsequent serological tests, including agar gel diffusion test. This lack of interfering antibodies is even true in the face of calf hood vaccination with strain 19 and subsequent adult vaccination with RB51 (68).

Although, sera from RB51 vaccinated cattle do not respond to standard diagnostic tests, they do contain antibodies that react to a dot-blot ELISA containing RB51 antigen (65). As these antigens are common to both RB51 and 2308, the dot-blot ELISA test cannot differentiate between vaccinated and infected animals; it is, therefore, relegated to assessing the humoral, non-protective immune response of cattle post-inoculation (69). In addition, there are two molecular methodologies that may be used to differentiate RB51 from other isolates: pulse field gel electrophoresis (PFGE) and polymerase chain reaction (PCR). RB51 possesses a unique fingerprint using the pulsed-field gel electrophoresis patterns of genomic DNA digested with restrictive endonuclease *Xba* I. The fingerprint of RB51 contains a unique band at 104 kb, as opposed to a 109-kb fragment within genomic DNA samples of *B. abortus* isolates from naturally infected cattle, bison, and elk (70). In addition, there is a specific PCR test that can differentiate RB51 isolates from all other *Brucella* isolates tested. This PCR method is based on the interruption of the *wboA* gene by an insertion element (IS711), a unique mutation present only in RB51 (71). In a murine model, *B. abortus* strain RB51 has been shown to confer protection against challenge with *B. melitensis*, *B. suis*, and *B. ovis*. However, in rams this vaccine did not induce protection against *B. ovis* challenge. Field trials indicate that *B. abortus* strain RB51 is also protective against swine brucellosis.

In addition to domesticated species, *B. abortus* strain RB51 has also been used to vaccinate wild animals such as bison and elk. Oral vaccination of mice and cattle with RB51 has been shown to be effective in inducing protective immune responses. These results are encouraging and highlight the feasibility of oral vaccination of wild life on a large scale. RB51 may appear to be a safe vaccine with respect to human exposure (72,73).

7.4 *Brucella melitensis* vaccines

7.4.1 *B. melitensis* Rev. 1.

B. melitensis Rev. 1 (Rev1) is currently the only approved vaccine available for protection against *B. melitensis* infection. In 1957, a smooth attenuated strain of *B. melitensis* was isolated from a streptomycin-dependent population that had been grown in a streptomycin deficient medium. In experimental challenge trials in goats, this strain was found to induce significant protection against the virulent challenge strain without shedding the organism. The organism was later designated *B. melitensis* Rev. 1. Use of the Rev1 vaccine has both advantages and disadvantages. Vaccination with Rev1 induces significant protection in sheep and goats. Rev1 has been found to be much more protective in goats and sheep challenged with virulent *B. melitensis* than those animals vaccinated with S19. The Rev1 vaccine does have some disadvantages. It can cause abortions if used in pregnant animals. Vaccination with Rev1 can result in persisting agglutinins that can interfere with various serological diagnostic tests. Rev1 is pathogenic to humans via aerosol exposure or self-inoculation causing generalized brucellosis in affected individuals. Like all other *Brucella* vaccines, Rev1 can cause local hypersensitivity reactions in cases of accidental inoculation (12,74,75,76,77,78).

8. *Brucella* R mutants for vaccine studies

8.1 *B. abortus* 45/20

This R vaccine was obtained after twenty passages in guinea pigs of a field isolate (*B. abortus* strain 45) in 1938. However, the original 45/20 strain was reported to revert to S pathogenic forms when injected into cattle. Alton reports of experiments with several 45/20 stocks which, after repeated passages in guinea pigs, showed either S-intermediate and R colonies or only R forms depending on the origin of the stocks. This suggests that the original strain contained in fact several different clones so that the S-intermediate ones were selected when injected into cattle. Also, it seems likely that different laboratory variants of this strain have coexisted for years. The genetic defects in this strain are unknown and the vaccine is not presently marketed (65,79).

8.2 *B. abortus* RB51

Strain RB51 is a spontaneous R mutant selected after repeated in vitro passages of *B. abortus* 2308 on media containing rifampin and penicillin. Selection was performed using crystal violet and acryflavin tests. RB51 carries an IS711 spontaneously inserted into *wboA* (putatively coding for a glycosyltransferase). However, a *wboA* transposon mutant obtained from strain 2308 is not as attenuated as RB51 and the protection afforded by *wboA* mutant vaccines in mice is better than that provided by RB51, which shows that RB51 carries additional and unknown defects. In the complete sequence of *B. melitensis, B. suis* and *B. abortus* genomes (an annotated *B. abortus* complete sequence is not available) *wboA* maps outside of the main *wbk** O-PS genetic region. RB51 accumulates small amounts of O-PS. This is noteworthy because, accepting that the current model of the *B. abortus* LPS structure is correct, mutation in a *wb*** gene should prevent O-PS synthesis. Complementation of RB51 with *wboA* increases O-chain expression but does not restore the S phenotype suggesting that other LPS genes are affected. In addition, although sodium dodecyl sulfate (SDS) polyacrylamide gel electrophoresis (SDS-PAGE) migration patterns have been interpreted to mean that RB51 carries a LPS with a complete core, chemical analyses showed that this R-LPS contains 2.5 times less mannose than the *B. abortus* RA1 *wboA* mutant. The presence of additional mutations in genes of strain RB51 are not involved in LPS synthesis and cannot be excluded either (80,81). On the contrary to 45/20, RB51 is stable and it is currently being used in some countries instead of S19. Although it should show very low or no virulence in humans, there is little information on this point and there has been at least one case of RB51 infection in a veterinarian demonstrated by bacteriological isolation and typing of the strain. It has to be stressed that RB51 is resistant to rifampin, an antibiotic currently used in the groups of brucellosis patients that cannot be treated with streptomycin (pregnant women, children of young age, and endocarditis and neurobrucellosis cases) (34).

RB51 has been used as the starting strain in two genetic manipulations. First, the *wboA* defect has been complemented with a functional *wboA* gene to generate strain *RB51Wboa.* This strain keeps the R phenotype manifested in the crystal violet and acryflavin tests, but expresses increased amounts of O-PS which by immuno-electron microscopy seems to be accumulated in the cytoplasm. However, at least part of this O-PS may be linked to a lipid to give an immunogenic form because it migrates in SDS-PAGE and vaccination of mice with RB51WboA elicits IgG antibodies of at least C specificity. Second, the *Brucella* Cu/Zn superoxide dismutase gene has been introduced in RB51 to obtain strain RB51SOD which over expresses (tenfold) this protein. The aim of this manipulation is to increase the expression of a *Brucella* antigen and a possible virulence factor on the RB51 background (33,82,83).

8.3 *wboA* mutants other than RB51

Mutants in this putative glycosyltransferase gene have been obtained from *B. melitensis* 16M and B. suis 2579 by allelic exchange to generate the strains VTRM1 and VTRS1, respectively. Both are kanamycin resistant since they carry a *Tn5* element. Although, it was originally named *rfbU,* blast analysis of the *Salmonella typhi* RfbU prototype against the *B. melitensis* genome shows the highest similarity (E value 1e–16) with *WbkA,* and more recently the gene has been renamed *wboA* (E value for *RfbU* versus *WboA* is only 2e–04). The VTRM1 and VTRS1 mutants are stable in mice, lack reactivity with monoclonal antibodies of C specificity and have an R phenotype but they have not been tested for the absence of core defects or expression of cytoplasmic O-PS (84,85,86).

8.4 Mutants in the *wbk* region

Several mutants in this cluster of O polysaccharide genes have been describe, and two have been analyzed as vaccines. *B. abortus* 2.17 and B. abortus 9.49 have been obtained from B. abortus 2308 by transposon mutagenesis and selection for polymyxin B sensitivity, and they carry the Tn5 insert (they are kanamycin resistant) in *wbkA* and per, respectively. Both are resistant to the S *Brucella* specific phages, sensitive to the R *Brucella* specific R/C phage and positive in the crystal violet and acryflavin tests and do not express O-PS. As judged by the electrophoretic mobility and the reactivity with monoclonal antibodies specific for the inner and outer core epitopes, the R-LPS of both mutants keeps an intact core oligosaccharide, which is consistent with the position of wbkA in the major O-PS genetic region and the putative role of Per. 4.6. Mutants in genes affecting the LPS core structure (27,28,29).

8.5 *B. abortus* B2211 *pgm*

This mutant carries a gentamicin-resistance non polar cassette in the *pgm* (phosphoglucomutase) gene of B. abortus 2308. It is resistant to the S-*Brucella* specific Tb phage and carries R-LPS as judged by SDS-PAGE analysis. The central role of this enzyme in the synthesis of hexoses derived from glucose makes pleiotropic effects on the synthesis of oligo- and polysaccharides likely and, at least, the pgm mutant is also blocked in the synthesisof the periplasmic β(1,2) cyclic glucans . Mutation in the homologous gene of B. melitensis causes a core defect as judged by the electrophoretic mobility in SDS-PAGE of its R-LPS (30,87,88)).

8.6 *B. abortus* mutant 80.16 wa**

This is a mutant in a putative glycosyltransferase gene involved in core synthesis (hence its provisional denomination as wa**) as shown by SDS-PAGE and Western blots with monoclonal antibodies to core epitopes. Like B. abortus 9.49, it was obtained by Tn5 transposon mutagenesis of B. abortus 2308 and selection for polymyxin B sensitivity. This mutant is resistant to kanamycin, to the S *brucella* phages, sensitive to phage R/C and does not express O-PS. A remarkable feature of the R-LPS of this mutant is that while keeping a fully reactive outer core epitope, it shows a reduced reactivity with monoclonal antibodies to the inner core epitope suggestive of a branch in the inner core in which the missing sugar(s) would be placed (29).

8.7 *B. abortus manB*core mutants

Two different mutants in this gene, both from B. abortus 2308, have been described: the *rfbK* mutant and mutant 55.30.

The mutated gene (formerly *rfbK* but *manB* according to recent nomenclature) putatively codes for a phosphomannomutase and is thus predicted to be involved in the synthesis of mannose-1-P. Although mannose-1-P is a precursor of perosamine (the O-PS sugar), the mutated gene is not homologous to the *manB* of the *wbk* region (manBOAg) and its location , the lack of reactivity with monoclonal antibodies of outer core specificity and the SDS-PAGE profile of the corresponding R-LPS show that it acts as a manBcore. This is consistent with the presence of mannose in the core of *B. abortus* (12,29,89).

9. Can proteomics help in developing vaccines to protect animals or humans against brucellosis?

The identification of immunogenic proteins will also be a further step towards the understanding of the humoral immune response during *Brucella* infections. Most studies on the antigenicity of *Brucella* proteins are either hampered by the limited number of proteins investigated or the complexity of the protein mixtures used. Differences in the seroreactivity of various protein classes are well known, e.g. cytoplasmic proteins induce a higher antibody response than outer membrane proteins. Additionally, the production of antibodies directed against proteins may be host specific, e.g. anti-OMP28 antibodies were detected in *Brucella* infected humans and goats, but not in pigs and cattle (90).

Immunoproteomics is the approach to identify specific immunogenic proteins in high resolution in the wide range of proteins expressed by *Brucella.* Previous studies of the *Brucella* proteome mainly focused on *B. melitensis* and the protein map of *B. melitensis* 16M (htpp://www.proteome.scranton.edu) may be used as a reference map for other *Brucella* spp.. However, crucial phenotypic differences responsible for host specificity, virulence, and immunogenicity may exist despite the close genetic relatedness within the genus *Brucella.* Five hundred fifty-seven protein spots representing 232 discrete ORFs were identified in B. melitensis using 2-D and MALDI-MS. Protein expression profiles of B. melitensis under various growth conditions, in wild type and attenuated vaccine strains have also been investigated. *B. abortus* proteomic studies have primarily been directed at the identification of virulence factors (Sowa et al., 1992; Lin and Ficht, 1995; Rafie-Kolpin et al., 1996). However, only one immunoproteomic study of *Brucella* has been published so far. In this, Teixeira- Gomes et al. (1997a) identified immunogenic proteins of B. ovis (91,92).

A lot of experiences have been involved in a comprehensive analysis of the *B. melitensis* 16M proteome, and initial results have been published recently. Previous proteomics studies using *B. melitensis* cells grown under different conditions have been reported, and initial work on the *B. abortus* proteome has been described. A comparative study was conducted with *B. abortus* vaccine strains S19 and RB51 and virulent strain 2308. recently, Eschenbrenner *et al.* compared the proteome of laboratory-grown strain Rev 1 to that of strain 16M by using two-dimensional (2-D) gel electrophoresis and matrix-assisted laser desorption/ionization (MALDI)-mass spectrometry (MS) to elucidate differences between the protein expression patterns of the two strains. Differentially expressed proteins were identified and grouped into three major classes: (i) protein spots unique to either 16M or Rev 1, (ii) proteins overexpressed in Rev 1, and (iii) proteins underexpressed in Rev 1 (93,94).

Comparative proteome analysis of vaccine strain Rev 1 and virulent strain 16M of *B. melitensis* indicates that the two strains have significant metabolic differences. Differentially expressed proteins involved in iron metabolism, sugar transport, lipid metabolism, and protein synthesis were identified. The expression of proteins essential for both low and high iron availability suggests a misregulated system for iron metabolism and capture, leading to possible unnecessary expenditure of energy. This may be a consequence of successive in vitro passages of *B. melitensis* in the presence of streptomycin. It is difficult to state what changes were directly or indirectly effected by this stressful growth condition. However, one plausible theory is that to compensate for these changes in gene expression, Rev 1 may have up-regulated other pathways, such as those involved in the _ oxidation of fatty acids and protein synthesis, to generate more reducing equivalents, ultimately for use in the production of ATP. These alterations would compensate for the energy loss due to misregulation of iron metabolism (72,95).

Brifly,The proteomes of selected *Brucella* spp. have been extensively analyzed by utilizing current proteomic technology involving 2-DE and MALDI-MS. In *B.* melitensis, more than 500 proteins were identified. The rapid and large-scale identification of proteins in this organism was accomplished by using the annotated *B. melitensis* genome which is now available in the GenBank. Coupled with new and powerful tools for data analysis, differentially expressed proteins were identified and categorized into several classes. A global overview of protein expression patterns emerged, thereby facilitating the simultaneous analysis of different metabolic pathways in B. melitensis. Such a global characterization would not have been possible by using time consuming and traditional biochemical approaches. The era of post-genomic technology offers new and exciting opportunities to understand the complete biology of different *Brucella* species (93,95,96).

Comprehensive proteome maps of all six *Brucella* species will be generated in order to obtain vital information for vaccine development, identification of pathogenicity islands, and establishment of host specificity and evolutionary relatedness.

10. *Brucella* subunit vaccine

Different studies have evaluated surface structures and antigens of *Brucella* as immunopotent components to design an efficient brucellosis subunit vaccine.

Currently subunit vaccines are being considered to develop effective vaccines for human which has been evidenced by vaccines currently available against the infections such as meningococcal diseases and influenza. In parallel, subunit vaccines are hot topics in the development and design of human brucellosis vaccine. Jacques et al., showed the efficacy of *Brucella* O-polysaccharide-BSA conjugate in protection against *Brucella melitensis* H38 (97). Other studies have been carried out to design subunit vaccines using other components and conjugated compounds such as porins and smooth lipopolysaccharide, recombinant ribosomal proteins and anti-OPS specific monoclonal antibodies (98, 99, 100, 101). *Brucella* antigens have been applied along with different adjuvants to augment immune responses against this organism.

The latest studies in the field of brucellosis subunit vaccines have been carried out by Bhattacharjee et al (102) and Sharifat et al. (103) have evaluated the (Group B Outer Membrane Proteins) GBOMP _ *B. melitensis* strain 16M LPS non-covalent complex to elicit the immunity against brucellosis in mice. In order to explore the efficacy of *Brucella abortus* LPS combined with different adjuvants and proteins (as a vaccine candidate) in the induction of response as an effective and long-lasting immunity against *Brucella*, Sharifat et al., evaluated and reported the outer membrane vesicles of *Neisseria meningitidis* serogroup B (GBMOMV) as a potent subcutaneous adjuvant and a part of a brucellosis candidate vaccine to induce high titres of specific anti-*Brucella abortus* S99 LPS in animal model.

The other candidate antigens are *Brucella* proteins with different cellular locations (Table 1). Four proteins are outer membrane proteins. The other nine proteins are located in cytoplasm (5 proteins), periplasm (4 proteins), and cytoplasmic membrane (1 protein) (104).

Symbol	Protein Description	Location
BLS	Brucella lumazine synthase	Cytoplasm
L7/L12	Ribosomal protein L7/L12	Cytoplasm
P39	sugar-binding 39-kDa protein	Periplasm
Bfr	Ferritin:Bacterioferritin	Cytoplasm
Bp26	Periplasmic immunogenic protein	Periplasm
DnaK	Molecular chaperone DnaK	Cytoplasm
IalB	Invasion protein B	Cytoplasmic membrane
Omp16	Outer membrane protein MotY	Outer membrane
Omp19	Lipoprotein Omp19	Outer membrane
Omp25	25 kDa outer-membrane immunogenic protein precursor	Outer membrane
Omp31	OmpA-like transmembrane domain	Outer membrane
SodC	Cu/Zn superoxide dismutase	Periplasm
SurA	Peptidyl-prolyl cis-trans isomerase	Periplasm
Tig	Trigger factor	Cytoplasm

Table 1. Brucella proteins studied as sub-unit vaccines

11. Bioinformatic application and reverse vaccinoloy

Reverse vaccinology is an emerging vaccine development approach that starts with the prediction of vaccine targets using bioinformatics screening of an entire genome of a pathogenic organism (105). Vaxign is the first web-based vaccine design program that predicts vaccine targets based on reverse vaccinology. The Vaxign computational pipeline includes the following features: subcellular localization, topology (transmembrane helices and beta barrel structure), adhesin probability, similarity to other pathogen sequences, similarity to host genome sequences (e.g., human or mouse), and MHC class I and II epitope predictions. Vaxign has been used to predict Brucella outer membrane proteins (OMP) as potential vaccine targets using B. abortus strain 2308 genome as the seed genome (106). Vaxign has identified 46 *Brucella* periplasmic proteins that are conserved in all *B. abortus, B. melitensis,* and *B. suis* genomes and lack sequence similarity with proteins in human or mouse genomes. The values of these proteins for vaccine development also deserve further analysis.

Using the same criteria (sequence conservation and dissimilarity from human or mouse proteins), Vaxign has detected approximately 1,000 cytoplasmic proteins. It is impractical to individually test this high number of proteins for vaccine development. Considering only five cytoplasmic proteins have been experimentally confirmed to be protective antigens out of 1,000 conserved cytoplasmic proteins, it is much less likely that cytoplasmic proteins serve as protective antigens compared to outer membrane and periplasmic proteins. Vaxign also contains an epitope prediction component that can predict MHC class I and II binding epitopes (107). The addition of epitope prediction allows further analysis for the existence of potential Brucella vaccine targets.

12. *Brucella* DNA vaccines

DNA vaccination is a novel and powerful method of immunization that induces both humoral and cellular (Th1 and CTL) immune responses and protection against a variety of pathogens (104). Based on the results obtained with DNA vaccines against other pathogenic intracellular bacteria, many studies of brucellosis have been conducted (108, 109, 110, 111, 112, 113, 114). These vaccines induced strong Th1 responses, and some of them conferred protection against challenge with *B. abortus* (108, 110, 112, 113, 114).

Immunization of BALB/c mice with *B. melitensis* Omp31 gene cloned in the pCI plasmid (pCIOmp31) conferred protection against *B. ovis* and B. melitensis infection. Mice vaccinated with pCIOmp31 developed a very weak humoral response, and in vitro stimulation of their splenocytes with recombinant Omp31 did not induced the secretion of gamma interferon. Splenocytes from Omp31-vaccinated animals induced a specific cytotoxic-T-lymphocyte activity, which leads to the in vitro lysis of *Brucella*-infected macrophages. pCIOmp31 immunization elicited mainly CD8_ T cells, which mediate cytotoxicity via perforins, but also CD4_ T cells, which mediate lysis via the Fas-FasL pathway. In vivo depletion of T-cell subsets showed that the pCIOmp31-induced protection against *Brucella* infection is mediated predominantly by CD8_ T cells, although CD4_T cells also contribute. Our results demonstrate that the Omp31 DNA vaccine induces cytotoxic responses that have the potential to contribute to protection against Brucella infection. The protective response could be related to the induction of CD8_ T cells that eliminate Brucella-infected cells via the perforin pathway (115).

Kurar and Splitter (110) showed that DNA vaccination with the *B. abortus* ribosomal L7/L12 gene elicits humoral and cellular immune responses and partial protection. Thus, plasmid DNA vaccination may be a successful alternative method for conferring protection against Brucella. In addition, a genetic vaccine, by inducing an immune response to a single protein, would make possible the development of diagnostic tests that could differentiate vaccinated animals from infected animal.

Velikovsky *et al.*,(113) showed that injection of plasmid DNA carrying the *Brucella abortus* lumazine synthase (BLS) gene (pcDNA-BLS) into BALB/c mice elicits both humoral and cellular immune responses. Antibodies to the encoded BLS included immunoglobulin G1 (IgG1) IgG2a, IgG2b, IgG3, and IgM isotypes. Animals injected with pcDNA-BLS exhibited a dominance of IgG2a over IgG1. pcDNA-BLS is a good immunogen for the production of humoral and cell-mediated responses in mice and is a candidate for use in future studies of vaccination against brucellosis.

Gonzalez-Smith et al (116) showed that Injection of mice with a plasmid DNA carrying the gene for superoxide dismutase (pSecTag-SOD) leads to the development of significant protection against *B. abortus* challenge. They also evaluated the effect of delivering IL-2 on the efficacy of SOD DNA vaccine by generating a plasmid (pSecTag-SOD-IL2) that codes for a secretory fusion protein of SOD and IL-2. Although mice immunized with pSecTag-SOD-IL2 showed increased resistance to challenge with *B. abortus* virulent strain 2308, this increase was not statistically significant from that of pSecTag-SOD vaccinated mice. These results suggest that a SOD DNA vaccine fused to IL2 did not improve protection efficacy (116).

DNA vaccination approaches offer the possibility of inducing both cellular and humoral responses. Approaches have varied from use of a whole library from *B. abortus* (117), overcoming the need for prior knowledge and selection of specific antigens to selection of specific candidates and their subsequent evaluation as DNA vaccines against brucellosis. Various candidates have been explored for their value as DNA vaccines against brucellosis providing various levels of protective efficacy in the mouse model (108, 111, 114, 113, 112). Disadvantages of the DNA vaccination approach are the amount of DNA required to elicit the required response, and the often disappointing results obtained following assessment of the vaccines in the target animal (118). Investigation of enhanced delivery mechanisms may overcome these issues.

The availability of the genome sequences and the application of postgenomic approaches to identify potential vaccine candidate antigens, together with the improving knowledge of the protective immune response would provide an efficient nonliving vaccine.

13. Conclusion

Brucellosis is a disease which causes economic disadvantages in developed as well as developing/ underdeveloped countries. However to overcome such economic disaster, it is essential by employing various techniques ranging from conventional techniques to advanced ones such as genetic , proteomics, metabolic engineering. However by employing such techniques it will be possible to develop a vaccine against Brucellosis either for animals or humans.

14. References

[1] Jinkyung K.,and A. S. Gary. 2003. Molecular Host-Pathogen Interaction in Brucellosis: Current Understanding and Future Approaches to Vaccine Development for Mice and Humans . Clin. Microb. Rev. 65-78

[2] Moriyon I, M.J. Grillo, D. Monreal,D. Gonzalez, C. Marin,I. Lopez-Gonii, . R.C. Mainar-Jaime, E. Moreno, and J.M. Blasco. 2004. Rough vaccines in animal brucellosis: Structural and genetic basis and present status. Vet. Res. 35 :1 38
[3] Boschiroli, M. L., V. Foulongne, and D. O Callaghan. 2001. Brucellosis: a worldwide zoonosis. Curr. Opin. Microbiol. 4:58 64.
[4] Adlimoghadam A, Hedayati M, Siadat SD, Ahmadi H, Norouzian D. 2008.Optimization of PCR Conditions for Detection of Human Brucellosis from Human Serum Samples. Res J Microbiol., 3(5):325-358.
[5] Pappas G., N. Akritidis , M. Bosilkovski , and E. Tsianos. 2005. Brucellosis. N Engl J Med .352:2325-36.
[6] Corbel, M. J., and W. J. Brinley-Morgan. 1984. Genus *Brucella*, p. 377-388. *In* N. R. Krieg (ed.), Bergey's manual of systematic bacteriology, vol. 1. Williams & Wilkins, Baltimore.
[7] Gargani G. and Lo´ pez-Merino A. 2006. International Committee on Systematic Bacteriology.Subcommittee on the taxonomy of *Brucella*. International Journal of Systematic and Evolutionary Microbiology 56: 1167 1168.
[8] Allen, C. A., L. G. Adams, and T. A. Ficht. 1998. Transposon-derived *Brucella abortus* rough mutants are attenuated and exhibit reduced intracellular survival. Infect Immun.66:1008-16.
[9] Hong, P. C., R. M. Tsolis, and T. A. Ficht. 2000. Identification of genes required for chronic persistence of *Brucella* abortus in mice. Infect. Immun. 68:4102 4107.
[10] Cloeckaert, A. 1997. Antigens of *Brucella*. The 50th Anniversary Meeting of Brucellosis Research Conference. 35-36.
[11] Cloeckaert, A., I. Jacques, R. A. Bowden, G. Dubray, and J. N. Limet. 1993. Monoclonal antibodies to *Brucella* rough lipopolysaccharide: characterization and evaluation of their protective effect against *B. abortus*. Res Microbiol. 144:475-84.
[12] Hinsdillr R.D.,Berman D.T. 1967. Antigens of *Brucella* abortus. J.Bacteriol.93(2):544-549.
[13] Cloeckaert, A., I. Jacques, N. Bosseray, J. N. Limet, R. Bowden, G. Dubray, and M. Plommet. 1991. Protection conferred on mice by monoclonal antibodies directed against outer-membrane-protein antigens of *Brucella*. J Med Microbiol. 34:175-80.
[14] Cloeckaert, A., A. Tibor, and M. S. Zygmunt. 1999. *Brucella* outer membrane lipoproteins share antigenic determinants with bacteria of the family Rhizobiaceae. Clin Diagn Lab Immunol. 6:627-9.
[15] Cloeckaert A., M.S. Zygmunt, and L.A. Guilloteau. 2002. *Brucella* abortus vaccine strain RB51 roduces low levels of M-like O-antigen, Vaccine. 20: 1820–1822.
[16] Sharifat Salmani A, Siadat SD, Fallahian MR, Ahmadi H, Norouzian D, Yaghmai P, Aghasadeghi MR, Izadi Mobarakeh J, Sadat SM, Zangeneh M, Kheirandish M. 2009. Serological Evaluation of *Brucella abortus* S99 Lipopolysaccharide Extracted by an Optimized Method. American Journal of Infectious Disease. 5(1): 11-16.
[17] Diaz, R., L. M. Jones, D. Leong, and J. B. Wilson. 1968. Surface antigens of smooth *Brucellae*. J Bacteriol. 96:893-901.
[18] Reeves P.R., M. Hobbs, M.A. Valvano, M.Skurnik, C. Whitfiled, D. Coplin, N. Kido, J. Klena, D. Klena, D. Masklell, C.R. Raetz, and P.D. Rick. 1996.Bacterial polysaccharide synthesis and gene nomenclature, Trends Microbiol.4:495-503.
[19] Godfroid F., B. Taminiau, I. Danese , P.A. Denoel , A. Tibor , V.E. Weynants, A. loeckaert A.,J. Godfroid, and J.J. Letesson , Identification of the perosamine synthetase gene of *Brucella* melitensis 16M and involvement of lipopolysaccharide

O side chain in *Brucella* survival in mice and in macrophages, Infect. Immun. 66 (1998) 5485–5493.

[20] Godfroid F., A. Cloeckaert, B. Taminiau, I. Danese, A. Tibor, X. de Bolle, P. Mertens, and J.J. Letesson. 2000. Genetic organisation of the lipopolysaccharide O-antigen biosynthesis region of *Brucella* melitensis 16M (wbk), Res. Microbiol. 151 : 655–668.

[21] Monreal D., M.J. Grillo, D. Gonzalez, C.M. Marin, M.J. de Miguel, I. Lopez-Goni, J.M. Blasco, A. Cloeckaert, and I. Moriyon. 2003. Characterization of *Brucella* abortus O-Polysaccharide and core lipopolysaccharide mutants and demonstration that a complete core is required for rough vaccines to be efficient against *Brucella* abortus and *Brucella* ovis in the mouse model, Infect. Immun. 71: 3261–3271.

[22] Sharifat Salmani A, Siadat SD, Norouzian D, Nejati M, Izadi Mobarakeh J, Kheirandish M, Zangeneh M, Aghasadeghi MR, Mehdi Nejati, Hedayati MH, Arfa Moshiri A, Sadat SM. 2009. Outer Membrane Vesicle of *Neisseria meningitidis* Serogroup B as an Adjuvant to Induce Specific Antibody Response against the Lipopolysaccharide of Brucella abortus S99. Annals of Microbiology. 59(1): 145-149.

[23] Bachrach, G., M. Banai, S. Bardenstein, G. Hoida, A. Genizi, and H. Bercovier. 1994. *Brucella* ribosomal protein L7/L12 is a major component in the antigenicity of brucellin INRA for delayed-type hypersensitivity in *Brucella* sensitized guinea pigs. Infect Immun. 62:5361-6.

[24] Bachrach, G., D. Bar-Nir, M. Banai, and H. Bercovier. 1994. Identification and nucleotide sequence of *Brucella melitensis* L7/L12 ribosomal protein. FEMS Microbiol Lett. 120:237-40.

[25] Bae, J. 1999. Generation of baculovirus-*Brucella abortus* heat shock protein recombinants; mice immune responses against the recombinants, and *B. abortus* superoxide dismutase and L7/L12 recombinant proteins. Ph.D. dissertation. Virginia Polytechnic Institute and State University, Blacksburg, VA.

[26] Karami S1, Siadat SD, Tabaraie B, Norouzian D, Harzandi N, Aghasadeghi MR, Razavi MR, Sadat SM , Sharifat Salmani A, Nejati M , Kordafshari AR , Moshiri A. 2009.Extraction and Molecular Determination of Major Outer Membrane Proteins of Brucella abortus S99. Feyz, Journal of Kashan University of Medical Sciences, 13(3): 174-179.

[27] Ekaza, E., L. Guilloteau, J. Teyssier, J. P. Liautard, and S. Kohler. 2000. Functional analysis of the ClpATPase ClpA of *Brucella* suis, and persistence of a knockout mutant in BALB/c mice. Microbiology 146:1605 1616.

[28] Robertson, G. T., M. E. Kovach, C. A. Allen, T. A. Ficht, and R. M. Roop, Jr. 2000. The *Brucella* abortus Lon functions as a generalized stress response protease and is required for wild-type virulence in BALB/c mice. Mol. Microbiol. 35:577 -588.

[29] Adams, L. G. 1997. Pathology of brucellosis in domestic animals: a minireview. 50th Anniversary Meeting of Brucellosis Research Conference.44-49.

[30] Sangari, F. J., and J. Aguero. 1996. Molecular basis of *Brucella* pathogenicity: an update. Microbiologia 12:207 218.

[31] Pizarro-Cerda, J., S. Meresse, R. G. Parton, G. van der Goot, A. Sola-Landa, I. Lopez-Goni, E. Moreno, and J. P. Gorvel. 1998. *Brucella abortus* transits through the autophagic pathway and replicates in the endoplasmic reticulum of nonprofessional phagocytes. Infect Immun. 66:5711-24.

[32] Pizarro-Cerda, J., E. Moreno, V. Sanguedolce, J. L. Mege, and J. P. Gorvel. 1998. Virulent *Brucella abortus* prevents lysosome fusion and is distributed within autophagosome-like compartments. Infect Immun. 66:2387-92.

[33] Lin, J., and T. A. Ficht. 1995. Protein synthesis in *Brucella abortus* induced during macrophage infection. Infect Immun. 63:1409-14.

[34] Zygmunt, M. S., F. B. Gilbert, and G. Dubray. 1992. Purification, characterization, and seroactivity of a 20-kilodalton *Brucella* protein antigen. J. Clin. Microbiol. 30:2662-2667.

[35] Tatum, F. M., N. F. Cheville, and D. Morfitt. 1994. Cloning, characterization and construction of *htrA* and *htrA*-like mutants of *Brucella abortus* and their survival in BALB/c mice. Microb Pathog. 17:23-36.

[36] Tatum, F. M., P. G. Detilleux, J. M. Sacks, and S. M. Halling. 1992. Construction of Cu-Zn superoxide dismutase deletion mutants of *Brucella* abortus: analysis of survival in vitro in epithelial and phagocytic cells and in vivo in mice. Infect. Immun. 60:2863-2869.

[37] Sola-Landa, A., J. Pizarro-Cerda, M. J. Grillo, E. Moreno, I. Moriyon, J. M. Blasco, J. P. Gorvel, and I. Lopez-Goni. 1998. A two-component regulatory system playing a critical role in plant pathogens and endosymbionts is present in *Brucella abortus* and controls cell invasion and virulence. Mol Microbiol. 29:125-38.

[38] Canning, P. C., J. A. Roth, and B. L. Deyoe. 1986. Release of 5'-guanosine monophosphate and adenine by *Brucella abortus* and their role in the intracellular survival of the bacteria. J Infect Dis. 154:464-70.

[39] O Callaghan, D., C. Cazevieille, A. Allardet-Servent, M. L. Boschiroli, G. Bourg, V. Foulongne, P. Frutos, Y. Kulakov, and M. Ramuz. 1999. A homologue of the Agrobacterium tumefaciens VirB and Bordetella pertussis Pt1 type IV secretion systems is essential for intracellular survival of *Brucella* suis. Mol. Microbiol. 33:1210 -1220.

[40] Caron, E., T. Peyrard, S. Kohler, S. Cabane, J. P. Liautard, and J. Dornand. 1994. Live *Brucella* spp. fail to induce tumor necrosis factor alpha excretion upon infection of U937-derived phagocytes. Infect Immun. 62:5267-74.

[41] Cheville, N. F., A. E. Jensen, S. M. Halling, F. M. Tatum, D. C. Morfitt, S. G.Hennager, W. M. Frerichs, and G. Schurig. 1992. Bacterial survival, lymph node changes, and immunologic responses of cattle vaccinated with standard and mutant strains of *Brucella abortus*. Am J Vet Res. 53:1881-8.

[42] Alton, G. G., S. S. Elberg, and D. Crouch. 1967. Rev. 1 *Brucella melitensis* vaccine. The stability of the degree of attenuation. J Comp Pathol. 77:293-300.

[43] Alton, G. G., L. A. Corner, and P. Plackett. 1983. Vaccination of cattle against brucellosis using either a reduced dose of strain 19 or one or two doses of 45/20 vaccine. Aust Vet J. 60:175-7.

[44] Chukwu, C. C. 1985. Serological investigation on cattle vaccinated with a killed *Brucella abortus* strain 45/20 adjuvant vaccine. Int J Zoonoses. 12:14-21.

[45] Cloeckaert, A., H. S. Debbarh, M. S. Zygmunt, and G. Dubray. 1996. Production and characterisation of monoclonal antibodies to *Brucella melitensis* cytosoluble proteins thatare able to differentiate antibody responses of infected sheep from Rev. 1 vaccinated sheep. J Med Microbiol. 45:206-13.

[46] Wyn-Jones, G., J. R. Baker, and P. M. Johnson. 1980. A clinical and immunopathological study of *Brucella abortus* strain S19 induced arthritis in cattle. Vet Rec. 107:5-9.

[47] Nielsen, K., and J. R. Duncan. 1988. Antibody isotype response in adult cattle vaccinated with *Brucella abortus* S19. Vet Immunol Immunopathol. 19:205-14.

[48] Herr, S., and L. A. Te Brugge. 1985. Profiles of serological reactions following adult cow inoculation with standard dose *Brucella abortus* strain 19 vaccine. J S Afr Vet Assoc. 56:93-6.

[49] Alton, G. G., L. A. Corner, and P. Plackett. 1980. Vaccination of pregnant cows with low doses of *Brucella abortus* strain 19 vaccine. Aust Vet J. 56:369-72.

[50] Corner, L. A., and G. G. Alton. 1981. Persistence of *Brucella abortus* strain 19 infection in adult cattle vaccinated with reduced doses. Res Vet Sci. 31:342-4.

[51] Beckett, F. W., and S. C. MacDiarmid. 1987. Persistent serological titres following reduced dose *Brucella abortus* strain 19 vaccination. Br Vet J. 143:477-9.

[52] Erasmus, J. A., and M. C. Erasmus. 1987. The use of reduced-dose *Brucella abortus* strain 19 vaccine in the control of bovine brucellosis. J S Afr Vet Assoc. 58:71-5.

[53] Campero, C. M., P. W. Ladds, D. Hoffmann, B. Duffield, D. Watson, and G. Fordyce. 1990. Immunopathology of experimental *Brucella abortus* strain 19 infection of the genitalia of bulls. Vet Immunol Immunopathol. 24:235-46.

[54] Gulasekharam, J. 1970. Illness following accidental self-inoculation of *Brucella abortus* strain 19 vaccine. Med J Aust. 2:642-3.

[55] Pivnick, H., H. Worton, D. L. Smith, and D. Barnum. 1966. Infection of veterinarians in Ontario by *Brucella abortus* strain 19. Can J Public Health. 57:225-31.

[56] Vincent, P., L. Joubert, and M. Prave. 1970. [2 occupational cases of *Brucella* infection after inoculation of B 19 vaccine]. Bull Acad Vet Fr. 43:89-97.

[57] Cheville, N. F., M. G. Stevens, A. E. Jensen, F. M. Tatum, and S. M. Halling. 1993. Immune responses and protection against infection and abortion in cattle experimentally vaccinated with mutant strains of *Brucella abortus*. Am J Vet Res. 54:1591-7.

[58] Schurig, G. G., R. M. d. Roop, T. Bagchi, S. Boyle, D. Buhrman, and N. Sriranganathan. 1991. Biological properties of RB51; a stable rough strain of *Brucella abortus*. Vet Microbiol. 28:171-88.

[59] USDA-APHIS. 1998. Brucellosis eradication: uniform methods and rules APHIS 91-45-011.

[60] Lord, V. R., G. G. Schurig, J. W. Cherwonogrodzky, M. J. Marcano, and G. E.Melendez. 1998. Field study of vaccination of cattle with *Brucella abortus* strains RB51and 19 under high and low disease prevalence. Am J Vet Res. 59:1016-20.

[61] Olsen, S. C., M. G. Stevens, N. F. Cheville, and G. Schurig. 1997. Experimental use of a dot-blot assay to measure serologic responses of cattle vaccinated with *Brucella abortus* strain RB51. J Vet Diagn Invest. 9:363-7.

[62] Jensen, A. E., N. F. Cheville, D. R. Ewalt, J. B. Payeur, and C. O. Thoen. 1995. Application of pulsed-field gel electrophoresis for differentiation of vaccine strain RB51 from field isolates of *Brucella abortus* from cattle, bison, and elk. Am J Vet Res. 56:308- 12.

[63] Vemulapalli, R., J. R. McQuiston, G. G. Schurig, N. Sriranganathan, S. M. Halling, and S. M. Boyle. 1999. Identification of an IS711 element interrupting the wboA gene of *Brucella abortus* vaccine strain RB51 and a PCR assay To distinguish strain RB51 from other *Brucella* species and strains. Clin Diagn Lab Immunol. 6:760-4.

[64] DelVecchio V.G., M.A. Wagner, M. Eschenbrenner, T.A. Horn, J.A. Kraycer, F. Estock, P. Elzer,and C.V. Mujer, 2002. *Brucella* proteomes a review. Vet. Microbiol. 90, 593.

[65] Jimenez de Bagues, M. P., P. H. Elzer, S. M. Jones, J. M. Blasco, F. M. Enright, G. G. Schurig, and A. J. Winter. 1994. Vaccination with *Brucella abortus* rough mutant RB51 protects BALB/c mice against virulent strains of *Brucella abortus*, *Brucella melitensis*, and *Brucella ovis*. Infect Immun. 62:4990-6.

[66] Alton, G. G. 1987. Control of *Brucella melitensis* infection in sheep and goats-a review. Trop Anim Health Prod. 19:65-74.
[67] Alton, G. G. 1966. Duration of the immunity produced in goats by the Rev. 1 *Brucella melitensis* vaccine. J Comp Pathol. 76:241-53.
[68] Blasco, J. M. 1997. A review of the use of B. melitensis Rev 1 vaccine in adult sheep and goats. Prev. Vet. Med. 31:275 283.
[69] Hoover, D. L., R. M. Crawford, L. L. Van De Verg, M. J. Izadjoo, A. K. Bhattacharjee, C. M. Paranavitana, R. L. Warren, M. P. Nikolich, and T. L. Hadfield. 1999. Protection of mice against brucellosis by vaccination with *Brucella* melitensis WR201(16M purEK). Infect. Immun. 67:5877 5884.
[70] Sharifat Salmani A, Siadat SD, Norouzian D, Ahmadi H, Nejati M, Tabaraie B, Atyabi SM , Zangeneh M, Mohabati Mobarez A ,Shapouri R, Mehdi Abbasi M and Karbasian M.2008. Optimization of Brucella abortus S99 Lipopolysaccharide Extraction by Phenol and Butanol Methods. Res J Bio Sci. 3(6): 576-580.
[71] Boschiroli, M. L., S. L. Cravero, A. I. Arese, E. Campos, and O. L. Rossetti. 1997. Protection against infection in mice vaccinated with a *Brucella abortus* mutant. Infect Immun. 65:798-800.
[72] Anonymous. 1998. Human exposure to *Brucella abortus* strain RB51--Kansas, 1997. MMWR Morb Mortal Wkly Rep. 47:172-5.
[73] Brew, S. D., L. L. Perrett, J. A. Stack, A. P. MacMillan, and N. J. Staunton. 1999.Human exposure to *Brucella* recovered from a sea mammal [letter]. Vet Rec. 144:483.
[74] Bricker, B. J., L. B. Tabatabai, B. A. Judge, B. L. Deyoe, and J. E. Mayfield. 1990.Cloning, expression, and occurrence of the *Brucella* Cu-Zn superoxide dismutase. Infect Immun. 58:2935-9.
[75] Fernandez-Prada, C. M., M. Nikolich, R. Vemulapalli, N. Sriranganathan, S. M. Boyle, G. G. Schurig, T. L. Hadfield, and D. L. Hoover. 2001. Deletion of wboA enhances activation of the lectin pathway of complement in *Brucella* abortus and *Brucella* melitensis. Infect. Immun. 69:4407 4416.
[76] Van, M. D., G. A. Kennedy, S. C. Olsen, G. R. Hansen, and D. R. Ewalt.1999. Brucellosis induced by RB51 vaccine in a pregnant heifer. J. Am. Vet.Med. Assoc. 215:1491 1493, 1449.
[77] Schurig G.G., N. Sriranganathan and M.J Corbel. Brucellosis vaccines: past, present and future. Vet Microbiol 2002;90:479-96.
[78] Winter, A. J., G. G. Schurig, S. M. Boyle, N. Sriranganathan, J. A. Bevins, F. M. Enright, P. H. Elzer, and J. D. Kopec. 1996. Protection of BALB/c mice against homologous and heterologous species of *Brucella* by rough strain vaccines derived from *Brucella* melitensis and *Brucella* suis biovar 4.Am. J. Vet. Res. 57:677- 683.
[79] Briones G.C., Iñón de Iannino N., Roset M., Vigliocco A.M., Paulo P.S., Ugalde R.A.,2001. *Brucella* abortus cyclic beta-1,2-glucan mutants have reduced virulence in mice and are defective in intracellular replication in HeLa cells, Infect. Immun. 69 4528- 4535.
[80] Ciuchini F., Adone R., Pasquali P. 2002. Coombs antiglobulin test using *Brucella* abortus 99 as antigen to detect incomplete antibodies induced by *B. abortus* RB51 vaccine in cattle, Clin. Diagn. Lab. Immunol. 9 : 1398- 1399.
[81] Adams L.G., Ficht T.A., Allen C.A., 1999. Derivation and evaluation of the rough rfbk brucellosis vaccine in cattle, in: Anonymous (Ed.), Memorias del III Foro Nacional de Brucelosis (20–21 July 1998), Acapulco, México, pp. 141–158.
[82] Dahouk S.A, , No¨ ckler K, Scholz H. C., H. Tomaso, R. Bogumil, and H .Neubauer. 2006. Immunoproteomic characterization of *Brucella* abortus 1119-3 preparations

used for the serodiagnosis of *Brucella* infections. J Immu. Mthods 309:34- 47.5. 91. Araya, L. N., and A. J. Winter. 1990. Comparative protection of mice against virulent and attenuated strains of *Brucella abortus* by passive transfer of immune T cells or serum. Infect Immun. 58:254-6.

[83] Chirhart-Gilleland, R. L., M. E. Kovach, P. H. Elzer, S. R. Jennings, and R. M.Roop, 2nd. 1998. Identification and characterization of a 14-kilodalton *Brucella abortus* protein reactive with antibodies from naturally and experimentally infected hosts and T lymphocytes from experimentally infected BALB/c mice. Infect Immun. 66:4000- 3.

[84] Teixeira-Gomes, A. P., A. Cloeckaert, G. Bezard, R. A. Bowden, G. Dubray, and M. S. Zygmunt. 1997. Identification and characterization of *Brucella* ovis immunogenic proteins using two-dimensional electrophoresis and immunoblotting. Electrophoresis 18:1491-1497.

[85] Cheville, N. F., S. C. Olsen, A. E. Jensen, M. G. Stevens, A. M. Florance, H. S. Houng, E. S. Drazek, R. L. Warren, T. L. Hadfield, and D. L. Hoover. 1996. Bacterial persistence and immunity in goats vaccinated with a *purE* deletion mutant or the parental 16M strain of *Brucella melitensis*. Infect Immun. 64:2431-9.

[86] Eschenbrenner, M., Wagner, M.A., Horn, T.A., Kraycer, J.A., Mujer, C.V., Hagius, S., Elzer, P., DelVecchio, V.G., 2002. Comparative proteome analysis of *Brucella* melitensis vaccine strain Rev 1 and a virulent strain 16M. J. Bacteriol. 184, 4962.

[87] Wagner, M.A., Eschenbrenner, M., Horn, T.A., Kraycer, J.A., Mujer, C.V., Hagius, S., Elzer, P., DelVecchio, V.G., 2002. Global analysis of the *Brucella* melitensis proteome: identification of proteins expressed in laboratory-grown culture. Proteomics 2,1047.

[88] Jacques I., Olivier-Bernardin V., Dubray G.1991. Induction of antibody and protective responses in mice by Brucella O-polysaccharide-BSA conjugate. Vaccine, 9:896-900.

[89] Cloeckaert A., Jacques I., De Wergifosse P., Dubray G., Limet J.N, 1992. Protection against Brucella melitensis and Brucella abortus in mice with immunoglobulin G (IgG), IgA, and IgM monoclonal antibodies specific for a common epitope shared by the Brucella A and M smooth lipopolysaccharide. Infect. Immun., 60: 312-315.

[90] Cloeckaert A., Zygmunt M.S., Dubray G., Limet J.N, 1993. Characterization of O-polysaccharide-specific monoclonal antibodies derived from mice infected with the rough Brucella melitensis strain B115. J. Gen. Microbiol., 139: 1551-1556.

[91] Oliveira S.C., Splitter G.A, 1996. Immunization of mice with recombinant L7/L12 ribosomal protein confers protection against Brucella abortus infection. Vaccine, 14: 959-962.

[92] Winter A.J., Rowe G.E., Duncan J.R., Eis M.J., Widom J., Ganem B., Morein B, 1988. Effectiveness of natural and synthetic complexes of porin and O-polysaccharide as vaccines against Brucella abortus in mice. Infect. Immun., 56: 2808-2817.

[93] Bhattacharjee A.K., Van De Verg L.V., Izadjoo M.J., Yuan L., Hadfield T.L., Zollinger W.D., Hoover D.L. 2002. Protection of mice against brucellosis by intranasal immunization with *Brucella melitensis* lipopolysaccharide as a noncovalent complex with *Neisseria meningitidis* group B outer membrane protein. Infect. Immun., 70: 3324-3329.

[94] Sharifat Salmani A, Siadat S.D, Norouzian D, Izadi Mobarakeh J, Kheirandish M, Zangeneh M, Aghasadeghi M.R, Nejati M, Hedayati M.H, Moshiri A, Sadat S.M, 2009. Outer membrane vesicle of Neisseria meningitidis serogroup B as an adjuvant to induce specific antibody response against the lipopolysaccharide of Brucella abortus S99. Annals of Microbiol, 59 (1) 145-149.

[95] He Y and Xiang Z. 2010.Bioinformatics analysis of Brucella vaccines and vaccine targets using VIOLIN. Immunome Research 2010, 6(Suppl 1):S5
[96] Rappuoli R: Reverse vaccinology. 2000. Curr Opin Microbiol, 3(5):445-450.
[97] Chain PS, Comerci DJ, Tolmasky ME, Larimer FW, Malfatti SA, Vergez LM, Aguero F, Land ML, Ugalde RA, Garcia E: Whole-genome analyses of speciation events in pathogenic Brucellae. Infect Immun 2005, 73(12):8353-8361.
[98] He Y, Xiang Z, Mobley HL: Vaxign: the first web-based vaccine design program for reverse vaccinology and applications for vaccine development. 2010. J of Biomed and Biotech,Article ID 297505, 15 pages.
[99] Gurunathan, S., C. Y. Wu, B. L. Freidag, and R. A. Seder. 2000. DNA vaccines: a key for inducing long-term cellular immunity. Curr. Opin. Immunol. 12:442–447.
[100] Al-Mariri, A., A. Tibor, P. Mertens, X. De Bolle, P. Michel, J. Godfroid, K. Walravens, and J. J. Letesson. 2001. Induction of immune response in BALB/c mice with a DNA vaccine encoding bacterioferritin or P39 of Brucella spp. Infect. Immun. 69:6264–6270.
[101] Cassataro, J., C. A. Velikovsky, G. H. Giambartolomei, S. Estein, L. Bruno, A. Cloeckaert, R. A. Bowden, M. Spitz, and C. A. Fossati. 2002. Immunogenicity of the Brucella melitensis recombinant ribosome recycling factor-homologous protein and its cDNA. Vaccine 20:1660–1669.
[102] Kurar, E., and G. A. Splitter. 1997. Nucleic acid vaccination of Brucella abortus ribosomal L7/L12 gene elicits immune response. Vaccine 15:1851–1857.
[103] Leclerq, S., J. S. Harms, G. M. Rosinha, V. Azevedo, and S. C. Oliveira. 2002. Induction of a Th1-type of immune response but not protective immunity by intramuscular DNA immunisation with Brucella abortus GroEL heat-shock gene. J. Med. Microbiol. 51:20–26.
[104] Munoz-Montesino, C., E. Andrews, R. Rivers, A. Gonzalez-Smith, G. Moraga-Cid, H. Folch, S. Cespedes, and A. A. Onate. 2004. Intraspleen delivery of a DNA vaccine coding for superoxide dismutase (SOD) of Brucella abortus induces SOD-specific CD4_ and CD8_ T cells. Infect. Immun. 72:2081–2087.
[105] Onate, A. A., S. Cespedes, A. Cabrera, R. Rivers, A. Gonzalez, C. Munoz, H. Folch, and E. Andrews. 2003. A DNA vaccine encoding Cu, Zn superoxide dismutase of Brucella abortus induces protective immunity in BALB/c mice. Infect. Immun. 71:4857–4861.
[106] Velikovsky, C. A., J. Cassataro, G. H. Giambartolomei, F. A. Goldbaum, S. Estein, R. A. Bowden, L. Bruno, C. A. Fossati, and M. Spitz. 2002. A DNA vaccine encoding lumazine synthase from Brucella abortus induces protective immunity in BALB/c mice. Infect Immun. 70:2507–2511.
[107] Cassataro J, A. Velikovsky C,De la Barrera S, M. Estein S, Bruno L, Bowden R, A. Pasquevich K, A. Fossati C and H. Giambartolomei G. 2005. A DNA Vaccine Coding for the Brucella Outer Membrane Protein 31 Confers Protection against B. melitensis and B. ovis Infection by Eliciting a Specific Cytotoxic Response. INFECT IMMUN. 6537–6546.
[108] González-Smith A, Vemulapalli R, Andrews E and Oñate A. 2005. Evaluation of Brucella abortus DNA vaccine by expression of Cu–Zn superoxide dismutase antigen fused to IL-2. Immunobiology. 2006; 211(1-2):65-74.
[109] Leclercq, S.Y. and Oliveira, S.C. (2003) Protective immunity induced by DNA-library immunization against an intracellular bacterial infection. J Drug Target 11, 531–538.
[110] Babiuk, L., Pontarollo, R., Babiuk, S., Loehr, B. and van Drunen Littel-van den Hurk, S. 2003. Induction of immune responses by DNA vaccines in large animals. Vaccine 21, 649–658.

10

Insights into Leptospirosis, a Neglected Disease

Manjula Sritharan
*Department of Animal Sciences,
University of Hyderabad, Hyderabad,
India*

1. Introduction

Leptospirosis is a zoonotic disease affecting man and animals worldwide. The causative organisms are the pathogenic members of the spirochetes belonging to the genus *Leptospira* [Bharti et al., 2003; Levett, 2001]. The disease, more prevalent in tropical regions, especially in developing and under-developed countries has remained largely unnoticed due to poor diagnosis. This zoonotic disease is predominantly an occupational disease affecting farmers and others working in close association with animals. It has also been reported in events like water sports, swimming and other recreational activities. In the past decade there were several outbreaks of the disease occurring globally after natural calamities like floods and cyclones. Leptospirosis occurs both in rural and urban environments with wet and humid conditions favouring its transmission. Humans are accidental hosts whereas wild, domestic and peri-domestic animals serve as reservoir hosts with rodents playing a major role in the transmission of the disease. The infected animals shed the organisms via urine into the immediate environment and humans acquire the infection, either directly from the animals or indirectly from the contaminated environment.

In 1886, Adolf Weil first reported leptospirosis (see Box 1 for a historical perspective of the disease) as a syndrome characterized by splenomegaly, jaundice and nephritis that is now commonly reported as Weil's disease and is synonymous with leptospirosis [Levett, 2001]. In several countries in the Southeast Asia region, the disease is endemic but is grossly under-reported as the protean clinical manifestations are difficult to differentiate from other diseases like influenza (commonly called 'flu'), dengue and malaria and due to the lack of simple, rapid and efficient tests for early diagnosis. The need of the hour is a better understanding of host-pathogen interactions; unravelling the complex mechanisms elaborated by the pathogen to establish infection and the diverse efforts of the mammalian host to contain the pathogen and prevent disease development will aid in the identification of potential vaccine and diagnostic candidates. This is now possible with significant advances in the field of leptospirosis, especially the sequencing of several leptospiral genomes providing better insights into the biology of the causative organisms and the development of better genetic tools for *Leptospira* spp.

Box 1: Leptospira and leptospirosis: a historical reflection

Several years after the first clinical reporting of the disease by Adolf Weil (1886), Inada and Ido (1915) demonstrated leptospires as the causative organisms for this disease [Inada et al., 1995]. Unfortunately, the sentinel observations made by Stimson [Stimson, 1907] went unrecognized. He demonstrated the presence of spirochetes in renal tubule specimens from a patient diagnosed to have died of yellow fever and called them *Spirocheta interrogans,* as the hook at the ends resembles a question mark. The free-living or the saprophytic counterparts of these organisms were found in fresh water and were called as *Spirocheta biflexa* [Walbach and Binger, 1914]. Ido and his group (1917) unequivocally proved the role of rats in the transmission of the disease to humans that led to the establishment of leptospirosis as a zoonotic disease. The disease came to be recognised as an occupational disease and was referred to as *'akiyami'* the harvest fever in Japan, cane cutter's disease in Australia, rice field leptospirosis in Indonesia and so on. The disease was reported in India, as early as 1903 by Chowdry (as reported by [Vijayachari et al., 2008]. An extensive and detailed account of the disease was documented by Taylor & Goyle [Taylor and Goyle, 1931] in the Andaman archipelago. Today, the leptospiral etiology of the 'Andaman fever' or 'Andaman haemorrhagic fever' (AHF) accounting for several deaths in the Andaman & Nicobar Islands, India is well known. The contribution of Faine and his group in the understanding of the basic biology of these organisms, identification of multitude of serovars and the range of mammalian hosts, including humans, wild and domestic animals contributed significantly to the field of leptospirosis. Subsequent years focused on leptospiral proteins, including LipL41 & Omp1 [Haake et al., 1993; Haake et al., 1999], LipL32 [Haake et al., 2000], LigA & LigB proteins [Koizumi and Watanabe, 2004; Matsunaga et al., 2003], HbpA [Sritharan et al., 2005], [Asuthkar, 2007]. Ren et al [Ren et al., 2003] was the first to sequence the genome of the pathogenic *L. interrogans* serovar Lai to be followed by others deciphering the genome of Copenhageni [Nascimento et al., 2004], two strains of serovar Hardjo belonging to *L. borgpetersenii* [Bulach et al., 2006] and the non-pathogenic *L. biflexa* serovar Patoc [Picardeau et al., 2008]. Today we have before us a vast amount of information on these organisms that needs to be mined towards development of better control measures.

2. Biology of leptospires

2.1 General features

Leptospires are obligate aerobic spirochetes with characteristic hooks at their ends. They are thin (0·25 μm) and long (6-25 μm) and can easily pass through 0.2 μM filters. These highly motile organisms showing the characteristic cork-screw movement include the pathogenic and saprophytic members (see Box 2 for classification); the former are usually shorter than the non-pathogenic members.

As these organisms are too thin, it is difficult to visualise them by the conventional stains, though occasionally silver staining is used. The characteristic cork-screw movement of these organisms in thin wet preparations makes it possible to view these organisms by dark field and phase-contrast microscopy.

Box 2: Classification of *Leptospira* spp.
Taxonomically, *Leptospira* are classified as Gracillicutes (Division), Scotobacteria (Class), Spirochaetales (Order), *Leptospiraceae* (Family) and *Leptospira* (Genus) [Paster and Dewhirst, 2000]. In addition to the genus *Leptospira*, the genera *Leptonema* and *Turneria* are included in the family *Leptospiraceae*. The different members of the genus *Leptospira* are classified based on their antigen-relateness (serological) or DNA-relatedness (molecular) as detailed below:

- **Serological classification:** Earlier classification, still used in epidemiological studies was based on antigen-relatedness. Broadly, pathogenic *Leptospira* were grouped as belonging to *Leptospira interrogans* and the non-pathogenic as *Leptospira biflexa*. The former includes more than 200 serovars, classified on the basis of structural heterogeneity in the carbohydrate component of the lipopolysaccharide [Bharti et al., 2003; Levett, 2001; Vijayachari et al., 2008] that resulted in the generation of specific antibodies in the mammalian host. The non-pathogenic *L. biflexa* consists of about 60 serovars. The newly added members include the serovars Sichvan (serogroup Sichvan), Hurstbridge (serogroup Hurstbridge) and Portblairi (serogroup Sehgali) [Brenner et al., 1999; Vijayachari et al., 2004].
- **Molecular / genotypic classification:** The current classification is based on DNA-relatedness. In the Subcommittee on the Taxonomy of *Leptospiraceae* held in Quito, Ecuador in 2007, it was decided to group them as species [Adler and Moctezuma, 2010]. The saprophytic species include *Leptospira biflexa, Leptospira wolbachii, Leptospira kmetyi, Leptospira meyeri, Leptospira vanthielii, Leptospira terpstrae* and *Leptospira yanagawae*. The pathogenic species include *Leptospira interrogans, Leptospira kirschneri, Leptospira borgpetersenii, Leptospira santarosai, Leptospira noguchii, Leptospira weilii, Leptospira alexanderi* and *Leptospira alstoni*. An additional group comprising of *Leptospira inadai, Leptospira broomii, Leptospira fainei, Leptospira wolffii* and *Leptospira licerasiae* consisted of species of unclear pathogenicity [Ko et al., 2009].

Molecular classification allows for the clear identification of distinct subtypes. For example, Hardjoprajitno and Hardjobovis, grouped earlier under serovar Hardjo now belong to *L. interrogans* and *L. borgpetersenii*.

**Historically, the first leptospiral strain reported by Inada and Ido (1915) was called as Spirochaeta Icterohaemorrhagiae japonica.*

2.2 Growth and culture conditions

Leptospires grow relatively slowly with a doubling time of approximately 6 - 8 hours. *In vitro* cultures are usually maintained at temperatures between 28° - 30°C. They have simple, but unique nutritional requirements. They utilize long-chain fatty acids as the carbon and energy source and require vitamins B1 & B12 as growth factors. Tween 80 is commonly used in artificial culture media as the source of carbon and it is necessary to include bovine serum albumin (BSA) to bind the free fatty acids that are toxic to these organisms. 10% rabbit serum is added in certain media, as a rich source of vitamins and albumin promotes the growth of these organisms [Ellis and Michno, 1976; Johnson and Gary, 1963a, b]. The conventional media for growing leptospires include the bovine serum albumin-based Ellinghausen-McCullough-Johnson-Harris (EMJH) medium [Ellinghausen and McCullough, 1965] and serum-containing Korthof's and Fletcher's media. Liquid media is used for propagating the organisms and long-term maintenance is done in semi-solid medium containing 0.1 - 0.2% agar, in which the organisms grow sub-surface and appear as an opaque mass called the 'Dinger's ring'. Leptospira are not affected by 5-fluorouracil and thus media can be made selective for the growth of leptospires from clinical specimens by the addition of 5-fluoruracil and neomycin sulphate [Ellis and Michno, 1976].

2.3 Membrane architecture and membrane proteins

Leptospira exhibits a surface architecture that resembles Gram-negative bacteria and consists of the outer membrane, the periplasmic region and the inner cytoplasmic membrane (Fig. 1). The peptidoglycan layer however is closely associated with the cytoplasmic membrane, unlike in other Gram-negative bacteria where it is located close to the outer membrane [Adler and Moctezuma, 2010]. The two internal flagella (endoflagella), arising from each

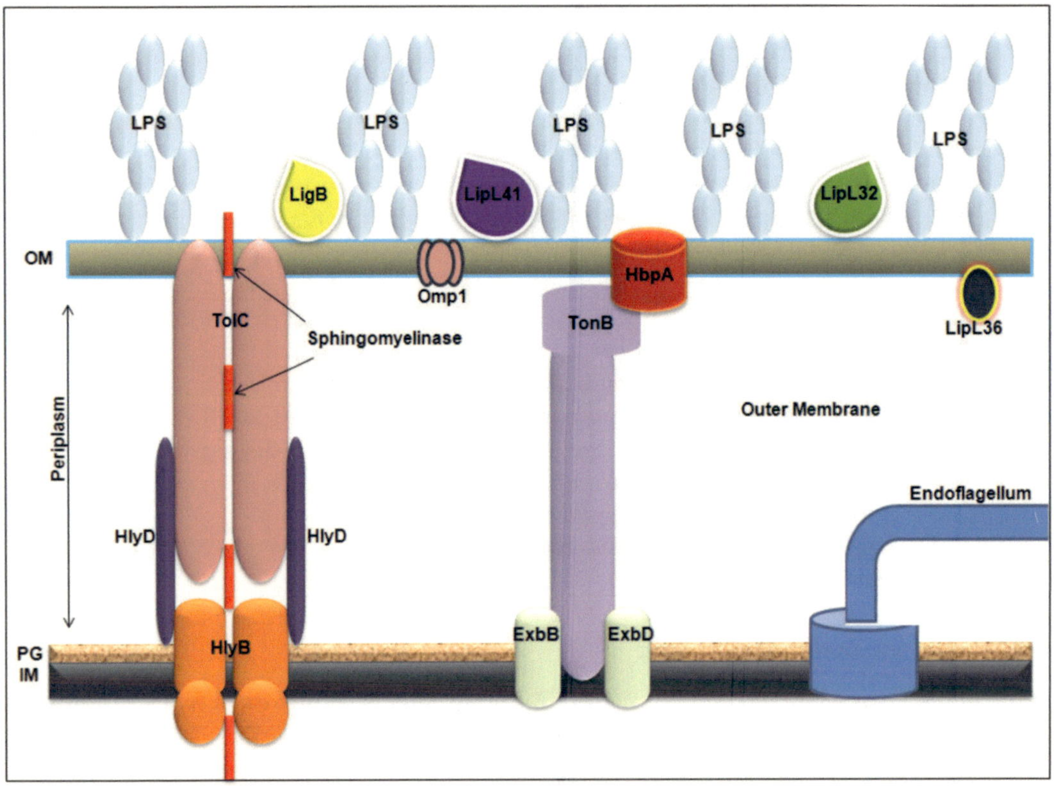

Fig. 1. Leptospiral membrane architecture and distribution of membrane proteins. The outer membrane (OM) with the associated lipopolysaccharide (LPS) and outer membrane proteins, including the lipoproteins LipL32, LipL41 and LigB protein are in contact with the immediate environment. The hemin-transporter HbpA is an example of a TonB-dependant outer membrane receptor that mediates the transport of hemin via the TonB protein located in the inner membrane (IM) along with ExbB and ExbD. TolC, in association with HlyC and HlyD forms a channel from the IM to the OM that possibly mediates the export of sphingomyelinase from the cytoplasm to the outside. The peptidoglycan (PG) is associated with IM.

end of the spirochete and extending towards the centre [Hovind-Hougen, 1976; Li et al., 2000] are responsible for the cork-screw movement of these organisms. The lipopolysaccharides (LPS), located within the outer membrane are highly antigenic and their structural variations give rise to the large diversity of the serovars and serotypes seen among the leptospiral species. Haake and his group [Haake et al., 1993; Haake et al., 2000; Haake et al., 1998; Haake and Matsunaga, 2002, 2005; Haake et al., 1999; Haake et al., 2004; Haake et al., 1991; Lo et al., 2006] contributed significantly to the identification and isolation of the leptospiral membrane proteins. They used different isolation techniques and classified the outer membrane proteins into transmembrane, lipoprotein and peripheral membrane proteins. The porin OmpL1, the first leptospiral OMP to be described [Haake et al., 1993] is a transmembrane protein present as a trimer. The second class of leptospiral OMPs, the lipoproteins, constitute the most abundant of the leptospiral proteins in the outer membrane, to which they are anchored by fatty acids.

The leptospiral lipoproteins include LipL32 (also called as hemolysis-associated protein-1; Hap-1), LipL36, LipL41, LipL31, LipL21, LipL45 and LipL48. LipL31 is located on the inner membrane whereas LipL21 [Cullen et al., 2002; Cullen et al., 2003; Cullen et al., 2005], LipL32 [Haake et al., 2000], LipL41, LipL36 [Haake et al., 1998], LipL45 [Matsunaga et al., 2002] and LipL48 are found in the outer membrane. Some of these proteins, namely LipL32 and LipL41 are conserved among many pathogenic *Leptospira* serovars and are also expressed during infection. Among the third class of proteins, classified as peripheral membrane proteins, the protein $P31_{LipL45}$ can be released from membranes by urea and can be partitioned into both Triton X - 114 detergent and aqueous phases [Haake et al., 2000; Haake and Matsunaga, 2002].

Other proteins that need mention here include the TonB-dependant outer membrane proteins and the TolC proteins. The former, present on the outer membrane of Gram-negative organisms mediate the transport of several important nutrients like iron and vitamin B12. Our search for iron transporters led us to the identification of the TonB-dependant hemin-binding protein HbpA in the pathogenic *L. interrogans* serovar Lai [Asuthkar, 2007; Sritharan et al., 2005]. It is an iron-regulated hemin-binding protein with the characteristic β - barrel structure composed of 22 anti-parallel β-sheets and a globular N-terminal region. This cell surface protein, expressed in low iron organisms mediates the transport of iron (discussed in detail in Section). TolC proteins are bacterial efflux proteins; in *E. coli* they are associated with the transport of α-hemolysin [Thanabalu et al., 1998]. A 63 kDa protein of *L. interrogans* serovar Lai, partitioning into the Triton X-114 detergent phase [Velineni et al., 2009] proved to be TolC efflux protein encoded by LA0957. The three-dimensional structure of the protein is identical to the corresponding homologue in *E. coli*. It is a trimeric molecule with each monomer consisting of 4 strands with β barrel and 4 α helices (Fig. 2a & b). There are two structural repeats (Fig. 2c), namely repeat 1 consisting of amino acid residues 16 - 294 and repeat 2 consisting of amino acid residues 295 - 557 respectively. The sequence and structures of the N and C terminal halves of the protein monomer are thus identical, as revealed by the alignment of these repeats (Fig. 2d).

2.4 Organization of the leptospiral genome

Whole genome sequencing of different leptospiral species is a major contribution to the advancement of knowledge about these organisms. The genome sequence of *L. interrogans*

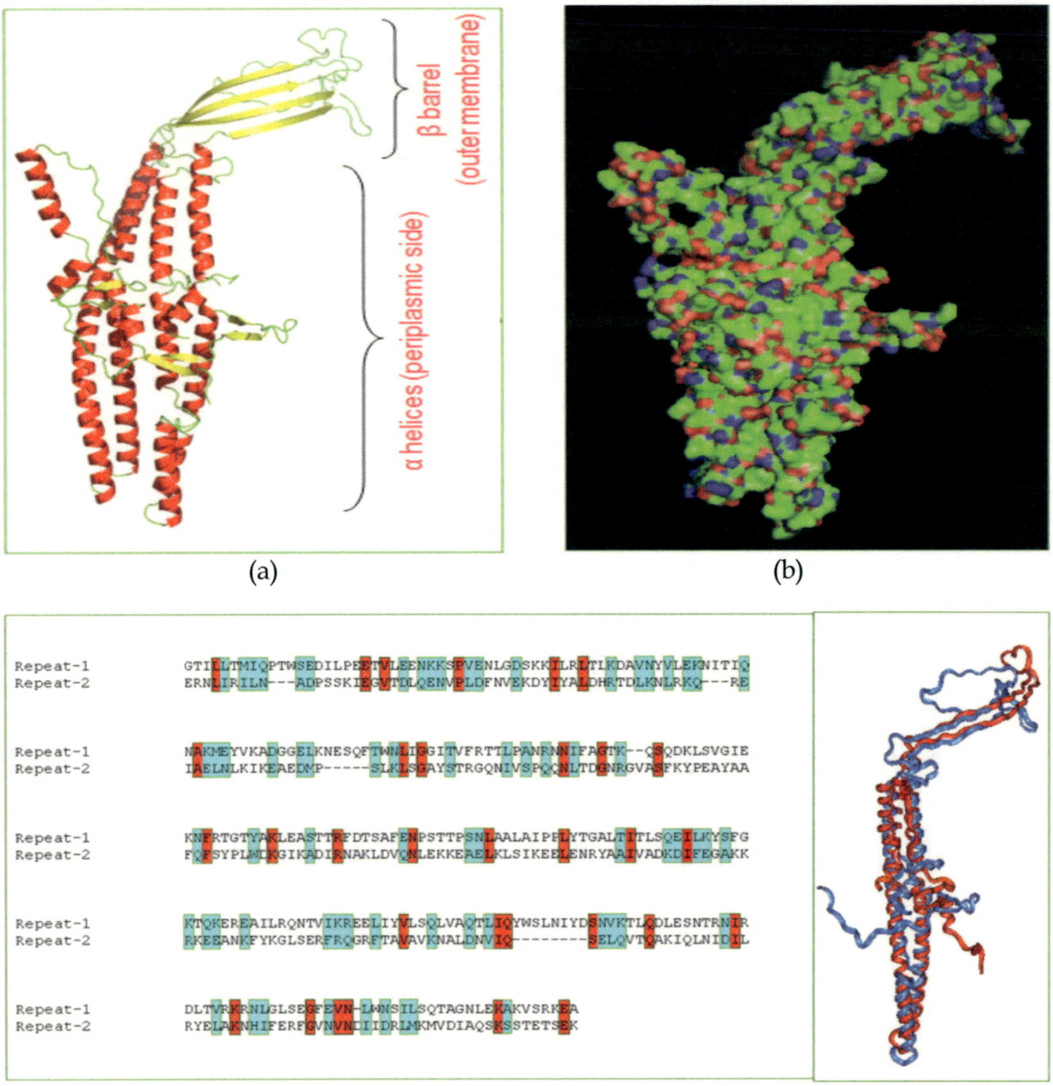

(a) (b)

(c) (d)

([Velineni et al., 2009], *Reproduced with permission from Online J Bioinformatics*)

Fig. 2. Structural organization of the efflux protein TolC in serovar Lai. Panel (a) shows the folding of the monomeric unit of TolC, with the β barrel and 4 α helices positioned in the outer membrane and periplasmic regions. Panel (b) shows the charge distribution on the surface of the molecule, with red, blue and green regions representing the electronegative, electropositive and the non polar residues respectively. Panels (c) and (d) show the two structural repeats in the molecule and the superimposed secondary structure of these structural repeats respectively.

serogroup Icterohaemorrhagiae serovar Lai strain 56601 was first made available in 2003 [Ren et al., 2003] closely followed by that of serovar Copenhageni strain Fiocruz L1-130 belonging to the same species [Nascimento et al., 2004]. Both these genomes are larger and differ considerably from those of the related spirochetes, *Treponema pallidum* and *Borrelia burgdorferi*, indicating their divergence from the phylum. Today, two additional genome sequences, namely that of *L. borgpetersenii* serovar Hardjo strains L550, JB197 [Bulach et al., 2006] and *L. biflexa* serovar Patoc strain Patoc 1 (Ames strain) [Picardeau et al., 2008] are available

With the exception of the non-pathogenic *L. biflexa* with three chromosomes, the others have genomes that consist of two chromosomes, the larger chromosome CI (approximately 4 Mb) and the relatively smaller chromosome CII (300 Kb). The non-pathogenic *L. biflexa* also shows the presence of the 74 kb leptospiral bacteriophage LE1 [Bourhy et al., 2005]. Re-annotation [Bulach et al., 2006] in both the serovars Lai and Copenhaginii has now made the number of recognized CDS to be 3613 and 3530 respectively. *Leptospira borgpetersenii* genome is 16% (approximately 700 Kb) smaller than *L. interrogans* and the reduction in the CDS (3166) is due to insertion sequence-mediated genome reduction.

Comparative genome analysis [Ko et al., 2009] provides insights into the role of specific gene products that enable the organisms to survive in their natural environment. For eg., the genome of *L. biflexa*, a free-living organism with 3590 CDS uses the additional genes to thrive in aquatic environments. Among the two pathogenic species, *L. borgpetersenii* can survive only within the mammalian host as against the additional advantage of survival of *L. interrogans* in wet and moist environments outside the mammalian host. Thus the higher gene density seen in *L. interrogans* confers properties for the successful survival, if not growth, in the outside environment. It may be recalled that *L. biflexa* lacks orthologs for LipL32, LipL41, HbpA, sphingomyelinases, Lig proteins, LipL21 and LipL36 seen in the pathogenic species. The vast wealth of data from genome analysis coupled with the modern tools for data analysis offers great opportunities for getting a better insight into the host-pathogen interactions.

3. Epidemiology

Leptospirosis is one of the most wide-spread zoonosis in the world. The global epidemiological data are extensively discussed elsewhere [Bharti et al., 2003; Levett, 2001]. The higher incidence in tropical countries is due to several reasons: one, the warm, wet and humid climatic conditions favour the survival and multiplication of the organisms; second, the close contact between the reservoir animal hosts and humans favour direct transmission between them and third, human practices such as walking barefoot and working in agricultural wet fields without protection allow indirect transmission from the contaminated environment. Rodents serve as major reservoirs of infection and rodent control must be considered as one of the important control measures. Pathogenic leptospires from the animal reservoirs are shed via the urine into the immediate environment. They can be transported from the immediate site of deposition to other areas during rainy / monsoon seasons; the heavy and torrential rains not only spread these organisms to new locations but also aid their survival in the environment for long periods of time. A reservoir of infection is thus established, with the movement of the infecting serovars among rodents, animals and humans; the latter are only accidental hosts and do not contribute to the transmission of the disease.

3.1 The Indian scenario

Historically, leptospirosis is not new to India with the disease reported in the 1930s in the Andaman & Nicobar islands [Taylor and Goyle, 1931]. In the 1960s, there were occasional reports of leptospiral etiology as seen in patients with PUO (Pyrexia of Unknown Origin) in whom the disease was attributed to the leptospiral serovars Icterohaemorrhagiae, Pomona and Canicola [Joseph and Kalra, 1966] and in a case of hepatitis due to *L. pyrogenes* [Bhatnagar et al., 1967]. In India, the incidence of the disease closely links to the rainy / monsoon seasons with higher incidence in the coastal states.

In South India, the states of Tamil Nadu and Kerala have reported several outbreaks of the disease, especially during rainy seasons [Natarajaseenivasan et al., 2004; Ratnam et al., 1993; Ratnam et al., 1983a; Ratnam et al., 1983b, 1986; Ratnam et al., 1987a; Ratnam et al., 1983c; Ratnam et al., 1987b; Sumathi et al., 2008]. The state of Kerala, called the Venice of the East, receiving heavy rainfall during several months of the year shows high prevalence of the disease, with the districts of Kottayam, Alleppey and Kozhikode being the worst affected [Vijayachari et al., 2008]. Patients present symptoms including history of fever, vomiting, jaundice, abdominal pain [Venkataraman et al., 1991], renal dysfunction [Muthusethupathi et al., 1995] and the involvement of the eye [Priya et al., 2007; Priya et al., 2008; Rathinam, 2002; Rathinam et al., 1997]. In 1994, there was an outbreak of leptospiral uveitis at Aravind Eye hospital, Madurai following severe flooding of the state of Tamil Nadu in the autumn of 1993; out of 46 patients, 80% of them were positive for leptospiral DNA and 72% were positive by serological tests. These studies clearly showed that leptospirosis is a significant health problem in coastal Tamil Nadu.

Other coastal regions include Mumbai, a heavily populated part of the country on the west coast of India. This city receives heavy rainfall during monsoon seasons and due to poor sanitation and unhygienic conditions is prone to the disease [Bal et al., 2002; Bharadwaj et al., 2002]. Several deaths due to leptospirosis were reported after the serious outbreak in 2005 [Sehgal, 2006]; around 310 cases of leptospirosis, with 27 deaths were reported, giving an incidence of 7.85 per 0.1 million population and a case fatality rate of 8.7%. The outbreak during the 2005 flooding in Mumbai clearly demonstrates the need for a proper surveillance and control measures during such times of need.

Leptospirosis is endemic in the Andaman Islands. After the report in 1931 [Taylor and Goyle, 1931], there were no reports of the disease till 1988. Following the monsoon of 1988, a mysterious febrile illness with hemorrhagic manifestations, named as 'Andaman haemorrhagic fever' (AHF) caused several deaths. Unfortunately for about 5 years the causative organism was not identified and it was in 1993 [Sehgal et al., 1995] the leptospiral etiology was identified. This important finding and several other notable contributions [Roy et al., 2003; Sehgal et al., 1999; Sehgal et al., 2000; Sharma et al., 2006; Sharma et al., 2003; Vijayachari et al., 2003] have been made by the National Leptospirosis Reference Centre located at Port Blair, Andamans. Pulmonary involvement in leptospirosis, observed in outbreaks in this part of India has been attributed to strain Valbuzzi serovar Valbuzzi of serogroup Grippotyphosa [Vijayachari et al., 2003]. Today, the disease is endemic and the whole population is at risk due to the climatic conditions and the occupation of the people living in these islands. There is high seroprevalence in manual laborers working in agricultural lands, sewage workers, animal handlers, personnel in slaughterhouses, making this disease a truly occupational nightmare.

In the state of Andhra Pradesh, there is no systematic study on human leptospirosis and the disease remains largely under-reported. We conducted a retrospective study in a hospital in Hyderabad, capital of Andhra Pradesh [Velineni et al., 2007]. 55 sera samples from patients who came from nearby villages with symptoms of leptospirosis were screened by MAT, Lepto-Tek Dri Dot and IgM ELISA. MAT identified 90% of the cases as positive and Icterohemorrhagiae emerged as the prevalent serogroup (68%). We also conducted a seroprevalence study in cattle in Mahbubnagar district, located about 100 km from Hyderabad. Agriculture is the major occupation in several villages in this district and the farmers live in close contact with the domestic animals that serve as a good source of income by way of milk and meat. We screened 107 sera from cattle from the villages of Ankur, Rajanagaram and Palakonda in this district and observed an overall seroprevalence of approximately 36.4% (Fig. 3a); the predominant serovar was Pomona (Fig. 3b).

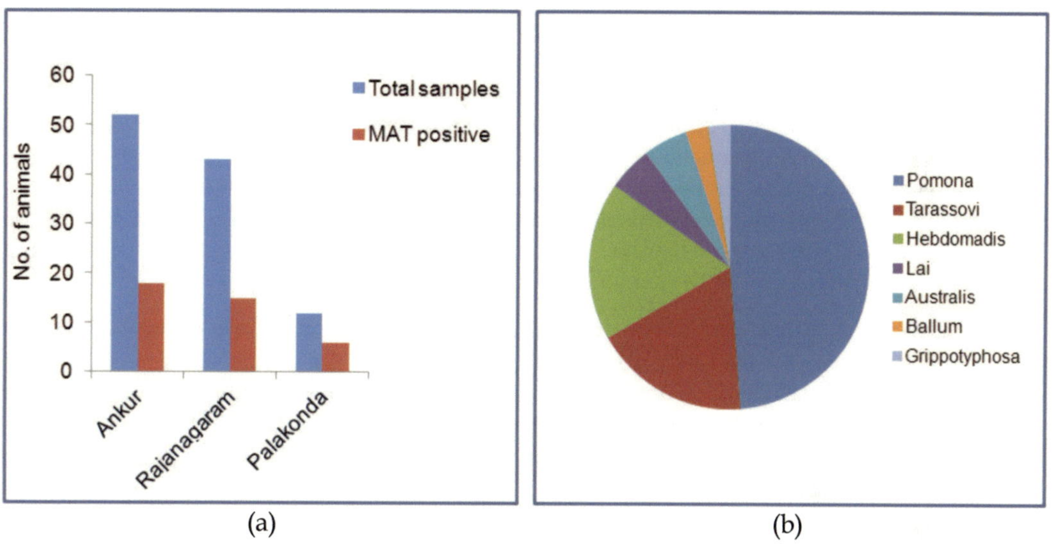

Fig. 3. Seroprevalence of leptospirosis in Mahbubnagar district. Panel (a) shows the MAT positive samples in the villages of Ankur, Rajanagaram and Palakonda in Mahbubnagar district in Andhra Pradesh. Panel (b) shows Pomona as the prevalent serovar (funding for the study by the Andhra Pradesh- Netherlands Program is acknowledged).

There are no reports of leptospirosis from the states of Jammu and Kashmir. Also, in general, there were few cases of the disease in North India due to the relatively dry weather. But now, a detailed study [Sethi et al., 2010] project the alarming increase in the incidence of the disease. The study aims to correlate predisposing factors like living conditions, human habits, exposure to animals, occupation etc to the observed disease prevalence as well as the severity of symptoms in these patients. An alarming increase in the severity of symptoms with the involvement of the liver and kidneys was seen. This may reflect a changing disease pattern in the Indian subcontinent or merely better diagnostic measures. There is a need for systematic and planned study to understand the prevalence of the disease, identification of the predominant serovars and recording of the symptoms associated with the disease. This will help to develop suitable control measures, especially in times of outbreaks.

4. Clinical features

It is beyond the scope of this review to detail the clinical features of leptospirosis in animals. The clinical manifestations in humans are discussed briefly. In humans, it is not easy to diagnose clinically because of the large spectrum of symptoms associated with it that overlaps other diseases, especially in tropical countries. The disease presents itself first as the acute phase that may progress into the severe phase. In a vast majority of patients, it is usually self limiting and the infected individuals recover from the acute phase symptoms of fever, headache, chills and severe myalgia. As these symptoms overlap with viral flu (influenza), malaria and dengue, the patients are often treated symptomatically initially. The majority of patients recover without other complications, but in 5 -10% of the patients, the disease can progress into the severe Weil's disease. This is the hemorrhagic or icteric form of the disease [Levett, 2001] involving several organs including the liver, lungs and kidneys; the patients quickly deteriorate and the disease is often fatal.

The involvement of the liver is associated with jaundice with high levels of serum bilirubin. The jaundice is attributed to be due to the failure in the secretion of the bilirubin into the bile canaliculi and not due to hepatocellular necrosis [Bharti et al., 2003]. Acute renal failure, resulting in oliguria often leads to death. In patients with the classical AHF (Andaman Hemorrhagic Fever) symptoms, hemoptysis leads to adult respiratory distress syndrome. This disease also causes damage to the heart. In India, there are well documented evidences for the involvement of the eye in leptospirosis. Patients attending the Uvea Clinic in Aravind Eye Hospital have been diagnosed as suffering from leptospiral uveitis with symptoms including conjunctival suffusion and muscle tenderness that can result in blindness.

Treatment includes parenteral administration of benzyl penicillin (5 million units) per day for five days. Doxycycline can also be administered 100 mg twice daily for 10 days [Vijayachari et al., 2008]. It is however important to note that timely treatment is required for the prompt elimination of the pathogen before the disease progresses into the second phase leading to hemorrhage and tissue damage in the vital organs. This emphasizes clearly the need for timely diagnosis.

5. Pathogenicity and virulence

In the majority of individuals, leptospirosis is often self-limiting as the host immune system efficiently clears the invading *Leptospira*. But, in a small percentage of infected individuals, the clinical manifestations can progress to the severe Weil's disease with jaundice, renal failure and potentially lethal pulmonary haemorrhage. While the pathogenesis and tissue damage is well documented in leptospirosis, mechanistic details like the pathogenic virulence determinants, their expression within the mammalian host and the damage inflicted due to immune mechanisms of the host are not completely understood. Extensive information on host tissue damage, involvement of specific leptospiral proteins and the host immune response are available [Bharti et al., 2003; Ko et al., 2009; Levett, 2001]

While 'pathogenicity' refers to the ability of a pathogen to cause disease, the term 'virulence', often used interchangeably with pathogenicity, refers to the degree of damage caused by the organism. Pathogens have adapted to the hostile environment of the mammalian host and elaborate several host-directed components for their survival. It is now becoming increasing evident that the expression of many of the toxins / virulence determinants of pathogenic bacteria is environmentally regulated in response to specified conditions. One of the contributing factors to virulence is iron limitation as the mammalian limits iron to an invading pathogen and the latter not only adapts to acquire this essential micronutrient but also expresses toxins upon iron limitation [Sritharan, 2000]. Iron is an essential micronutrient for *Leptospira* and they fail to grow in the absence of iron in culture media [Faine, 1959]. Nothing was known about how iron is acquired by these organisms, especially under conditions of iron deprivation. We first reported the high affinity transport system in *L. interrogans* serovar Lai [Asuthkar, 2007; Sritharan et al., 2005] and studied the role of iron as a regulatory molecule in the expression of the virulence factors sphingomyelinases [Velineni et al., 2009].

5.1 Adaptation of *Leptospira* to iron limitation

5.1.1 Low bioavailability of iron

Iron oscillates between ferrous (Fe^{2+}) and ferric (Fe^{3+}) states and by virtue of its wide redox potential plays an important role in biological systems. It transfers reducing equivalents in the electron transport chain and acts as a cofactor for several enzymes in biochemical reactions. Most bacteria, including *Leptospira* require iron for growth. However, the inherent insolubility of the metal ion at biological pH makes it unavailable to bacteria, as it exists as insoluble ferric hydroxides and oxyhydroxides. Nature has perhaps made iron highly insoluble, as excess iron is toxic, due to its catalytic role in the Fenton reaction, resulting in the formation of free radicals [Sritharan, 2000]. At physiological pH, the major form of iron is $Fe(OH)_2^+$ with a solubility of approximately 1.4 X 10^{-9} M [Chipperfield, 2000] that is too low to support the growth of microorganisms. The mammalian host further limits iron to pathogenic bacteria by holding the metal ion as protein-bound iron; most of the free iron is bound by transferrin and lactoferrin and the excess iron is stored as ferritin.

5.1.2 Infection, iron-withholding & 'nutritional immunity' of the mammalian host

The mammalian host limits iron to an invading pathogen by a process called 'nutritional immunity' [Kochan, 1976]. In response to infection, the mammalian host lowers the level of circulating iron by decreasing the intestinal absorption of iron and increasing synthesis of transferrin. Other mechanisms [Weinberg, 2009] aimed at depriving iron to the actively multiplying pathogen include increased synthesis of hepcidin and lipocalin, the former inhibiting the release of iron by macrophages and the latter inhibiting bacterial growth by binding to the bacterial siderophores. Haptoglobulins and hemopexins are proteins expressed in the liver that come into play during conditions such as hemorrhage when there is high level of hemoglobin the circulation. While haemoglobin constitutes nearly two-thirds of the total iron in the human body, it is not readily available to pathogens because of its compartmentalization within the erythrocytes. When the level of free haemoglobin increases in the circulation, consequent to host cell lysis by bacterial toxins, the mammalian host immediately responds by triggering increased synthesis and release of haptoglobin and hemopexin in the liver as a part of the host defense mechanism [Sassa and Kappas, 1995].

5.1.3 How do *Leptospira* acquire iron?

Bacterial pathogens have evolved novel machinery to acquire the tightly-bound iron from the mammalian host. Box 3 summarizes the two general strategies for acquiring this essential micronutrient.

Box 3: Bacterial adaptation to iron limitation
High affinity bacterial iron acquisition systems include

- a) **Siderophore-mediated system:** Siderophores are Fe^{3+}-specific low molecular weight ligands (~1000 Da) that chelate iron from the immediate environment (from sources including insoluble iron and protein-bound iron in the mammalian host) and deliver the metal ion to the organism by active transport mediated by specific cell-surface receptors called iron-regulated membrane proteins.
- b) **Direct acquisition:** Pathogenic bacteria directly chelate Fe^{3+} via specific cell-surface receptors for host transferrin / lactoferrin / heme / hemoglobin.

(for detailed reviews see [Braun et al., 1998.; Sritharan, 2000])

Leptospira do not produce siderophores, suggesting that direct acquisition from the host iron-containing molecules must occur. We identified the hemin-binding protein HbpA and demonstrated iron acquisition from hemin. First, using in *silico* tools we identified HbpA as the leptospiral homologue of the ferric enterobactin receptor *FepA* of *E. coli*. Structural elucidation and bioinformatic analysis confirmed the protein to be a TonB-dependant protein with the TonB box in its N terminal region [Sritharan et al., 2005]. As in other bacterial iron transporters, HbpA possibly transports the hemin molecule via the TonB system, comprising of the cytoplasmically localised TonB, ExbB and ExbD proteins; the TonB protein, extending through the periplasm to the outer membrane mediates the transfer of the proton motive force of the cytoplasmic membrane to the outer membrane iron transporters, followed by the internalization of the Fe^{3+}- complexes. It is not clear if the entire hemin molecule is internalized or the iron is released at the cell surface. The former probably occurs as *Leptospira* spp. possesses a heme oxygenase, encoded by *hemO*, than can degrade the tetrapyrrole ring of the heme molecule, thereby releasing ferrous iron.

The hemin-binding property of HbpA was proved in several ways [Asuthkar, 2007]. The presence of the conserved FRA/PP-NPNL motif in the primary sequence of the protein reflected its ability to bind hemin. Experimentally, hemin-binding was demonstrated both by assaying the inherent heme-dependent peroxidase activity of the bound hemin and by spectrofluorimetry. Addition of hemin resulted in the quenching of the emitted light and notably a spectral shift to light of a lower wavelength (blue shift), a characteristic feature of receptor-ligand binding.

HbpA is up-regulated by iron limitation and increase in temperature; both these conditions are noteworthy as they will be encountered by the pathogen inside the mammalian host. The expression of HbpA *in vivo* [Sridhar et al., 2008] and its absence in the non-pathogenic *L. biflexa* highlights its role in pathogenic Leptospira. It is not clear if all leptospiral species elaborate this mechanism of iron acquisition as the *hbpA* gene could not detected by PCR in several leptospiral species. The latter probably express receptors for other host iron-containing proteins; we identified a transferrin-binding protein in iron-limited *L. kirschneri* serovar Grippotyphosa strain Moskva V (unpublished observations in our lab).

Intracellular iron acts at the molecular level to regulate the expression of the components of the iron acquisition machinery in bacteria [Sritharan, 2000, 2006]. In most Gram negative bacteria, iron binds to the Fur regulator (DtxR in Gram positive organisms) and this dimeric Fur-Fe^{2+} complex binds to Fur / iron box with the consensus sequence 5'-GATAATGATAATCATTATC present upstream of iron-regulatable genes. Iron must act via the Fur protein in *Leptospira* as they show the presence of Fur homologs and Fur box.

Several *fur* genes are present in the serovar Lai that however remains to be experimentally proved as iron regulators. Table 1 lists the *fur* genes in serovar Lai and their corresponding homologues in the other leptospiral species. Fur, encoded by LB183, one of the *fur* genes present in the vicinity of *hbpA* (LB191) possibly acts by binding to the Fur box (5′ GATAATCATAATAATTT) located upstream of *hbpA* [Sritharan et al., 2005].

Leptospira interrogans		*L. borgpetersenii* Serovar Hardjo-bovis[3]		*L. biflexa*
Serovar Lai[1]	Serovar Copenhageni[2]	Strain L550	Strain JB197	Serovar Patoc[4]
LB183 (II)	LIC 20147 (II)	-	-	LEPBI_I2152 (I)
LA 3094 (I)	LIC 11006 (I)	LBL_2245 (I)	LBJ_0837 (I)	LEPBI_I2330 (I)
LA1857 (I)	LIC 12034 (I)	LBL_1818 (I)	LBJ_1600 (I)	LEPBI_I2461 (I)
LA2887 (I)	LIC11158 (I)	LBL_1012 (I)	LBJ_2038 (I)	-
-	-	-	-	LEPBI_I2849 (I)

Table 1. The *fur* genes in *Leptospira* spp.

- References represented by 1, 2, 3 & 4 include [Bulach et al., 2006; Nascimento et al., 2004; Picardeau et al., 2008; Ren et al., 2003].
- The *fur* genes, as annotated in the respective genomes are represented by their locus tag and the chromosome in which they are present is indicated within parenthesis. When the corresponding orthologue is absent, it is indicated by (-) sign.

5.2 Iron levels and expression of the leptospiral sphingomyelinases

The ability of pathogens to utilize heme compounds is particularly important as heme is one of the most abundant forms of organic iron in animals. Acquisition of iron from heme or hemoglobin may be facilitated by the production of hemolysins or cytotoxins which lyse host cells and release the intracellular iron. Cytotoxin production coupled with the capability to utilize heme and/or hemoglobin could serve as an effective iron acquisition strategy during the progression of infection. It is well known that leptospires cause localized damage to the endothelium of the small blood vessels that leads to severe damage in tissues like kidneys, liver and lungs. The necrosis in the renal tubules, hepatocellular and pulmonary hemorrhage is irreversible and is often fatal.

5.2.1 Leptospiral hemolysins

The hemorrhage and the ensuing symptoms observed in leptospirosis are due to the lysis of the host cells by the hemolysins. The hemolytic activity of these toxins was reported as early as 1956 [Alexander et al., 1956]. Later, several researchers implicated these molecules in the pathogenesis of the disease [Bernheimer and Bey, 1986; del Real et al., 1989; Kasarov, 1970; Segers et al., 1990; Thompson and Manktelow, 1989]. The phospholipase and sphingomyelinase activities of these molecules were clearly demonstrated in some of the studies. However, it was not easy to correlate all these findings as they were variously called and demonstrated in different serovars. Today, with the information from genome data there is clarity on the types and numbers of hemolysin genes in the two pathogenic species and the saprophytic *L. biflexa*.

There are nine hemolysin genes in *L. interrogans* serovar Lai (Table 2) encoding four sphingomyelinase, one pore-forming and four non-sphingomyelinase types of hemolysins. Fig. 4 shows the corresponding orthologues in *L. borgpetersenii* serovar Hardjo and it may be noted that it lacks the pore-forming hemolysin SphH. The sphingomyelinase orthologs are absent in the non-pathogenic *L. biflexa*, suggesting that their expression in the pathogenic *Leptospira* are likely to confer additional advantages for their survival within the mammalian host. The role of the five non-sphingomyelinase genes in *L. biflexa* (LEPBIa0082, LEPBIa0717, LEPBIa2015, LEPBIa2375 & LEPBIa2477) is however not clear.

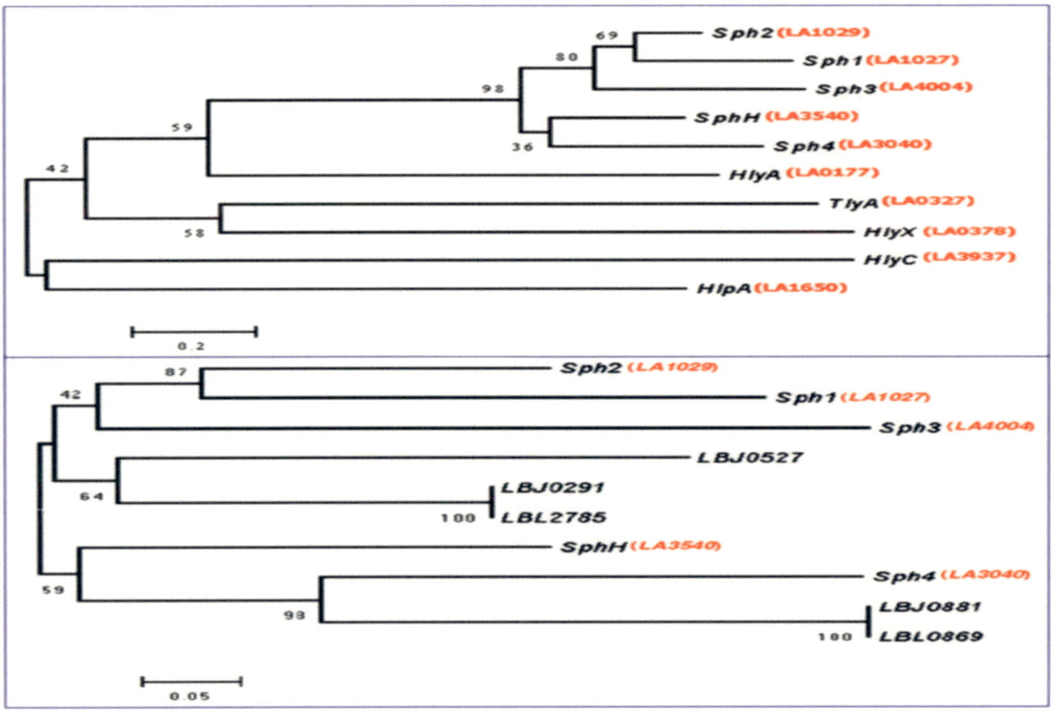

Fig. 4. Phylogenetic analysis of leptospiral hemolysins. Panel (a) shows the phylogenetic tree of the sphingomyelinase and the non-sphingomyelinase hemolysins of *L. interrogans* serovar Lai and Panel (b) shows the corresponding orthologues in *L. borgpetersenii* serovar Hardjo (strains L550 and JB197). The tree was generated using Clustal X and Mega 3.1 software. The phylogenies generated by neighborhood joining with 400 bootstrap replicates, rooted at midpoint and bootstrap values, are shown as percentages. The numbers refer to the divergence between the sequences.

There are reports on the biological activity of recombinant hemolysins including the hemolytic, enzymatic (sphingomyelinase and phospholipase) and pore-forming activity of these molecules [Artiushin et al., 2004; Lee et al., 2000; Lee et al., 2002]. Studies in our lab are also focused in the structural elucidation and functional characterization of the sphingomyelinases (under communication).

Type of hemolysin	Gene	Locus Tag	Approximate molecular mass (kDa)
Sphingomyelinases	*sph1*	LA1027	68.19
	sph2	LA1029	71.03
	sph3	LA4004	65.33
	sph4	LA3050	27.92
Pore-forming hemolysin	*sphH*	LA3540	64.43
Non-sphingomyelinase hemolysins	*hlyC*	LA3937	50.53
	hlyX	LA0378	44.95
	tlyA	LA0327	31.67
	hlpA	LA1650	36.53

Table 2. Hemolysins in the genome of *L. interrogans* serovar Lai [Ren et al., 2003]

5.2.2 Expression of sphingomyelinase(s) in *L. interrogans* serovar Lai upon iron limitation

In *L. interrogans* serovar Lai, a 42 kDa protein was detected in the outer membrane vesicles (OMVs) of low iron organisms that was absent in the OMVs from high iron cultures [Velineni et al., 2009]. This protein was recognized by antibodies against the common domain shared by the sphingomyelinases Sph1, Sph2 and Sph3 (Fig. 5).

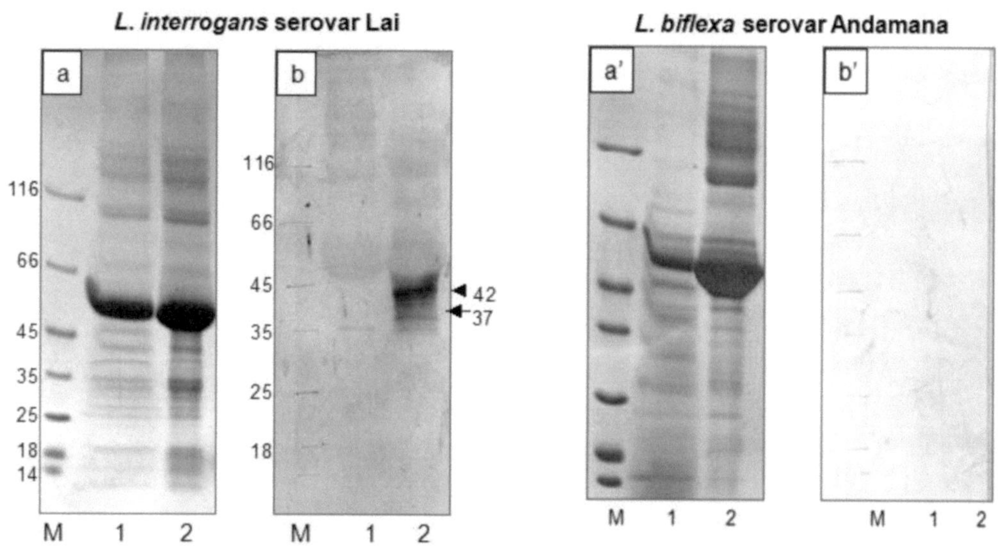

Fig. 5. Expression of sphingomyelinase in iron-limited serovar Lai. Anti-sphingomyelinase antibodies identified a major 42 kDa band in the OMVs of low iron serovar Lai (lane 2, Panel b); the band was absent in OMVs of high iron organisms (lane 1, Panel b). The Panel (a) shows the corresponding SDS-PAGE profile of high and low iron organisms. The panels a′ and b′ represent the corresponding samples from the non-pathogenic *L. biflexa* that does not show any reactivity with anti-sphingomyelinase antibodies. (Reproduced with permission from Online Journal of Bioinformatics)

As all the three sphingomyelinases encode bigger products, it clearly indicates that the 42 kDa protein is a cleavage product. This raises several questions, including the role of iron in the expression of one or more of these sphingomyelinase precursors, the proteolytic cleavage of the precursor and functional characterization of the 42 kDa protein.

Anti-sphingomyelinase antibodies, primarily used in the pull-down assay for the identification of sphingomyelinases from outer membranes, surprisingly led to the identification of the 63 kDa efflux protein TolC encoded by LA0957 [Velineni et al., 2009]. Structurally it is identical to the α- hemolysin-transporting TolC protein of *E. coli* [Balakrishnan et al., 2001]. Based on the structural similarity and the presence of the associated ATP-binding protein HlyB (LA0150) and HlyD (LA3737) in the leptospiral genome, we predict that the leptospiral TolC acts as a transporter of sphingomyelinase. However, unlike the cistronic organization of the genes *hlyCABD* responsible for α hemolysin (HlyA) secretion seen in *E. coli*, the leptospiral *hlyB* and *hlyD* are not organized as an operon. This is similar to the organization seen in *Neisseria meningitides* in which *hlyD* and *tolC* genes are adjacent but unlinked to *hlyB*, with the three genes being expressed independently (Wooldridge et al., 2005).

6. Diagnosis

6.1 Leptospiremic or antigenic phase: Culture, DFM and PCR

The organisms gain entry into a host through skin via cuts or abrasions or mucous membranes such as the conjunctiva. They enter the blood circulation where they can be detected for about a week. This period, called the septicemic or leptospiremic phase allows the direct detection of the pathogen either by culture, dark field microscopy or by molecular methods such as PCR (Fig. 6). Culture can be done by directly inoculating semi-solid media

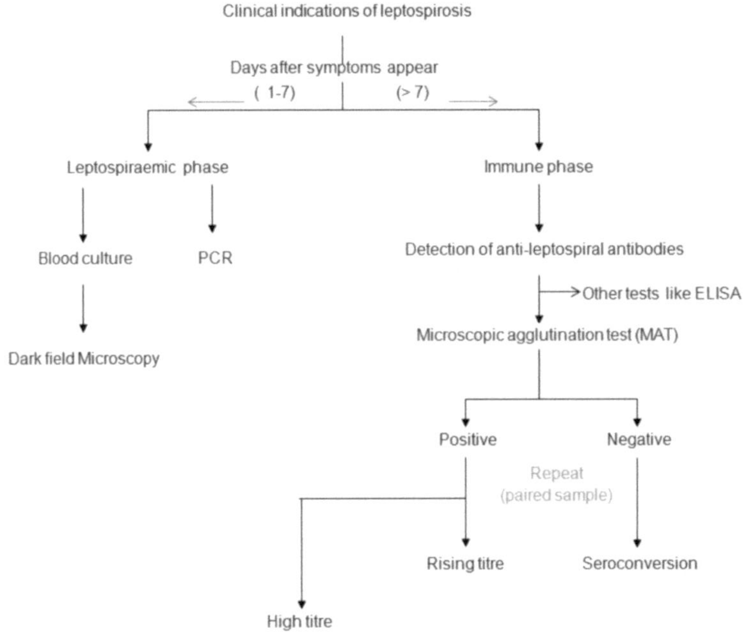

Fig. 6. Diagnosis of leptospirosis – a schematic representation.

with a few drops of blood, care taken not to include citrate as an anticoagulant as it inhibits growth of the organisms (Wolff, 1954). The media should be inoculated within 24 hours upon collection and incubated at 28 - 30°C for several weeks. The main disadvantage of blood culture is that it requires several weeks of incubation, has low sensitivity and is not useful during epidemics. Dark field microscopy, though reported as a method for diagnosis is not advisable as artifacts in biological samples can be mistaken for the organisms, leading to false positivity.

Molecular diagnosis by PCR has been used as a tool to detect pathogenic leptospires in biological fluids. Several targets specific for pathogenic serovars have been used. One of them is the 16s rDNA from which a 631 bp product [Hookey, 1992] or a 330 bp product (Senthilkumar *et al.* 2001) can be amplified. A real-time PCR method based on 16S rDNA was developed that could be used on samples without the need for prior isolation and culture [Smythe et al., 2002]. Another popularly used method [Gravekamp et al., 1993] is based on 2 sets of PCR primers, namely G1 / G2 and B64-I / B64-II that amplify products of 285 bp and 563 bp respectively. The former detected *L. interrogans, L. borgpetersenii, L. weilii, L. noguchii, L. santarosai and L. meyeri*, while the later identified *L. kirschneri.* Other variations included 'Magnetic Immuno PCR Assay' (MIPA) [Taylor et al., 1997] that consists of the immuno-magnetic separation of leptospires from inhibitors in frozen formalin-fixed bovine urine prior to PCR detection that resulted in a marked improvement in the detection of leptospires in urine samples. PCR based on *ompL1* [Reitstetter, 2006] detected serovars belonging to *L. interrogans, L. borgpetersenii, L. kirschneri, L. santarosai, L. weilli* and *L. noguchii.* We used *hbpA* as a target for PCR [Sridhar et al., 2008] and detected all serovars belonging to *L. interrogans* from clinical isolates obtained from different geographical locations around the world. A detailed study to identify the presence of *hbpA* in other species, sequence analysis and the design of suitable primers is required to use *hbpA* as a target for the identification of other leptospiral species.

6.2 Immune phase: Assay of anti-leptospiral antibodies by MAT, ELISA, lateral flow devices

High levels of anti-leptospiral antibodies of the IgM class appear 7-10 days after infection (Fig. 6) as a strong humoral immune response is mounted by the mammalian host [Fennestad and Borg-Petersen, 1957; Fennestad et al., 1968; Levett, 2001; Ratnam et al., 1983b; Ratnam et al., 1983c]. The mammalian host strives to eliminate the pathogen via the antibody-complement system. However, the leptospires may migrate into the organs, with a predilection for liver, lungs and kidneys. In the latter, they may settle in the convoluted tubules of the kidneys thus evading the antibody-complement system of the host. In humans and more characteristically in animals, where the infection tends to be chronic, leptospires are shed via urine. Thus detection of the pathogen in the urine by dark field microscopy, PCR or culture may be attempted, though it may be noted that the shedding is not uniform and occurs randomly and intermittently, with periods of nil shedding, when the testing for the pathogen will yield negative results.

The antibody response is classical, with peak IgM levels appearing first, followed by IgG antibodies. The IgM antibodies however remain in circulation for considerably long periods, even upto 2 months. It has also been observed that anti-leptospiral antibodies can be detected even after several years of infection. This, coupled to the endemicity of the infection may result in relatively high levels of antibodies within a population. Thus, it is common to collect a second serum sample from a suspected case of leptospirosis, 3 - 4 days after the first sample. Sero-conversion with a four-fold rise in titre in paired serum samples in the presence of clinical symptoms is an important criterion for the definitive diagnosis of leptospirosis. Anti-leptospiral antibodies can be detected by several methods, including the microscopic agglutination test, ELISA, lateral flow devices, latex bead agglutination tests etc.

6.2.1 Microscopic agglutination test

Microscopic agglutination test (MAT) is the 'gold standard' for leptospiral diagnosis [Cumberland et al., 1999]. This highly specific and sensitive test is based on the agglutination of live organisms in the presence of serum containing anti-leptospiral antibodies. The agglutination results in the formation of highly refractive spheroids of various sizes and with time, when maximal degree of agglutination is seen, no free leptospires are visible due to the disintegration of the organisms. The degree of agglutination is usually assessed in terms of the proportion of free leptospires. The accepted endpoint of an agglutination reaction is the final dilution of serum at which 50% or more of the leptospires are agglutinated. As per WHO guidelines, agglutination at dilution of 100 is considered positive for MAT. Antibodies in the serum of infected patients / animals, predominantly against the surface-exposed lipopolysacharides are serovar-specific, although cross-reactivity may be recorded against other serovars within the same serogroup. It is thus necessary to include several serovars, including the prevalent local isolates for screening by this method. As mentioned earlier, paired samples are to be considered for diagnosis. However, a positive diagnosis can also be made with a titre of more than 800 with single samples [Ko et al., 2009].

MAT has been used as the test of choice in outbreaks and sporadic cases. It has also been useful in retrospective studies in confirming leptospirosis cases and identifying the prevalent serovar during that period. Ismail *et al.* (2006) used MAT in a retrospective study on serum samples from patients with undiagnosed acute febrile illness (AFI) and hepatitis cases from Egypt and showed leptospiral etiology in 16% of AFI (141/886) and 16% of acute hepatitis cases (63/392). A retrospective hospital-based study done in our lab [Velineni et al., 2007] on serum samples collected from suspected cases of leptospirosis identified Icterohaemorrhagiae as the predominant serogroup.

MAT can be used to study the seroprevalence in domestic animals. In a study on 424 sow's sera from the Mekong delta in Vietnam [Boqvist et al., 2002], including 283 sows from small-scale family farms and 141 from large-scale state farms, the overall seroprevalence was 73 and 29% respectively; the predominant infecting serovars in the respective farms were *L. interrogans* serovar Bratislava and *L. interrogans* serovars Icterohaemorrhagiae. As mentioned earlier, in a seroprevalence study on cattle in Mahbubnagar district in the state of Andhra Pradesh, MAT identified Pomona as the predominant serovar (Fig. 3).

6.2.2 Enzyme Linked Immunosorbent Assay (ELISA)

Antigens used in ELISA include whole cell sonicate, formalin-extract of a culture of leptospires [Terpstra et al., 1985] and whole leptospires coated on polysterene microtitre plates [McBride et al., 2007]. Outer membrane proteins like rLipL32 [Fernandes et al., 2007; Flannery et al., 2001] , rLipL41 [Flannery et al., 2001; Mariya et al., 2006] and immunoglobulin (Ig)-like Lig proteins (Croda *et al.*, 2007; Srimanote *et al.*, 2008) have been used as antigens in ELISA.

Antibodies against the iron-regulated hemin-binding protein HbpA are present in the serum of patients with leptospirosis [Sridhar et al., 2008]. It shows considerable potential as a candidate antigen in ELISA for the screening of sera from cattle and in humans with leptospiral uveitis (both under communication). ELISA-based testing will be less expensive than MAT as it does not require the maintenance of live organisms and can be performed in any routine laboratory and further, unlike MAT, does not require trained personnel and can be quantitated and is not prone to inter-observer and intra-observer errors as in MAT.

7. Future perspectives

Timely diagnosis of leptospirosis will result in a significant reduction in the mortality. This is possible with better insights into the pathogenesis and host-pathogen interactions. The great strides made in the past decade in understanding the basic biology has certainly broadened our efforts and approaches towards better control measures. Studies in our lab are focused on the development of a simple, easy-to-do ELISA test based on anti-HbpA antibody detection for sero-diagnosis. This will facilitate screening for the disease, not only in well-established hospitals and labs but also in rural centers for the early diagnosis of the disease.

8. Acknowledgements

The author thanks several funding agencies (Government agencies including DBT, DRDE, DRDO and the Andhra Pradesh-Netherlands Program) for financial assistance towards research that is presented in this review.

9. References

Adler B, Moctezuma AdlP: Leptospira and leptospirosis. Veterinary Microbiology 2010;27:287-296.

Alexander AD, Smith OH, Hiatt CW, Gleiser CA: Presence of hemolysin in cultures of pathogenic leptospires. Proc Soc Exp Biol Med 1956;91:205-211.

Artiushin S, Timoney JF, Nally J, Verma A: Host-inducible immunogenic sphingomyelinase-like protein, lk73.5, of leptospira interrogans. Infect Immun 2004;72:742-749.

Asuthkar S: Expression and characterization of an iron-regulated hemin-binding protein, hbpa, from leptospira interrogans serovar lai. Infection Immunity 2007;75:4582-4591.

Bal AM, Bharadwaj RS, Joshi SA, Kagal AS, Arjunwadkar VP: Common infecting leptospiral serovars in and around pune, maharashtra. Indian J Med Res 2002;115:14-16.

Balakrishnan L, Hughes C, Koronakis V: Substrate-triggered recruitment of the tolc channel-tunnel during type i export of hemolysin by escherichia coli. Journal of Molecular Biology 2001;313:501 - 510.

Bernheimer AW, Bey RF: Copurification of leptospira interrogans serovar pomona hemolysin and sphingomyelinase c. Infect Immun 1986;54:262-264.

Bharadwaj R, Bal AM, Joshi SA, Kagal A, Pol SS, Garad G, Arjunwadkar V, Katti R: An urban outbreak of leptospirosis in mumbai, india. Jpn J Infect Dis 2002;55:194-196.

Bharti AR, Nally JE, Ricaldi JN, Matthias MA, Diaz MM, Lovett MA, Levett PN, Gilman RH, Willig MR, Gotuzzo E, Vinetz JM: Leptospirosis: A zoonotic disease of global importance. Lancet Infect Dis 2003;3:757-771.

Bhatnagar RK, Sant MV, Jhala HI: Prevalence of leptospirosis in bombay. Studies in man and animals. Indian J Pathol Bacteriol 1967;10:324-331.

Boqvist S, Thu HT, Vagsholm I, Magnusson U: The impact of leptospira seropositivity on reproductive performance in sows in southern viet nam. Theriogenology 2002;58:1327-1335.

Bourhy P, Frangeul L, Couve E, Glaser P, Saint Girons I, Picardeau M: Complete nucleotide sequence of the le1 prophage from the spirochete leptospira biflexa and characterization of its replication and partition functions. J Bacteriol 2005;187:3931-3940.

Braun V, Hantke K, Koster W: Bacterial iron transport: Mechanisms, genetics and regulation. . In Metal Ions in Biological systems Iron transport and storage in Microorganisms, Plants and Animals pp 1998.;Ed. Sigel, A & Sigel, H. New York, Marcel Dekker. ISBN 0-8247-9984-4. :67- 145.

Brenner DJ, Kaufmann AF, Sulzer KR, Steigerwalt AG, Rogers FC, Weyant RS: Further determination of DNA relatedness between serogroups and serovars in the family leptospiraceae with a proposal for leptospira alexanderi sp. Nov. And four new leptospira genomospecies. Int J Syst Bacteriol 1999;49 Pt 2:839-858.

Bulach DM, Zuerner RL, Wilson P, Seemann T, McGrath A, Cullen PA, Davis J, Johnson M, Kuczek E, Alt DP, Peterson-Burch B, Coppel RL, Rood JI, Davies JK, Adler B: Genome reduction in leptospira borgpetersenii reflects limited transmission potential. Proc Natl Acad Sci U S A 2006;103:14560-14565.

Chipperfield JR: Salicylic acid is not a bacterial siderophore: A theoretical study. BioMetals 2000;13:165-168.

Cullen PA, Cordwell SJ, Bulach DM, Haake DA, Adler B: Global analysis of outer membrane proteins from leptospira interrogans serovar lai. Infect Immun 2002;70:2311-2318.

Cullen PA, Haake DA, Bulach DM, Zuerner RL, Adler B: Lipl21 is a novel surface-exposed lipoprotein of pathogenic leptospira species. Infect Immun 2003;71:2414-2421.

Cullen PA, Xu X, Matsunaga J, Sanchez Y, Ko AI, Haake DA, Adler B: Surfaceome of leptospira spp. Infect Immun 2005;73:4853-4863.

Cumberland P, Everard CO, Levett PN: Assessment of the efficacy of an igm-elisa and microscopic agglutination test (mat) in the diagnosis of acute leptospirosis. Am J Trop Med Hyg 1999;61:731-734.

del Real G, Segers RP, van der Zeijst BA, Gaastra W: Cloning of a hemolysin gene from leptospira interrogans serovar hardjo. Infect Immun 1989;57:2588-2590.

Ellinghausen HC, Jr., McCullough WG: Nutrition of leptospira pomona and growth of 13 other serotypes: Fractionation of oleic albumin complex and a medium of bovine albumin and polysorbate 80. Am J Vet Res 1965;26:45-51.

Ellis WA, Michno SW: Bovine leptospirosis: A serological and clinical study. Vet Rec 1976;99:387-391.

Faine S: Iron as a growth requirement for pathogenic leptospira. Journal of General Microbiology 1959;20:246 - 251.

Fennestad KL, Borg-Petersen C: Leptospira antibody production by bovine foetuses. Nature 1957;180:1210-1211.

Fennestad KL, Borg-Petersen C, Brummerstedt E: Leptospira antibody formation by porcine foetuses. Res Vet Sci 1968;9:378-380.

Fernandes CP, Seixas FK, Coutinho ML, Vasconcellos FA, Seyffert N, Croda J, McBride AJ, Ko AI, Dellagostin OA, Aleixo JA: Monoclonal antibodies against lipl32, the major outer membrane protein of pathogenic leptospira: Production, characterization, and testing in diagnostic applications. Hybridoma (Larchmt) 2007;26:35-41.

Flannery B, Costa D, Carvalho FP, Guerreiro H, Matsunaga J, Da Silva ED, Ferreira AG, Riley LW, Reis MG, Haake DA, Ko AI: Evaluation of recombinant leptospira antigen-based enzyme-linked immunosorbent assays for the serodiagnosis of leptospirosis. J Clin Microbiol 2001;39:3303-3310.

Gravekamp C, Van de Kemp H, Franzen M, Carrington D, Schoone GJ, Van Eys GJ, Everard CO, Hartskeerl RA, Terpstra WJ: Detection of seven species of pathogenic leptospires by pcr using two sets of primers. J Gen Microbiol 1993;139:1691-1700.

Haake DA, Champion CI, Martinich C, Shang ES, Blanco DR, Miller JN, Lovett MA: Molecular cloning and sequence analysis of the gene encoding ompl1, a transmembrane outer membrane protein of pathogenic leptospira spp. J Bacteriol 1993;175:4225-4234.

Haake DA, Chao G, Zuerner RL, Barnett JK, Barnett D, Mazel M, Matsunaga J, Levett PN, Bolin CA: The leptospiral major outer membrane protein lipl32 is a lipoprotein expressed during mammalian infection. Infect Immun 2000;68:2276-2285.

Haake DA, Martinich C, Summers TA, Shang ES, Pruetz JD, McCoy AM, Mazel MK, Bolin CA: Characterization of leptospiral outer membrane lipoprotein lipl36: Downregulation associated with late-log-phase growth and mammalian infection. Infect Immun 1998;66:1579-1587.

Haake DA, Matsunaga J: Characterization of the leptospiral outer membrane and description of three novel leptospiral membrane proteins. Infect Immun 2002;70:4936-4945.

Haake DA, Matsunaga J: Leptospiral membrane proteins--variations on a theme? Indian J Med Res 2005;121:143-145.

Haake DA, Mazel MK, McCoy AM, Milward F, Chao G, Matsunaga J, Wagar EA: Leptospiral outer membrane proteins ompl1 and lipl41 exhibit synergistic immunoprotection. Infect Immun 1999;67:6572-6582.

Haake DA, Suchard MA, Kelley MM, Dundoo M, Alt DP, Zuerner RL: Molecular evolution and mosaicism of leptospiral outer membrane proteins involves horizontal DNA transfer. J Bacteriol 2004;186:2818-2828.

Haake DA, Walker EM, Blanco DR, Bolin CA, Miller MN, Lovett MA: Changes in the surface of leptospira interrogans serovar grippotyphosa during in vitro cultivation. Infect Immun 1991;59:1131-1140.

Hookey JV: Detection of leptospiraceae by amplification of 16s ribosomal DNA. FEMS Microbiol Lett 1992;69:267-274.

Hovind-Hougen K: Determination by means of electron microscopy of morphological criteria of value for classification of some spirochetes, in particular treponemes. Acta Pathol Microbiol Scand Suppl 1976:1-41.

Inada R, Ido Y, Kaneko R, Hoki R, Ito H, Wani H, Okuda K: [scientific raisins from 125 years smw (swiss medical weekly). A brief report on the discovery of the pathogen (spirochaeta icterohaemorrhagiae nov. Sp.) of so-called weil's disease in japan and on current studies of the disease. 1916]. Schweiz Med Wochenschr 1995;125:816-826.

Johnson RC, Gary ND: Nutrition of leptospira pomona. Iii. Calcium, magnesium, and potassium requirements. J Bacteriol 1963a;85:983-985.

Johnson RC, Gary ND: Nutrition of leptospira pomona. Ii. Fatty acid requirements. J Bacteriol 1963b;85:976-982.

Joseph KM, Kalra SL: Leptospirosis in india. Indian J Med Res 1966;54:611-614.

Kasarov LB: Degradiation of the erythrocyte phospholipids and haemolysis of the erythrocytes of different animal species by leptospirae. J Med Microbiol 1970;3:29-37.

Ko A, Goarant C, Picardeau M: Leptospira: The dawn of the molecular genetics era for an emerging zoonotic pathogen. Nature Reviews Microbiology 2009;7 736-747.

Kochan I: Role of iron in the regulation of nutritional immunity. Bioorganic Chemistry 1976;2:55-57.

Koizumi N, Watanabe H: Leptospiral immunoglobulin-like proteins elicit protective immunity. Vaccine 2004;22:1545-1552.

Lee SH, Kim KA, Park YG, Seong IW, Kim MJ, Lee YJ: Identification and partial characterization of a novel hemolysin from leptospira interrogans serovar lai. Gene 2000;254:19-28.

Lee SH, Kim S, Park SC, Kim MJ: Cytotoxic activities of leptospira interrogans hemolysin sphh as a pore-forming protein on mammalian cells. Infect Immun 2002;70:315-322.

Levett PN: Leptospirosis. Clin Microbiol Rev 2001;14:296-326.

Li C, Motaleb A, Sal M, Goldstein SF, Charon NW: Spirochete periplasmic flagella and motility. J Mol Microbiol Biotechnol 2000;2:345-354.

Lo M, Bulach DM, Powell DR, Haake DA, Matsunaga J, Paustian ML, Zuerner RL, Adler B: Effects of temperature on gene expression patterns in leptospira interrogans serovar lai as assessed by whole-genome microarrays. Infect Immun 2006;74:5848-5859.

Mariya R, Chaudhary P, Kumar AA, Thangapandian E, Amutha R, Srivastava SK: Evaluation of a recombinant lipl41 antigen of leptospira interrogans serovar canicola in elisa for serodiagnosis of bovine leptospirosis. Comp Immunol Microbiol Infect Dis 2006;29:269-277.

Matsunaga J, Barocchi MA, Croda J, Young TA, Sanchez Y, Siqueira I, Bolin CA, Reis MG, Riley LW, Haake DA, Ko AI: Pathogenic leptospira species express surface-exposed proteins belonging to the bacterial immunoglobulin superfamily. Mol Microbiol 2003;49:929-945.

Matsunaga J, Young TA, Barnett JK, Barnett D, Bolin CA, Haake DA: Novel 45-kilodalton leptospiral protein that is processed to a 31-kilodalton growth-phase-regulated peripheral membrane protein. Infect Immun 2002;70:323-334.

McBride AJ, Santos BL, Queiroz A, Santos AC, Hartskeerl RA, Reis MG, Ko AI: Evaluation of four whole-cell leptospira-based serological tests for diagnosis of urban leptospirosis. Clin Vaccine Immunol 2007;14:1245-1248.

Muthusethupathi MA, Shivakumar S, Suguna R, Jayakumar M, Vijayakumar R, Everard CO, Carrington DG: Leptospirosis in madras--a clinical and serological study. J Assoc Physicians India 1995;43:456-458.

Nascimento AL, Ko AI, Martins EA, Monteiro-Vitorello CB, Ho PL, Haake DA, Verjovski-Almeida S, Hartskeerl RA, Marques MV, Oliveira MC, Menck CF, Leite LC, Carrer H, Coutinho LL, Degrave WM, Dellagostin OA, El-Dorry H, Ferro ES, Ferro MI, Furlan LR, Gamberini M, Giglioti EA, Goes-Neto A, Goldman GH, Goldman MH, Harakava R, Jeronimo SM, Junqueira-de-Azevedo IL, Kimura ET, Kuramae EE, Lemos EG, Lemos MV, Marino CL, Nunes LR, de Oliveira RC, Pereira GG, Reis MS, Schriefer A, Siqueira WJ, Sommer P, Tsai SM, Simpson AJ, Ferro JA, Camargo LE, Kitajima JP, Setubal JC, Van Sluys MA: Comparative genomics of two leptospira interrogans serovars reveals novel insights into physiology and pathogenesis. J Bacteriol 2004;186:2164-2172.

Natarajaseenivasan K, Prabhu N, Selvanayaki K, Raja SS, Ratnam S: Human leptospirosis in erode, south india: Serology, isolation, and characterization of the isolates by randomly amplified polymorphic DNA (rapd) fingerprinting. Jpn J Infect Dis 2004;57:193-197.

Paster BJ, Dewhirst FE: Phylogenetic foundation of spirochetes. J Mol Microbiol Biotechnol 2000;2:341-344.

Picardeau M, Bulach DM, Bouchier C, Zuerner RL, Zidane N, Wilson PJ, Creno S, Kuczek ES, Bommezzadri S, Davis JC, McGrath A, Johnson MJ, Boursaux-Eude C, Seemann T, Rouy Z, Coppel RL, Rood JI, Lajus A, Davies JK, Medigue C, Adler B: Genome sequence of the saprophyte leptospira biflexa provides insights into the evolution of leptospira and the pathogenesis of leptospirosis. PLoS One 2008;3:e1607.

Priya CG, Hoogendijk KT, Berg M, Rathinam SR, Ahmed A, Muthukkaruppan VR, Hartskeerl RA: Field rats form a major infection source of leptospirosis in and around madurai, india. J Postgrad Med 2007;53:236-240.

Priya CG, Rathinam SR, Muthukkaruppan V: Evidence for endotoxin as a causative factor for leptospiral uveitis in humans. Invest Ophthalmol Vis Sci 2008;49:5419-5424.

Rathinam SR: Ocular leptospirosis. Curr Opin Ophthalmol 2002;13:381-386.

Rathinam SR, Rathnam S, Selvaraj S, Dean D, Nozik RA, Namperumalsamy P: Uveitis associated with an epidemic outbreak of leptospirosis. Am J Ophthalmol 1997;124:71-79.

Ratnam S, Everard CO, Alex JC, Suresh B, Thangaraju P: Prevalence of leptospiral agglutinins among conservancy workers in madras city, india. J Trop Med Hyg 1993;96:41-45.

Ratnam S, Subramanian S, Madanagopalan N, Sundararaj T, Jayanthi V: Isolation of leptospires and demonstration of antibodies in human leptospirosis in madras, india. Trans R Soc Trop Med Hyg 1983a;77:455-458.

Ratnam S, Sundararaj T, Subramanian S: Serological evidence of leptospirosis in a human population following an outbreak of the disease in cattle. Trans R Soc Trop Med Hyg 1983b;77:94-98.

Ratnam S, Sundararaj T, Subramanian S: Role of bandicoots in human leptospirosis in madras city. An epidemiological approach. Indian J Public Health 1986;30:167-169.

Ratnam S, Sundararaj T, Subramanian S, Adinarayanan N: Experimental study with leptospires in bandicoot bandicota bengalensis. Indian J Exp Biol 1987a;25:105-107.

Ratnam S, Sundararaj T, Thyagarajan SP, Rao RS, Madanagopalan N, Subramanian S: Serological evidence of leptospirosis in jaundice and pyrexia of unknown origin. Indian J Med Res 1983c;77:427-430.

Ratnam S, Venugopal K, Kathiravan V: Evidence of leptospiral infections in human samples in madras city. Indian J Med Res 1987b;85:516-518.

Reitstetter RE: Development of species-specific pcr primer sets for the detection of leptospira. FEMS Microbiol Lett 2006;264:31-39.

Ren SX, Fu G, Jiang XG, Zeng R, Miao YG, Xu H, Zhang YX, Xiong H, Lu G, Lu LF, Jiang HQ, Jia J, Tu YF, Jiang JX, Gu WY, Zhang YQ, Cai Z, Sheng HH, Yin HF, Zhang Y, Zhu GF, Wan M, Huang HL, Qian Z, Wang SY, Ma W, Yao ZJ, Shen Y, Qiang BQ, Xia QC, Guo XK, Danchin A, Saint Girons I, Somerville RL, Wen YM, Shi MH, Chen Z, Xu JG, Zhao GP: Unique physiological and pathogenic features of leptospira interrogans revealed by whole-genome sequencing. Nature 2003;422:888-893.

Roy S, Biswas D, Vijayachari P, Sugunan AP, Sehgal SC: Antigenic and genetic relatedness of leptospira strains isolated from the andaman islands in 1929 and 2001. J Med Microbiol 2003;52:909-911.

Sassa S, Kappas A: Disorders of heme production and catabolism. In Blood, Principles and Practice of Hematology 1995;Handlin, R.I., Lux, S.E., and Stossel, T.P. (eds). Philadelphia: J.B. Lippincott,:1473.

Segers RP, van der Drift A, de Nijs A, Corcione P, van der Zeijst BA, Gaastra W: Molecular analysis of a sphingomyelinase c gene from leptospira interrogans serovar hardjo. Infect Immun 1990;58:2177-2185.

Sehgal S, Murhekar M, Sugunan A: Outbreak of leptospirosis with pulmonary involvement in north andaman. Indian J Med Res 1995;102:9-12.

Sehgal SC: Epidemiological patterns of leptospirosis. Indian J Med Microbiol 2006;24:310-311.

Sehgal SC, Vijayachari P, Murhekar MV, Sugunan AP, Sharma S, Singh SS: Leptospiral infection among primitive tribes of andaman and nicobar islands. Epidemiol Infect 1999;122:423-428.

Sehgal SC, Vijayachari P, Smythe LD, Norris M, Symonds M, Dohnt M, Korver H, v d Kemp H, Hartskeerl RA, Terpstra WJ: Lai-like leptospira from the andaman islands. Indian J Med Res 2000;112:135-139.

Sethi S, Sharma N, Kakkar N, Taneja J, Chatterjee S, Banga S, Sharma M: Increasing trends of leptospirosis in northern india: A clinico-epidemiological study. PloS Neglected Tropical Diseases 2010;12:e579.

Sharma S, Vijayachari P, Sugunan AP, Natarajaseenivasan K, Sehgal SC: Seroprevalence of leptospirosis among high-risk population of andaman islands, india. Am J Trop Med Hyg 2006;74:278-283.

Sharma S, Vijayachari P, Sugunan AP, Sehgal SC: Leptospiral carrier state and seroprevalence among animal population--a cross-sectional sample survey in andaman and nicobar islands. Epidemiol Infect 2003;131:985-989.

Smythe LD, Smith IL, Smith GA, Dohnt MF, Symonds ML, Barnett LJ, McKay DB: A quantitative pcr (taqman) assay for pathogenic leptospira spp. BMC Infect Dis 2002;2:13.

Sridhar V, Manjulata Devi S, Ahmed N, Sritharan M: Diagnostic potential of an iron-regulated hemin-binding protein hbpa that is widely conserved in leptospira interrogans. Infect Genet Evol 2008;8:772-776.

Sritharan M: Iron as a candidate in virulence and pathogenesis in mycobacteria and other microorganisms. World Journal of Microbiology and Biotechnology 2000;16:769-780.

Sritharan M: Iron and bacterial virulence. Indian Journal of Medical Microbiology 2006;24:163-164.

Sritharan M, S.Ramadevi, Pasupala N, Tajne S, S.Asuthkar: In-silico identification and modelling of a putative iron-regulated tonb-dependant outer membrane receptor protein from the genome of leptospira_interrogans serovar lai. . Online Journal of Bioinformatics 2005;6:74-90.

Stimson: Note on an organism found in yellow-fever tissue. Public health reports Washington 1907;**22**:541 - 555.

Sumathi G, Narayanan R, Shivakumar S: Leptospirosis laboratory, madras medical college: Review of our experience (2004-2006). Indian J Med Microbiol 2008;26:206-207.

Taylor J, Goyle A: Leptospirosis in the andamans. Indian Journal of Medical Research Memoirs Supplementary series 1931;20:55-56.

Taylor MJ, Ellis WA, Montgomery JM, Yan KT, McDowell SW, Mackie DP: Magnetic immuno capture pcr assay (mipa): Detection of leptospira borgpetersenii serovar hardjo. Vet Microbiol 1997;56:135-145.

Terpstra WJ, Ligthart GS, Schoone GJ: Elisa for the detection of specific igm and igg in human leptospirosis. J Gen Microbiol 1985;131:377-385.

Thanabalu T, Koronakis E, Hughes C, Koronakis V: Substrate-induced assembly of a contiguous channel for protein export from *e.Coli*: Reversible bridging of an inner-membrane translocase to an outer membrane exit pore. Embo Journal 1998;17:6487 - 6496.

Thompson JC, Manktelow BW: Pathogenesis of renal lesions in haemoglobinaemic and non-haemoglobinaemic leptospirosis. J Comp Pathol 1989;101:201-214.

Velineni S, Asuthkar S, Umabala P, Lakshmi V, Sritharan M: Serological evaluation of leptospirosis in hyderabad andhra pradesh: A retrospective hospital-based study. Indian J Med Microbiol 2007;25:24-27.

Velineni S, S R, Asuthkar S, M.Sritharan: Effect of iron deprivation on expression of sphingomyelinase in pathogenic serovar lai. Online Journal of Bioinformatics 2009;10 (2):241-258.

Venkataraman KS, Ramkrishna J, Raghavan N: Human leptospirosis: A recent study in madras, india. Trans R Soc Trop Med Hyg 1991;85:304.

Vijayachari P, Sehgal SC, Goris MG, Terpstra WJ, Hartskeerl RA: Leptospira interrogans serovar valbuzzi: A cause of severe pulmonary haemorrhages in the andaman islands. J Med Microbiol 2003;52:913-918.

Vijayachari P, Sugunan AP, N.Shriram A: Leptospirosis: An emerging global public health problem. J Biosci 2008;**33**:557-569.

Vijayacharit P, Hartskeerl RA, Sharma S, Natarajaseenivasan K, Roy S, Terpstra WJ, Sehgal SC: A unique strain of leptospira isolated from a patient with pulmonary haemorrhages in the andaman islands: A proposal of serovar portblairi of serogroup sehgali. Epidemiol Infect 2004;132:663-673.

Walbach, Binger: Notes on filterable spirochaete from fresh water, *spirochaeta biflexa* (new species). The Journal of Medical Research 1914;**30**:3023 - 3026.

Weinberg E: Iron availability and infection Biochimica et Biophysica Acta 2009;1790:600-605.

11

Crimean-Congo Hemorrhagic Fever (CCHF)

Sadegh Chinikar, Ramin Mirahmadi, Maryam Moradi,
Seyed Mojtaba Ghiasi and Sahar Khakifirouz
Pasteur Institute of Iran
(Laboratory of Arboviruses and Viral Hemorrhagic Fevers)
(National Reference Laboratory)
Iran

1. Introduction

CCHF name derives from the separate regions in Asia and Africa where severe and often fatal human cases of hemorrhagic disease and fever were recognized in the 1940s and 1950s. Virus isolates from the two regions are antigenetically indistinguishable. The disease come to people's attention in the Crimea where about 200 military personnel become ill while helping peasants to harvest gain.

Russian scientists, led by Professor M.P.Chumakov, isolated the virus from human patients and from ticks. The same virus was isolated by C.Courtoise in 1956 from a 13 years old patient in the Belgium Congo. However, Crimean-Congo haemorrhagic Fever has a much longer history, with the first record in the early 12th century. Although ticks transmit CCHF virus to a wide variety of animal species, the severe disease only affects humans. Cattle, sheep and small mammals, such as hares may develop mild fever following infection. The disease in humans is comparatively rare but a cause for concern because of high mortality and transmission through contact with patients. Handling the virus requires the highest degree of laboratory containment (Knipe (2001), Chinikar(2009), Chinikar(2007)).

2. History of the virus in the world and in Iran

CCHF is a tick- borne Viral Zoonosis widely distributed in Africa, Asia and Eastern Europe within the ranges of ticks belonging to the genus *Hyalomma*. The virus is a member of the Nairovirus genus of the family Bunyaviridae. It causes mild fever and virema in cattle, sheep and small mammals such as hares.

Humans become infected by contact with infected blood or other tissues of livestock or human patients or from tick bite. Human infection is usually characterized by a febrile illness with headache, myalgia and petechial rash, frequently followed by a hemorrhagic state with necrotic hepatitis. The case fatality rate is approximately40%, but it can range from 20% to 80 %(Goodman (2005), Knipe (2001)).

A hemorrhagic disease with symptoms suggestive of CCHF infection was described in Eastern Europe and Asia as far back as the 12th century (Hoogstraal 1979). However, a disease given the name Crimean hemorrhagic fever was first described in people bitten by ticks while harvesting crops and sleeping outdoors on the Crimean Peninsula in 1944. In the following year, it was demonstrated by inoculation of human subjects that the disease was caused by a filterable agent present in the blood of patients during the acute stage of illness and that the agent was also present in suspension prepared from ticks, suspected to be the vectors of the agent. The causative virus was finally isolated in a laboratory host, suckling mice, in 1967 (Chumakov 1974). In 1968 it was found that the agent of Crimean hemorrhagic fever was identical to a virus named Congo which had been isolated in 1956 from the blood of a febrile child in what was then the Belgian Congo (now democratic Republic of Congo), and since that time the two names have been used in combination (Casals 1980, Casals 1969, Chumakov 1970, Simpson 1976).

The first evidence that CCHF virus circulated in Iran was investigated by Chumakov et al in 1970, when 45% of a shipment of sheep sent from Tehran abattoir to Moscow tested positive for CCHF antigen. Although human infection with CCHF was suspected in areas close to the Azerbaijan border, the first confirmed human cases were not reported until 1974-1975. This lead to a large-scale serological study performed in collaboration with Yale University (New Haven, Connecticut, USA), focusing on the northern half of Iran. Using classic agar gel diffusion precipitation assays this study demonstrated high levels of seroconversion for humans (13%), cattle (38%) and sheep (18%).

In 1978, CCHF virus was isolated for the first time from engorged specimens of the ornithodoros tick Alveonasus lahorensis in the north eastern region of Iran. Since this early period to 1999 reports of CCHF were uncommon in Iran, the disease has however increased in prevalence since 2000 warranting new surveys and study (Chinikar2010, Chinikar2009 and Chinikar2007).

3. Etiology agent and biology

Crimean-Congo Hemorrhagic Fever virus is classified as a member of the genus Nairovirus, of the family Bunyaviridae (Knipe 2001).

The genus, consisting of 33 viruses, is divided into seven serogroups on the basis of antigenic relationships.

The CCHF serogroup contains CCHF virus, Hazara virus from Pakistan, and Khasan virus from the former USSR.

Apart from CCHF virus, the only members of the genus known to be pathogenic from humans are Nairobi sheep disease virus and Dugbe virus. Nairobi sheep disease virus of East Africa is believed to be identical to Ganjam virus of India and is a tick-borne pathogen of sheep and goats which sporadically causes benign illness in humans (Davies 1978).

Dugbe virus is a tick-borne virus commonly associated with mild infection of cattle and sheep in West Africa and infrequently causes benign human disease (Burt1996). The classification of the Nairoviruses was originally based on their antigenic relatedness; however, the groupings have subsequently been substantiated through demonstration of morphological and molecular affinities between the viruses (Calisher 1989).

Viewed using an electron microscope, CCHF virus appears spherical, approximately 100nm in diameter (buoyant density1.17 $g.ml^{-1}$) with a dense core (capsid) surrounded by a lipid envelope, through which protrude spikes, 5-10 mm in length. The viral genome is segmented, comprising three circular, single strands of negative sense RNA.

All three genomic RNA segments have a unique 3'end sequence of 3'AGAG (A/U) UUCU.

The small (S) segment (approximately 1.7 Kb) has a single open reading frame encoding the nucleocapsid (N) protein.

In contrast, the medium (M) segment (approximately 5Kb) encodes a large polyprotein, which is processed into the two surface glycoproteins, G_1 and G_2, and several mon-structural proteins. The large (L) segment encodes a single L protein of approximately 460 KD_a, which is probably the viral polymerase (Fig. 1).

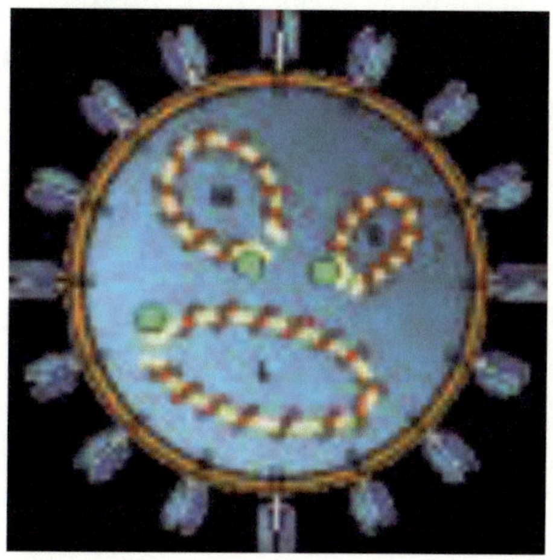

Fig. 1. CCHF virus Schema

Virus infection of cells is probably through receptor-mediated endocytosis, followed by fusion of the viral envelope with endosomal membranes. Monoclonal antibodies directed against G_1 (but not against the N protein) neutralized viral infectivity, suggesting an important role for G_1in the infection process. All stages of viral replication occur in the cell cytoplasm, although comparatively little is known of these events. As the viral RNA is negative-sense, the first step in replication is the transcription of the incoming genomic RNA into viral complementary RNA. The transcriptase has not yet been identified. Viral messengers RNA (mRNA) has host derived primer sequences, indicating a cap-snatching mRNA priming mechanism, as found with influenza viruses. Virion assembly occurs in the Golgi complex.

Nucleocapsids acquire their outer envelope by budding into the Golgi lumen. Virions are then transported to the cell membrane and released from the infected cell by exocytosis. (Richman 2002, Krasus2003, Isba2004, Van der Giessen 2004, Chhabra2003, M.W Service.2001, Goodman 2005, Fields2001).

Little information is available on the stability of the CCHF virus, but once enveloped, it is sensitive to lipid solvents (Karabatsos 1985), and it is known that its infectivity is destroyed by low concentration of formalin and B-propriolactone. The virus is labile in infected human tissues after host death (Hoogstraal 1979), but the examination of specimens from human patients appears to show that infectivity is preserved for at least a few days at ambient temperature in separated serum.

Infectivity is destroyed by boiling in autoclaving, but the virus is stable at temperatures below-60°C.

CCHF virus replicates in a wide variety of primary cell and line cell cultures, including Vero, CER, and BHK21 cells, but not usually to high titer. The virus is poorly cytopathic, so that titers of infectivity are demonstrated by plaque production or immunoflorescence in infected cells (Hoogstraal1979, Calisher 1989 and Clerx 1981).

The virus has been isolated and titers have been determined most frequently by intracerebral inoculation of suckling mice (Hoogstraal 1979).

Because of its propensity for human-to-human transmission, its ability to cause infections in laboratory workers, and the severity of the disease in humans, CCHF is placed in biohazard class IV in countries which have relevant biosafety guidelines. This dictates that culture of the virus is permitted only in maximum-security biosafety level 4 (BSL-4) laboratories (Richman 2002, Knipe 2001).

4. Transmission and zoonotic hosts

Vectors are ixodid (hard) ticks. Although CCHF virus has been isolated from at least 31 different tick species and subspecies (including two argasid (soft) species), the primary vectors are *Hyalomma* species, particularly *H. marginatum marginatum, H. marginatum rufipes* (the African representative of the *H. marginatum* complex), and *H. anatolicum anatolicum*.

All three species are two-host ticks: immature stage (larvae and nymphs) feed on the same individual host before dropping off to mouth to the adult stage which then feeds on a second host.

Both immature stages and adults of *H. a. anatolicum* feed on domesticated mammals, whereas *H. m. marginatum* and *H. m. rufipes* immature stage and adults feed on dissimilar hosts: immature stages on birds, hares and hedgehogs, and adults on cattle and other large mammals. Adult ticks successfully attack humans, only being detected after a few days of feeding when they become enlarged with blood. Humans do not contribute to the transmission cycle. *Hares* (*Lepus* species), hedgehogs (*Erinaceus* and *Hemiechinus* species) and cattle are probably important amplifying hosts.

Feeding on viraemic animals may provide the source of infection for ticks. However, screening domestic and wild vertebrates for CCHF viremia has often failed to identify viraemic host species that maintain the viral enzootic cycle. Sheep and ground-feeding birds, such as Hornbills and Ostriches may act as non-viremic hosts. Otherwise birds play an important role in disseminating ticks, particularly those of the *H. marginatum* complex.

Virus can be transmitted sexually, from infected male to uninfected female ticks during mating (venereal transmission), and trans-ovarially, from infected females to their offspring. The epidemiologal significance of vertical (transovarial) transmission is unknown. However it could provide an important amplification mechanism if virus is transmitted from infected to uninfected larvae co-feeding on the same host. Virus survival in infected ticks and the ability of *Hyalomma* species to survive at least 800 days without a blood meal indicate that ticks act as virus reservoirs (Fig. 2).

Direct transmission through contact with infected blood and body fluids and, possibly, crushed ticks are an important route of human infectious (M.W Service.2001, Goodman 2005, Knipe 2001). The virus causes in apparent infection or mild fever in livestock (Swanepoel 1985 S.Af.Med 68:638-641 - Swanepoel 1985.Af.Med 68:635-637).

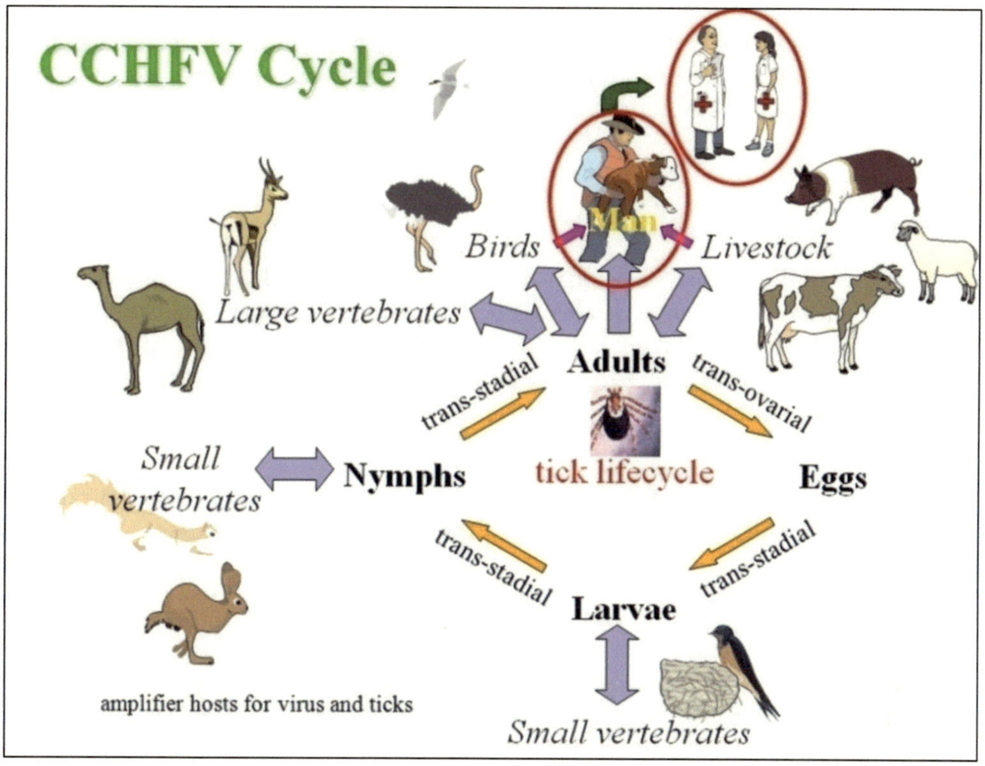

Fig. 2. CCHF virus Cycle in nature

Young ruminants, including calves and lambs, acquire maternal antibody from colostrums, but it has not been determined whether this is protective, and many animals seroconvert early in life after the occurrence of natural infection. Consequently, humans commonly become infected when they come into contact with the viremic blood of young animals in the course of performing procedures such as castrations, vaccination, insertion of ear tags, or slaughter of animals (Hoogstraal1979, Swanepoel1985). The evidence suggests that the infection in humans is acquire through contact of viremic blood with broken skin, and this is consistent with the observations that nosocomial infection in medical personnel usually results from accidental pricks with needles contaminated with the blood of patients or similar mishaps (Hoogstraal1979, Shepherd,A.J 1985).

In view of the serological evidence that infection of livestock occurs on a wide scale in areas infested by *Hyalomma* ticks, it is surprising that so few human infections are diagnosed. This raises the possibility that many human infections are asymptomatic or mild and pass unnoticed, but the low prevalence of antibody generally detected in surveys and the sparse evidence of infection encountered among cohorts of cases of the disease suggest that a high proportion of CCHF infections does, in fact, come to medical attention (Fisher-Hock 1992).

Possible explanation for the low incidence of infection which occurs in humans include the fact that viremia in livestock is short lived and of low intensity compared to that in other zoonotic disease such as Rift Valley fever, which is more readily acquired from contact with infected tissues.

Furthermore, despite the fact that a high proportion of patients acquire infection from ticks, humans are not the preferred hosts of *Hyalomma* ticks and are infrequently bitten in comparison to livestock (M.W.Service 2001, Goodman2005 and Knipe 2001).

5. Epidemiology

5.1 CCHF in the world

The distribution of the disease coincides with that of the principal vectors of the virus, ticks of the genus *Hyalomma*. Cases of the naturally acquired human infection have been documented in the former Soviet Union, China ,Bulgaria, Yugoslavia, Albania, Kosovo, Pakistan, Iran, Iraq, United Arab Emirates, Saudi Arabia, Oman, Tanzania, Central African Republic, DRC(former Zaire) Uganda, Kenya, Mauritania, Burkina Faso, South Africa and Namibia.

In addition, virus has been isolated from ticks or non-human mammals in Madagascar, Senegal, Nigeria, Central African Republic, Ethiopia, Afghanistan, Greece and Hungary (Swanepoel 1987).

The initial outbreaks of CCHF recognized on the Crimean Peninsula in 1944 and 1945 occurred under conditions of war when large members of soldiers and peasant farmers were exposed to tick bites while harvesting crops and sleeping outdoors (Hoogstraal 1979). Subsequent recognition of the presence of the disease in many countries in Eastern Europe and Asia similarly came about through the occurrence of highly visible epidemics or nosocomial outbreaks occasioned by human intervention , resulting in multiple exposure of people to infection. These include the institution of major land reclamation schemes or abrupt changes in animal husbandry practices in the former Soviet Union and Bulgaria in the 1950s and 1960s,nosocomial outbreaks of infection in Pakistan in 1976 and in Iraq and Dubai in1979, large - scale exposure of war refugees to outdoor conditions in Kosovo in 2000,Albania in 2001,and Pakistan in2001-2002, and multiple exposure of people to blood and ticks from the handling and slaughter of livestock imported from Africa and Asia to Saudi Arabia in1990,the United Arab Emirates in1994-1995 and Oman in1995.

The occurrence of these epidemics led to the perception that CCHF was an emerging disease. However, in many other countries in Eurasia and Africa the presence of the viruses was discovered because prospective laboratory investigations were undertaken, not because a specific clinical entity had been recognized, antibody surveys indicate that there is widespread circulation of virus in nature in many countries that have not yet recognized the occurrence of human disease (Hoogstraal 1979, Swanepoel 1987).

Hoogstraal pointed out that mechanisms for the dissemination of ticks and hence viruses, which include the movement of birds migrating annually on a north-south axis (Hoogstraal 1961, Hoogstral 1963) must have operated in Eurasia and Africa for millennia.

In addition, ticks can be dispersed between continents by movement of livestock. Although there is evidence that recent outbreaks of CCHF in the Arabian Peninsula resulted from trade of tick -infected livestock from Africa and Asia, long -established CCHF endemicity in the region cannot be excluded. Despite the potential for dispersal of the virus between the continents, it appears from phylogenetic analyses of CCHF isolates that the circulation of the virus is largely compartmentalized within the two land masses of Africa and Eurasia where the distribution of strains of the virus is probably related to the distribution and dispersal of the virus vectors.

The implication is not that there is continuing spread of CCHF from its present range, but that further investigation would reveal the presence of the virus and disease in the remaining countries of Africa, Eastern Europe and Asia, which lie within the distribution range of *Hyalomma* ticks.

Although the incidence of recognized cases of human infection is generally extremely low in countries where CCHF is endemic, it should be borne in mind in assessing the socioeconomic impact of the virus that the disease affects particular segments of the population, including those involved in the livestock industry and in health care. Hence, the occurrence of outbreaks can have dire consequences. For instance, the dedication of highly trained staff and expensive facilities and equipment to the intensive care of a single patient in isolation can prove to be very costly and disruptive of normal medical services .Bans imposed on the importation of slaughter livestock can seriously affect the economies of exporting countries (Goodman 2005).

5.2 CCHF in Iran

Although sporadic surveys of CCHF in livestock and humans have been undertaken since 1970, it was not however until the 1999 outbreak that CCHF was recognized as one of the country's major public health problems.

In consequence the laboratory of Arboviruses and Viral Hemorrhagic Fevers was established as a National Reference laboratory in the Pasteur Institute of Iran (a member of National Expert Committee on Viral Hemorrhagic Fevers).

The mission of the institution is to test all human, livestock and ticks suspected to be infected with CCHF viruses from all provinces of Iran with a rapid and charge free service. Thus since 2000, the percentage of CCHF infections throughout the country has been closely monitored. Twenty three (23) out of 30 provinces of Iran are endemic for CCHF virus and Sistan-Va-Baluchistan, Isfahan, Fars, Khuzestan are respectively the most heavily infected provinces.

In 2002 the CCHF virus genome was detected in 22.3% of ticks collected from Chaharmahal-va-Bakhtiari province, southwest of Iran.

In 2004, after a report of a human CCHF confirmed case in Hamadan province, western region of Iran, similar studies showed CCHF virus in 11.3% of ticks and nearly 30% of the livestock were IgG positive.

A study in 2003-2004 in Sistan-va-Balouchistan province, demonstrated that among 285 human volunteers, 6.3% were seropositive for CCHF infection. A seroepidemiological survey among livestock in Isfahan province between 2004 and 2005, showed seropositivity in almost 56% of the animals.

During the years 2003-2005, of 448livestock sera collected from Khorassan province, northeast part of Iran, 77.5% of 298 sheep samples and 46% of 150 goat samples were seropositive which implied a hyper enzootic region for CCHF. Other work that has focused on isolating and analyzing the CCHF viruses genome has led to the discovery of interesting phylogenetic relationship of the virus strains circulating in Iran. Thus Iran strains are very similar to the Matin strain of Pakistan (Chinikar 2010, Chinikar 2004).

In December 2008, a reemerging outbreak of CCHF occurred in the southern part of Iran. Five people were hospitalized with sudden fever and hemorrhaging, and CCHF was confirmed by RT-PCR and serological assays.

One of the cases had a fulminant course and died. Livestock was identified as the source of infection, all animals in the incriminated herd were serologically analyzed and more than half of them were positive for CCHF. Two routes of transmission played a role in this outbreak: contact with tissue and blood of infected livestock, and nosocomial transmission.

Phylogenetic analyses helped to identify the origin of this transmission. It is possible that a new strain occurred in the outbreak region, and future phylogenetic analyses are required to identify the precise origin of this genetic variant (Chinikar 2010).

In 2006, recombinant CCHF Virus antigen (nuclear protein) was produced by the Semliki Forest Virus expression system. The recombinant antigen is used in Elisa for serological diagnosis of CCHF, and is a useful advantage in that its production does not need biosafety level4 facilities.

In very recent years, new research projects focused on expression of a recombinant antigen to develop a subunit vaccine are being performed at the National Reference Laboratory as well as the previously mentioned projects (Chinikar 2005, Chinikar 2002, and Garsia 2006).

From June 2000 to 20 September2011, 2382 serum samples from CCHF probable patients have been collected from different provinces and transferred according to safety procedures to the laboratory of Arboviruses and Viral Hemorrhagic Fevers (National Reference Laboratory).

Among these 2382 probable cases, 853 were confirmed as positive CCHF either serologically and/or molecularly, and between these 853 confirmed cases 122 have died (Fig. 3.)

The data showed that the disease has been seen in a majority of Iranian regions, i.e. 23 out of 30 provinces of Iran (Fig. 4.).

More than one decade experience on CCHF in Iran has conducted to the following conclusions:

Sistan-va-Baluchistan is the most infected province (in the southeast of Iran, near the border of Pakistan and Afghanistan, where the disease is endemic) with 70% of positive cases.

The phylogenetic studies showed that the Iranian CCHF strain is very similar to the Matin (Pakistan) CCHF strain.

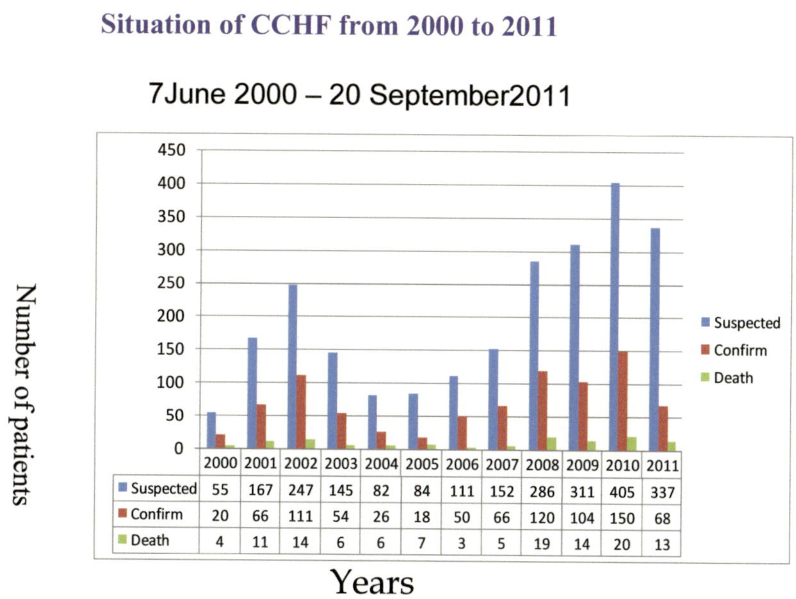

	2000	2001	2002	2003	2004	2005	2006	2007	2008	2009	2010	2011
Suspected	55	167	247	145	82	84	111	152	286	311	405	337
Confirm	20	66	111	54	26	18	50	66	120	104	150	68
Death	4	11	14	6	6	7	3	5	19	14	20	13

Fig. 3. Situation of CCHF from 2000 to September2011

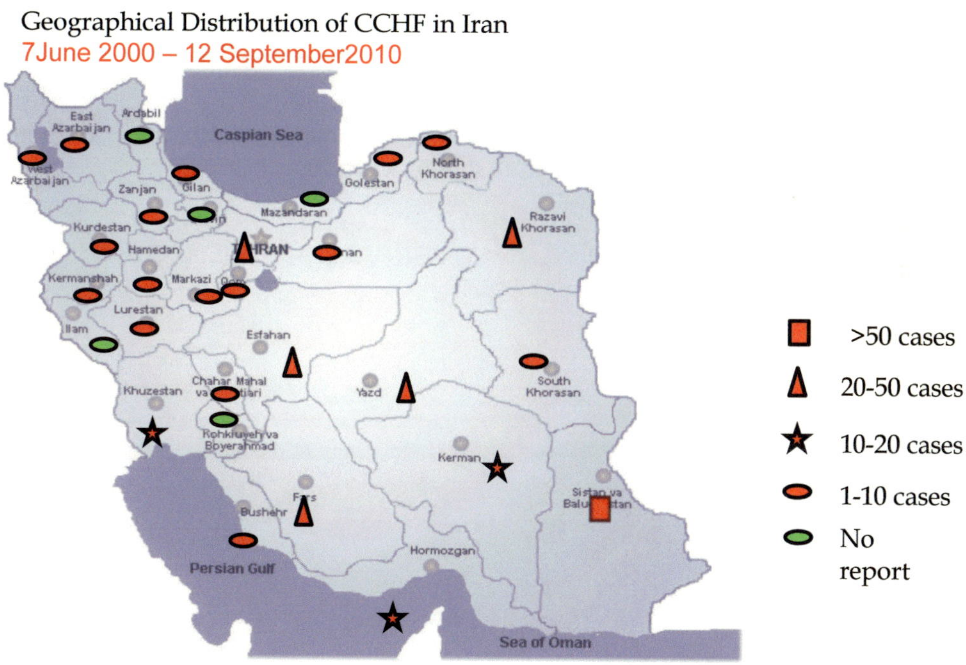

Fig. 4. Geographical Distribution of CCHF in Iran

The khorassan province and the Fars province are respectively the second and third infected province after Sistan-va-Baluchistan province (Fig. 5.).

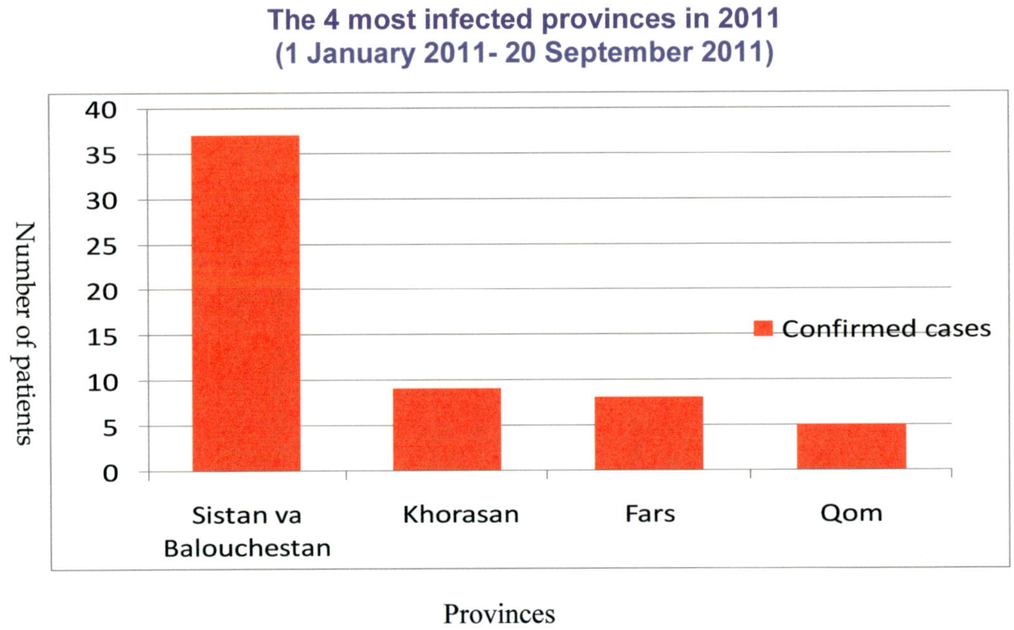

Fig. 5. The 4 most infected province in 2011

The epidemiological data showed that severity of the disease and also mortality rate of CCHF in different years and different provinces are different, so it seems more phylogenetic and pathogenesis studies should be done in this regard.

The majority of confirmed cases in Iran have profession like butchers, slaughterers, slaughter house workers, which have to deal with infected livestock blood or organs (Fig. 6.).

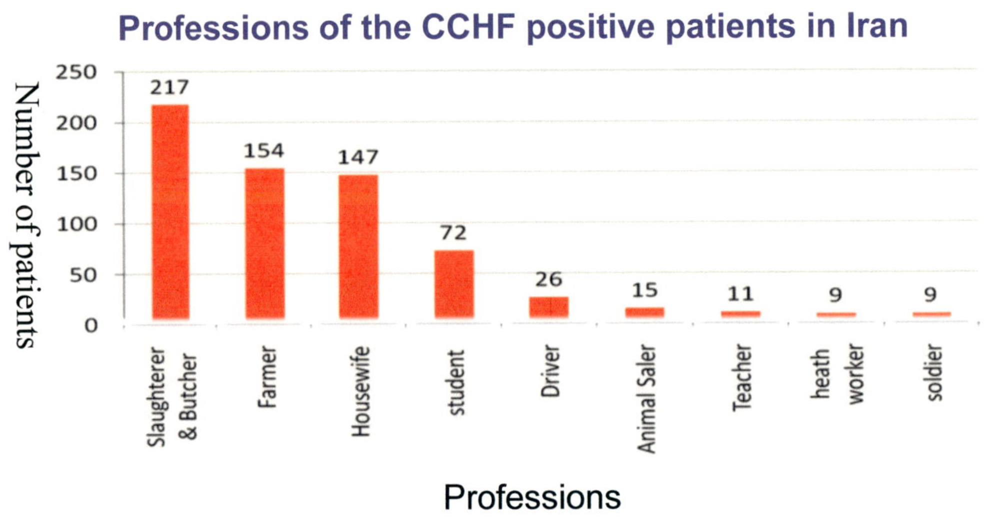

Fig. 6. Profession of the CCHF Positive patients in Iran

The majority of the positive cases in all the study years are seen in June and July (in warm months in which ticks population and their activity is high) (Fig. 7.).

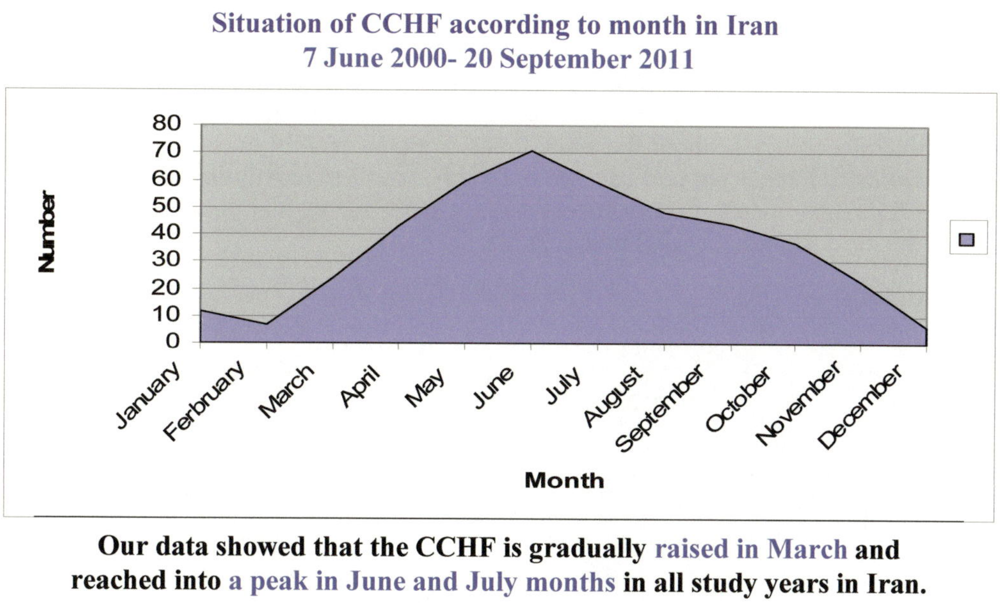

Fig. 7. Situation of CCHF according to month in Iran

The sex distribution of CCHF in Iran is a 3:1 ratio (male/female).

Age distribution: the majority of Iranian patients are between 20-40years (working age) (Fig. 8.).

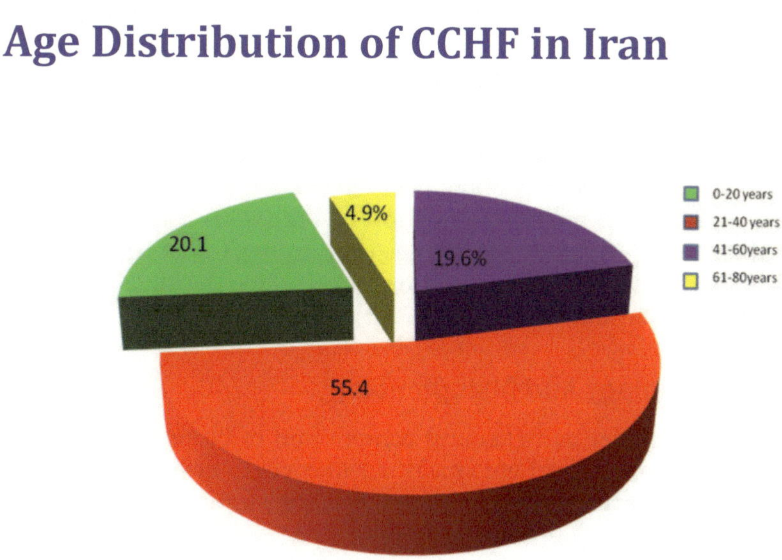

Fig. 8. Age Distribution of CCHF in Iran

6. Clinical manifestations

6.1 Symptoms

Disease severity appears similar wherever Crimean-Congo haemorrhagic fever occurs. Clinical signs of the disease follow an incubation period of 1-7 days but this may be longer when infection is by contagion rather than by tick bite. The disease is characterized by a sudden onset with severe headache, dizziness, neck pain and stiffness and photophobia. Fever with chills occurs at about the same times. Patients rapidly develop general myalgia and malaise, with intense leg and back pain. By the second to fourth day of illness, patients may have a flushed appearance. In severe cases, a petechial rash appears on the trunk and limbs by the third to sixth day of illness (Fig. 9.).

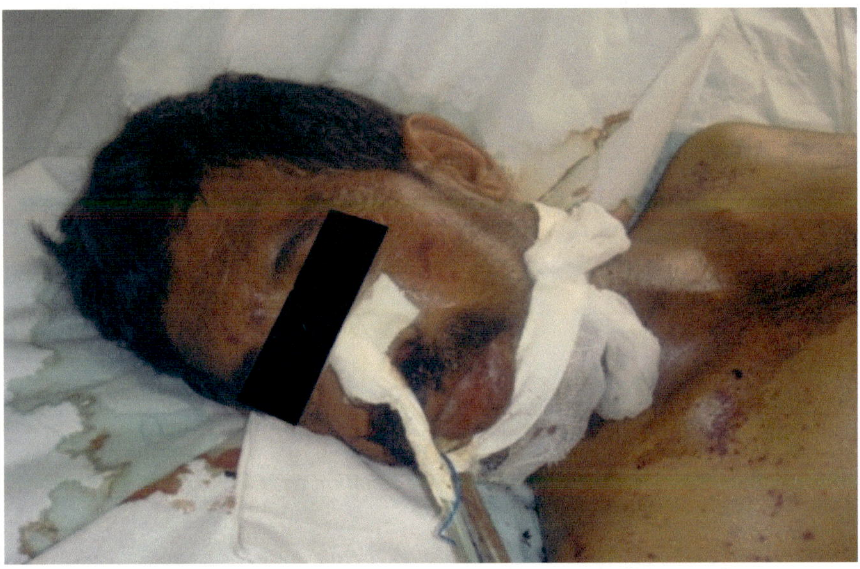

Fig. 9. CCHF Patient

Internal and external bleedings are common, although sometimes a tendency to haemorrhage is apparent only from the oozing of blood from injection or venepuncture sites. Severely ill patients may show hepatorenal and pulmonary failure from about day 5 onwards, and become progressively drowsy, stuporous and comatose. Deaths generally occur on the 5th to 14th day of illness. Recovery from CCHF begins on day 9 or 10 with the abatement of the rash and general improvement, although convalescence may continue for a month or longer (Richman 2002, Knipe 2001).

7. Clinical pathology and histopathology

Changes in the cellular and chemical composition of blood recorded during the first few days of illness in human patients include leukocytosis or leukopenia and elevated serum aspartate transaminase, alanine transaminase, gamma-glutamyl transferase, lactic dehydrogenase, alkhaline phosphatase, and creatine kinase levels, while bilirubin, creatinine and urea levels increase and serum protein levels decline during the second week (Swanepoel 1989). Thrombocytopenia, elevation of the prothrombin ratio, increased thrombin time, and elevated levels of fibrin degradation products, as well as depression of fibrinogen and hemoglobin values, are evident during the first few days of illness.

Complete autopsies are seldom performed on patients who die of CCHF, and examination of tissue is often confined to liver samples taken with biopsy needles. Lesions in the liver vary from disseminated foci of necrosis, to massive necrosis involving over 75% of hepatocytes and a variable degree of hemorrhage (Swanepoel 1985).

Inflammatory cell infiltrates in necrotic areas are absent or mild and unrelated to the extent of hepatocellular damage.

Limited observations of splenic tissue show lymphoid depletion, focal necrosis, and scattered lymphoblasts in periarterial sheaths. In addition, diffuse alveolar damage, intra-alveolar hemorrhage, hyaline membrane formation, and a mononuclear interstitial pneumonitis have been observed in the lungs, and congestion and slight interstitial edema have been noted in the heart. Lesions in other organs include congestion, hemorrhage, and focal necrosis in the central nervous system, kidneys, and adrenal glands, and general depletion of lymphoid tissue. None of the histopathologic features is pathognomonic, and similar features can be seen in other viral, rickettsial, and bacterial infections, as well as toxic exposures. Hence, a definitive diagnosis can be established only by immunohistochemical or virological tests (Richman 2002, Goodman 2005, and Knipe 2001).

7.1 Pathogenesis

The Pathogenesis of the disease is incompletely understood (Shepherd, A.J 1989), but by analogy with other arthropod-borne virus infections it can be surmised that CCHF virus undergoes some replication at the site of inoculation and that there is hematogeneous and lymph-borne spread of infection to organs such as the liver, which are major sites of replication. Localization of CCHF virus in tissues by immunohistochemistry has shown that mononuclear phagocytes and endothelial cells are also major targets of virus infection (Burt 1997). A similar tropism is exhibited by many lethal hemorrhagic fever viruses. The mononuclear phagocyte system may constitute a mechanism for viral clearance in some patients, but in others replication of virus in these cells may enhance viremia. Infection of mononuclear phagocytes and depletion of lymphoid cells may protect the virus from phagocytosis and immune inactivation and enhance the spread of virus. In addition it may play a role in the pathogenesis of CCHF through the release of physiologically active substances, including cytokines, tumor necrosis factor and other inflammatory mediators and procoagulants.

The occurrence of disseminated intravascular coagulation (DIC) appears to be an early and central event in the pathogenesis of the disease. The hepatocytes are a major target of the virus, and the occurrence of minimal inflammatory infiltration suggests that hepatocellular necrosis may be mediated by a direct viral cytopathic effect. Hepathocellular necrosis leads to further release of tumor necrosis factor and other procoagulation into the circulation, and ultimately to impairment of the synthesis of coagulation factors to replace those which are consumed in DIC. Wide spread infection of endothelium with degenerative change rather than necrosis is associated with capillary dysfunction, which contributes to the occurrence of a hemorrhagic diathesis and the generation of a petechial rash (Richman 2001, Krasus 2003, Goodman 2005, Knipe 2001).

8. Diagnosis

8.1 Generalities

A diagnosis of CCHF should be suspected when severe influenza-like illness with sudden onset and short incubation period, usually less than 1 week, occurs in persons exposed to tick bites or fresh blood and other tissues of livestock or human patients. The disease is easier to recognize once a rash appears and there are hemorrhagic signs such as epistaxis, hematemesis and melena.

Etiologic investigation of suspected CCHF infections should be performed in a BSL-4 laboratory (Krasus 2003, Isba 2004, Van der Giessan2004 and Chhabra 2003).

Confirmation of the diagnosis in the acute phase of illness consists of detection of viral nucleic acid by reverse transcriptase PCR (RT-PCR), demonstration of viral antigen by enzyme-linked immunoassay (ELISA) of serum samples, or isolation of the virus (Burt 1994 and Burt 1998).

In samples collected later, the diagnosis is confirmed by demonstration of an immune response. RT-PCR using conventional thermocycling or real-time PCR constitutes a rapid and sensitive technique for diagnosing CCHF infection during the early stage of infection before an antibody response is demonstrable or in fatal cases where an antibody response is frequently not demonstrable (Burt 1998). Virus may be isolated in cell cultures, commonly of vero cells or by intracerebral inoculation of 1- day- old mice. The virus is detected and identified in cell cultures by performing an immunofluorescence (IF) test.

Isolation of the virus in cell cultures can be achieved in 1 to 5 days, compared to 5 to 8 days in mice, but mouse inoculation is more sensitive for isolating virus that is present at low concentrations. Nairoviruses in general, including CCHF, induce a weak neutralizing antibody response, and serum samples frequently contain nonspecific inhibitors of virus infectivity. Hence, neutralization test have found limited application for demonstrating antibody response. In contrast, indirect IF has proved to be a rapid and sensitive technique for detecting an immune response to CCHF virus. The Elisa is also a sensitive technique, and both Elisa and IF can distinguish between immunoglobulin G (IgG) and IgM antibodies.

Both IgG and IgM antibodies become demonstrable by IF from about day 5 of illness onwards and are present in the sera of all survivors of the disease by day 9 at the latest. The IgM antibody activity declines to undetectable levels by the fourth month after infection, and IgG titers may begin to decline gradually at this stage but remain demonstrable for at least 5 years. Recent or current infection is confirmed by demonstrating seroconversion, a fourfold or greater increase in antibody activity in paired serum samples, or IgM activity in a single specimen.

Patients who succumb rarely develop a demonstrable antibody response, and the diagnosis is confirmed by isolation of virus or detection of viral nucleic acid in serum samples, liver samples taken after death, or demonstration of CCHF antigen by immunohistochemical techniques with paraffin embedded liver sections. Virus antigen may sometimes be demonstrated in liver impression smears by IF or in serum or liver homogenate by Elisa.

Observation of necrotic lesions compatible with CCHF in sections of liver provides presumptive evidence in support of the diagnosis. (Richman 2002, Chhabra 2003, Goodman 2005, Knipe 2001)

8.2 Differential diagnosis

The vast majority of suspected cases of CCHF prove to be severe infections with more common agents, including bacterial septicemias, malaria, viral hepatitis, rickettsioses and complications of human immunodeficieng virus AIDS. In arriving at a diagnosis, it is important to take into account an accurate history of possible exposure to infection, signs and symptoms of illness and clinical pathology findings (Richman 2002, Knipe 2001).

In Africa, CCHF should be distinguished from other febrile diseases associated with ticks (Burt 1996) and particularly from tick borne typhus which has an incubation period of 7 to 10 days and a more insidious onset than CCHF. Tick-borne typhus is associated with a petechial rash and is capable of causing a fatal disease in humans with hemorrhagic manifestations similar to CCHF, but it is amenable to treatment with appropriate antibiotics. Other tick-borne diseases occurring in Africa which could be considered include Q fever and relapsing fever borreliosis. In addition, there are a number of tick-borne viruses in Africa apart from CCHF, which have been associated with human disease such as Dughe and Nairobi sheep disease viruses (M.W. Service 2001).

Rift-Valley fever can also be acquired from contact with the tissues of livestock in Africa, but it usually occurs in the context of massive epidemics involving abortion and death of sheep and cattle at irregular intervals in years when heavy rains favor the breeding of the mosquito vectors of the virus.

Particular consideration should be given to the other viral hemorrhagic fevers of Africa. In brief, they include Marburg disease and Ebola fever, caused by members of the family Filoviridae, and Lassa fever, caused by a virus of the family Arenaviridae. Marburg and Ebola viruses cause sporadic outbreaks of highly lethal disease in tropical Africa, often in association with similar disease in non-human primates, but the source of these viruses in nature remains unknown. Lassa fever virus causes chronic renal infection of rodents in West Africa and transmission to humans occurs through contamination of food and house dust with rodent urine.

Another group of rodent-associated viruses which belongs to the Hantavirus genus of the family Bunyaviridae are found in Europe, Asia and the Americas.

Diseases caused by the Hantaviruses of Europe and Asia are known collectively as hemorrhagic fever with renal syndrome, and these could conceivably be confused with CCHF on occasion. The Hantaviruses of north and South America are associated with the so-called Hantaviruses pulmonary syndrome, which is less likely to be confused with CCHF. There is inconclusive evidence for the presence of Hantaviruses in Africa.

Yellow fever and dengue virus (of which there are four serotypes) are mosquito-borne flaviviruses capable of causing fatal hemorrhagic disease in humans within defined geographic ranges.

Chikungunya virus is a mosquito-borne alphavirus which has been associated with hemorrhagic disease in Asia, although in Africa it is reported as a benign febrile illness with severe joint pain. Although not found in Africa, Omsk hemorrhagic fever and Kyasanur forest disease (tick-borne flavivirus infections) might also be considered in the differential diagnosis in their respective ranges.

Distinguishing between the various possible causes of suspected viral hemorrhagic fever is a specialized task, normally undertaken in laboratories dedicated to the purpose (Goodman 2005).

9. Common laboratory diagnostic methods

9.1 Serological assay

Serological methods have been developed to diagnose CCHF using either inactivated virus or extract from infected suckling mouse brain. Since CCHF is highly pathogenic for humans and the available therapeutical means are limited to the use of ribavirin when administered early upon onset of syndromes, it must be handled in BSL4 containment, rendering difficult the production of native antigen. Due to these limitations, recombinant antigens were produced, replacing native antigen in Elisa and other antigen dependent assays. As the nucleoprotein of CCHF virus is recognized as the predominant antigen inducing a high immune response in most Bunyavirus infection, the recombinant nucleoprotein of the CCHF virus has been produced through Semliki Forest virus and baculovirous expression systems and used to detect IgM and IgG in human and animal serum.

9.1.1 IgG Elisa (Swanepoel, R 1987)

The wells were coated overnight at 4°C with the mouse hyper immune ascetic fluid diluted at1:1000 in 0.05% Tween 20-PBS containing 5% skim milk as a saturating reagent. This solution was used to dilute antigen and sera. The native or the recombinant antigen at a 1:100 dilution was added for 1h 37°C. Peroxydase labeled antihuman or anti- animal immunoglobulin was added at 1:1000 for 1h at 37°C.After 10min of incubation with the TMB substrate (KDL, Gaithersburg MD,USA),the OD was read at 450and 620nm (Chinikar 2005, Chinikar 2002, Chinikar 2010).

9.1.2 IgM Elisa

The Elisa plates are coated with the goat IgG fraction to human IgM (anti μ chain) diluted in PBS 1x and incubate over night at4°C.After addition of diluted recombinant or native antigen, diluted immune-ascite is then added .After a definite incubation , peroxydase - labeled anti - mouse immunoglobulin is added and incubated in 37°C. The plates then are washed three times with PBST containing 0.5% Tween. Finally, hydrogen peroxyde and TMB (3, 3', 5, 5' tetra methyl benzedrine) are added and after a short incubation, the enzymatic reaction is stopped by the addition of 4N sulfuric acid. Then, the plates are read by one Elisa reader at 450nm (Chinikar 2005, Chinikar 2002, and Chinikar 2010).

9.2 Molecular assay

Viral RNA is extracted from 140μl of serum or phenol extracted tick suspensions using QIAamp RNA mini kit according to the instructions of the manufactures (QIAgen GmbH, Hilden, Germany). The extracted viral RNA is analyzed by gel - based and Real -Time RT - PCR using a one -step RT-PCR kit(QIAgen GmbH , Hilden ,Germany) and specific primers F2 5′TGGACACCTTCACAAACTC 3′and R3 5′GACAATTCCCTACACC 3′,which amplify a 536 bp fragment of the S segment of CCHF virus genome. The PCR reaction is done in 50μl total volume and 30min at 50°C, 15min at 95°C, and 40cycles including 30s at95°C, 30s at 50°C, 45s at 72°C, and finally10 min in 72°C as a final extension. (Chinikar 2010, Chinikar 2004)

10. Prevention, control and treatment

Nosocomial infections have been associated with needle stick injuries or contact of broken skin with infected blood, tissues, and body fluids of patients.

Aerosol transmission is not considered a primary mode of transmission, in situations where infection with CCHF virus is suspected, patients should be isolated and subjected to barrier nursing techniques until the diagnosis is confirmed or excluded, to protect health care workers from potential exposure to infection.

In brief, the patient should be isolated in a room with an adjoining anteroom, if possible, for storage of supplies required for barrier nursing and patient care. Health care workers should wear protective clothing such as disposable gowns, gloves, masks, goggles and overshoes, which are discarded on leaving the isolation room via the anteroom.

All items removed from the isolation ward should be safety disposed of or suitably disinfected. Blood samples should be wrapped in absorbent material such as paper towels and placed in secondary leak-proof containers, such as rigid metal or plastic screw-cap containers or sealed plastic bags for safe transport to the laboratory.

Clinical laboratory tests should be kept to a maximum security and performed by experienced staff wearing protective clothing, and automated analyzers must be decontaminated after use, commonly with dilute chlorine disinfectants, CCHF virus is classified as a biohazard class IV pathogen, hence, specific diagnostic tests and culture of the virus are undertaken only in BSL-4 laboratories in countries which have relevant biosafety regulations.

Acaricide treatment of livestock and controlling the numbers of hares are effective in reducing the populations of infected ticks and hence the risk of infection. However, tick control is impractical in many regions of the world where *Hyalomma* ticks are most prevalent.

Clothing impregnated with pyrethroid acaricides can give some protection against tick bites. Wearing gloves and limiting exposure of naked skin to fresh blood and other tissues of animals are practical control measures that should be undertaken by veterinarians, slaughter workers and others involved with potentially infected livestock, and by medical staff treating patients.

Treatment of the disease consists essentially of supportive and replacement therapy with blood products .Immune plasma has been used, but the efficacy of this treatment is not clear, since there has been no systematic investigation with a uniform product of known virus-neutralizing activity.

Promising results were obtained in limited trials with the chemotherapeutic drug Ribavirin, but the disease is often recognized only at a late stage, ideally, treatment should commence before day 5of illness.

Owing to the occurrence of vomiting and hemorrhagic gastroenteritis, oral ribavirin is not very useful in severely ill patients who need treatment most, and the intravenous form of the drug is often difficult to obtain, since it is produced on a limited scale owing to the lack of demand, and it is not available in Iran.

Oral ribavirin can be used prophylactically in instances of known exposure to infection, such as in needle stick injuries with the blood of patients with a confirmed diagnosis.

Inactivated vaccines prepared from infected mouse brain were used for the protection of humans in Eastern Europe and the former Soviet Union in the past, but no commercial vaccines are currently available (Richman 2002, M.W.Service 2001, Goodman 2005).

11. References

Burt F.J., P.A.Leman, J.F.Smith, R.Swanepoel. (1998). The use of a reverse transcription - polymerase chain reaction for the ection of viral nucleic acid in the diagnosis of Crimean-Congo haemorrhagic fever. *Virol. Methods* 70:129-137.

Burt, F.J., Swanepoel, R., Shieh, W.J., Smith, J.F., Leman P.A., Geer, P.W., Coffield, L.M., Rollin, P.E., Ksiazek T.G. Peters, C.J., Zaki, S.R. (1997). Immunohistochemical and in situ localization of Crimean-Congo Hemorrhagic fever (CCHF) virus in human tissues and implications for CCHF pathogensis. *Arch. Pathol. Lab. Med.* 121: 839-846.

Burt,F.J, Spencer, D.C., leman, P.A. Patterson, B. Swanepoel, R.(1996) Investigation of tick-borne viruses as pathogens of humans in South Africa and evidence of Dugbe virus infection in patients with prolonged thrombocytopenia. *Epidemiol. Infect.* 116: 353-361.

Burt, F.J., Leman, P.A., Abbott, J.C., Swanepoel, R., (1994) "Serodiagnosis of Crimean-Congo haemorrhagic fever". Epidemiol. Infect. 113: 551-562.

Calisher, C.H & karabatsos N. (1989). "Arbovirus serogroups: definition and geographic distribution, p 19-57. In T.P. Monath *(ed.)*". The *Arboviruses: Epidemiology*, vol1. CRC Press, Inc, Boca Raton, Flc.

Casals, J and Tignor G.H(1980) "The Nairivirus genus" *Intrvirology* 14: 144-147.

Casalas, J. (1969) "Antigenic similarity between the virus causing Crimean Haemorrhagic fever and Congo virus". Proc.*Soc.Exp.Biol.HED* 131: 233-236.

Chhabra, Daljeet & Arora, Sushrut (2003) "*Atext book on General and Microzoonoses*"(first editon),JAYPEE BROTHERS, ISBN 81-8061-043-8, New Delhi.

Chinikar.S, Ghiasi.S.M,Hewson.R, Moradi.M, Haeri.A (2010) "Crimen-Congo hemorrhagic fever in Iran and neighboring countries" *Journal of Clinical Virology47* (2010) 110-114.

Chinikar.S, Ghiasi.S, Moradi.M,et al . (2010) "Phylogenetic analysis in a recent controlled outbreak of Crimean_ Congo haemorrhagic fever in the south of Iran" . *Eurosureveill, 2010;*15 (47):pii=19720. December 2008.

Chinikar.S, Ghiasi.S, et al. (2009) An overview of Crimean_ Congo haemorrhagic fever in Iran. *Iranian journal of Microbiology* (spring 2009) 7-12

Chinikar.S, Mirahmadi R., Mazaheri V., Nebeth P., Saron MF., Salehi P. (2005) "A serological survey in suspected human patients of Crimean-Congo haemorrhagic fever in Ira by determination of IgM specific ELISA method during2000-2004". Arch. *Iranian Med* 2005: 8: 52-55.

Chinikar.S., Persson Stine-Mari, Johansson Marie, Bladh Linda, Goya Mehdi, Houshmand Badakhshan, Mirazim Ali, Plyusnin Alexander,et al.(2004) "Genetic Analysis of Crimean- Congo Hemorrhagic Fever Virus in Iran".*Journal of Medical Virology 73*:404–411

Chinikar S., Fayaz A., Mirahmadi R., Mazaheri V., Mathiot C., Saron M.F.(2002) "The specific serological investigation of suspected human and domestic animals to Crimean-Congo haemorrhagic fever in various parts of Iran using Elisatechniques". *Hakin J* 2002: 4: 294-300.

Chinikar.S (2007). Crimean_ Congo haemorrhagic fever *"A Global Perspective Book"* (Published by springer,Onder Ergonul ChrisA.Whitehouse Editors) (89-99) ISBN 978-1-4020-6106-6 (e-book)

Chumakov, M.P(1974) "*Contribution to 30years of investigation of Crimean-Congo haemorrhagic fever*"Abad.Hed.Naul SSR 22:5-18.

Chumakov, M.P, Smirnova, S.E and tkachenho, E.A. (1970) "*Relationship between strains of Crimen haemorrhagic fever and Congo viruses*" Acta Virol. 14:82-85.

Clerx J.P. Casals, J. Bioshop, D.H.(1981) "*structural characteristics of nairoviruses (genus Nairovirus, Bunyaviridae*". J.Gen.Viral. 55:165-178.

Davies, F.G, casals J, Jesset D.M., and Ochieng, P.(1978). "*The serological relationships of Nairobi sheep disease virus*.J.Camp.Pathol. 88:519-523.

Fisher-Hock S.P, Mc Cormick, J.B., Swanepoel, R., Van Middle loop, A. Harvey , S. Kustner H.G.(1992) "Risk of human infections with Crimean-Congo haemorrhagic fever virus in a South African rural community". *An.J. Trop. Med. Hyg*. 47:337-345

Garsia.S, Chinikar.S, Coudrier.D, et al: "Evaluation of a Crimean-Congo Hemorrhagic fever virus recombinant antigen expressed by Semliki Forest suicide virus for IgM and IgG antibody detection in human and animal sera collected in Iran". *Journal of Clinical Virology 35* (2006) 154-159.

Goodman, L.Jesse.(T.Dennis David, and Shine E.Sonen)(Ed). (2005) "*Tick-Borne Disease of Humans* " ASM Press, ISBN1-55581- 238-4, Washington,DC.

Hoogstraal, H. (1979). "The epidemiology of tick-borne Crimean-Congo hemorrhagic fever in Asia, Europe and Africa". *J.Med.Entomol*.15: 307-417.

Hoogstral, H. Kaiser, M.N., Traylor, M.A., Guindy, E., Gaber, S. (1963). "Ticks (Ixodidae) on bird's migratig from Europe and Asia to Africa" 1959-61. *Bull.W.H.O*. 28: 235-262.

Hoogstraal, H., Kaiser, MN., Traylor, M.A., Gaber , S. and Guindy, E. (1961). "Ticks (Ixodidae) on bird's migration from Africa to Euroupe and Asia". *Bull.W.H.O*.24: 197-212

Isba Rachel (2004)"*Rapid infectious Disease and Tropical Medicine*" (First edition) Blackwell, ISBN 1-4051-1325-1, Massachusetts,USA.

Karabatsos, N.(1985) "*International Catalogue of Arboviruses (including certain other viruses of vertebrates*" (3rd ed) American Society of tropical Medicine and Hygiene, San Antonio, Tex.

Knipe, David M. Howely, Peter M. (Eds) (2001) Bunyaviridae, In: *Fields Virology* ,LIPPINCOTT WILLIAMS & WILKINS, ISBN 0-7817-1832-5, USA .

Krasus, Harmut., Weber, Albert., Appel, Max., Enders, Burkhards., D.Isenberg, Henry., Gerd Schifer, Hans. Slenczka, Werner., Von Graevenitz,Alexander., Zahner, Horst. (2003) *ZOONOSES Infectious Disease Transmissible from Animals to Humans* (Third edition)ASM Press,ISBN: 155812368,Washington DC.

M.W. Service.(Ed) (2001) "*The Encyclopedia of Arthropod_transmitted Infectious of Man and Domesticated Animals* "CABI Publishing, ISBN 0851994733New York,USA

Richman, Douglas D .(WHITLey ,Richard J. and Hayden, Frederick G.)(Ed) (2002) *Clinical Virology*. ASM Press, ISBN 1 55581- 226-0, Washington,D.c.

Shepherd, A.J., Swanepoel, R., Leman, P.A. (1989). "Antibody response in Crimean-Congo haemorrhagic fever". *Rev. Infect. Dis.* 11: 806-811

Shepherd,A.J, Swanepoel, R. Shepherd, S.P. leman, P.A, Blachbun , N.K. and Hallett, A.F.(1985) "A nosocomial outbreak of Crimean-Congo haemorrhagic fever at Tygenberg Hospital". *S.Af.Med.J.* 68: 733-736.

Simpson, D.K, Knight, M.C, G.Courtois, Weinbren , M.P and Kibuhanusoke, J.W. (1976.) Congo virus a hitherto undescribed virus occurring in Africa.*E.Af.Med.J* 44:87-92.

Swanepoel, R., Gill, D.E., Shepherd, A.J., Leman, P.A., Mynhardt, J.H., Harvey, S. (1989). "The clinical pathology of Crimean- Congo haemorrhagic fever". *Rev. Infect. Dis.* 11:794-800.

Swanepoel, R., shepherd, A.J. leman, P.A. shepherd, S.P, Mc Gillivray, G.M. Erasmus ,M.J. Seark, L.A. Gill ,D.E.(1987). "Epidemiology and clinical features of Crimean-Congo haemorrhagic fever in southern Africa" .*Am.J.Trop.Med.Hyg*:36:120-132.

Swanepoel, R., shepherd, A.J, leman, P.A. shepherd , S.P. Miller, G.B. (1985) "A common-source outbreak of Crimean- Congo haemorrhagic fever on a diary farm". *S.Af.Med*.J. 68:635-637.

Swanepoel, R. , shepherd A.J. leman,P.A . Shepherd, S.P. (1985). "Investigation foolowing initial recognition of Crimean-Congo haemorrhagic fever in South Africa". *S.Af.Med*.J.68:638-641.

Van der Giessen, J.W.B., Isken L.D., Tiemersma E.W. (2004) *Zoonoses in Europe :A risk to public Health* (First Edition National Institute for public health and the environment, Bilthoven, The Netherlands.

Watts, D.M. Ksiazek, T.G. Linthicum ,K.J. Hoogstraal, H. (1989). "Crimean-Congo haemorrhagic fever". In Month, T.P. (ed), the *Arboviruse: Epidemiology and Ecology,* (p 177-222) vol2, CRCPress, Inc. Boca Raton, Fle.

12

Epidemiology, Surveillance and Laboratory Diagnosis of Leptospirosis in the WHO South-East Asia Region

Chandika D. Gamage[1,2], Hiko Tamashiro[1], Makoto Ohnishi[3] and Nobuo Koizumi[3]

[1]*Department of Global Health and Epidemiology, Hokkaido University Graduate School of Medicine*

[2]*Faculty of Veterinary Medicine and Animal Science, University of Peradeniya*

[3]*Department of Bacteriology, National Institute of Infectious Diseases*

[1,3]*Japan*

[2]*Sri Lanka*

1. Introduction

Leptospirosis is a serious spirochete zoonotic disease of increasing worldwide prevalence and distribution (Bharti et al., 2003; Levett, 2001). The disease especially occurs in tropical areas with high rainfall and severe human cases may cause multi-organ failure leading to death. The World Health Organization (WHO) has estimated that approximately 10-100 cases per 100,000 people are infected annually in tropics (WHO, 2003). Although leptospirosis has been recognized for many years, it is considered a re-emerging disease of humans in many regions, exemplified by recent outbreaks in Brazil (Romero et al., 2003), India (Chaudhry et al., 2002), Malaysia (Sejvar et al., 2003), Nicaragua (Ashford et al., 2000; Trevejo et al., 1998), Sri Lanka (Epidemiology Unit-Sri Lanka, 2009a) and Thailand (Thaipadungpanit et al., 2007). It also causes substantial domestic livestock losses annually (Faine et al., 1999).

The disease occurs mainly in areas where humans or other animals come into contact with the urine of infected animals or a urine-polluted environment. Secondary human-to-human transmission occurs rarely (WHO, 2003). In tropics, approximately 10% of hospital admissions case attributes to leptospirosis infection, particularly following rains or floods (Kenneth et al., 2010). True incidence of leptospirosis is under-estimated due to lack of appropriate diagnostic capacity, and case finding and reporting in both human and veterinary medicine have been limited and biased (Cachay and Vinetz, 2005).

The clinical diagnosis of leptospirosis is complicated due to the varied and non-specific manifestations of its symptoms which resemble those of other infectious diseases in tropics, such as dengue fever or dengue hemorrhagic fever, malaria and scrub typhus. Inadequate and poor laboratory facilities tend to hamper the accurate identification of leptospirosis, thus the disease remains largely under-diagnosed and therefore under-estimated (WHO, 2003).

At present, 26.5 % of the 6.8 billion (2010) of the world population live in the WHO South-East Asia (WHO SEA) Region and 57% of the 774 million workforce is engaged in agriculture (WHO, 2009a). In the last few decades, tropical diseases continue to have crippling effects on the inhabitants especially people who live in poverty. The WHO SEA Region possess a high burden of tropical diseases such as lymphatic filariasis, soil transmitted helminthiasis, visceral leishamaniasis, trachoma, yaws, schistosomiasis, dengue, rabies, leprosy, Japanese encephalitis and leptospirosis, which are reported from one or more of the Member States of this region (Table 1) (WHO, 2011). The WHO SEA Region is a hotspot for emerging infectious diseases especially zoonoses and vector-borne diseases. Continuous population growth, mobility, rapid urbanization, environmental changes, deforestation, and climate change are acting as major factors that lead to increase the infectious diseases incidence in the region.

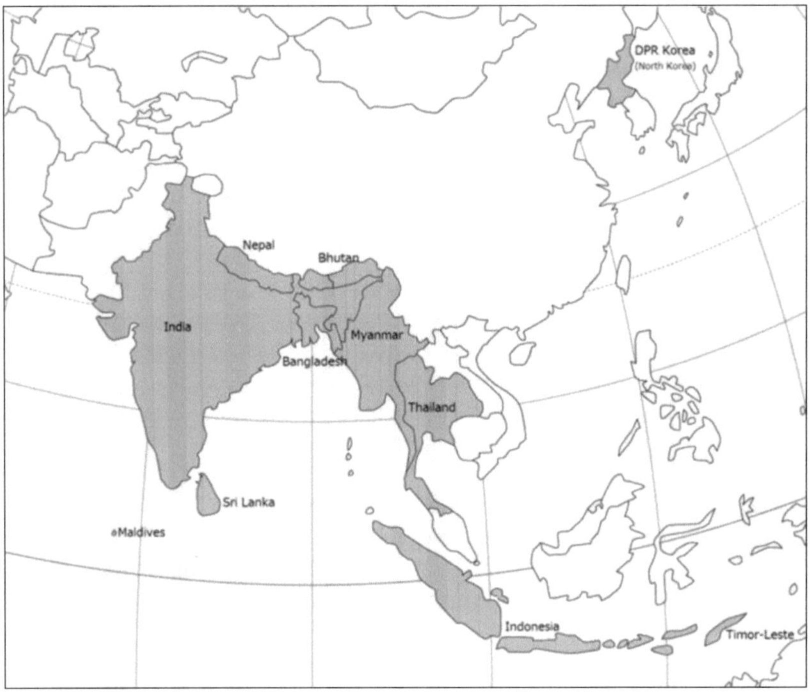

Fig. 1. Map of the WHO South-East Asia Region. The WHO South-East Asia (SEA) Region has eleven Member States: Bangladesh, Bhutan, Democratic People's Republic (DPR) of Korea, India, Indonesia, Maldives, Myanmar, Nepal, Sri Lanka, Thailand, and Timor-Leste.

Despite the high prevalence of many infectious diseases in the region, up-to-date information is not sufficiently available to make an estimation of the burden of diverse diseases and any cross-country comparison difficult. Laboratory diagnosis and surveillance are crucial to generate proper epidemiological information on the diseases in a country or a region (WHO, 2002). However, most of the Member States are lacking proper diagnostic laboratories despite the continuation of endemics of these diseases for many decades.

The aim of this chapter is to summarize the current situations of epidemiology, surveillance and laboratory diagnosis of leptospirosis in the WHO SEA Region. We reviewed the literature for the past two decades published in the PubMed (NLM) database. The combination of keywords <Country name> and <Leptospirosis> were used as search criteria. Appropriate publications were selected and summarized in subsequent sections. Furthermore, we used the Google search engine to locate the documents on leptospirosis of the WHO SEA Region.

Disease Name	Member country name										
	Bangladesh	Bhutan	DPR Korea	Inida	Indonesia	Maldives	Myanmar	Nepal	Sri Lanka	Thailand	Timor-Leste
1 Chikungunya				◆	◆	◆	◆		◆		
2 Dengue	◆	◆		◆	◆	◆	◆	◆	◆	◆	◆
3 Japanese Encephalitis				◆	◆		◆	◆	◆	◆	
4 Leprosy	◆	◆	◆	◆	◆	◆	◆	◆	◆	◆	◆
5 Leptospirosis	◆			◆	◆			◆	◆	◆	
6 Lymphatic filariasis	◆			◆	◆	◆	◆	◆	◆	◆	◆
7 Rabies	◆	◆		◆	◆		◆	◆	◆	◆	
8 Schistosomiasis					◆						
9 Soil Transmitted helminthaiasis	◆	◆	◆	◆	◆	◆	◆	◆	◆	◆	◆
10 Trachoma				◆			◆	◆			
11 Visceral Leishmaniasis	◆	◆		◆				◆			
12 Yaws				◆	◆						◆

(Adopted from Communicable Disease Newsletter, World Health Organization Regional Office for South-East Asia January 2011 Volume 8 issue 1; and revised accordingly leptospirosis situation in the WHO South-East Asia Region, World Health Organization Regional Office for South-East Asia)

Table 1. Distribution of reported tropical diseases in South-East Asia region.

2. Epidemiology

Leptospirosis is an important public health problem in resource-poor countries in tropics. In tropical regions, cases are reported year-round but predominantly during the rainy season (Sarkar et al., 2002; Trevejo et al., 1998). The increased risk during the rainy season becomes higher after flooding that accompanies natural disasters, when the human population may be exposed to water contaminated with urine from infected animals. Outbreaks associated with flooding and natural disasters have occurred in Nicaragua in 1995 (Trevejo et al., 1998), in Brazil in 1996 (Barcellos & Sabroza, 2000), and in India in 2002 (Karande et al., 2002). Seasonality of leptospirosis would be related to agricultural cycles.

It has been shown that people who are engaged in agriculture and animal husbandry have high risk of leptospirosis in comparison to other occupations (WHO, 2011a). A case-control study in Thailand revealed an increased risk of leptospiral infection among persons that performed various agricultural activities in wet fields for > 6 hours/day (Tangkanakul et al., 2005). In tropical areas such as SEA Region, annual incidence rates ranges from 10–100 per 100,000 people (WHO, 2003) and the disease is endemic in almost all Member States for many decades. Recent outbreaks were reported from Sri Lanka, India and Thailand. Epidemiology of leptospirosis in SEA Region mainly depends on various socio-cultural, occupational, behavioral and environmental factors. Unfortunately, national incidence data is not available other than outbreak reports or research based case series studies in many SEA Member States (Table 2). Among the Member States, Bangladesh, Bhutan, DPR of Korea, Maldives, Myanmar, Nepal and Timor-Leste has limited or no published epidemiological information compared to Thailand, Sri Lanka, India and Indonesia (WHO, 2008). In SEA region, the most recent large leptospirosis outbreak occurred in Sri Lanka in 2008, with 7,423 clinically diagnosed leptospirosis cases (Incidence rate 35.7 per 100,000 people) and 207 deaths reported according to leptospirosis case definition (Epidemiology Unit-Sri Lanka, 2009b). Although the number of leptospirosis cases and deaths were reduced in 2009 and 2010, Sri Lanka still reported the highest annual leptospirosis cases among the SEA Member States (4,980 in 2009 and 4,545 cases in 2010). Based on hospital-based sentinel surveillance data, nearly half of the cases are aged between 30-49 years and 80% are male. Two thirds of the patients were exposed to paddy fields and muddy areas either accidently or due to the nature of occupation. During the 2008 outbreak, 37% of 1,414 clinically diagnosed cases were positive for genus specific MAT using the Patoc strain of *Leptospira biflexa*. Agampodi et al (2011) and Koizumi et al (2009) have investigated portions of the 2008 outbreak serum samples by MAT using a panel of pathogenic strains. The results revealed that serogroups Pyrogenes and Sejroe were predominant in Kegalle and Kandy, respectively.

Leptospirosis is an important public health issue in Thailand. From 1995 to 2000, the disease incidence rate increased from 0.3 to 23.7 per 100,000 people, although the incident rate has dropped in recent years (2009a). In 2009 Bureau of Epidemiology Department of Disease Control, Ministry of Public Health Thailand reported that 5,439 leptospirosis cases and 64 deaths due to leptospirosis (incidence rate of 8.57 per 100,000 people and fatality rate of 0.1 per 100,000 people) with the male to female ratio of 4:1. Of the 5,439 cases, 72.9% were aged between 25 - 64 years and 72.4% were occupied in agriculture and labor sectors. Most infections occur in agricultural workers, primarily rice producers (Bureau of Epidemiology Department of Disease Control, 2009).

In India, outbreaks of leptospirosis have increasingly been reported from the coastline: Gujarat (Clerke et al., 2002), Mumbai (Karande et al., 2002), Kerala (Kuriakose et al., 2008), Chennai (Ratnam et al., 1993) and Andaman Islands (Sehgal et al., 1995). A 5 year consecutive sero-epidemiological study conducted in Kerala state has shown that 29.6% inhabitants possessed anti-leptospiral antibodies and the prevalent serogroups were Autumnalis, Louisiana, Australis, and Grippotyphosa (Kuriakose et al., 2008). In another study conducted by Sehgal and colleagues as part of a multi-centric study on disease burden due to leptospirosis (initiated by the Indian Council of Medical Research in 2000), 3,682 patients with acute febrile illness, from 13 different centers in India, were investigated for the presence of current leptospiral infection using the Lepto-dipstick test. Of these patients, 469 (12.7%) were found to possess anti-leptospiral IgM. The positivity rate ranged from 3.27% in the central zone to 28.16% in the southern zone. Fever, body aches and chills were the common symptoms observed. Urinary abnormalities, such as oliguria, yellow discoloration of urine and hematuria were found in 20%-40% of patients. (Sehgal et al., 2003).

In Indonesia, human leptospirosis cases were reported first in 1952, when it had been known as Canicola fever (Smit et al., 1952). There was a marked increase in human leptospirosis cases between 2003 (85 cases) to 2007 (666 cases). The outbreak in 2007, approximately 93% of the cases were laboratory confirmed and the case fatality rate was 8% (WHO, 2009a). However, a recent outbreak in Bantul regency in Indonesia's central Java region had a 27% case fatality (Netnewspublisher, 2011). Prevalence of rickettsioses and leptospirosis was investigated among urban residents in Semarang, revealing that 13 out of 137 febrile patients were confirmed as leptospirosis (Gasem et al., 2009).

Although data on leptospirosis in Bangladesh is limited, LaRocque R. C., et al. (2005) reported 18% of dengue-negative febrile patients at two Dhaka hospitals were positive for leptospirosis by PCR in a 2000 dengue outbreak. In a serosurvey conducted in rural Bangladesh in 1994 revealed high prevalence of anti-leptospiral antibodies among both patients with jaundice and healthy controls (Morshed et al., 1994).

There is no published information on human leptospirosis in Bhutan and Myanmar. However, leptospirosis in animal populations has been reported from both countries (WHO, 2009a). In 2000 Maldives reported their first human leptospirosis case (WHO, 2009a). In Nepal, no national surveillance program for leptospirosis exists. However, Myint, K. S., et al (2010) detected anti-leptospiral antibodies in military personnel participating in an efficacy study of a hepatitis E virus vaccine in Nepal. Among the 1,566 study volunteers, the prevalence of leptospirosis was 9% among hepatitis cases and 8% among febrile cases. The predominant serogroups were Bratislava, Autumnalis, Icterohaemorrhagiae, and Sejroe. Timor-Leste and DPR Korea have no published data about human leptospirosis.

Considering the urgent necessity of obtaining proper and up-to-date leptospirosis burden data to formulate and revise ongoing control and prevention activities, the WHO convened an international consultation to assess potential methods to determine a global burden of leptospirosis in October 2006. As an outcome of this meeting, the Leptospirosis Burden Epidemiology Reference Group (LERG), established in partnership with other international organizations, has started conducting global research that provides the necessary data for designing an appropriate policy targeted towards decreasing the burden of leptospirosis. LERG conducted an informal expert consultation on surveillance, diagnosis and risk reduction of leptospirosis in SEA Region, in Chennai, India on 17-18 September 2009. The experts recommended necessary measures to improve surveillance, estimation of burden of the disease, advocacy, awareness and education, diagnosis and vaccination (WHO, 2009b). Although WHO's LERG mainly focuses on human leptospirosis and its burden, future models which estimate the burden of the disease should pay attention to animal reservoirs, climate change and other environmental factors that may have an effect on particular regions of the world (Abela-Ridder et al., 2010)

3. Surveillance systems

Disease surveillance is a critical component of the health system in generating essential epidemiological information for a cost-effective healthcare delivery (WHO, 2002). Through surveillance, incidences and distributions of diseases (e.g., leptospirosis) and the implications for effective public health strategies are identified. Although surveillance of leptospirosis has been in place in many SEA Member States for decades now, it has yet to be adopted and implemented as a monitoring tool to address issues related to control and prevention of the disease (WHO, 2002). Surveillance of leptospirosis has been proven to be an effective and economical disease control tool in detecting and preventing large outbreaks (Jena et al., 2004). The WHO provides standards and guidelines for leptospirosis surveillance (WHO, 1999). Only a few SEA Member States adopted these standards (*e.g.*, Sri Lanka and Thailand). Most of the Member States are lacking specific government policies and legal frameworks to support surveillance and have inadequate laboratory facilities and reporting systems. Furthermore, there is poor interaction between human and veterinary health sectors for better coordination and collaboration toward surveillance and control of leptospirosis (Narain and Bhatia, 2010).

Among the WHO SEA Member States, Maldives, Myanmar, Sri Lanka and Thailand include leptospirosis as one of the notifiable diseases in the country. In India, although leptospirosis is not listed as a target disease in the National Surveillance Program for Communicable Diseases (NSPCD) or in the Integrated Disease Surveillance Program (IDSP) under the core diseases, it is included in 5 endemic States (Maharashtra, Karnataka, Kerala, Gujarat, Tamil Nadu) (Regional Medical Research Centre, 2006).

Sri Lanka's national disease reporting system, which is empowered by the quarantine and prevention of diseases ordinance enacted in 1897 with subsequent amendments, identifies 28 notifiable diseases including leptospirosis, and provides the guidelines for their reporting to physicians and other healthcare personnel (Figure 2). In 2004, in parallel to the notifiable diseases reporting system, the government implemented the hospital-based sentinel site

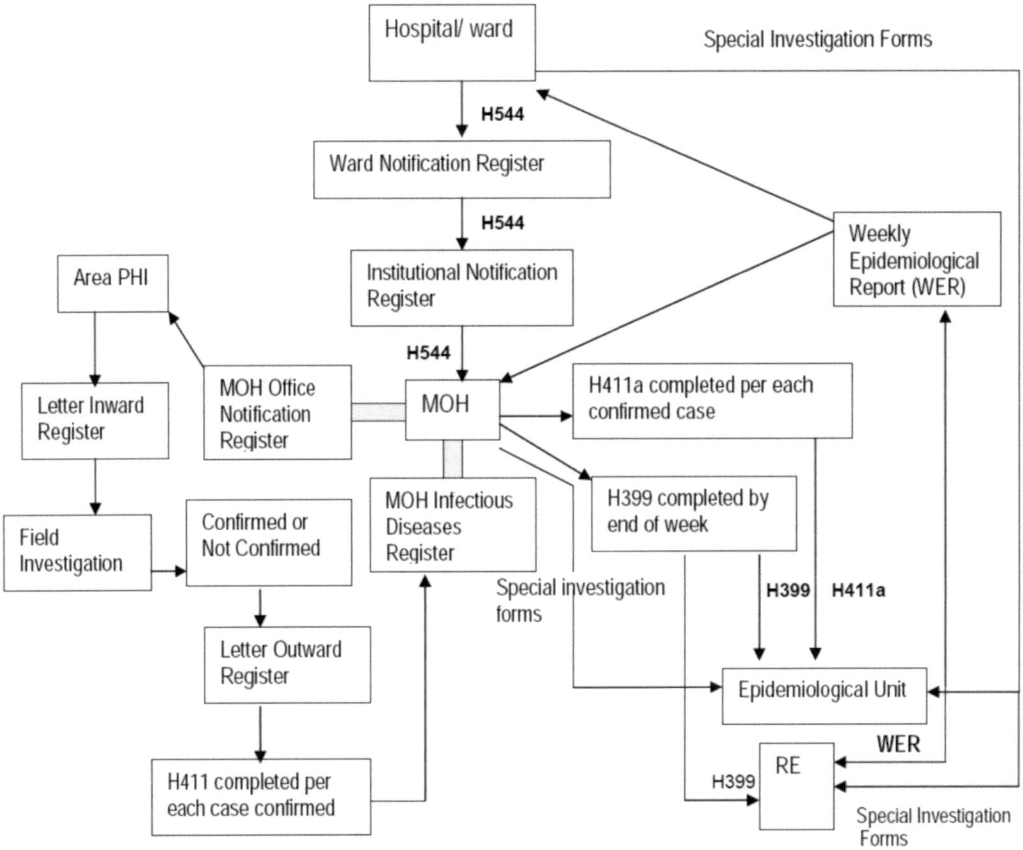

MOH: Medical Office of Health; RE: Regional Epidemiologist; WER: Weekly Epidemiological Report; PHI: Public Health Inspector; H544, H399, H411a : specific forms for reporting process.

Fig. 2. Flow chart on the reporting system of notifiable diseases in Sri Lanka (Source: Sentinel site surveillance guidelines (2010), Epidemiology Unit, Ministry of Health, Sri Lanka).

surveillance for leptospirosis. The sentinel surveillance seeks to obtain clinical (e.g. signs and symptoms), epidemiological (e.g. exposures), laboratory (e.g. infected serogroup) and prophylactic treatment (e.g. use of antibiotics) information among those suspected of having an infection (Epidemiology Unit-Sri Lanka, 2009a).

Surveillance of leptospirosis and other 49 diseases is currently (2009) undertaken in Thailand by the Bureau of Epidemiology, Department of Disease Control, Ministry of Public Health. The disease surveillance data such as morbidity rate, mortality rate, gender, age group, occupation, place of treatment and type of patient (for death and cure cases) are published weekly and annually through the homepage of Bureau of Epidemiology, Thailand (http://www.boe.moph.go.th/).

Leptospirosis is one of the most economically important diseases in the livestock sector and possesses a zoonotic hazard towards the people who are involved in this sector. However, leptospirosis is drastically neglected in most of the WHO SEA Member States, although its surveillance in rodents and domestic animals is important for developing its appropriate control and prevention strategies. It is not a priority disease in the veterinary sector and there is no systematic surveillance among livestock in the WHO SEA Region. Furthermore, there is no veterinary and medical institutional arrangement to estimate the burden of leptospirosis in most of the Member States of the WHO SEA region.

4. Laboratory diagnosis

Leptospirosis has diverse clinical manifestations that resemble many other tropical infectious diseases such as dengue fever, malaria, and scrub typhus which are prevalent in the region. Though a large number of fever of unknown origin are reported to the health facilities, investigation for leptospirosis is not carried out partly due to poor knowledge of clinical manifestations of the disease or lack of proper laboratory diagnostic facilities. Thus a large number of leptospirosis cases are reported without laboratory confirmation which directly affects the estimated disease burden in the region. Laboratory diagnosis of leptospirosis involves two groups of tests. One group is designed to detect anti-leptospiral antibodies, while the other group is to detect leptospires, leptospiral antigens, or leptospiral nucleic acid in body fluids or tissues (Levett, 2001). Culture and microscopic agglutination test (MAT) are the gold standard methods for its laboratory diagnosis. However, these methods are laborious for the routine use.

The MAT is the most widely used diagnostic serological test. Although MAT detects serogroup-specific antibodies, it appeared to be of little value for predicting infecting serogroup (serovar) of patients (Levett, 2003; Katz et al., 2003; Smythe et al., 2009). MAT requires paired sera for definitive diagnosis of leptospirosis. Seroconvension or at least fourfold increase in the titer must be observed between acute and convalescent serum samples. Anti-leptospiral antibodies detected by MAT are present for months to years after infection. Thus, it is difficult to confirm acute infection from a single serum sample. In endemic areas, a high titer of 400 or more in a symptomatic patient is generally accepted as a criterion for disease confirmation (Levett, 2001). Furthermore, MAT requires maintenance of a panel of *Leptospira* cultures prevalent in a particular geographical area, and appropriate quality control must be employed.

Several whole *Leptospira* cell-based rapid screening tests for antibody detection in acute infection have been developed, including enzyme linked immunosorbent assay (ELISA), latex agglutination test, lateral flow assay, and IgM dipstick (Bharti et al., 2003; Levett, 2001; McBride et al., 2005, Toyokawa et al., 2011). These assays have been used as alternatives to MAT but have low sensitivity especially during the acute phase (Smits et al., 2001; Effler et al., 2002; Hull-Jackson et al., 2006; McBride et al., 2007). Furthermore, the diagnostic accuracies of these techniques are poor in some areas where leptospirosis is endemic (Blacksell et al., 2006; Myint et al., 2007).

PCR is demonstrably useful for early diagnosis of leptospirosis before its antibody production has commenced. PCR protocols for detection of leptospiral DNA in clinical materials have been developed (Ahmed et al., 2009). Conventional or real time PCR assays targeting a range of genes, such as 16SrRNA, 23SrRNA, LipL32, LipL21, RpoB, GyrB, OmpL1, LigA and B, and flagellin, have been described (Slack et al., 2006; Stoddard et al., 2009; Reitstetter et al., 2006; Kawabata et al., 2001). However, PCR may not be widely applied in resource-poor countries due to its high operational cost (Sehgal et al., 2003). Thus, diagnostic methods that not only have higher sensitivity and accuracy for early-phase leptospirosis but also are applicable widely in resource-poor countries remain to be developed.

Country* (reference)	Area	Study duration	No of study participants	Diganostic methods used	Point prevalence	Demographics	Rsik factors	Prevalent serogroup
India (Chauhan et al., 2010)	Sub-Himalayan state of North India (i.e. Himachal Pradesh)	August 1 - October 31, 2009	13 leptospirosis suspected patients	IgM ELISA and PCR (G1 and G2 primers)	10 were IgM positive, One positive by PCR	Male: 77% Age: ranged 24-78years, mean 44years old	Contacted with animals or contaminat ed water	NA
Sri Lanka (Agampodi et al., 2011)	Kandy, Kegalle and Matale districts	August 20 2008 - January 6 2009	Of 746 patients with acute febrile illness 401 probable cases of leptospirosis were examined	ELISA, MAT and PCR	NA	NA	NA	Pyrogenes, Javanica, Sejroe and Hebdomadis
Indonesia (Gasem et al., 2009)	Semaranga in central Java	Feb 2005 - Feb 2006	137 acute undeferentiated fever patients	Lepto Tek Dri Dot (a commercial prodcut), MAT and IgG ELISA	10%	NA	NA	Bataviae
Thailand (Wuthiekanun et al., 2007)	9 provinces located in north, northeast, central and southern regions	March 2003 - November 2004	700 leptospirosis suspected patients	MAT and culture	20% were laboratory confirmed leptospirosis patients	Among confirmed cases median age was 35 years (range 10-68 years). 85% were men	NA	Autumnalis, Bataviae, Pyrogenes, Javanika, Hebdomadis, Grippotyphosa
Bangladesh (Kendall et al., 2010)	Kamalapur, Dhaka	Jan 1 - Dec 31, 2001	878 febrile patients. Only 584 had paired sera samples	Sceening by IgM ELIA. Confirmation by MAT	8.4% (definite + probable infection)	Male 41% Age: 17.8+-13.1 years		Sarmin and Mini
Nepal (Myint et al., 2010)	Army unit stationed in Kathmandu	July-August 2001	2000 volunteers from the Nepalese Army	IgM ELISA and MAT	9% among clinical hepatitis cases 11% among non hepatic febrile cases	All male, mean age (+-SD) 25.2+-6.25	NA	Bratislava, Icterohaemorrhagiae, Autumnalis and Sejroe

*No publication were found from Bhutan, DPR Korea, Madives Myanmar and Timor-Leste for the period of January, 2009 – October, 2011.

Table 2. Leptospinosis in WHO South-East Asian Member States bases on the publucation published form 2007 to 2011.

Inadequate and poor laboratory facilities available in the WHO SEA Region, tend to hamper the accurate identification of leptospirosis, thus remaining largely under-diagnosed and therefore under-estimated (WHO, 2003). Among the WHO SEA Member States, only India, Indonesia, Sri Lanka and Thailand have fully or partially implemented laboratory facilities to diagnose leptospirosis (WHO, 2009b). However, those laboratories need to be strengthened and standardized to produce countrywide services and to perform more accurate and specific diagnostic procedures.

In Sri Lanka, two governmental institutions, namely the Medical Research Institute (MRI), the Ministry of Health and the Veterinary Research Institute (VRI), Department of Animal Health and Production, have the capacity to diagnose leptospirosis using MAT. However, MRI is capable of a limited genus level serological diagnosis using only *L. biflexa* Patoc I strain (Dassanayake et al., 2009). In 2008, 37% of 1,414 suspected leptospirosis human cases were serological positive, but no information on infective serogroup was available (Epidemiology Unit, Ministry of Health, 2009a).

In India, the isolation of pathogenic leptospires from human and animal hosts in several parts of India has been reported (WHO, 2006). Because there are only limited facilities for serotyping in the country, most of the isolates were typed to the serogroup level only (Gangadhar et al., 2008).

Diagnosis of leptospirosis in Indonesia has been performed at the Pasteur Institute located in Ho Chi Minh (HCM) City, Vietnam (Laras et al., 2002). In-house developed ELISA, MAT and PCR methods are employed in Thailand (Kee et al., 1994; Tangkanakul et al., 2005). In Thailand, local institutes collaborate with the Collaborating Center for Reference and Research on Leptospirosis, Brisbane, Queensland, Australia (Wuthiekanunet al., 2007).

5. Conclusion

Leptospirosis is an emerging zoonotic disease of public health importance in countries of the WHO's South-East Asia Region. In some Member States, the disease has been endemic for many decades and causes sporadic outbreaks. The disease epidemiology is tightly linked to regional climatic factors and major occupational sectors such as agricultural and livestock workers. Interventions need to give special attention to at-risk geographic areas with a high case fatality rate and to individuals of particular socio-demographic characteristics (*e.g.*, men and agricultural workers). Further research needs to be carried out concerning more patho-physiological information of the disease to prevent leptospirosis deaths that could be prevented with proper and timely treatment after an early and accurate diagnosis of the disease. However, adequate laboratory tests for early diagnosis are still lacking (Toyokawa et al, 2011). Diagnostic methods that not only have higher sensitivity and accuracy for early-phase leptospirosis but also are applicable widely in resource-poor countries need urgently to be developed. The existence of large numbers of reservoir animals and route of disease transmission make activities in prevention and control of leptospirosis in WHO SEA Region difficult, especially with financial constraints. The quality of data on which the control and prevention of leptospirosis in the region is based will hinge upon a periodic assessment of the efficacy with which the sentinel surveillance system captures, analyzes and disseminates information. Data quality along with accurate results from laboratory investigations will determine the true burden of leptospirosis infection in each member country and the region.

6. References

Abela-Ridder, B.; Sikkema, R. & Hartskeerl, R. A. "Estimating the burden of human leptospirosis." Int J Antimicrob Agents 36 Suppl 1: S5-7 Epub Date 2010/08/07

Agampodi, S. B.; Peacock, S. J.; Thevanesam, V.; Nugegoda, D. B.; Smythe, L.; Thaipadungpanit, J.; Craig, S. B.; Burns, M. A.; Dohnt, M.; Boonsilp, S.; Senaratne, T.; Kumara, A.; Palihawadana, P.; Perera, S. & Vinetz, J. M. "Leptospirosis Outbreak in Sri Lanka in 2008: Lessons for Assessing the Global Burden of Disease." Am J Trop Med Hyg 85(3): 471-478 Epub Date 2011/09/08

Ahmed, A.; Engelberts, M. F.; Boer, K. R.; Ahmed, N. & Hartskeerl, R. A. (2009). "Development and validation of a real-time PCR for detection of pathogenic leptospira species in clinical materials." PLoS One 4(9): e7093.

Ashford, D. A.; Kaiser, R. M.; Spiegel, R. A.; Perkins, B. A.; Weyant, R. S.; Bragg, S. L.; Plikaytis, B.; Jarquin, C.; De Lose Reyes, J. O. & Amador, J. J. (2000). "Asymptomatic infection and risk factors for leptospirosis in Nicaragua." Am J Trop Med Hyg 63(5-6): 249-54.

Barcellos, C. & Sabroza, P. C. (2000). "Socio-environmental determinants of the leptospirosis outbreak of 1996 in western Rio de Janeiro: a geographical approach." Int J Environ Health Res 10(4): 301-13.

Bharti, A. R.; Nally, J. E.; Ricaldi, J. N.; Matthias, M. A.; Diaz, M. M.; Lovett, M. A.; Levett, P. N.; Gilman, R. H.; Willig, M. R.; Gotuzzo, E. & Vinetz, J. M. (2003). "Leptospirosis: a zoonotic disease of global importance." Lancet Infect Dis 3(12): 757-71.

Blacksell, S. D.; Smythe, L.; Phetsouvanh, R.; Dohnt, M.; Hartskeerl, R.; Symonds, M.; Slack, A.; Vongsouvath, M.; Davong, V.; Lattana, O.; Phongmany, S.; Keolouangkot, V.; White, N. J.; Day, N. P. & Newton, P. N. (2006). "Limited diagnostic capacities of two commercial assays for the detection of Leptospira immunoglobulin M antibodies in Laos." Clin Vaccine Immunol 13(10): 1166-9.

Bureau of Epidemiology Department of Disease Control (2009). "Annual Epidemiology Surveillance Report" Ministry of Public Health, Thailand 09.08.2011, Available from: http://http://epid.moph.go.th/Annual/Annual%202552/AESR52_Part2/Ranking/Ranking_TABLE%2015_52.pdf.

Cachay, E. R. & Vinetz, J. M. (2005). "A global research agenda for leptospirosis." J Postgrad Med 51(3): 174-8.

Chaudhry, R.; Premlatha, M. M.; Mohanty, S.; Dhawan, B.; Singh, K. K. & Dey, A. B. (2002). "Emerging leptospirosis, North India." Emerg Infect Dis 8(12): 1526-7.

Chauhan, V.; Mahesh, D. M.; Panda, P.; Mokta, J. & Thakur, S. "Profile of patients of leptospirosis in sub-Himalayan region of North India." J Assoc Physicians India 58: 354-6 Epub Date 2010/12/04

Clerke, A. M.; Leuva, A. C.; Joshi, C. & Trivedi, S. V. (2002). "Clinical profile of leptospirosis in South gujarat." J Postgrad Med 48(2): 117-8.

Dassanayake, D. L.; Wimalaratna, H.; Agampodi, S. B.; Liyanapathirana, V. C.; Piyarathna, T. A. & Goonapienuwala, B. L. (2009). "Evaluation of surveillance case definition in the diagnosis of leptospirosis, using the Microscopic Agglutination Test: a validation study." BMC Infect Dis 9: 48.

Effler, P. V.; Bogard, A. K.; Domen, H. Y.; Katz, A. R.; Higa, H. Y. & Sasaki, D. M. (2002). "Evaluation of eight rapid screening tests for acute leptospirosis in Hawaii." J Clin Microbiol 40(4): 1464-9.

Epidemiology Unit - Sri Lanka (2009a). An Interim Analysis of Leptospirosis Outbreak in Sri Lanka– 2008, Ministry of Health, Sri Laka. Available from: http://www.epid.gov.lk/Disease%20Situations.htm.

Epidemiology Unit - Sri Lanka (2009b). Surveillance report on leptospirosis - 2008. Epidemiology Bulletin, Ministry of Health, Sri Lanka 50:14-8

Faine, S.; Adler, B.; Bolin, C., & Perolat, P. (1999). Leptospira and Leptospirosis. (MediSci, Melbourne, Australia.).

Gangadhar, N. L.; Prabhudas, K.; Bhushan, S.; Sulthana, M.; Barbuddhe, S. B. & Rehaman, H. (2008). "Leptospira infection in animals and humans: a potential public health risk in India." Rev Sci Tech 27(3): 885-92.

Gasem, M. H.; Wagenaar, J. F.; Goris, M. G.; Adi, M. S.; Isbandrio, B. B.; Hartskeerl, R. A.; Rolain, J. M.; Raoult, D. & van Gorp, E. C. (2009). "Murine typhus and leptospirosis as causes of acute undifferentiated fever, Indonesia." Emerg Infect Dis 15(6): 975-7

Hull-Jackson, C.; Glass, M. B.; Ari, M. D.; Bragg, S. L.; Branch, S. L.; Whittington, C. U.; Edwards, C. N. & Levett, P. N. (2006). "Evaluation of a commercial latex agglutination assay for serological diagnosis of leptospirosis." J Clin Microbiol 44(5): 1853-5.

Jena, A. B.; Mohanty, K. C. & Devadasan, N. (2004). "An outbreak of leptospirosis in Orissa, India: the importance of surveillance." Trop Med Int Health 9(9): 1016-21.

Karande, S.; Kulkarni, H.; Kulkarni, M.; De, A. & Varaiya, A. (2002). "Leptospirosis in children in Mumbai slums." Indian J Pediatr 69(10): 855-8.

Katz, A. R.; Effler, P. V. & Ansdell, V. E. (2003). "Comparison of serology and isolates for the identification of infecting leptospiral serogroups in Hawaii, 1979 - 1998." Trop Med Int Health 8(7): 639-42.

Kawabata, H.; Dancel, L. A.; Villanueva, S. Y.; Yanagihara, Y.; Koizumi, N. & Watanabe, H. (2001). "flaB-polymerase chain reaction (flaB-PCR) and its restriction fragment length polymorphism (RFLP) analysis are an efficient tool for detection and identification of Leptospira spp." Microbiol Immunol 45(6): 491-6.

Kee, S. H.; Kim, I. S.; Choi, M. S. & Chang, W. H. (1994). "Detection of leptospiral DNA by PCR." J Clin Microbiol 32(4): 1035-9.

Kendall, E. A.; LaRocque, R. C.; Bui, D. M.; Galloway, R.; Ari, M. D.; Goswami, D.; Breiman, R. F.; Luby, S. & Brooks, W. A. "Leptospirosis as a cause of fever in urban Bangladesh." Am J Trop Med Hyg 82(6): 1127-30 Epub Date 2010/06/04

Kenneth J. Ryan; C. George Ray (2003). Sherris Medical Microbiology: An Introduction to Infectious Diseases. New York: McGraw-Hill Medical Publishing Division. ISBN 0-8385-8529-9.

Koizumi, N.; Gamage, C. D.; Muto, M.; Kularatne, S. A.; Budagoda, B. D.; Rajapakse, R. P.; Tamashiro, H. & Watanabe, H. (2009). "Serological and genetic analysis of leptospirosis in patients with acute febrile illness in kandy, sri lanka." Jpn J Infect Dis 62(6): 474-5.

Kuriakose, M.; Paul, R.; Joseph, M. R.; Sugathan, S. & Sudha, T. N. (2008). "Leptospirosis in a midland rural area of Kerala State." Indian J Med Res 128(3): 307-12.

Laras, K.; Cao, B. V.; Bounlu, K.; Nguyen, T. K.; Olson, J. G.; Thongchanh, S.; Tran, N. V.; Hoang, K. L.; Punjabi, N.; Ha, B. K.; Ung, S. A.; Insisiengmay, S.; Watts, D. M.; Beecham, H. J. & Corwin, A. L. (2002). "The importance of leptospirosis in Southeast Asia." Am J Trop Med Hyg 67(3): 278-86.

LaRocque, R. C.; Breiman, R. F.; Ari, M. D.; Morey, R. E.; Janan, F. A.; Hayes, J. M.; Hossain, M. A.; Brooks, W. A. & Levett, P. N. (2005). "Leptospirosis during dengue outbreak, Bangladesh." Emerg Infect Dis 11(5): 766-9.

Levett, P. N. (2001). "Leptospirosis." Clin Microbiol Rev 14(2): 296-326.

Levett, P. N. (2003). "Usefulness of serologic analysis as a predictor of the infecting serovar in patients with severe leptospirosis." Clin Infect Dis 36(4): 447-52.

McBride, A. J.; Athanazio, D. A.; Reis, M. G. & Ko, A. I. (2005). "Leptospirosis." Curr Opin Infect Dis 18(5): 376-86.

McBride, A. J.; Santos, B. L.; Queiroz, A.; Santos, A. C.; Hartskeerl, R. A.; Reis, M. G. & Ko, A. I. (2007). "Evaluation of four whole-cell Leptospira-based serological tests for diagnosis of urban leptospirosis." Clin Vaccine Immunol 14(9): 1245-8.

Morshed, M. G.; Konishi, H.; Terada, Y.; Arimitsu, Y. & Nakazawa, T. (1994). "Seroprevalence of leptospirosis in a rural flood prone district of Bangladesh." Epidemiol Infect 112(3): 527-31.

Myint, K. S.; Gibbons, R. V.; Murray, C. K.; Rungsimanphaiboon, K.; Supornpun, W.; Sithiprasasna, R.; Gray, M. R.; Pimgate, C.; Mammen, M. P., Jr. & Hospenthal, D. R.(2007). "Leptospirosis in Kamphaeng Phet, Thailand." Am J Trop Med Hyg 76(1): 135-8.

Myint, K. S.; Murray, C. K.; Scott, R. M.; Shrestha, M. P.; Mammen, M. P., Jr.; Shrestha, S. K.; Kuschner, R. A.; Joshi, D. M. & Gibbons, R. V. "Incidence of leptospirosis in a select population in Nepal." Trans R Soc Trop Med Hyg 104(8): 551-5 Epub Date 2010/05/25

Narain, J. P. & Bhatia, R. "The challenge of communicable diseases in the WHO South-East Asia Region." Bull World Health Organ 88(3): 162.

Netnewpublisher (2011). Leptospirosis Outbreak in Indonesia Prompts Emergency Action, In: Netnewspublisher/Asia, 10.08.2011, Available from: http://www.netnewspublisher.com/leptospirosis-outbreak-in-indonesia-prompts-emergency-action/

Ratnam, S.; Everard, C. O.; Alex, J. C.; Suresh, B. & Thangaraju, P. (1993). "Prevalence of leptospiral agglutinins among conservancy workers in Madras City, India." J Trop Med Hyg 96(1): 41-5.

Regional Medical Research Centre (2006). Report of the Brainstorming Meeting on Leptispirosis Prevention and Control, 10.08.2011, Available from: http://www.whoindia.org/LinkFiles/Communicable_Diseases_Report_of_the_Leptospirosis_meeting_Final.pdf .

Reitstetter, R. E. (2006). "Development of species-specific PCR primer sets for the detection of Leptospira." FEMS Microbiol Lett 264(1): 31-9.

Romero, E. C.; Bernardo, C. C. & Yasuda, P. H. (2003). "Human leptospirosis: a twenty-nine-year serological study in Sao Paulo, Brazil." Rev Inst Med Trop Sao Paulo 45(5): 245-8.

Sarkar, U.; Nascimento, S. F.; Barbosa, R.; Martins, R.; Nuevo, H.; Kalofonos, I.; Grunstein, I.; Flannery, B.; Dias, J.; Riley, L. W.; Reis, M. G. & Ko, A. I. (2002). "Population-based case-control investigation of risk factors for leptospirosis during an urban epidemic." Am J Trop Med Hyg 66(5): 605-10

Sehgal, S. C.; Murhekar, M. V. & Sugunan, A. P. (1995). "Outbreak of leptospirosis with pulmonary involvement in north Andaman." Indian J Med Res 102: 9-12.

Sehgal, S. C.; Sugunan, A. P. & Vijayachari, P. (2003). "Leptospirosis disease burden estimation and surveillance networking in India." Southeast Asian J Trop Med Public Health 34 Suppl 2: 170-7.

Sejvar, J.; Bancroft, E.; Winthrop, K.; Bettinger, J.; Bajani, M.; Bragg, S.; Shutt, K.; Kaiser, R.; Marano, N.; Popovic, T.; Tappero, J.; Ashford, D.; Mascola, L.; Vugia, D.; Perkins, B. & Rosenstein, N. (2003). "Leptospirosis in "Eco-Challenge" athletes, Malaysian Borneo, 2000." Emerg Infect Dis 9(6): 702-7.

Slack, A. T.; Symonds, M. L.; Dohnt, M. F. & Smythe, L. D. (2006). "Identification of pathogenic Leptospira species by conventional or real-time PCR and sequencing of the DNA gyrase subunit B encoding gene." BMC Microbiol 6: 95.

Smit, A. M.; Wolff, J. W. & Bohlander, H. (1952). "A human case of canicola fever in Indonesia." Doc Med Geogr Trop 4(3): 265-7.

Smits, H. L.; Eapen, C. K.; Sugathan, S.; Kuriakose, M.; Gasem, M. H.; Yersin, C.; Sasaki, D.; Pujianto, B.; Vestering, M.; Abdoel, T. H. & Gussenhoven, G. C. (2001). "Lateral-flow assay for rapid serodiagnosis of human leptospirosis." Clin Diagn Lab Immunol 8(1): 166-9

Smythe, L. D.; Wuthiekanun, V.; Chierakul, W.; Suputtamongkol, Y.; Tiengrim, S.; Dohnt, M. F.; Symonds, M. L.; Slack, A. T.; Apiwattanaporn, A.; Chueasuwanchai, S.; Day, N. P. & Peacock, S. J. (2009). "The microscopic agglutination test (MAT) is an unreliable predictor of infecting Leptospira serovar in Thailand." Am J Trop Med Hyg 81(4): 695-7.

Stoddard, R. A.; Gee, J. E.; Wilkins, P. P.; McCaustland, K. & Hoffmaster, A. R. (2009). "Detection of pathogenic Leptospira spp. through TaqMan polymerase chain reaction targeting the LipL32 gene." Diagn Microbiol Infect Dis 64(3): 247-55.

Tangkanakul, W.; Smits, H. L.; Jatanasen, S. & Ashford, D. A. (2005). "Leptospirosis: an emerging health problem in Thailand." Southeast Asian J Trop Med Public Health 36(2): 281-8.

Thaipadungpanit, J.; Wuthiekanun, V.; Chierakul, W.; Smythe, L. D.; Petkanchanapong, W.; Limpaiboon, R.; Apiwatanaporn, A.; Slack, A. T.; Suputtamongkol, Y.; White, N. J.; Feil, E. J.; Day, N. P. & Peacock, S. J. (2007). "A dominant clone of Leptospira interrogans associated with an outbreak of human leptospirosis in Thailand." PLoS Negl Trop Dis 1(1): e56

Toyokawa, T.; Ohnishi, M. & Koizumi, N. (2011) "Diagnosis of acute leptospirosis." Expert Rev Anti Infect Ther 9(1): 111-21.

Trevejo, R. T.; Rigau-Perez, J. G.; Ashford, D. A.; McClure, E. M.; Jarquin-Gonzalez, C.; Amador, J. J.; de los Reyes, J. O.; Gonzalez, A.; Zaki, S. R.; Shieh, W. J.; McLean, R. G.; Nasci, R. S.; Weyant, R. S.; Bolin, C. A.; Bragg, S. L.; Perkins, B. A. & Spiegel, R. A. (1998). "Epidemic leptospirosis associated with pulmonary hemorrhage-Nicaragua, 1995." J Infect Dis 178(5): 1457-63.

WHO (1999). Leptospirosis, In: WHO Recommended Surveillance Standards. Second edition, 30.06.2011, Available from:
http://www.who.int/csr/resources/publications/surveillance/whocdscsrisr992.pdf

WHO (2002). Regional Strategy for Integrated Disease Surveillance, In: Report of an Inter-country Consultation Yangon. Myanmar, 14.07.2011, Available from:

http://www.searo.who.int/LinkFiles/Publication_130_RSI-Disease-Surveillance.pdf

WHO (2003). Human Leptospirosis: Guidance for Diagnosis, Surveillance and Control, World Health Organization, 04.08.2011, Available from: http://whqlibdoc.who.int/hq/2003/WHO_CDS_CSR_EPH_2002.23.pdf

WHO (2008). Leptospirosis in South-East Asia. The tip of the iceberg?, World Health Organization Regional Office for South-East Asia, 05.08.2011, Available from: http://www.searo.who.int/LinkFiles/Communicable_Diseases_Surveillance_and_response_Leptospirosis_in_South_East_Asia.pdf.

WHO (2009a). Leptospirosis situation in the WHO South-East Asia Region. World Health Organization Regional Office for South-East Asia, 07.08.2011, Available from: http://www.searo.who.int/LinkFiles/Communicable_Diseases_Surveillance_and_response_SEA-CD-216.pdf.

WHO (2009b). Informal Expert consultation on Surveillance, Diagnosis and Risk Reduction of Leptospirosis. World Health Organization Regional Office for South-East Asia, 05.08.2011 Available from: http://www.searo.who.int/LinkFiles/Communicable_Diseases_Surveillance_and_response_SEA-CD-217.pdf.

WHO (2011). Mapping of Neglected Tropical Diseases in the South-East Asia Region, In: Communicable Disease Newsletter, 20.08.2011, Available from: http://www.searo.who.int/LinkFiles/CDS_News_letter_vol-8_issue-1.pdf.

Wuthiekanun, V.; Sirisukkarn, N.; Daengsupa, P.; Sakaraserane, P.; Sangkakam, A.; Chierakul, W.; Smythe, L. D.; Symonds, M. L.; Dohnt, M. F.; Slack, A. T.; Day, N. P. & Peacock, S. J. (2007). "Clinical diagnosis and geographic distribution of leptospirosis, Thailand." Emerg Infect Dis 13(1): 124-6

Part 3

Protozoan Zoonosis

13

Toxoplasma gondii in Meat and Food Safety Implications – A Review

Susana Bayarri, María Jesús Gracia, Regina Lázaro, Consuelo Pérez-Arquillué and Antonio Herrera
University of Zaragoza, Veterinary Faculty, Spain

1. Introduction

In contrast to the important global advance in the last decades in the food availability, hundreds of million people anywhere in the world suffer diseases caused by the food consumption, maintaining effective today, an important problem for the public health and an extraordinary cause of reduction of the productive economy.

Foodborne diseases are caused by a number of agents, varying their severity from weak to chronic or acute disturbances that can affect or compromise the life of the consumer, and being the agents of biological origin (bacteria, viruses, parasites) the major cause of these diseases.

The important advances accomplished regarding personal hygiene, basic cleaning, potable water supply, food control structures, and the increase of the systems of technological control that assure the elimination or destruction of food pathogens to safe limits, have led to a practically null number of cases of classic food diseases at the present time in the industrialized countries.

Nevertheless, there are many reasons for foodborne disease remaining a global public health challenge. As some diseases are controlled, others emerge as new threats. New agents of risk have occupied the ecological niche of those on which control pressure has been exerted, replacing the previous ones. The proportions of the population who are elderly, immunosuppressed or otherwise disproportionately susceptible to severe outcomes from foodborne diseases are growing in many countries. Globalization of the food supply has led to the rapid and widespread international distribution of foods. This fundamental fact has motivated a radical change in the modern systems of management of the food safety, forced to the search of new methods of risk assessment, more effective preventive systems, permanent research of new systems of identification of these agents, to the development of the epidemiology applied to the food hygiene and the application of much more effective methods in the complex world of the decision making.

A recent publication from the United States concludes that more than 90 percent of the health burden is caused by five pathogens: *Salmonella* spp., *Campylobacter* spp., *Listeria monocytogenes*, *Toxoplasma gondii* and norovirus. *Toxoplasma gondii* is not a "front page" foodborne pathogen, but it is very important from a public health standpoint (Batz et al., 2011). The CDC (Centers for Disease Control and Prevention) estimates that foodborne toxoplasmosis is surpassed only by *Salmonella* in the number of annual deaths it causes. Although toxoplasmosis is conventionally associated with cats and kitty litter, curently it is estimated that 50% of cases are foodborne (Scallan et al., 2011).

Parasites, including *Toxoplasma gondii,* are reported less frequently in humans, and have caused fewer outbreaks than bacteria and viruses in the European Union (EU). However, in many instances, their impact (severe illness, disability, death, and costs related to diagnostic procedures, hospitalization and treatment) on vulnerable groups of the population, and often in immunocompetent persons, has been considerable (EFSA, 2007).

Toxoplasmosis is a common infection in animals and humans. It is caused by an obligate intracellular protozoan parasite, *Toxoplasma gondii.* The life cycle of *Toxoplasma* includes asexual multiplication in the intermediate host and sexual reproduction in the definitive host. Many species of warm-blooded animals can act as intermediate hosts and, seemingly, most animal species may be carriers of tissue cysts of this parasite. Cats and wild felids are the only definitive hosts that may pass oocysts with their faeces and these needs to sporulate in the environment before becoming infective.

In intermediate hosts, *Toxoplasma* undergoes two phases of asexual development. In the first phase, tachyzoites multiply rapidly in many different types of host cells. Tachyzoites of the last generation initiate the second phase of development which results in the formation of tissue cysts containing bradyzoites, which multiply only infrequently. All hosts, including humans, can be infected by three different life cycle stages: tachyzoites, bradyzoites contained in tissue cysts and sporozoites contained in sporulated oocysts (Dubey, 2007).

The organotropism of tissue cysts varies in different intermediate host species. In many hosts, tissue cysts have a high affinity for neural and muscular tissues. They are located predominantly in the central nervous system, the eye as well as skeletal and cardiac muscles. However, to a lesser extent they may also be found in visceral organs, such as lungs, liver, and kidneys (Dubey, 1993; Dubey et al., 1998). Tissue cysts are the terminal life-cycle stage in the intermediate host and are immediately infective. In some intermediate host species, including most livestock, they may persist for the life of the host, being consumption of raw or undercooked meat products containing tissue cysts a major risk factor associated with human toxoplasmosis (Dubey & Beattie, 1988; García et al., 2006; Hill, 2007; Mie et al., 2008). *Toxoplasma* has historically been associated with pork meat but a recent case-control study by CDC found the leading foodborne risks to be eating raw ground beef, rare lamb or locally-produced cured, dried or smoked meat (Jones et al., 2009).

Consumption of food and water contaminated with sporulated oocysts and congenital infection, are another main modes of transmission of *T. gondii*. In humans, the majority of infections is asymptomatic or cause mild flu-like symptoms. However, infection may produce a severe disease in immunocompromised people, and abortions in pregnant women, as well as adverse effects such as perinatal death, fetal abnormalities, or reduced quality of life in children who survive a prenatal infection. *T. gondii* can cause permanent and devastating damage to developing fetuses, including stillbirths, serious hospitalization during infancy, and permanent, lifelong mental and physical disabilities (EFSA, 2011 b).

Batz et al. (2011) estimate that congenital toxoplasmosis acquired through food results in 16 stillbirths or neonatal deaths annually in USA, as well as in 216 infants born with mild to serious permanent impairments, ranging from blurry vision, mental impairment and neurological problems such as partial paralysis and abnormal movement.

There is a globalisation in the trade of animals and food worldwide, so rules for trade of meat and meat products seek to guarantee that all imports and exports fulfil high standards to guarantee food safety. This should also be addressed to the animal health status and high standard of meat and meat products in order to avoid human toxoplasmosis. Besides measures focussing on pre-harvest food safety (*e.g.* surveillance and monitoring in animals), post-harvest strategies at slaughter and during food processing have become more and more important in recent years.

With regard to meat processing, demands of consumers for pathogen free meat products have focused the attention of the meat industry on food safety and the necessity to produce meat that is wholesome, safe, and of high quality, using the appropriate technological treatments. Scientific studies have indicated that *T. gondii* tissue cysts in meat are susceptible to various physical procedures such as heat treatment, freezing, irradiation or high hydrostatic pressures, and some authors have suggested that tissue cysts are killed by commercial procedures of curing with salt.

Improved surveillance is needed to better estimate the true incidence of foodborne toxoplasmosis, and significant increases in data collection, epidemiologic studies and scientific research are needed to understand the relative importance of routes of toxoplasmosis transmission. Addressing the risk of the foodborne disease requires the implementation of a well functioning and integrated food control system, and this necessitates collaboration among all the components of a food control system, including food law and regulations, food control management, inspection services, epidemiological and food monitoring (laboratory services), education, and communication with the consumer (WHO, 2008). Under this consideration, surveillance and monitoring in food and food products could provide important information for a better risk assessment on *Toxoplasma* and toxoplasmosis from the consumer protection point of view (EFSA, 2007).

Considering the importance for the risk assessment process, the aim of this review is to show the state of the art for data implicating meat as a source of infection and to describe studies focused on the effect of technological processes of meat products in the inactivation of *Toxoplasma gondii*.

2. Surveillance and monitoring in animals used for human consumption. Meat as a source of *Toxoplasma gondii* infection in humans

There is a widespread distribution of *Toxoplasma* infection in a variety of livestock, wild animals and pets. Ingestion of environmentally robust stages (sporozoites in oocysts) or eating raw or undercooked meat or meat products containing tissue stages (tachyzoites or bradyzoites in tissue cysts), are the main transmission routes for *T. gondii* to humans (EFSA, 2007).

Some authors assume that about 50% of all human toxoplasmosis cases are related to foodborne infection (Slifko et al., 2000), and retrospective epidemiological analyses of human toxoplasmosis outbreaks suggest that many are associated with consumption of raw or undercooked meat or other edible parts of animals. Tenter et al. (2000) and Schlundt et al. (2004) estimated that the percentage of meat-borne cases was approximately 30% to 63%, depending on eating habits.

However, the relative importance of the risk factor and the type of meat associated with it varied among different countries (Cook et al., 2000). For example, in France and Norway consumption of undercooked lamb was a stronger risk factor than consumption of undercooked pork (Kapperud et al., 1996; Baril et al., 1999), whereas in Poland consumption of undercooked pork was the principal risk factor identified in the study (Paul, 1998). These findings may reflect differences in eating habits of consumers or different prevalences of infection in meat producing animals in these regions.

In response to natural infection, most farm animals are seropositive for *T. gondii* and serological studies have found evidence of widespread *T. gondii* infection in meat-producing animals. It is important to note that the organotropism of *Toxoplasma* and the number of tissue cysts produced in a certain organ vary with the intermediate host species. In livestock, tissue cysts of *Toxoplasma* are most frequently observed in various tissues of infected pigs, sheep, and goats, and less frequently in infected poultry, rabbits, and horses (Tenter et al., 2000). Although tissue cysts are less resistant to environmental conditions than oocysts, they are relatively resistant to changes in temperature and remain infectious in refrigerated (1 to 4°C) carcasses or minced meat for up to 3 weeks, *i.e.* probably as long as the meat remains suitable for human consumption (Dubey, 1988; Tenter et al., 2000).

Experimental infections of food animals such as cattle, pigs, sheep and goats, have shown that these animals are susceptible to *T. gondii* contamination by intake of oocysts or tissue cysts, and that following experimental infection *T. gondii* can be isolated from their tissues, with the exception of beef (Dubey et al., 1980, 1984; Dubey, 1983, 1986a, 1988; Blewett et al., 1982; McColgan et al., 1988; Lunden & Uggla, 1992; Dubey & Thulliez, 1993; Esteban-Redondo et al., 1999; Tenter et al., 2000; Zia-Ali et al., 2007).

It is very important the impact of farming systems on the risk of *Toxoplasma* infections. Recent data show that it is possible to significantly reduce the risk of *Toxoplasma* infection in livestock using intensive farm management with adequate measures of hygiene, confinement, and prevention. These measures include: (A) keeping meat-producing animals indoors throughout their life-time, (B) keeping the sheds free of rodents, birds, and insects, (C) feeding meat producing animals on sterilised food, and (D) controlling access to sheds and feed stores, *i.e.* no pet animals should be allowed inside them. On the contrary, production of free-ranging livestock will inevitably be associated with *Toxoplasma* infection. Animals kept on pastures with an increased pressure of infection due to contamination of the environment with oocysts, such as goats and sheep, show a high level of seropositives in many areas of the world, *i.e.* up to 75% to 92% respectively (EFSA, 2007).

The observed decline in *Toxoplasma* seroprevalence as noted in many developed countries over past decades has been attributed to the introduction of modern farming systems resulting in a lower prevalence of *Toxoplasma* cysts in meat in combination with an increased use of frozen meat by consumers (Tenter et al., 2000; Kortbeek et al., 2004; AFSSA, 2005; Diza et al., 2005; Jones et al., 2007).

Another important aspect is the age of the animals. In a recent study (Berger-Schoch et al., 2011), a P-30-ELISA was used to detect *T. gondii*-specific antibodies and to determine seroprevalences in meat juice of slaughtered animals in Switzerland. The study included pigs, cattle, sheep and wild boar of different age groups and housing conditions. The results show that the seropositivity increased with the age of the assessed animals. Independent of the age-group, the overall seroprevalence was lowest in wild boars (6.7%), followed by pigs (23.3%), cattle (45.6%) and sheep (61.6%). Conventional fattening pigs and free-ranging pigs surprisingly had comparable seroprevalences (14.0% and 13.0%, respectively). Unlike in other European countries, where generally a decrease in the number of seropositive animals had been observed, these authors found that the prevalence of seropositive animals, when compared with that of 10 years ago, had increased for most species/age groups. Conclusively, the results demonstrated a high seroprevalence of *T. gondii* in animals slaughtered for meat production and revealed that increasing age of the animals is a more important risk factor than housing conditions in this country.

Sheep, rather than pigs, are the main source of infected meat in Southern European countries (EFSA, 2007). Data from a number of different European countries showing that, whilst seroprevalence of *Toxoplasma* amongst pigs has fallen in the last three decades, to around 1%, the measured values for sheep have remained significantly higher at 20–30% (Tenter et al., 2000). Relevant to this apparent increase in the potential of sheep to serve as a route of human infection is the fact that, like pigs, they do not generally develop overt clinical symptoms upon *T. gondii* infection (Owen & Trees, 1999).

In sheep and goats, seropositives reported in different countries vary widely. Dubey (2009) reviewed serological surveys in various countries conducted since 1988, and found 3–96% positive results. This author also concluded that in general most sheep acquired infection before 4 years of age. Congenitally-infected lambs that survive the first week after birth usually grow normally and can be a source of infection for humans. In Europe, data available in sheep report seropositive rates of 16-66% (Tenter et al., 2000; Dumètre et al., 2006; Pinheiro et al., 2009; Panadero et al., 2010; Pikka et al., 2010). High seroprevalences were found also in Bangladesh (40%) (Shahiduzzaman et al., 2011), and in New Zealand (61%) (Dempster et al., 2011). Seropositivity is found correlated with age, increasing from lambs (22%) to ewes (65.6%) (Dumetre et al., 2006) and also differences among different geographical areas were found (Panadero et al., 2010).

Prevalence of *T. gondii* in lambs can be high but the role of ingestion of infected lamb in the epidemiology of toxoplasmosis in humans remains to be determined (Dubey & Jones, 2008). Raw or undercooked lamb meat is considered a delicacy in certain countries such as France and is therefore considered an important source of infection in that country (AFSSA, 2005). Adult sheep meat is often well cooked and therefore probably poses a smaller risk of infection to the consumer than lamb meat. All case-control studies have identified the consumption of mutton/lamb meat as a highly significant risk factor for contracting *T. gondii* infection in pregnant women. Symptomatic toxoplasmosis in a family in New York City was circumstantially linked to eating rare lamb (Masur et al., 1978). Recently a large-scale screening of sheep farms has shown that 3.4% of sheep were shedding *T. gondii* in their milk (Fusco et al., 2007).

Although abortion and neonatal mortality are the main clinical signs, adult goats can develop clinical toxoplasmosis involving liver, kidneys and brain (Dubey & Beattie, 1988). Seroprevalence is dependent on the presence of oocysts in the environment, housing and climatic conditions (Tenter et al., 2000). Seropositivities reported in Europe in farmed goats vary from 4% to 77% and data in slaughtered goats in non-European countries range from 0% to 40% (data reviewed by Tenter et al., 2000). Recently, a high seroprevalence was found in goats in Bangladesh (32%) (Shahiduzzaman et al., 2011).

Although studies have reported the isolation of *T. gondii* from caprine tissues, no large-scale prevalence data are available on the presence of parasites in goat meat products (Dubey, 1980, 1981; Sharma et al., 2003). Small ruminants such as goats are an important source of meat (very popular in several ethnic groups, especially from Asia) and milk in many undeveloped countries and may play a role as a source of infection for humans residing in these areas (Shrestha & Fahmy, 2005). As well, consumption of raw goat's milk and milk products has been linked to cases of toxoplasmosis in humans (Riemann et al., 1975; Sacks et al., 1982; Skinner et al., 1990; Meerburg et al., 2006).

Numerous serologic surveys on prevalence of *T. gondii* in pigs from different countries have been performed. The results showed wide variation in the prevalence values among countries and between regions within the same country (Tenter et al., 2000; Dubey, 2009; Dubey & Jones, 2008; Alvarado-Esquivel et al., 2011; Yu et al., 2011). *T. gondii* infection is widespread in pigs raised in Spain and a seroprevalence of 16.6% was obtained in a recent study (Garcia-Bocanegra et al., 2010). Similar seroprevalences were obtained in studies carried out in Italy (Villari et al., 2009; Veronesi et al., 2011), Portugal (De Sousa et al., 2006) and Germany (Damriyasa et al., 2004). Lower seroprevalence levels were found in USA (2.6%) (Hill et al., 2010), Sweden (5.2%) (Lundén et al., 2002), the Netherlands (10.9%) (Kijlstra et al., 2004) and Mexico (12.7%) (Alvarado-Esquivel et al., 2011); while higher values were observed in Serbia (28.9%) (Klun et al., 2006) and Argentina (37.8%) (Venturini et al., 2004). Analysis of swine management practices indicated that rodent control methods and carcass disposal methods were associated with differences in the number of *T. gondii* positive samples on farm (Hill et al., 2010).

Also, prevalence of *T. gondii* varies dramatically among the classes of pigs surveyed (market pigs *versus* sows, indoor pigs with a biosecurity system *versus* free-range) (Dubey& Jones, 2008). Seropositivities in swine reared in Europe (Tenter et al., 2000) vary from null to 64% for fattening/ slaughter pigs and from 3 to 31% for sows.

Seropositivity in general is a good indicator of the presence of viable parasites in tissues (Dubey et al., 1995, 2002; Dubey & Jones, 2008) and the level of isolation increased with antibody titre in the pig (Dubey et al., 1995). However, the antibody titre that should be considered indicative of latent infection in pigs is not always certain because viable *T. gondii* has been isolated from seronegative pigs (Hejlíček & Litérak, 1993; Omata et al., 1994; Dubey et al., 1995, 2002; De Sousa et al., 2006). These results indicates that either these pigs were recently infected and had not yet developed *T. gondii* antibodies, or that the antibody titres had declined to undetectable levels (Dubey et al., 1995). In this regard, Hill et al. (2006) suggest that the antibody response may be independent of parasite burden.

Toxoplasma cysts in pork can persist for a long time, and has been considered an important source of infection for humans (EFSA, 2007). A qualitative risk assessment identified

Toxoplasma gondii and *Trichinella* spp., as well as *Salmonella* spp. and *Yersinia enterocolitica*, as the most relevant biological hazards in the context of meat inspection of swine (EFSA, 2011a). However, due to major changes in animal production hygiene, the prevalence of *T. gondii* in pork meat has decreased (Tenter et al., 2000; Dubey & Jones, 2008), and currently, modern production systems, especially those in which intensive management has been adapted, have virtually eliminated *T. gondii* infection in pigs (van Knapen et al., 1995; Davies et al., 1998; Kijlstra et al., 2004; van der Giessen et al., 2007; Kijlstra & Jongert, 2008b).

Several epidemiological studies conducted in The Netherlands show that the prevalence of antibodies specific for *Toxoplasma* antigens in industrially kept fattening pigs is declining over the years. In 1969, a seroprevalence of 54% for *Toxoplasma* antibodies was observed in fattening pigs, while in 1982 this was only 1.8% (van Knapen et al., 1995). In a survey conducted in 1983–1984, seroprevalence was 23% in market pigs and 42% in breeder pigs (sows) (Dubey et al., 1991). When pigs from these same areas were tested in 1992, prevalence had dropped to 20.8% in breeders and 3.1% in finisher pigs (Dubey et al., 1995). In Brazil, the seroepidemiological investigation of *T. gondii* on farms revealed a prevalence of 37.8% in the early 1990s, ten years later this rate had decreased to 15.4% (Vidotto et al., 1990; Tsutsui, 2000). This downward tendency has been observed worldwide and is presumed to be related to the indoor housing system of pigs, where contact with cats is prevented and vermin in the stables is under control (van Knapen et al., 1995). However if bio security standards are low, the prevalence could increase up to 51-55% (Dubey et al., 2005).

Although modern meat production has reduced the prevalence of *T. gondii* in young pigs in Europe and North America (Tenter et al., 2000), a higher seroprevalence of *T. gondii* has been observed in sows compared to fattening pigs (Dubey, 1986a; Weigel et al., 1995; Lundén et al., 2002; Damriyasa, et al., 2004; Villari et al., 2009; García-Bocanegra et al., 2010; Alvarado-Esquivel et al., 2011). The higher seroprevalence in sows compared with market age pigs is epidemiologically relevant with respect to transmission of *T. gondii*. Market age pigs are sold for use in fresh, unprocessed pork products whereas meat from breeding sows is usually processed (such as sausages, salami, etc.) and processing kills or reduces *T. gondii* in pork (Dubey, 2009).

Recent trends in consumer habits indicate a shift towards consumption of "animal-friendly" or "organic" pigs. This animal production system of rearing pigs outdoors increased risk of exposure to *T. gondii* and it is likely to increase *T. gondii* seroprevalence. A study on seroprevalence of *Toxoplasma* antibodies conducted in 2001-2002 in The Netherlands indeed demonstrated a prevalence of 2.9% in pigs kept in animal-friendly housing systems, while 0% of the indoor pigs were seropositive (Kijlstra et al., 2004). Moreover, a seroprevalence study in indoor, organic and free ranging pigs carried out in 2004 in the Netherlands showed an overall prevalence of antibodies specific for *Toxoplasma* of 2.6%. In this study the seroprevalence in intensively raised pigs was close to nil (0.38%), whereas in organic pigs was 2.74%, and in free-range pigs the prevalence was 5.62%. The risk of detecting *Toxoplasma* antibodies in a free-range farm is statistically higher (almost 16 times higher) than in an intensive farm (van der Giessen, 2007). Pigs reared in organic farms and free-ranging pigs have indeed increased opportunities of contact with *Toxoplasma* compared to animals reared in close confinement, as they may be more exposed to contact with soil contaminated with *Toxoplasma* oocysts or to ingestion of infected preys, like rodents harbouring tissue cysts. In addition, farm management practices in organic farms such as feeding goat whey to pigs and allowing contact between pigs and cats may influence the prevalence of *Toxoplasma* infection in the herd (Meerburg et al., 2006). In fact, increasingly popular animal friendly production systems may cause a re-emergence of pork meat as an infectious meat source (Kijlstra et al., 2004; Schulzig & Fehlhaber, 2006; van der Giessen et al., 2007).

Any part of infected pork can be a source of infection because the parasite has been found in most edible tissues or cuts of meat, both in experimentally and naturally-infected pigs (Kijlstra & Jongert, 2008a). However, Dubey et al. (1996) have estimated that less than 1 cyst per 50g of tissue is likely to be found in *Toxoplasma*-infected pigs. Tissue cysts have a high affinity for neural and muscular tissues. They are located predominantly in the central nervous system, the eye as well as skeletal and cardiac muscles, and to a lesser extent they may also be found in visceral organs, such as lungs, liver, and kidneys (Dubey, 1993; Dubey et al., 1998).

Examinations were conducted on the presence of *Toxoplasma* cysts in fresh pork sausages, produced in factories in Londrina (Parana State, Brazil). After bioassay in mice, 13 (8.7%) sausage samples were positive, in one of them *Toxoplasma* was isolated and in the other 12 the mice seroconverted (Dias et al., 2005). Lower detection was obtained by Galván-Ramírez et al. (2010) who analyzed meat samples of pork meat from butcher shops in Ocotlán (Jalisco, Mexico), detecting *T. gondii* in 1 of the 48 samples analyzed (2.1% positivity).

Bayarri et al. (in press), carried out a study on the prevalence of viable *T. gondii* in retail fresh pork meat collected in the city of Zaragoza (Northeast Spain). To ensure that samples were not from the same animal, sampling was carried out in different weeks and in different shops (supermarkets and butchers) distributed in different quarters of the city. More in detail, 25 pieces of fresh pork meat were sampled, corresponding to tongue, rib, loin, and shoulder loin. A mouse concentration bioassay technique was used, and the presence of the parasite in mice was determined by indirect immunofluorescence assay (IFA). *T. gondii* were detected in two samples of rib, reflecting a frequency of 8% positive fresh pork meat. Brains of seropositive mice were analyzed by histology and PCR, although the parasite was not isolated in the seroconverted mice. No viable forms were detected either in other type of fresh meat.

Aspinall et al. (2002) analyzed 58 pork meat product samples obtained from United Kingdom retail outlets, and obtained that 20 were *T. gondii* positive by PCR detection (34.5%). The higher positivity obtained may be because unlike the previously mentioned studies, detection of *Toxoplasma* in this work was purely by PCR, and they only demonstrated the presence of *T. gondii* and not the presence of viable parasites capable of initiating a human infection.

Birds can serve as a potential source of infection for humans. In chickens, *T. gondii* was found in skeletal muscles, heart, brain, ovary, oviduct, kidney, spleen, liver, lung, pancreas, gizzard, proventriculus, intestine and retina, and even in eggs (Jacobs & Melton, 1966; Kaneto et al., 1997). Several surveys in different non-European countries have shown that seropositivities to *Toxoplasma* in poultry can be moderate to high. Seroprevalence of up to 65% in free ranging chickens has been reported and the presence of the parasite in meat could be shown in 81% of seropositive animals (Da Silva et al., 2003; Lehmann et al., 2006). Recently, Bártová et al. (2009) found very low antibody prevalence in gallinaceous birds.

Seropositivity to *Toxoplasma* and isolation of the parasite has been reported in free-range chickens reared in Austria (Dubey et al., 2005) and in Portugal (Dubey et al., 2006). Viable *T. gondii* from ovaries, oviducts and leg muscle were isolated by Jacobs & Melton (1966) and viable *T. gondii* was isolated from 27% to 100% of chickens from backyard operations on small farms in USA (Dubey et al., 2003, 2004). Tissue cysts of *T. gondii* were found in breast and leg muscles, heart, brain, liver and stomach of experimentally infected domestic ducks (Bártová et al., 2004).

Free ranging chickens, especially in developing countries, may be considered as an important source of *T. gondii* infection in humans. In the Western world, commercially produced free ranging chickens intended for meat consumption (broilers) have a limited life span and to date no recent data are available concerning *T. gondii* seroprevalence in these chickens, however it can be expected that poultry kept outside has a higher chance of being infected with the parasite (Dubey et al., 2004). The recent trend of consumers demanding meat from organically grown free-range poultry will increase the prevalence of *T. gondii* in chickens consumed by humans and it will be necessary to cook the meat properly to protect consumers from infection. However, chicken meat is mostly well cooked for consumption (Dubey & Jones 2008).

Due to their habit of feeding close to the ground, poultry is considered a good indicator of environmental contamination by *Toxoplasma* oocysts and to identify *Toxoplasma* strains throughout the world (Lehman et al., 2006).

In a comprehensive study, the prevalence of *Toxoplasma* was determined in 2,094 meat samples of different species from 698 retail meat stores of the United States (Dubey et al., 2005). None of cats fed chicken samples became positive. There are several reasons why the results of this study do not negate the possibility that infected chickens may be important sources of infection for humans. In this study, chicken breasts were selected for sampling because of the experimental design that required testing of 1 kg of boneless meat for each sample, although the authors were aware that the prevalence of *T. gondii* in chicken breast is lower than in other tissues. Further, many of the chicken breasts had been injected with enhancing solutions that have a deleterious effect on *T. gondii*. Finally, some of the samples collected might have been frozen or hard chilled, although the labels indicated otherwise. Standards of hard chill are vague and *T. gondii* is highly susceptible to freezing. In contrast to the bioassay results, antibodies to *T. gondii* were found in 1.3% of the juice extracted from the breast meat using an ELISA, with values six times higher than in control chicken sera. These data suggest that *T. gondii* does occur in commercially marketed chickens in the USA but processing and handling procedures inactivate the organisms prior to sale to consumers.

Several surveys have also reported the finding of antibodies to *Toxoplasma* in horses. Seropositivities reviewed by Tenter et al. (2000) ranged from <1% to 8% in EU, up to 32% in non-EU countries, even in certain regions of the world, up to 90% of the animals were shown to be seropositive (Tassi, 2007). Presence of cysts has been shown in edible tissues from horses (Alkhalidi & Dubey, 1979). The role of horses as a source of *T. gondii* infection depends on regional preferences for horse meat, the preparation method and the seroprevalence of horses used for consumption (Gill, 2005; Tassi, 2007). Raw or undercooked horse meat is frequently consumed in countries such as Belgium, Italy, France and Japan (Gill, 2005).

Cattle are considered a poor host for *T. gondii*. Although cattle can be successfully infected with *T. gondii* oocysts, the parasite is eliminated or reduced to undetectable levels within a few weeks (Dubey, 1983, 1986b), perhaps due to innate resistance. For cattle, resistance to *Toxoplasma* infection and the ability to clear the infection has been suggested (Munday & Corbould, 1979).

Seroprevalence can be high in bovine (up to 92% has been reported) (van Knapen et al., 1995; Tenter et al., 2000; Sroka, 2001; More et al., 2008; Santos et al., 2009). Recent surveys show prevalences of 7.3% in Spain (Panadero et al., 2010) and 12% in Bangladesh (Shahiduzzaman et al., 2011). However, despite the high seropositivity reported in some studies, this may not correlate with presence of parasites in the meat. Isolation of infective tissue cysts from beef is rarely reported (Hellmann & Tauscher, 1967; Canada et al., 2002). However, we cannot be sure that beef does not play a role in *T. gondii* transmission as only relatively small amounts of beef have been tested for viable *T. gondii* parasites (Dubey & Jones, 2008).

The relationship between a seropositive calf or cow and the presence of infective tissue cysts needs to be clarified, because although food habits differ between European countries, eating raw beef or beef products is common in many regions of Europe. Epidemiological studies have shown that the consumption of raw or undercooked beef is considered a risk for *T. gondii* infection in humans (Baril et al., 1999; Cook et al., 2000). Outbreaks have been reported following consumption of raw beef, although doubt was raised whether the meat was unadulterated (Dubey & Jones, 2008). Drinking unpasteurized cow milk was not associated with *T. gondii* infections (Kapperud et al., 1996).

Few surveys have been carried out in farmed rabbits, reporting seropositivities between 6% and 53% in Europe (Hejlíček & Literák, 1994; Sroka et al., 2003).

3. Detection methods in meats

T. gondii cannot be macroscopically detected during current meat inspection of livestock either *ante-* or *post-mortem*. The hazard can be detected only through laboratory testing. The testing methods are based on direct detection of *T. gondii* in tissues or on the indirect detection of specific antibodies in serum.

It is difficult to find *T. gondii* tissue cysts in large animal species for several reasons, including sampling bias and preferred parasite sites. Dubey et al. (1996) have estimated that less than 1 tissue cyst/50 g of tissue is likely to be found in *T. gondii*-infected pigs. Thus, it is possible that when performing any test for tissue cyst detection, false-negatives can result from insufficient sample size or improper sample acquisition (Esteban-Redondo et al., 1999).

The established reference method for the isolation of *Toxoplasma* from foodstuffs is gavage or inoculation into animals. These tests (bioassays) are carried out in laboratory mice or in cats. Mice are either inoculated by the intraperitoneal or subcutaneous route or fed with a homogenate of tissues and maintained in observation for 6-8 weeks, when they are tested for antibodies to *Toxoplasma* and their brain is examined for the detection of tissue cysts. Cats are fed with muscle tissue and their faeces are examined for oocysts 3 days after inoculation. The sensitivity of bioassay is good, since it allows the detection of 1 cyst in 100 grams of tissue (Dubey et al., 1995). Bioassay in cats is more likely to detect *Toxoplasma* in meat than bioassay in mice, because cats are more susceptible than mice to the infection, and more tissue can be fed (Dubey et al., 2005). However, mouse and cat bioassays require use of live animals, which are not desirable for screening large numbers of samples from an animal ethics point of view, are time-consuming and not suitable for slaughterhouse testing (Warnekulasuriya et al., 1998; Opsteegh et al., 2010).

Therefore, PCR-based methods to detect *T. gondii* in meat samples have been developed. However, although the PCR itself is usually sensitive in detecting *T. gondii* DNA, when used on meat samples, these methods lack sensitivity in comparison to the bioassay (Da Silva & Langoni, 2001; Garcia et al., 2006). This lack of sensitivity of PCR-based methods is likely due to the inhomogeneous distribution of *T. gondii* tissue cysts, in combination with the small size of the sample. For PCR, DNA is usually isolated from 50 mg of sample at maximum, while in the bioassay either up to 500 g of meat is fed to a cat, or digestion extract from 50-100 g of meat is inoculated into mice. As a consequence, taking fifty milligrams of the homogenate of a large sample, instead of taking a fifty milligram sample randomly, will increase the probability of isolating *T. gondii* DNA. However, it will be present at a low concentration in a high background of host DNA, which might lead to inhibition of the PCR (Bellete et al., 2003).

Opsteegh et al. (2010) have developed a method for detection and quantification of *T. gondii*. The method involved preparation of crude DNA extract from hundred gram samples of meat, magnetic capture of *T. gondii* DNA and, quantitative real-time PCR targeting the *T. gondii* 529-bp repeat element. The detection limit of this assay was approximately 230 tachyzoites per 100 g of meat sample. Results obtained with the PCR method were comparable to bioassay results for experimentally infected pigs, and to serological findings for sheep. The authors state that the PCR method can be used as an alternative to bioassay for detection and genotyping of *T. gondii*, and to quantify the organism in meat samples of various sources.

In a study on detection of *Toxoplasma* in ready-to-eat cured meat samples by amplification of the parasite's P30 gene, PCR was able to detect parasite contamination down to a level of $5x10^3$ trophozoites/g while viable *Toxoplasma* could be detected in tissue culture at a level of 10^3 trophozoites/g cured meat. The high salt content of some cured meats limited sensitivity of the PCR assay by inhibition of the polymerase enzyme and reduced the sensitivity of tissue culture due to osmotic pressure causing cytopathic effect (Warnekulasuriya et al., 1998).

The presence of DNA shows that the meat originates from a *Toxoplasma*-infected animal but does not necessarily mean that the product contains infectious organisms (Aspinall et al., 2002). To address this problem, Zintl et al. (2009) have developed a robust method for the assessment of *Toxoplasma* tissue cyst viability that combines an in vitro culture approach with quantitative PCR.

Hill et al. (2006) compared the efficacy of serum serology, tissue extract serology, real time PCR, nested PCR, and direct PCR for the detection of *T. gondii* in pork using samples from 25 naturally infected pigs from a farm, 10 experimentally infected pigs, and 34 retail meat samples, and then ranked detection methods in the following descending order of sensitivity: serum ELISA (test sensitivity 100%), serum MAT

(80.6%), tissue fluid ELISA (76.9%), real time PCR (20.5%), semi-nested PCR (12.8%), and direct PCR (0%). Neither ELISA nor MAT reliably detected antibodies in frozen and thawed muscle samples (Hill et al., 2006). Garcia et al. (2006) compared PCR, bioassay, and histopathology in 10 pigs fed *T. gondii* oocysts and killed 60 days later; *T. gondii* was detected in 55.1% of 98 muscle samples by bioassay in mice, in 16.6% of 150 muscle samples by PCR and in 0 samples by histopathology. Tsutsui et al. (2007) compared distribution of *T. gondii* in commercial cuts of pork by bioassay and PCR in 10 pigs 59 days after feeding them oocysts; *T. gondii* was found in 67.5% by bioassays in mice and 22.5% of samples by PCR.

The European Food Safety Authority (EFSA) states that the analytical methods to be used to detect and identify *Toxoplasma* in food and animals need to be characterised in terms of sensitivity, specificity and other performance parameters associated with the reliability and consistency of such methodologies. In order for such characteristics to be attained, there is an absolute requirement for reference materials and reagents (EFSA, 2007).

4. Influence of processing of meat products on the viability of *Toxoplasma gondii*

Approaches to meat safety assurance in respect to tissue cysts of *T. gondii* have to be considered, particularly for high risk populations. They are primarily based on meat treatments with aim to inactivate the cysts. Studies have indicated that *T. gondii* tissue cysts in meat are susceptible to various physical procedures (thermal and non-thermal) such as heat treatment, freezing, irradiation, high-pressure, among others. All these technologies try to be mild, guarantee natural appearance, energy saving and environmentally friendly while knocking the parasites (Aymerich et al., 2008). Their combination, as in the hurdle theory proposed by Leistner (2000) may improve their effectiveness.

It seems that currently, the most reliable cyst inactivation treatments are based on application of either adequate meat heating or meat freezing treatments, and some temperature-time regimes of these treatments have been assayed. According to the opinion adopted in 2007 by the Scientific Panel on Biological Hazards of the EFSA, to prevent foodborne transmission of *Toxoplasma* to humans, meat and other edible parts of animals should not be consumed raw or undercooked, *i.e.* they should be cooked thoroughly (at 67°C or higher) before consumption. Although freezing alone is not a reliable means of rendering all tissue cysts non-infective, deep-freezing meat (-12°C or lower) before cooking can reduce the risk of infection. In addition, meat should not be tasted during preparation or cooking (Paul, 1998; Cook et al., 2000).

It is also essential that preventive measures to reduce the risk of horizontal transmission of *Toxoplasma* to humans via tissue cysts include a high standard of kitchen hygiene. Thus, in a case-control study in Norway, washing kitchen knives infrequently after preparation of raw meat was independently associated with an increased risk of primary infection during pregnancy (Kapperud et al., 1996). Both tissue cysts and tachyzoites are killed by detergents and, thus, hands and all kitchen utensils used for the preparation of uncooked meat or other food from animals should be cleaned thoroughly with hot water and soap (Dubey, 2000).

The first experiments describing the inactivation of tissue cysts of *T. gondii* examined the effects of storage conditions on parasite survival and showed that parasite tissue cysts could be lysed in distilled water (Jacobs et al., 1960), but survived for several weeks in the presence of physiological saline (0.85%) and storage at 4 °C (Jacobs et al., 1960; Dubey et al., 1990). Raising the salt concentration or the temperature led to inactivation of the parasite (Kijlstra & Jongert, 2008a).

4.1 Thermal technologies

4.1.1 Heating and microwave cooking

The primary control factor for prevention of *T. gondii* infection via meat consumption is adequate cooking and prevention of cross-contamination (McCurdy et al., 2006). Limited data are available concerning consumer cooking habits and it is certainly possible that parts of meat being grilled or barbecued do not reach sufficiently high-temperatures to kill the parasite.

Jacobs et al. (1960) were the first to show that heating could inactivate tissue cysts: at 50 °C it takes 1 h to inactivate tissue cysts. Studies on killing of tissue cysts in meat by cooking (49-67°C for 0.01-96 min) were conducted by Dubey (2000) and found that *T. gondii* was rendered nonviable when internal temperatures had reached at least 67 °C.

Survival of tissue cysts at lower temperatures depends on the duration of cooking. For example, under laboratory conditions tissue cysts remained viable at 60 °C for about 4 min and at 50 °C for about 10 min (Dubey et al., 1990). It is important to note that cooking for a prolonged period of time may be necessary under household conditions to achieve the temperatures that are required to kill all tissue cysts of *Toxoplasma* in all parts of the meat. For this reason, cooking infected meat in a microwave does not guarantee killing some tissue cyst, which can remain infective, most probably due to uneven heating (Lundén & Uggla, 1992).

4.1.2 Freezing

Freezing of meat by consumers is widely applied in westernized countries. The loss of sensory quality may be an important factor in consumers' attitudes towards freezing of meat. However, it is very valuable for food safety as, in general, freezing can inactivate the *T. gondii* tissue cysts, although proper timing and temperature are necessary for a 100% parasite killing efficiency.

The effect of freezing on *T. gondii* cyst viability was first described in 1965 (Sommer et al., 1965). It was observed that freezing for 2 days at -20 °C was sufficient to inactivate the parasite.

Experiments with meat from pigs that were fed with *T. gondii*-infected mice, showed that all meat samples were rendered non-infectious by freezing 6–35 days at -25 °C (Grossklaus & Baumgarten, 1968).

Freezing meat for 1 day in a household freezer rendered tissue cysts nonviable (Dubey, 1988). Kotula et al. (1991) carried out experiments using different freezing temperatures (from -1 °C to -171 °C for 1 second to 67 days) and found that an internal temperature of -12 °C was sufficient to render the parasite non-viable. In addition, *Toxoplasma gondii* tissue cysts remained viable up to 22 days at -1 and -3.9 °C and 11 days at -6.7 °C.

Kuticic and Wikerhauser (1996) reported that parasites in meat from experimentally infected pigs did not survive when frozen for 4 days at -7 °C to -12 °C. Other studies showed that at least 3 days at -20 °C were required to inactivate isolated tissue cysts (Djurkovic-Djakovic & Milenkovic, 2000).

4.2 Non-thermal technologies

4.2.1 Gamma irradiation

Several studies have demonstrated that *Toxoplasma gondii* was rendered nonviable by irradiation at doses of 0.4-1kGy (Song et al., 1993; Dubey & Thayer, 1994; Kuticic & Wikerhauser, 1996; Dubey, 2000), and the strain of *T. gondii* did not affect the killing of tissue cysts by irradiation under defined conditions (Dubey & Thayer, 1994).

However, the adverse effects of irradiation on colour have a major impact on the use of this technology and in certain countries large-scale implementation is restricted due to poor consumer acceptance (Brewer, 2004; Aymerich et al., 2008), in addition, irradiation of meat has not been approved in the EU.

4.2.2 High Hydrostatic Pressure (HHP)

Studies on the effectiveness of HHP in eliminating foodborne parasites show the sensitivity of parasites and their destruction is achieved with relatively low pressures.

High-pressure treatment using 300 MPa or higher can inactivate *T. gondii* tissue cysts under laboratory conditions (Lindsay et al., 2006) but negative effects on meat colour and texture have to be addressed before this method can be developed for routine decontamination (Cheftel & Culioli, 1997).

4.2.3 Curing

Curing treatments are used to preserve meat by the addition of a combination of salt, nitrates, nitrite or sugar. Many curing processes also involve smoking. Some researchers have suggested that tissue cysts are killed during commercial curing procedures with salt, but relatively few studies have been conducted to examine the efficiency of the curing process for the inactivation of *T. gondii*. One of the first experiments describing the inactivation of *T. gondii* tissue cysts was conducted by Sommer et al. in 1965. These authors found that encysted *T. gondii* survived for 4 days in 8% NaCl, but neither these researchers nor Work (1968) could find viable parasites in *T. gondii*-infected pork meat subjected to various curing processes.

Lundén & Uggla (1992) reported the absence of viable *Toxoplasma* in mutton meat after curing and smoking. Curing of lamb meat with salt and sugar for 64 h at 4°C or smoking salt-injected meat at temperatures not exceeding 50°C for 24 to 28 h was effective for killing *T. gondii*. However, these experiments do not reflect conditions under which commercial cured pork products are produced.

The survival time of tissue cysts is highly dependent on the concentration of the salt solution and the temperature of storage. Isolated tissue cysts can survive for 56 days in a solution of 0.85% salt, 49 days in 2% salt, and 21 days in 3.3% salt (Dubey, 1997). Under laboratory conditions, Dubey (1997) found that tissue cysts were killed in 6% NaCl solution at all temperatures examined (4 to 20°C) but survived for several weeks in aqueous solutions with lower salt concentrations. More recent data have indicated that injection of 2% NaCl and/or 1.4% lactate salt solutions into experimentally infected pig meat could kill the parasite. However, 1% NaCl solution provided variable results, and the addition of tripolyphosphate salts had no effect on parasite viability (Hill et al., 2004, 2006). Navarro et al. (1992), studying sausages manufactured from pigs experimentally inoculated with *T. gondii*, concluded that salt in concentration equal to 2.0% and 2.5% inactivated the parasite in 48 hours of the beginning of the curing process.

In order to evaluate the importance of swine sausages in toxoplasmosis epidemiology, Mendonça et al. (2004) investigated the presence of *T. gondii* in 70 samples of the meat product. Samples were analyzed by bioassay in mice and DNA amplification by PCR. Although the parasite was not isolated from any sample in the bioassay, 33 (47.14%) samples were positive in the PCR. The authors concluded that these swine sausages probably had low importance as a source of infection for human toxoplasmosis. Nevertheless, the great number of PCR positive samples showed that the protozoan may be present, but may be inactivated by salt added in sausage manufacture.

In contrast, other studies have indicated the potential failure of curing to inactivate *T. gondii* (Warnekulasuriya et al., 1998), and in epidemiological studies of risk factors for recent *Toxoplasma* infection in pregnant women, a strong association was found between infection and eating cured pork or raw meat (Buffolano et al., 1996; Cook et al., 2000; Kapperud et al., 1996). In addition, curing of meat products often involves the mixing of meat from various animals from different farms and sometimes from different farming systems (organic and regular), and thus a few infected animals may lead to the contamination of a whole batch of cured meat products. Warnekulasuriya et al. (1998) investigated the presence of *T. gondii* in cured meat samples by PCR, and using tissue culture in order to isolate viable parasites. The high salt content of some cured meats limited the sensitivity of PCR assay and reduced the sensitivity of tissue culture due to osmotic pressure causing cytopathic effect, but viable *T. gondii* was detected in one out of 67 ready-to-eat cured meat samples (1.5% contamination). However, these authors did not provide information about the time of curing and final salt concentrations, which could affect the viability of the parasite.

From all different meat products made with pork meat, dry-cured ham stands out among them as a high-quality product of increasing economic relevance. It is a nonsmoked product manufactured by curing with salt and nitrites and stabilized through decreasing water activity. It is greatly appreciated by consumers because of its flavor and texture and for its nutritional properties. The whole process takes several months (from 6 to 36 months) and it is consumed without heat treatment. In the market, it is possible to find several presentations of dry-cured ham. Consumers can buy unpackaged entire or sliced ham (sold on request), and we also can find refrigerated vacuum-packaged dry-cured hams cuts which may be either distributed to specialized butchery, or directly sold in supermarket displays. Due to the lack of information regarding the efficacy of meat curing for inactivating *T. gondii* and the inconsistency of results of epidemiological studies in which ingestion of cured meat was identified as a risk factor for acquiring acute *Toxoplasma* infection during pregnancy, Bayarri et al. (2010, in press) carried out some studies with the aim to provide data that could be used to estimate the risk of *T. gondii* infection from eating cured ham.

In a first study, the influence of processing of cured ham on the viability of *T. gondii* was evaluated using bioassay to assess the risk of infection from eating this meat product (Bayarri et al., 2010). Naturally infected pigs were selected for the study, and a mouse concentration bioassay technique was used to demonstrate viable bradyzoites of *T. gondii* in porcine tissues and hams. The selected pigs were slaughtered in a commercial abattoir. Both haunches were obtained for subsequent curing as is normal industry practice. At day 0 (before the curing process began), samples were obtained from the external surface of six haunches (one from each pig) to avoid quality loss of the final product. After 7 months of curing, the whole ham was analyzed for viable forms of *Toxoplasma*. The six remaining hams continued the curing process until 14 months, when samples were collected. They isolated viable parasites from hams after 7 months of curing, while no viable parasites were found in the final product (14 months of curing) based on results of IFA, histological, and PCR analyses. These authors evidenced that curing time is a major factor to ensure that the consumption of this meat product does not pose a risk of contracting toxoplasmosis.

However, both salt composition of the hams and curing time can vary according to the manufacturer or producer countries, and we can find in the market hams with different composition and curing times. Bayarri et al. (in press), carried out an investigation about the prevalence of viable *T. gondii* in commercially available cured ham. Twenty five samples of cured ham were randomly collected for analysis, corresponding to *paleta* and ham, white and Iberian, package sliced of different trade-mark and cut on request. The authors noted that not always information on the length of curing process was provided in the label. A mouse concentration bioassay technique was used, and the presence of the parasite in mice was determined by IFA. *T. gondii* was not detected in any of the samples of cured ham studied. Results reported in this paper are optimistic concerning food safety. However, in order to achieve a complete risk assessment on the viability of *T. gondii*, it is necessary to analyse a much larger number of samples, particularly those from organic farms, as well as cured ham considering different curing times and salt composition.

5. Acknowledgment

Funding by the University of Zaragoza (project UZ2006-CIE-04) and the Government of Aragón (Grupo de Investigación Consolidado A01, Fondo Social Europeo) is acknowledged.

6. References

AFSSA. (2005). Toxoplasmose: état des connaissances et évaluation du risque lié à l'alimentation – rapport du groupe de travail "*Toxoplasma gondii*" del'AFSSA. 328p.

Alkhalidi, N.W. & Dubey, J.P. (1979). Prevalence of *Toxoplasma gondii* infection in horses. *Journal of Parasitology*, 65, 331–334.

Alvarado-Esquivel, C.; García-Machado, C.; Alvarado-Esquivel, D.; González-Salazar, A.M.; Briones-Fraire, C.; Vitela-Corrales, J.; Villena, I. & Dubey JP. (2011).

Seroeroprevalence of *Toxoplasma gondii* infection in domestic pigs in Durango state, Mexico. *Journal of Parasitology*, 97(4), 616–619.

Aspinall, T.V.; Marlee, D.; Hyde, J.E. & Sims, P.F.G. (2002). Prevalence of *Toxoplasma gondii* in commercial meat products as monitored by polymerase chain reaction – food for thought? *International Journal of Parasitoogy*, 32, 1193–1199.

Aymerich, T.; Picouet, P.A. & Monfort, J.M. (2008). Decontamination technologies for meat products. *Meat Science*, 78, 114–129.

Baril, L.; Ancelle, T.; Goulet, V.; Thulliez, P.; Tirard-Fleury, V. & Carme, B. (1999). Risk factors for *Toxoplasma* infection in pregnancy: a case-control study in France. *Scandinavian Journal of Infectious Diseases*, 31, 305-309.

Bártová, E.; Dvoraková, H.; Bárta. J.; Sedlák, K. & Literák, I. (2004). Susceptibility of the domestic duck (*Anas platyrhynchos*) to experimental infection with *Toxoplasma gondii* oocysts. *Avian Pathology*, 33, 153-157.

Bártová, E.; Sedlák, K. & Litera, I. (2009). Serologic survey for toxoplasmosis in domestic birds from the Czech Republic. *Avian Pathology*, 38(4), 317-320.

Batz, M.; Hoffman, S. &.Morris Jr, J.G. (2011). Ranking the risk: The 10 pathogen-food combination with the greatest burden on public health. University of Florida.

Bayarri, S.; Gracia, M.J.; Lázaro, R.; Pérez-Arquillué, C.; Barberán, M. & Herrera, A. (2010). Determination of the Viability of *Toxoplasma gondii* in Cured Ham Using Bioassay: Influence of Technological Processing and Food Safety Implications. *Journal of food Protection*, 73(12), 2239–2243.

Bayarri, S.; Gracia, M.J.; Pérez-Arquillué, C.; Lázaro, R. & Herrera, A. *Toxoplasma gondii* in commercially available pork meat and cured ham: a contribution to risk assessment to consumers. *Journal of food Protection* (in press).

Bellete, B.; Flori, P.; Hafid, J.; Raberin, H. & Tran Manh Sung, R. (2003). Influence of the quantity of nonspecific DNA and repeated freezing and thawing of samples on the quantification of DNA by the Light Cycler. *Journal of Microbiological Methods*, 55, 213–219.

Berger-Schoch, A.E.; Bernet, D.; Doherr, M. G.; Gottstein, B. & Frey, C. F. (2011). *Toxoplasma gondii* in Switzerland: A Serosurvey Based on Meat Juice Analysis of Slaughtered Pigs, Wild Boar, Sheep and Cattle. *Zoonoses and Public Health*, 58, 472–478.

Blewett, D.A.; Miller, J.K. & Buxton, D. (1982). Response of immune and susceptible ewes to infection with *Toxoplasma gondii*. *Veterinary Record*, 111, 175–177.

Brewer, S. (2004). Irradiation effects on meat color – a review. *Meat Science*, 68, 1–17.

Buffolano, W.; Gilbert, R.E.; Holland, F.J.; Fratta, D.; Palumbo, F. & Ades, A.E. (1996). Risk factors for recent *Toxoplasma* infection in pregnant women in Naples. *Epidemiology and Infection*, 116, 347–351.

Canada, N.; Meireles, C.S.; Rocha, A.; da Costa, J.M.; Erickson, M.W. & Dubey J.P. (2002). Isolation of viable *Toxoplasma gondii* from naturally infected aborted bovine fetuses. *Journal of Parasitology*, 88 (6), 1247-1248.

Cheftel, J.C. & Culioli, J. (1997). Effects of high pressure on meat: a review. *Meat Science*, 46, 211–236.

Cook, A.J.C.; Gilbert, R.E.; Buffolano, W.; Zufferey, J.; Petersen, E.; Jenum, P.A.; Foulon, W.; Semprini, A.E. & Dunn, D.T. (2000). Sources of *Toxoplasma* infection in pregnant women: European multicentre case-control study. *British Medical Journal* 321, 142–147.

Da Silva, A.V. & Langoni, H. (2001). The detection of *Toxoplasma gondii* by comparing cytology, histopathology, bioassay in mice, and the polymerase chain reaction (PCR). *Veterinary Parasitology,* 97, 191–198.

Damriyasa, I.M.; Bauer, C.; Edelhofer, R.; Failing, K.; Lind, P.; Petersen, E.; Schares, G.; Tenter, A.M.; Volmer, R. & Zahner, H. (2004). Cross-sectional survey in pig breeding farms in Hesse, Germany: seroprevalence and risk factors of infections with *Toxoplasma gondii, Sarcocystis* spp. and *Neospora caninum* in sows. *Veterinary Parasitology,* 126, 271-286.

Davies, P.R.; Morrow, W.E.M.; Deen, J.; Gamble, H.R. & Patton, S. (1998). Seroprevalence of *Toxoplasma gondii* and *Trichinella spiralis* in finishing swine raised in different production systems in North Carolina, USA. *Preventive Veterinary Medicine,* 36, 67-76.

Dempster, R.P.; Wilkins, M.; Green, R. & de Lisle, G.W. (2011). Serological survey of *Toxoplasma gondii* and *Campylobacter fetus fetus* in sheep from New Zealand. *New Zealand Veterinary Journal,* 59(4), 155–159.

De Sousa, S.; Ajzenberg, D.; Canada, N.; Freire, L.; Correia da Costa, J.M.; Dardé , M.L.; Thulliez, P. & Dubey, J.P. (2006). Biologic and molecular characterization of *Toxoplasma gondii* isolates from pigs from Portugal. *Veterinary Parasitology,* 135, 133–136.

Dias, R.A.; Navarro, I.T.; Ruffolo, B.B.; Bugni, F.M.; de Castro, M.V. & Freire, R.L. (2005). *Toxoplasma gondii* in fresh pork sausage and seroprevalence in butchers from factories in Londrina, Paraná State, Brazil. *Revista do Instituto de Medicina Tropical de Sao Paulo,* 47(4), 185-189.

Diza, E.; Frantzidou, F.; Souliou, E.; Arvanitidou, M.; Gioula, G. & Antoniadis, A. (2005). Seroprevalence of *Toxoplasma gondii* in northern Greece during the last 20 years. *Clinical Microbiology and Infection,* 11, 719–723.

Djurkovic-Djakovic, O. & Milenkovic, V. (2000). Effect of refrigeration and freezing on survival of *Toxoplasma gondii* tissue cysts. *Acta Veterinaria Beograd,* 50, 375–380.

Dubey, J.P. (1980). Mouse pathogenicity of *Toxoplasma gondii* isolated from a goat. *American Journal of Veterinary Research,* 41, 427–429.

Dubey, J.P.; Sharma, S.P.; Lopes, C.W.G.; Williams, J.F.; Williams, C.S.F. & Weisbrode, S.E. (1980). Caprine toxoplasmosis - abortion, clinical signs, and distribution of *Toxoplasma* in tissues of goats fed *Toxoplasma gondii* oocysts. *American Journal of Veterinary Research,* 41, 1072–1076.

Dubey, J.P. (1981). Epizootic toxoplasmosis associated with abortion in dairy goats in Montana. *Journal of the American Veterinary Medical Association,* 178, 661–670.

Dubey, J.P. (1983). Distribution of cysts and tachyzoites in calves and pregnant cows inoculated with *Toxoplasma gondii* oocysts. *Veterinary Parasitology,* 13, 199–211.

Dubey, J.P.; Murrell, K.D. & Fayer, R. (1984). Persistence of encysted *Toxoplasma gondii* in tissues of pigs fed oocysts. *American Journal of Veterinary Research,* 45, 1941–1943.

Dubey, J.P.; Brake, RJ.; Murrell, KD. & Fayer, R. (1986). Effect of irradiation on the viability of *Toxoplasma gondii* cysts in tissues of mice and pigs. *American Journal of Veterinary Research*, 47, 518-522

Dubey, J.P. (1986a). A review of toxoplasmosis in pigs. *Veterinary Parasitology*, 19, 181–223

Dubey, J.P. (1986b). A review of toxoplasmosis in cattle. *Veterinary Parasitology*, 22, 177–202.

Dubey, J.P. (1988). Long-term persistence of *Toxoplasma gondii* in tissues of pigs inoculated with *T. gondii* oocysts and effect of freezing on viability of tissue cysts in pork. *American Journal of Veterinary Research*, 49, 910–913.

Dubey, J.P. & Beattie C.P. (1988). Toxoplasmosis of animals and man. CRC Press, Boca Raton.

Dubey, J.P.; Kotula, A.W.; Sharar, A.; Andrews, C.D. & Lindsay, D.S. (1990). Effect of high-temperature on infectivity of *Toxoplasma gondii* tissue cysts in pork. *Journal of Parasitology*, 76, 201–204.

Dubey, J.P.; Leighty, J.C.; Beal, V.C.; Anderson, W.R.; Andrews, C.D. & Thulliez, P. (1991). National seroprevalence of *Toxoplasma gondii* in pigs. *Journal of Parasitology*, 77, 517-521.

Dubey, J.P. (1993). *Toxoplasma, Neospora, Sarcocystis*, and other tissue cyst-forming coccidian of humans and animals. In: Kreier JP, editor. Parasitic Protozoa, 2nd edition, volume 6. San Diego: Academic Press, 1-158.

Dubey, J.P. & Thulliez, P. (1993). Persistence of tissue cysts in edible tissues of cattle fed *Toxoplasma gondii* oocysts. *American Journal of Veterinary Research*, 54, 270–273.

Dubey, J.P. & Thayer, D.W. (1994). Killing of different strains of *Toxoplasma gondii* tissue cysts by irradiation under defined conditions. *Journal of Parasitology*, 80, 764-767.

Dubey, J.P.; Weigel, R.M.; Siegel, A.M.; Thulliez, P.; Kitron, U.D.; Mitchell, M.A.; Mannelli, A.; Mateus-Pinilla, N.E.; Shen, S.K.; Kwok, O.C.H. & Todd, K.S. (1995). Sources and reservoirs of *Toxoplasma gondii* infection on 47 swine farms in Illinois. *Journal of Parasitology*, 81, 723–729.

Dubey, J.P.; Lunney, J.K.; Shen, S.K.; Kwok, O.C.H.; Ashford, D.A. & Thulliez, P. (1996). Infectivity of low numbers of *Toxoplasma gondii* oocysts to pigs. *Journal of Parasitology*, 82, 438-443.

Dubey, J. P. (1997). Survival of *Toxoplasma gondii* tissue cysts in 0.85–6% NaCl solutions at 4–20°C. *Journal of Parasitology*, 83, 946-949.

Dubey, J.P.; Lindsay, D.S. & Speer, C.A. (1998). Structures of *Toxoplasma gondii* tachyzoites,bradyzoites, and sporozoites and biology and development of tissue cysts. *Clinical Microbiology Reviews*, 11, 267-99.

Dubey, J.P. (2000). The scientific basis for prevention of *Toxoplasma gondii* infection: studies on tissue cyst survival, risk factors and hygiene measures. In: Ambroise-Thomas P, Petersen E, editors. Congenital Toxoplasmosis: Scientific Background, Clinical Management and Control. Paris: Springer-Verlag France, 271-275.

Dubey, J.P.; Gamble, H.R.; Hill, D.; Sreekumar, C.; Romand, S. & Thulliez, P. (2002). High prevalence of viable *Toxoplasma gondii* infection in market weight pigs from a farm in Massachusetts. *Journal of Parasitology*, 88, 1234–1238.

Dubey, J.P.; Graham, D.H.; Dahl, E.; Hilali, M.; El-Ghaysh, A.; Sreekumar, C.; Kwok, O.C.H.; Shen, S.K. & Lehmann, T. (2003). Isolation and molecular characterization of

Toxoplasma gondii from chickens and ducks from Egypt. *Veterinary Parasitology*, 114, 89-95.

Dubey, J.P.; Salant, H.; Sreekumar, C.; Dahl, E.; Vianna, M.C.B.; Shen, S.K.; Kwok, O.C.H.; Spira, D.; Hamburger, J. & Lehmann, T.V. (2004). High prevalence of *Toxoplasma gondii* in a commercial flock of chickens in Israel, and public health implications of free-range farming. *Veterinary Parasitology*, 121, 317–322.

Dubey, J.P.; Hill, D.E.; Jones, J.L.; Hightower, A.W.; Kirkland, E.; Roberts, J.M.; Marcet, P.L.; Lehmann, T.; Vianna, M.C.B.; Miska, K.; Sreekumar, C.; Kwok, O.C.H.; Shen, S.K. & Gamble, H.R. (2005). Prevalence of viable *Toxoplasma gondii* in beef, chicken, and pork from retail meat stores in the United States: risk assessment to consumers. *Journal of Parasitology*, 91,1082–1093.

Dubey, J.P.; Vianna, M.C.; Sousa, S.; Canada, N.; Meireles, S.; Correia da Costa, J.M.; Marcet, P.L.; Lehmann, T.; Darde, M.L. & Thulliez P. (2006). Characterization of *Toxoplasma gondii* isolates in free-range chickens from Portugal. *Journal of Parasitology*, 92 (1), 184-186.

Dubey, J.P. (2007). The history and life cycle of *Toxoplasma gondii*. Chapter 1 in *Toxoplasma gondii*. The model apicomplexan: perspectives and methods. Luis M. Weiss and Kami Kim Eds. Academia Press. Elsevier Ltd.

Dubey, J.P. & Jones, J.L. (2008). *Toxoplasma gondii* infection in humans and animals in the United States. *International Journal of Parasitology*, 38, 1257–1278.

Dubey, J.P. (2009). *Toxoplasmosis* in pigs-The last 20 years. *Veterinary Parasitology*, 164, 89-103.

Dumètre, A.; Ajzenberg, D.; Rozette, L.; Mercier, A. & Dardé, M.L. (2006). *Toxoplasma gondii* infection in sheep from Haute-Vienne, France: Seroprevalence and isolate genotyping by microsatellite analysis. *Veterinary Parasitology*, 142, 376–379.

EFSA, European Food Safety Authority. (2007). Scientific Opinion of the Panel on Biological Hazards on a request from EFSA on Surveillance and monitoring of *Toxoplasma* in humans, foods and animals. *The EFSA Journal*, 583, 1-64.

EFSA, European Food Safety Authority. (2011a). Scientific Opinion on the public health hazards to be covered by inspection of meat (swine). *The EFSA Journal*, 9(10), 2351.

EFSA, European Food Safety Authority. (2011b). Technical specifications on harmonised epidemiological indicators for public health hazards to be covered by meat inspection of swine. *The EFSA Journal*, 9(10), 2371.

Esteban-Redondo, I.; Maley, S.W.; Thomson, K.; Nicoll, S.; Wright, S.; Buxton, D. & Innes, E.A. (1999). Detection of *T. gondii* in tissues of sheep and cattle following oral infection. *Veterinary Parasitology*, 86, 155-171.

Fusco, G.; Rinaldi, L.; Guarino, A.; Proroga, Y.; Pesce, A.; Giuseppina de, M. & Cringoli, G. (2007). *Toxoplasma gondii* in sheep from the Campania region (Italy). *Veterinary Parasitology*, 149, 271–274.

Galván-Ramírez, M.L.; Madriz Elisondo, A.L.; Rico Torres, C.P.; Luna-Pastén, H.; Rodríguez Pérez, L.R.; Rincón Sánchez, A.R.; Franco, R.; Salazar-Montes, A. & Correa, D. (2010). Frequency of *Toxoplasma gondii* in Pork Meat in Ocotlán, Jalisco, Mexico. *Journal of Food Protection*, 73(6), 61121–1123.

Garcia, J.L.; Gennari, S.M.; Machado, R.Z. & Navarro, I.T. (2006). *Toxoplasma gondii*: detection by mouse bioassay, histopathology, and polymerase chain reaction in tissues from experimentally infected pigs. *Experimental Parasitology*, 113, 267–271.

García-Bocanegra, I.; Simon-Grifé, M.; Jitender, P.; Dubey, G.P.; Casal, J.; Gerard, E.; Martín, G.E.; Cabezón, O.; Perea A. & Almería A. (2010). Seroprevalence and risk factors associated with *Toxoplasma gondii* in domestic pigs from Spain. *Veterinary Parasitology*, 59, 421–426

Gill, C.O. (2005). Safety and storage stability of horse meat for human consumption. *Meat Science*, 71, 506–513.

Grossklaus, D. & Baumgarten, H.J. (1968). Die überlebensdauer von *Toxoplasma*-zysten in schweinefleisch I. Mitteilung: ergebnisse von lagerungsversuchen bei verschiedenen temperaturen. *Fleischwirtschaft*, 48, 930–932.

Hellmann, E. & Tauscher, L. (1967). Research into the occurrence of *Toxoplasma* in fresh beef and pork. *Berliner und Munchener Tierarztliche Wochenschrift*, 80, 209–212.

Hejlíček, K. & Literák, I. (1993). Prevalence of toxoplasmosis in pigs in the region of South Bohemia. *Acta Veterinaria Brno*, 62, 159-166.

Hejlíček, K. & Literák, I. (1994). Prevalence of toxoplasmosis in rabbits in South Boemia. *Acta Veterinaria Brno*, 63, 145-150.

Hill, D. E.; Sreekumar, C.; Gamble, H. R. & Dubey, J. P. (2004). Effect of commonly used enhancement solutions on the viability of *Toxoplasma gondii* tissue cysts in pork loin. *Journal of Food Protection*, 67,2230–2233.

Hill, D. E.; Benedetto, S. M.; Coss, C.; McCrary, J. L.; Fournet, V. M. & Dubey, J. P. (2006). Effects of time and temperature on the viability of *Toxoplasma gondii* tissue cysts in enhanced pork loin. *Journal of Food Protection*, 69, 1961–1965.

Hill, D. E. (2007). *Toxoplasma gondii*, p. 2887–2991. In Animal health production compendium. CAB International, Wallingford, UK.

Hill, D.E.; Haley, C.; Wagner, B.; Gamble, H.R. & Dubey J.P. (2010). Seroprevalence of and Risk Factors for *Toxoplasma gondii* in the US swine herd using sera collected during the National Animal Health Monitoring Survey (Swine 2006). *Zoonoses and Public Health*, 57(1), 53-59.

Jacobs, L.; Remington, J.S. & Melton, M.L. (1960). The resistance of the encysted form of *Toxoplasma gondii*. *Journal of Parasitology*, 46, 11–21.

Jacobs, L. & Melton, M.L. (1966). Toxoplasmosis in chickens. *Journal of Parasitology*, 52, 1158-1162.

Jones, J.L.; Kruszon-Moran, D.; Sanders-Lewis, K. & Wilson, M. (2007). *Toxoplasma gondii* infection in the United States, 1999–2004, declinen from the prior decade. *The American Journal of Tropical Medicine and Hygiene*, 77, 405–410.

Jones, J.L.; Dargelas, V.; Roberts, J.; Press, C.; Remington, J.S. & Montoya, J.G. (2009). Risk factors for *Toxoplasma gondii* infection in the United States. *Clinical Infectious Diseases*, 49(6), 878-884.

Kaneto, C.N.; Costa, A.J.; Paulillo, A.C.; Moraes, F.R.; Murakami, T.O. & Meireles, M.V. (1997). Experimental toxoplasmosis in broiler chicks. *Veterinary Parasitology*, 69, 203-210.

Kapperud, G.; Jenum, P.A.; Stray-Pedersen, B.; Melby, K.K.; Eskild, A. & Eng, J. (1996). Risk factors for *Toxoplasma gondii* infection in pregnancy. Results of a prospective case-control study in Norway. *American Journal of Epidemiology*, 144, 405–412.

Kijlstra, A.; Meerburg, B.G. & Mul, M.F. (2004). Animal-friendly production systems may cause re-emergence of *Toxoplasma gondii*. *Njas- Wageningen Journal of Life Sciences*, 52, 119–132.

Kijlstra, A. & Jongert, E. (2008a). *Toxoplasma*-safe meat: close to reality? *Trends in Parasitology*, 25, 18-21.

Kijlstra, A. & Jongert, E. (2008b). Control of the risk of human toxoplasmosis transmitted by meat. *International Journal of Parasitology*, 38, 1359–1370.

Klun, I.; Djurković-Djaković, O.; Katić-Radivojević, S. & Nikolić, A. (2006). Cross-sectional survey on *Toxoplasma gondii* infection in cattle, sheep and pigs in Serbia: seroprevalence and risk factors. *Veterinary Parasitology*, 135, 121-131.

Kortbeek, L. M.; De Melker, H.E.; Veldhuijzen, I. K.; & Conyn-Van Spaendonck, M.A.E. (2004). Population-based *toxoplasma* seroprevalence study in the Netherlands. *Epidemiology and Infection*, 132(5), 839-845.

Kotula, A.W.; Dubey, J.P.; Sharar, A.K.; Andrews, C.D.; Shen, S. & Lindsay, D.S. (1991). Effect of freezing on infectivity of *Toxoplasma gondii* tissue cysts in pork. *Journal of Food Protection*, 54, 687-690.

Kuticic, V. & Wikerhauser, T. (1996). Studies of the effect of various treatments on the viability of *Toxoplasma gondii* tissue cysts and oocysts. *Current Topics in Microbiology and Immunology*, 219, 261–265.

Lehmann, T.; Marcet, P.L.; Graham, D.H.; Dahl, E.R. & Dubey J.P. (2006). Globalization and the population structure of *Toxoplasma gondii*. *Proceedings of the National Academy of Sciences of the United States of America*, 103(30), 11423-11428.

Leistner, L. (2000). Basic aspects of food preservation by hurdle technology. *International Journal of Food Microbiology*, 55, 181–186.

Lindsay, D. S.; Collins, M. V.; Holliman, D.; Flick, G. J. & Dubey, J. P. (2006). Effects of high-pressure processing on *Toxoplasma gondii* tissue cysts in ground pork. *Journal of Parasitology*, 92(1), 195-196.

Lundén, A. & Uggla, A. (1992). Infectivity of *Toxoplasma gondii* in mutton following curing, smoking, freezing or microwave cooking. *International Journal of Food Microbiology*, 15, 357-363.

Lundén, A.; Lind, P.; Engvall, E.O.; Gustavsson, K.; Uggla, A. & Vågsholm, I. (2002). Serological survey of *Toxoplasma gondii* infection in pigs slaughtered in Sweden. *Scandinavian Journal of Infectious Diseases*, 34, 362-365.

Masur, H.; Jones, T.C.; Lempert, J.A. & Cherubini, T.D. (1978). Outbreak of toxoplasmosis in a family and documentation of acquired retinochoroiditis. *American Journal of Medicine*, 64, 396–402.

McColgan, C.; Buxton, D. & Blewett, D.A. (1988). Titration of *Toxoplasma gondii* oocysts in non-pregnant sheep and the effects of subsequent challenge during pregnancy. *Veterinary Record*, 123, 467–470.

McCurdy, S.M.; Takeuchi, M.T.; Edwards, Z.M.; Edlefsen, M.; Kang, D.H.; Mayes, V.E. & Hillers, V.N. (2006). Food safety education initiative to increase consumer use of food thermometers in the United States. *British Food Journal*, 108, 775–794.

Mendonça, A.O.; Domingues, P.F.; Silva, A.V.D.; Pezerico, S.B. & Langoni, H. (2004). Detection of *Toxoplasma gondii* in swine sausages. *Parasitologia Latinoamericana*, 59, 42–45.

Meerburg, B.G.; Van Riel, J.W.; Cornelissen, J.B.; Kijlstra, A. & Mul, M.F. (2006). Cats and goat whey associated with *Toxoplasma gondii* infection in pigs. *Vector Borne and Zoonotic Diseases*, 6, 266–274.

Mie, T.; Pointon, A. M.; Hamilton, D. R. & Kiermeier, A. (2008). A qualitative assessment of *Toxoplasma gondii* risk in ready-to-eat smallgoods processing. *Journal of Food Protection*, 71, 1442–1452.

More, G.; Basso, W.; Bacigalupe, D.; Venturini, M.C. & Venturini, L. (2008). Diagnosis of *Sarcocystis cruzi, Neospora caninum*, and *Toxoplasma gondii* infections in cattle. *Parasitology Research*, 102, 671–675.

Munday, B.L. & Corbould, A. (1979). Serological responses of sheep and cattle exposed to natural *Toxoplasma* infection. *Australian Journal of Experimental Biology & Medical Science*, 57 (2), 141-145.

Navarro, I.T.; Vidoto, O.; Giraldini, N & Mitsuka, R. (1992). Resistência do *Toxoplasma gondii* ao cloreto de sódio e aos condimentos em lingüiça de suínos. *Boletín de la Oficina Sanitaria de Panamá*, 112, 138-43.

Omata, Y.; Dilorenzo, C.; Venturini, C.; Venturini, L.; Igarashi, I.; Saito, A. & Suzuki, N. (1994). Correlation between antibody levels in *Toxoplasma gondii* infected pigs and pathogenicity of the isolated parasite. *Veterinary Parasitology*, 51 (3–4), 205–210.

Opsteegh, M.; Langelaar, M.; Sprong, H.; den Hartog, L.; De Craeye, S.; Bokken, G.; Ajzenberg, D.; Kijlstra, A. & van der Giessen, J. (2010). Direct detection and genotyping of *Toxoplasma gondii* in meat samples using magnetic capture and PCR. *International Journal of Food Microbiology*, 139, 193-201.

Owen, M.R. & Trees, A.J. (1999). Genotyping of *Toxoplasma gondii* associated with abortion in sheep. *Journal of Parasitology*, 85, 382-384.

Panadero, R.; Painceira, A.; López, C.; Vázquez, L.; Paz, A.; Díaz, P.; Dacal, V.; Cienfuegos, S.; Fernández, G.; Lago, N.; Díez-Baños, P. & Morrondo, P. (2010). Seroprevalence of *Toxoplasma gondii* and *Neospora caninum* in wild and domestic ruminants sharing pastures in Galicia (Northwest Spain). *Research in Veterinary Science*, 88, 111–11.

Paul, M. (1998). Potencjalne źródła zarażenia *Toxoplasma gondii* w przypadkach badanych w krótkim czasie po zarażeniu. *Przegl. Epidemiology*, 52, 447-454.

Pikka, J.; Näreaho, A.; Knaapi, S.; Oksanen, A.; Rikula, U. & Sukura, A. (2010). *Toxoplasma gondii* in wild cervids and sheep in Finland: North-south gradient in seroprevalence. *Veterinary Parasitoloy*, 171, 331-336.

Pinheiro, J.W.; Mot, R.A.; da Fonseca Oliveira, A.A.; Bento Faria, E.; Pita Gondim, L.F.; Vieira da Silva, A. & Aires Anderlini, G. (2009). Prevalence and risk factors associated to infection by *Toxoplasma gondii* in ovine in the State of Alagoas, Brazil. *Parasitology Research*, 105, 709–715.

Riemann, H.P.; Meyer, M.E.; Theis, J.H.; Kelso, G. & Behymer, D.E. (1975). Toxoplasmosis in an infant fed unpasteurized goat milk. *Journal of Pediatrics*, 87, 573–576.

Sacks, J.J.; Roberto, R.R. & Brooks, N.F. (1982). Toxoplasmosis infection associated with raw goat's milk. *The Journal of American Medical Association*, 248, 1728–1732

Santos, T.R.; Costa, A.J.; Toniollo, G.H.; Luvizotto, M.C.R.; Benetti, A.H.; Santos, R.R.; Matta, D.H.; Lopes, W.D.Z.; Oliveira, J.A. & Oliveira, G.P. (2009). Prevalence of anti-*Toxoplasma gondii* antibodies in dairy cattle, dogs, and humans from the Jauru micro-region, Mato Grosso state, Brazil. *Veterinary Parasitology*, 161, 324–326.

Sharma, S.P.; Baipoledi, E.K.; Nyange, J.F.C. & Tlagae, L. (2003). Isolation of *Toxoplasma gondii* from goats with a history of reproductive disorders and the prevalence of *toxoplasma* and chlamydial antibodies. *Onderstepoort Journal of Veterinary Research*, 70, 65–68.

Scallan, E.; Hoekstra, R.M.; Angulo, F.J.; Tauxe, R.V.; Widdowson, M.A.; Roy, S.L.; Jones, J.L. & Griffin, P.M. (2011). Foodborne Illness adquired in the United States. Major Pthogens. *Emerging Infections Diseases*, 17(1), 7-15.

Schulzig, H.S. & Fehlhaber, K. (2006). Seroprevalence of *Toxoplasma gondii* in conventionally and organically produced pork and pork-products. *Fleischwirtschaft*, 86, 106–108.

Shahiduzzaman, M.; Islam, R.; Khatun, M,; Batanova, T.A.; Kitoh, K. & Takashima Y. (2011). *Toxoplasma gondii* seroprevalence in domestic animals and humans in Mymensingh District, Bangladesh. *The Journal of Veterinary Medical Science*, 73(10), 1375–1376.

Schlundt, J.; Toyofuku, H.; Jansen, J. & Herbst, S.A. (2004). Emerging food-borne zoonoses. *Revue Scientifique et Technique de l'Office International des Epizooties*, 23, 513-533.

Shrestha, J.N.B. & Fahmy, M.H. (2005). Breeding goats for meat production: a review – 1. Genetic resources, management and breed evaluation. *Small Ruminant Research*, 58, 93–106.

Skinner, L.J.; Timperley, A.C.; Wightman, D.; Chatterton, J.M.W. & Hoyen, D.O. (1990). Simultaneous diagnosis of toxoplasmosis in goats and goatowners family. *Scandinavian Journal of Infectious Diseases*, 22, 359–361.

Slifko, T.R.; Smith, H.V. & Rose, J.B. (2000). Emerging parasite zoonoses associated with water and food. *International Journal of Parasitology*, 30, 1379-1393.

Sommer, R.; Rommel, M. & Levetzow, R. (1965). Die Uberlebensdauer von Toxoplasmazysten in fleish und fleishzubereitungen. *Fleischwirtschaf*, 5, 454–457.

Song, C.C.; Yuan, X.Z.; Shen, L.Y.; Gan, X.X. & Ding, J.Z. (1993). The effect of cobalt-60 irradiation on the infectivity of *Toxoplasma gondii*. *International Journal of Parasitology*, 23, 89-93.

Sroka, J. (2001). Seroepidemiology of toxoplasmosis in the Lublin region. *Annals of Agricultural and Environmental Medicine*, 8, 25-31.

Sroka, J.; Zwolinski, J.; Dutkiewicz, J.; Tos-Luty, S. & Latuszynska J. (2003). Toxoplasmosis in rabbits confirmed by strain isolation: a potential risk of infection among agricultural workers. *Annals of Agricultural and Environmental Medicine*, 10, 125-128.

Tassi P. (2007). *Toxoplasma gondii* infection in horses- a serological survey in horses slaughtered for human consumption in Italy. In Toxo & Food 2006, Palermo, Italy, pp. 96–97.

Tenter, A.M.; Heckeroth, A.R. & Weiss, L.M. (2000). *Toxoplasma gondii*: from animals to humans. *International Journal for Parasitology*, 30, 1217-1258.

Tsutsui, VS. (2000). Soroepidemiologia e fatores associados à transmissão do *Toxoplasma gondii* em suínos no norte do Paraná. Trabalho de Conclusão de Curso - Universidade Estadual de Londrina.

Tsutsui, V.S.; Freire, R.L.; Garcia, J.L.; Gennari, S.M.; Vieira, D.P.; Marana, E.R.M.; Prudencio, L.B. & Navarro, I.T. (2007). Detection of *Toxoplasma gondii* by PCR and mouse bioassay in commercial cuts of pork from experimentally infected pigs. *Arquivo Brasileiro de Medicina Veterinária e Zootecnia*, 11(1), 53-59.

Van der Giessen, J.; Fonville, M.; Bouwknegt, M.; Langelaar, M. & Vollema A. (2007). Seroprevalence of *Trichinella spiralis* and *Toxoplasma gondii* in pigs from different housing systems in The Netherlands. *Veterinary Parasitology*, 148, 371–374.

Van Knapen, F.; Kremers, A.F.T.; Franchimont, J.H. & Narucka, U. (1995). Prevalence of antibodies to *Toxoplasma gondii* in cattle and swine in the Netherlands: towards an integrated control of livestock production. *The Veterinary Quarterly*, 17, 87-91.

Venturini, M.C.; Bacigalupe, D.; Venturini, L.; Rambeaud, M.; Basso, W.; Unzaga J.M. & Perfumo CJ. (2004). Seroprevalence of *Toxoplasma gondii* in sows from slaughterhouses and in pigs from an indoor and an outdoor farm in Argentina. *Veterinary Parasitology*, 124, 161–165.

Veronesi, F.; Ranucci, D.; Branciari, R.; Miraglia, D.; Mammoli, R. & Fioretti DP. (2011). Seroprevalence and Risk Factors for *Toxoplasma gondii* Infection on Finishing Swine Reared in the Umbria Region, Central Italy. *Zoonoses Public Health*, 58, 178–184.

Vidotto, O.; Navarro, I.T.; Giraldi, N.; Mitsuka, R. & Freire, RL. (1990). Estudos epidemiológicos da toxoplasmose em suínos da Região de Londrina, Paraná. *Semina* (Londrina), 11(1), 53-59.

Villari, S.; Vesco, G.; Petersen, E.; Crispo, A. & Buffolano, W. (2009). Risk factors for toxoplasmosis in pigs bred in Sicily, Southern Italy. *Veterinary Parasitology*, 161, 1-8.

Warnekulasuriya, M.R.; Johnson, J.D. & Holliman, R.E. (1998). Detection of *Toxoplasma gondii* in cured meats. *International Journal of Food Microbiology*, 45, 211–215.

WHO (World Health Organization). (2008). Foodborne disease outbreaks : guidelines for investigation and control. WHO Library Cataloguing-in-Publication Data ISBN 978 92 4 154722 2.

Work, K. (1968). Resistance of *Toxoplasma gondii* encysted in pork. *Acta Pathologica Microbiologica Scandinavica*, 73, 85–92.

Weigel, R.M.; Dubey, J.P.; Siegel, A.M.; Kitron, U.D.; Mannelli, A.; Mitchell, M.A.; Mateuspinilla, N.E.; Thulliez, P.; Shen, S.K.; Kwok, O.C.H. & Todd, K.S. (1995). Risk-Factors for transmission of *Toxoplasma gondii* on swine farms in Illinois. *Journal of Parasitology*, 25, 736–741.

Yu, H.J.; Zhang, Z.; Liu, Z.; Qu, D.F.; Zhang, D.F.; Zhang, H.L.; Zhou Q.J. & Du AF. (2011). Seroprevalence of *Toxoplasma gondii* Infection in Pigs, in Zhejiang Province, China. *Journal of Parasitology*, 97(4), 748–749.

Zintl, A.; Halova, D.; Mulcahy, G.; O'Donovan, J.; Markey, B. & DeWaal, T. (2009). In vitro culture combined with quantitative TaqMan PCR for the assessment of *Toxoplasma gondii* tissue cyst viability. *Veterinary Parasitology,* 164, 167–172.

Zia-Ali, N.; Fazaeli, A.; Khoramizadeh, M.; Ajzenberg, D.; Darde, M. & Keshavarz-Valian, H. (2007). Isolation and molecular characterization of *Toxoplasma gondii* strains from different hosts in Iran. *Parasitology Research,* 101, 111–115.

14

Major Role for CD8+T Cells in the Protection Against *Toxoplasma gondii* Following Dendritic Cell Vaccination

Isabelle Dimier-Poisson
UMR ISP 1282 University-INRA,
Parasite Immunology, Vaccinology and Anti-Infectious Biotherapies,
University François Rabelais, Faculty of Pharmacy, Tours,
France

1. Introduction

Toxoplasma gondii is an obligate intracellular protozoan that infects one-third of the world population. Asymptomatic in immunocompetent hosts, toxoplasmosis has severe consequences in immunosuppressed individuals and can even lead to death.[1,2] Congenital toxoplasmosis causes development of sequelae later in life, including chorioretinitis, hearing loss or mental retardation.[3] *Toxoplasma gondii* is also recognized as being a major cause of abortion in farm animals, such as sheep and goats thus causing substantial reproductive and economic losses.[4] Additionally, these infected animals are a parasitic reservoir involved in human contamination. Recently it has been reported that *Toxoplasma gondii* has some degree of causal relation to Schizophrenia[5] because of the positive relationships between the prevalence of *Toxoplasma* antibodies and the development of schizophrenia. A recent article reports that *Toxoplasma* infection in rodents blocks the aversion toward predator odors and develop an attraction suggesting an integrating effect of the parasite.[6] This study provides an example of the behavioral effects of *Toxoplasma* in models of psychiatric and emotional conditions.

Once human beings or animals have been infected, no drug treatment available at present will eliminate the parasite. Nor is there any vaccine for human use to control the disease.

Primary infection with *T. gondii* results in the setting of both humoral and cell-mediated immune responses and confers long-term protection. This suggests that the development of an efficient vaccine is a realistic goal. Moreover because of the enormous estimated costs and social impact of *T. gondii* infection and the fact that primary infection with this parasite could give the host a protective immunity against re-infection, many studies have investigated possible solutions for an efficient vaccine.[7,8] However the immune response set following a *T. gondii* infection firstly needs to be clearly defined before a vaccine can be developed.

Host resistance seems to occur *via* synthesis of IFN-γ by NK cells and adaptive T lymphocytes.[9] Following infection, antigen-presenting cells synthesize TNF-α and IL-12 which induce NK cells to secrete IFN-γ. The combined action of IL-12 and IFN-γ induce a strong differentiation of T helper precursors into Th1 lymphocytes. These CD4+ T cells then synthesize large amounts of IFN-γ and IL-2. These two cytokines finally induce CD8+ T lymphocytes proliferation and IFN-γ secretion.[10] Thus protection against *T. gondii* infection is mainly attributed to cell-mediated immunity.

Previous studies have shown that both CD4+ and CD8+ T-cell subtypes are involved in the protection and the relative contribution of these two populations was investigated by adoptive transfer or *in vivo* depletion.[10] The transfer of T cells from infected or immunized mice to naïve mice provided protection against a lethal challenge of *T. gondii*, but this protection was abolished by depletion of CD8+ T cells prior to transfer but not by depletion of CD4+ T cells[11,12]. Similarly, transfer of $CD8^+$ T cells from chronically infected mice to naïve WT or nude mice was also able to provide protection from *T. gondii* challenge[11]. However, in response to *T. gondii*, the lack of $CD8^+$ T cells could be compensate by a potent NK cell response, though β2-m-deficient mice remained more susceptible than WT mice.[13] All these data suggest a prominent role of CD8+ cells with a supporting role for CD4+ cells during the acute phase as well as during the chronic phase of infection.

$CD8^+$ T lymphocytes mediated protection by IFN-γ which has been demonstrated to be crucial by studies using neutralizing antibody to IFN-γ or mice deficient in its production [14, 15, 16]. Evidence that production of this cytokine and subsequent protection against toxoplasmosis is dependent on $CD8^+$ T cells was demonstrated by showing that treatment of infected mice with anti-CD8 antibodies resulted in reduced production of IFN-γ and loss of IFN-γ-mediated protection. [17, 18] $CD8^+$ T cells can also mediate perforin-dependent cytotoxicity against target cells that present the correct peptide in the context of MHC on their cell surface. Several studies have shown that $CD8^+$ T cells isolated from immunized or infected mice lysed infected cells or targets pulsed with *Toxoplasma* antigens[19,20, 21,22]. All these data suggest a prominent role of CD8+ cells during the acute phase as well as during the chronic phase of infection.

If IFN-γ is the major cytokine of resistance to *T. gondii*, IL-12 is a crucial initiation cytokine to trigger an efficient cell-mediated immunity. Indeed, IL-12 is a major cytokine secreted in response to *T. gondii* by neutrophils[23], macrophages[24], plasmacytoid dendritic cells (pDCs) [25], conventional dendritic cells (cDCs) [26] and the subset of cDCs expressing CD8α[27]. Recently Mashayekhi et al have demonstrated the critical role of CD8α+ DCs for activation of innate immunity through IL-12 production during *T. gondii* infection and have shown that CD8α+ DCs are the only cells whose IL-12 production is required to control acute infection[28].

IL-12 is produced in response to Toll-like receptor (TLR) recognition of molecular structures broadly conserved across microbial species[29] that triggers the early IFN-γ secretion following *T. gondii* infection. IFN-γ activates various cell-intrinsic antiparasitic defense defense pathway within infected cells for intracellular elimination of *Toxoplasma*, including the activation of interferon-regulated GTPases (IRGs)[30,31], induction of reactive nitrogen intermediates[32], tryptophan degradation in human cells[33], and autophagy[34,35].

So DCs are the first producers of IL-12 in response to *T. gondii* antigens and several previous studies suggest that DCs play an important role in the setting of the immune response to the intracellular parasite *T. gondii* during the early and chronic phases of infection.

The central role of DCs in controlling immunity makes these cells ideal tools for priming functional immune responses. Many studies have proposed the use of DCs as vaccine vectors. For instance, *T. gondii* extract-pulsed splenic DCs administered *in vivo* induce a strong humoral and cellular immune response and promote protection against a virulent challenge.[36, 37] It has been also observed that *Toxoplasma* pulsed DCs induced protective immunity against *T. gondii* infection in both syngeneic and allogeneic mouse models. This protection was associated with the induction of humoral and cellular Toxoplasma-specific responses[38]. However, expensive treatments of this type, based on living cells, could be envisaged only for severe diseases, such as cancers, which are specific to the individual due to MHC restriction. For ethical reasons, it is not possible to use live cell lines in an immunisation protocol in humans. New approaches, involving the development of non-live and DNA-free vaccines, must therefore be pursued. Moreover, the use of DCs is limited by the difficulty of obtaining large numbers of cells suitable for vaccination purposes.

If DCs can effectively process *T. gondii* antigens for presentation *in vivo*, their use in a vaccine strategy is not acceptable. It is of interest to study the effector mechanisms induced by *T. gondii*-sensitized dendritic cells as a well-described protective immune response would help the development of new efficient vaccine strategies.

So the relative contribution of two main lymphocytic populations, CD4+ and CD8+, was investigated in a model of chronically infected mice, following dendritic cell vaccination and lymphocyte depletion.

We first determined the role of CD4+ T lymphocytes after an efficient depletion of over 90%. The results revealed a minor role for these cells since CD4-depleted or non depleted mice have similar cytokine secretion profiles in spleen as well as in MLNs. Moreover, depleted mice did not show any significant loss of protection in terms of brain cyst load. These results contrast with those obtained by Casciotti in 2002.[10] They demonstrated that CD4+ T cells are important for early IFN-γ production during *T. gondii* infection and that lack of CD4+ lymphocytes leads to parasite multiplication in the tissues. Moreover CD4 deficient mice exhibited parasite burdens in the brain. Johnson and Sayles also showed the implication of CD4+ cells as they induce CD8+ T cells through the production of IL-2 and maintain CD8+ T cells effector immunity.[39] CD4+ T lymphocytes also contributed significantly to protection against chronic infection *via* their role as helper cells for production of isotype-switched antibodies. The contradictory results obtained following infection alone or following vaccination plus infection could result from a particular orientation of the immune response. Indeed, in our protocol dendritic cells could directly prime CD8+ T lymphocytes *via* cross-presentation of *T. gondii* antigens, as previously demonstrated by Gubbels *et al.*[40]

So CD4+ T lymphocytes appeared to be not implicated either in spleen or mesenteric lymph node cytokine secretion or in long-term protection of mice.

We next studied the implication of CD8+ T lymphocytes after an efficient depletion of over 90%. In spleens CD8+ cells seem to be responsible for cytokine synthesis. Indeed, their depletion leads to a significant decrease of both Th1 (IFN-γ and IL-2) and Th2 (IL-10 and IL-4) cytokines. We further confirmed these data by identifying the CD8+ T cells as the IFN-γ-producing cells. These results are in accordance with another vaccination assay where Gazzinelli *et al.* got similar results. They vaccinated BALB/c mice with the mutant *T. gondii* strain TS-4 before depleting them of CD4+ or CD8+ lymphocytes and challenging them with a lethal dose of tachyzoites. They identified IFN-γ-producing CD8+ T cells as the major effectors of immunity *in vivo*.[41] Moreover, in our experiment, CD8+ cells depletion induced a loss of protection in mice previously immunized with pulsed dendritic cells, so CD8+ cells are crucial for CBA/J mice resistance to *T. gondii* infection. CD8+ cells also appear to play a major role in *Trypanosoma cruzi* infection. Mice lacking CD8+ T-cell function fail to control a normally non-lethal infection and die early in the acute phase. Moreover, depletion of CD8+ T cells in the chronic phase results in increased parasite load.[42]

In contrast to spleens, MLNs showed increased secretions of cytokines following CD8+ depletion suggesting that CD8+ T lymphocytes could act as regulatory cells. A recent review summarizes the current knowledge on CD8+ Tregs, a newly described CD8+ lymphocyte subtype with dedicated suppressor function.[43] Although not proven in parasitic infections, their importance in autoimmunity is well-documented and they could be responsible for the moderation of the immune response set in local lymph nodes. It would be of importance to determine which cell population is responsible for the MLN IFN-γ secretion. It has been demonstrated that splenic NK cells could produce this cytokine in response to *T. gondii* in MHC-I deficient mice thus unable to activate CD8+ T cells.[44]

So CD8+ T lymphocytes appeared as the main effectors, inducing a strong Th1 response in spleen while inhibiting both Th1 and Th2 responses in mesenteric lymph nodes.

This is the first study to point to CD8+ lymphocytes as the unique effector population responsible for the protection of mice following efficient DC vaccination and subsequent virulent challenge. This is partly in accordance with a previous description of CD8+ T cells as effector lymphocytes while CD4+ T cells were crucial for the regulation of the immune response in a very different vaccination assay.[17]

We provide further insight into the long-term immunity that protects mice against *T. gondii*, a ubiquitous parasite resulting in severe sequelae in immunocompromised individuals. Future studies will be needed to determine how *T. gondii* antigens are presented to CD8+ lymphocytes. A recent study showed encouraging results. Indeed, the authors demonstrated that CD8+ DCs were very efficient in processing and cross-presenting exogenous antigen to CD8+ T cells. They also highlighted CD24 as an essential co-stimulatory molecule required for CD8+ DCs to generate CD8+ and CD4+ T-cell responses.[45] The possible roles of various CD4+ lymphocyte subtypes and other immune cell populations during the chronic phase of the disease also need to be elucidated, with a view to developing an effective vaccine to be used in animals that serve as a natural reservoir for human contamination.

Finally, the next step to efficiently develop a vaccine strategy will be to identify which parasitic peptides are cross-presentated by DCs to CD8+ T cells to initiate the specific protective response to *T. gondii*. Blanchard *et al.* recently found that a decapeptide from the dense granule protein GRA6 could effectively induce such protection against *T. gondii*, as assessed by survival of mice.[46] However, their study was conducted using bone marrow-derived DCs. It could be of interest to target *in vivo* splenic CD8+ DCs, known to protect our mice, with such putative protective parasitic peptides.

Fully dissecting the cellular and molecular events leading to this protective response will allow for better design of vaccine strategies to enhance immunity and decrease morbidity and mortality associated with Toxoplasma infection.

Thus, transfer of Toxoplasma antigens to lymphoid resident DCs is a feature of DC vaccination that can be exploited to improve vaccine outcome.

2. References

[1] Hoffmann C, Ernst M, Meyer P, Wolf E, Rosenkranz T, Plettenberg A. Evolving characteristics of toxoplasmosis in patients infected with human immunodeficiency virus-1: clinical course and *Toxoplasma gondii*-specific immune responses. Clin. Microbiol. Infect. 2007; 13: 510-15.

[2] Barsoum RS. Parasitic infections in organ transplantation. Exp. Clin. Transplant. 2004; 2: 258-67.

[3] Elsheikha HM. Congenital toxoplasmosis: priorities for further health promotion action. Public Health. 2008; 122: 335-53.

[4] Bennett R, Christiansen K, Clifton-Hadley R. Preliminary estimates of the direct costs associated with endemic diseases of livestock in Great Britain. Prev. Vet. Med. 1999; 39: 155-71.

[5] Yolken RH, Bachmann S, Rouslanova I, Lillehoj E, Ford G, Fuller Torrey E *et al.* Antibodies to *Toxoplasma gondii* in individuals with first-episode schizophrenia. Clin. Infect. Dis. 2001; 32: 842-44.

[6] Vyas A, Kim SK, Giacomini N, Boothroyd JC, Sapolsky RM. Behavioral changes induced by *Toxoplasma* infection of rodents are highly specific to aversion of cat odors.Proc Natl Acad Sci U S A. 2007;104 (15):6442-6447.

[7] Buxton D, Thomson K, Maley S, Wright S, Bos HJ. Vaccination of sheep with a live incomplete strain (S48) of *Toxoplasma gondii* and their immunity to challenge when pregnant. Vet. Rec. 1991; 129: 89-93.

[8] Bourguin I, Chardès T, Bout D. Oral immunization with *Toxoplasma gondii* antigens in association with cholera toxin induces enhanced protective and cell-mediated immunity in C57BL/6 mice. Infect. Immun. 1993; 61: 2082-2088.

[9] Gazzinelli RT, Wysocka M, Hayashi S, Denkers EY, Hieny S, Caspar P *et al.* Parasite-induced IL-12 stimulates early IFN-γ synthesis and resistance during acute infection with *Toxoplasma gondii*. J. Immunol. 1994; 153: 2533-43.

[10] Casciotti L, Ely KH, Williams ME, Khan IA. CD8+-T-cell immunity against *Toxoplasma gondii* can be induced but not maintained in mice lacking conventional CD4+ T cells. Infect. Immun. 2002; 70: 434-43.

[11] Parker S.J., Roberts C.W. and Alexander J. $CD8^+$ T cells are the major lymphocyte subpopulation involved in the protective immune response to *Toxoplasma gondii* in mice. Clinical and Exp. Immunol, 1991; 84: 207–212.

[12] Suzuki Y. and Remington J.S. Dual regulation of resistance against *Toxoplasma gondii* infection by $Lyt\text{-}2^+$ and $Lyt\text{-}1^+$, $L3T4^+$ T cells in mice. J. Immunol. 1988; 140: 3943–3946.

[13] Denkers E.Y., Gazzinelli R.T., Martin D. and Sher A. Emergence of NK1.1+ cells as effectors of IFN-gamma dependent immunity to *Toxoplasma gondii* in MHC class I-deficient mice. J. Exp. Med., 1993; 178: 1465–1472.

[14] Scharton-Kersten, T.A. Wynn, E.Y. Denkers, S. Bala, E. Grunvald, S. Hieny, R.T. Gazzinelli and Sher A.. In the absence of endogenous IFN-gamma, mice develop unimpaired IL-12 responses to *Toxoplasma gondii* while failing to control acute infection. J. Immunol. 1096; 157 : 4045–4054

[15] Suzuki Y., Conley F.K. and Remington J.S. Importance of endogenous IFN-gamma for prevention of toxoplasmic encephalitis in mice. J. Immunol. 1989, 143: 2045–2050.

[16] Suzuki Y., Orellana M.A., Schreiber R.D. and Remington J.S. Interferon-gamma: the major mediator of resistance against *Toxoplasma gondii*. Science, 1988, 240 : 516–518.

[17] Gazzinelli R.T., Hakim F.T., Hieny S., Shearer G.M. and Sher A. Synergistic role of $CD4^+$ and $CD8^+$ T lymphocytes in IFN-gamma production and protective immunity induced by an attenuated *Toxoplasma gondii* vaccine. J. Immunol. 1991, 146 : 286–292.

[18] Shirahata T., Yamashita T., Ohta C., Goto H. and Nakane A. $CD8^+$ T lymphocytes are the major cell population involved in the early gamma interferon response and resistance to acute primary *Toxoplasma gondii* infection in mice. Microb and Immunol, 1994. 38 : 789–796.

[19] Denkers E.Y., Gazzinelli R.T., Hieny S., Caspar P. and Sher A., Bone marrow macrophages process exogenous *Toxoplasma gondii* polypeptides for recognition by parasite-specific cytolytic T lymphocytes. J. Immunol. 1993. 150 : 517–526.

[20] Hakim F.T., Gazzinelli R.T., Denkers E., Hieny S., Shearer G.M. and Sher A., $CD8^+$ T cells from mice vaccinated against *Toxoplasma gondii* are cytotoxic for parasite-infected or antigen-pulsed host cells. J. Immunol. 1991. 147 : 2310–2316.

[21] Subauste C.S., Koniaris A.H. and Remington J.S. Murine $CD8^+$ cytotoxic T lymphocytes lyse *Toxoplasma gondii*-infected cells. J. Immunol. 1991 147: 3955–3959.

[22] Jordan K.A., Wilson E.H., Tait E.D., Fox B.A., Roos D.S., Bzik D.J., Dzierszinski F. and Hunter C.A. Kinetics and phenotype of vaccine-induced $CD8^+$ T-cell responses to *Toxoplasma gondii*. Infect Immun. 2009. 77: 3894–3901.

[23] Bliss S.K., Zhang Y. and Denkers E.Y. Murine neutrophil stimulation by *Toxoplasma gondii* antigen drives high level production of IFN-gamma-independent IL-12. J. Immunol. 1999. 163 : 2081–2088.

[24] Robben P.M., Mordue D.G., Truscott S.M., Takeda K., Akira S. and Sibley L.D. Production of IL-12 by macrophages infected with *Toxoplasma gondii* depends on the parasite genotype. J. Immunol. 2004. 172 : 3686–3694.

[25] Pepper M., Dzierszinski F., E. Wilson, E. Tait, Q. Fang, F. Yarovinsky, T.M. Laufer, D. Roos and C.A. Hunter, Plasmacytoid dendritic cells are activated by *Toxoplasma gondii* to present antigen and produce cytokines. J. Immunol., 2008. 180 : 6229–6236.

[26] Liu C.H., Fan Y.T., Dias A., Esper L., Corn R.A., Bafica A., Machado F.S. and Aliberti J. Cutting edge: Dendritic cells are essential for in vivo IL-12 production and development of resistance against *Toxoplasma gondii* infection in mice. J. Immunol., 2006. 177 : 31–35.

[27] Reis e Sousa C., Hieny S., Scharton-Kersten T., Jankovic D., Charest H., Germain R.N. and Sher A. In vivo microbial stimulation induces rapid CD40 ligand-independent production of interleukin 12 by dendritic cells and their redistribution to T cell areas. J. Exp. Med., 1997. 186 : 1819–1829.

[28] Mashayekhi M, Sandau MM, Dunay IR, Frickel EM, Khan A, Goldszmid RS, Sher A, Ploegh HL, Murphy TL, Sibley LD, Murphy KM. CD8α(+) dendritic cells are the critical source of interleukin-12 that controls acute infection by *Toxoplasma gondii* tachyzoites. Immunity. 2011. 26;35(2):249-59.

[29] Pifer R. and Yarovinsky F. Innate responses to *Toxoplasma gondii* in mice and humans. Trends Parasitol. 2011. 27 : 388–393.

[30] Zhao Y.O., Khaminets A, Hunn JP, Howard JC. Disruption of the *Toxoplasma gondii* parasitophorous vacuole by IFNgamma-inducible immunity-related GTPases (IRG proteins) triggers necrotic cell death. PLoS Pathog., 2009. 5 (2):e1000288.

[31] Zhao Y, Ferguson DJ, Wilson DC, Howard JC, Sibley LD, Yap GS. Virulent *Toxoplasma gondii* evade immunity-related GTPase-mediated parasite vacuole disruption within primed macrophages. J. Immunol., 2009. 182 : 3775–3781

[32] Scharton-Kersten TM, Yap G, Magram J, Sher A. Inducible nitric oxide is essential for host control of persistent but not acute infection with the intracellular pathogen *Toxoplasma gondii*. J. Exp. Med., 1997. 185 : 1261–1273.

[33] Pfefferkorn E.R. Interferon gamma blocks the growth of *Toxoplasma gondii* in human fibroblasts by inducing the host cells to degrade tryptophan. Proc. Natl. Acad. Sci. U.S.A. 1984. 81 : 908–912.

[34] Andrade RM, Wessendarp M, Gubbels MJ, Striepen B, Subauste CS. CD40 induces macrophage anti-*Toxoplasma gondii* activity by triggering autophagy-dependent fusion of pathogen-containing vacuoles and lysosomes. J. Clin. Invest., 2006. 116 2366–2377.

[35] Ling YM, Shaw MH, Ayala C, Coppens I, Taylor GA, Ferguson DJ, Yap GS. Vacuolar and plasma membrane stripping and autophagic elimination of *Toxoplasma gondii* in primed effector macrophages. *J. Exp. Med.*, 2006. 203: 2063–2071.

[36] Dimier-Poisson I, Aline F, Mévélec MN, Beauvillain C, Buzoni-Gatel D, Bout D. Protective mucosal Th2 immune response against *Toxoplasma gondii* by murine mesenteric lymph node dendritic cells. Infect. Immun. 2003; 71: 5254-65.

[37] Ruiz S, Beauvillain C, Mévélec MN, Roingeard P, Breton P, Bout D *et al.* A novel CD4-CD8α+CD205+CD11b- murine spleen dendritic cell line: establishment, characterization and functional analysis in a model of vaccination to toxoplasmosis. Cell. Microbiol. 2005; 7: 1659-71.

[38] Beauvillain C, Ruiz S, Guiton R, Bout D, Dimier-Poisson I. A vaccine based on exosomes secreted by a dendritic cell line confers protection against *T. gondii* infection in syngeneic and allogeneic mice. Microbes Infect. 2007;9 (14-15):1614-22.

[39] Johnson LL, Sayles PC. Deficient humoral responses underlie susceptibility to *Toxoplasma gondii* in CD4-deficient mice. Infect. Immun. 2002 ; 70: 185-91.

[40] Gubbels MJ, Striepen B, Shastri N, Turkoz M, Robey EA. Class I major histocompatibility complex presentation of antigens that escape from the parasitophorous vacuole of *Toxoplasma gondii*. Infect. Immun. 2005 ; 73: 703-11.

[41] Gazzinelli RT, Hakim FT, Hieny S, Shearer GM, Sher A. Synergistic role of CD4+ and CD8+ T lymphocytes in IFN-γ production and protective immunity induced by an attenuated *Toxoplasma gondii* vaccine. J. Immunol. 1991; 146: 286-92.

[42] Martin D, Tarleton R. Generation, specificity, and function of CD8+ T cells in *Trypanosoma cruzi* infection. Immunol. Rev. 2004; 201: 304-17.

[43] Smith TR, Kumar V. Revival of CD8+ T reg-mediated suppression. Trends Immunol. 2008; 29: 337-42.

[44] Denkers EY, Gazzinelli RT, Martin D, Sher A. Emergence of NK1.1+ cells as effectors of IFN-γ dependent immunity to *Toxoplasma gondii* in MHC class I-deficient mice. J. Exp. Med. 1993; 178: 1465-72.

[45] Askew D, Harding CV. Antigen processing and CD24 expression determine antigen presentation by splenic CD4+ and CD8+ dendritic cells. Immunology. 2008; 123: 447-55.

[46] Blanchard N, Gonzalez F, Schaeffer M, Joncker NT, Cheng T, Shastri AJ *et al.* Immunodominant, protective response to the parasite *Toxoplasma gondii* requires antigen processing in the endoplasmic reticulum. 2008; 9: 937-44.

15

Visceral Leishmaniosis: An Old Disease with Continuous Impact on Public Health

Marcella Zampoli Troncarelli,
Deolinda Maria Vieira Filha Carneiro and Helio Langoni
University Estadual Paulista, School of Veterinary Medicine and Animal Science
Brazil

1. Introduction

Visceral Leishmaniasis (VL) is an important Zoonosis, caused by *Leishmania* spp. protozoa. VL is commonly present in tropical countries, due its complex epidemiological characteristics that involve environmental and climatic conditioning factors; phlebotomine vectors and several species of domestic and wild animals. These aspects determine high difficulty for the disease control.

VL is considered the second most important protozoosis and one of the six main infectious-parasitary diseases in the world (WHO). However, VL is a neglected disease that occurs in 80% of poor or miserable populations witch survive with less than two dollars per day (Desjeux, 2004). VL is considered an emergent/re-emergent Zoonosis with high mortality levels, with continuous and serious impact on Public Health.

2. Epidemiology

2.1 Definition and etiology

Visceral leishmaniasis (VL) is a worldwide zoonotic disease caused by flagellar protozoa (family Trypanosomatidae, order Kinetoplastida, genus *Leishmania* (*L. donovani* complex) (Farrel et al., 2002). *L. chagasi* is frequently reported in Americas (New World), genetically similar to *L. infantum* that is found in some countries of Mediterranean and Asia. *L. infantum* / *L. donovani* are the more prevalent species in Europe, Asia and Africa (Old World).

2.2 Distribution and classification

The VL origin in the New World is controversial. *L. chagasi* may be carried out by wild dogs some millions years ago, but some researches appoint that *L. infantum* may be disseminated after the European colonization. In a study of evolutive and geographical history of *L. donovani* complex, using specific molecular tests, it was possible to infer that *L. (L.) chagasi* and *L. (L.) infantum* are, in fact, different denominations of the same parasite specie, considering their molecular and biochemical similarity (Luke et al., 2007). It was possible to suggest that the primordial lineage of *Leishmania* spp. could be originated in South America.

VL was initially described in Greece, in 1835, and was called "ponos" or "hapoplinakon". The denomination "calazar" is proceeding from India, which means "black skin" due the clinical characteristic presented in severe cases of infection (Lainson et al, 1987).

VL is classified according to its clinical characteristics and epidemiology in five types: Indian, African, Mediterranean, Chinese and American. The Indian type is considered an antropozoonosis caused by L. donovani, mainly identified in children, adolescents and adults determining frequent outbreaks with high mortality levels. This VL type occurs in Afghanistan, Iran, Iraq, Jordan, Israel, Lebanon, Oman, Saudi Arabia, Syrian, Yemen and Bengala. The African type, similar to the Indian one, considering the susceptibility and clinical signs, is caused by L. donovani or L. infantum. The transmission areas of African type are next to forests. The Mediterranean type is a zooantroponosis mainly transmitted in the near-house place. This type is frequently identified in children with five year of age or less, and dogs. L. infantum is involved and also participates on the wild cycle infecting foxes and coyotes. It occurs in Mediterranean, the Middle East and the South of Russia. The Chinese type is another one antropozoonosis caused by L. infantum that complete its biological cycle in dogs, raccoons, coatis, and in children of China. The American type is an antropozoonosis in urbanization process. L. chagasi is enrolled predominantly in children of 15 years of age or less, being transmitted by Lutzomyia longipalpis. In Colombia, Lutzomyia evansi is considered a secondary vector. In Latin America, VL is present in 12 countries with 90% of cases occurring in Brazil. Great urban centers and capitals are being invaded by VL, including Belo Horizonte, Teresina, São Luís, Fortaleza and Rio de Janeiro, where autochthon cases are registered.

First VL human case in Brazil was reported in 1913, when Migone identified amastigotes forms in necropsy materials collected from a man from Boa Esperança, Mato Grosso state (Brasil, 2006). Until the 90`s, the main reported VL cases in human were from Northeast states. However, the recent and fast VL expansion to the Southeast, Midwest and North states has being verified. Northeast states presented the greatest number of VL cases in 2001 (81.7%), followed by North regions (8.8%), Southeast (7.6%) and Midwest (1.9%). However, in 2003, the disease was reported in 58%; 15%; 7% and 19% of the Northeast; North; Midwest and Southeast states, respectively, demonstrating VL urbanization in Brazil (Silva et al., 2001b; Lindoso & Goto, 2006).

Canine visceral leishmaniasis (CVL) prevalence is also high in Brazil, ranging 1% to 36% according to Brazilian region (Silva et al., 2001b). Araçatuba was the first city in Sao Paulo state where CVL was diagnosed (Luvizotto et al., 1999). Forty one cities in Sao Paulo state present the CVL transmission, and human VL transmission was reported in 28 cities, with 10% to 15% prevalence levels (Camargo-Neves, 2005).

2.3 Vectors

The vectors related with *Leishmania* dispersion are phlebotomines (mainly *Lutzomyia longipalpis*). Fleas and ticks are considered other possible leishmaniasis vectors. Reservoirs are infected by phlebotomine females biting during its blood feeding in the skin or the peripheral blood of the reservoirs (mainly in dogs).

In Brazil, the main country of VL transmission in Latin America, the vectors *L. longipalpis* or *L. cruzi* are enrolled on disease transmission.

Phlebotomines are small size insects (3-5 mm lenght) and present a straw coloration. They multiply on organic materials like humid soil, leaves, manure, etc. The action area of phlebotomines is of 150-300 meters (300-600m diameter). They usually fly in small salts and when the females are blood feeding, they keep their flies erect.

2.4 Reservoirs

The direct transmission (person-to-person) of VL is rare. In regions of the New World, where *L. chagasi* is endemic, the infection dispersion/maintenance in human beings had been also attributed to the canine reservoirs. They live closely to human and attract the vector to human houses. Dogs present elevate subcutaneous parasitism levels with high infectivity to the VL vector. The infectivity levels for phlebotomines are similar in asymptomatic and symptomatic dogs (Zivicnjak et al., 2005).

On the other hand, *Leishmania* can be also identified in wild animals as foxes (mainly *Lycalopex vetulus* and *Cerdocyon thous*) (De Lima et al., 2006), and opossums (*Didelphis albiventris*) (Santiago et al., 2007). Equines, cats and rodents have been also identified as reservoirs.

Cats are susceptible to both VL and integumentary leishmaniasis. Xenodiagnosis studies with experimental *Leishmania* infections in cats demonstrated the evidence of feline`s infectivity to the vector *L. longipalpis*. Skin lesions and protozoan distribution in organs were verified in infected cats, but the disease was self-limited after few months post-infection. Cats' eclectic habit as well as the vectors adaptation to different animal species would be favorable factors for VL transmission (Dantas-Torres et al., 2006).

VL in cats may be also associated with immunosuppressive diseases such as leukemia and feline immunodeficiency. Recent studies are been developed in order to investigate the real feline role on VL epidemiology: if they are important reservoirs or only accidental hosts.

2.5 *Leishmania* life cycle

Infected vertebrate hosts (reservoirs) are bitted by phlebotomine vectors during the blood feeding. Vectors acquire macrophages containing *Leishmania* amastigotes forms which multiply by binary division. Amastigotes differentiate to promastigote (flagellar) forms which colonize vectors` pharynges and esophagus and stay adhered to epithelium by their flagella. Then, these promastigotes forms differentiate to metacyclical promastigotes (infecting) forms.

Biological cycle is completed when vectors bite new vertebrate hosts and the infecting *Leishmania* forms are inoculated in the hosts` epidermis and phagocyted by macrophages. After phagocytosis, promastigotes change to amastigotes which intensively multiply by binary division. Macrophages become devitalized and break and release the amastigotes which are phagocyted by new macrophages in a continuous process. The haematogenic and lymphatic dissemination of protozoa for other tissues and organs occurs especially in mononuclear phagocytical system cells (Ikeda-Garcia & Marcondes, 2007).

2.6 Characteristics and risk factors

VL has been considered as a re-emergent disease in some countries and has assumed a new profile due economic and social changes in the two last decades. Initially, VL was considered a typical and sporadically agricultural disease (Nunes et al., 2001). It reached dogs and human beings that lived in close contact with forest regions (Gontijo & Melo, 2004). However, VL has been pointed currently as a re-emergent zoonosis, characterizing a clear process of epidemiological transition. LV has become an urban endemic disease that represents serious problems for Public Health due its zoonotic potential. The frequent deforestation has reduced the availability of original wild animals to vector. Then, dogs and human actually represents alternative sources for vector`s feeding (Desjeaux, 2004).

This zoonosis has demonstrated an increased prevalence in recent years, not only considering the number of registered cases, but also regarding its geographic distribution. The important social, political and environmental damages (Fig. 1), added to continuous population migrations for urban centers without sanitary structure (Fig. 2) and lack of educative programs, associated to the easy vector adaptability to new environments and to the high population of dogs which are potential reservoirs, had contributed to establish favorable conditions to the VL urbanization (Camargo-Neves, 2005). Reduction of the disease ecological space is also verified, leading to important outbreaks.

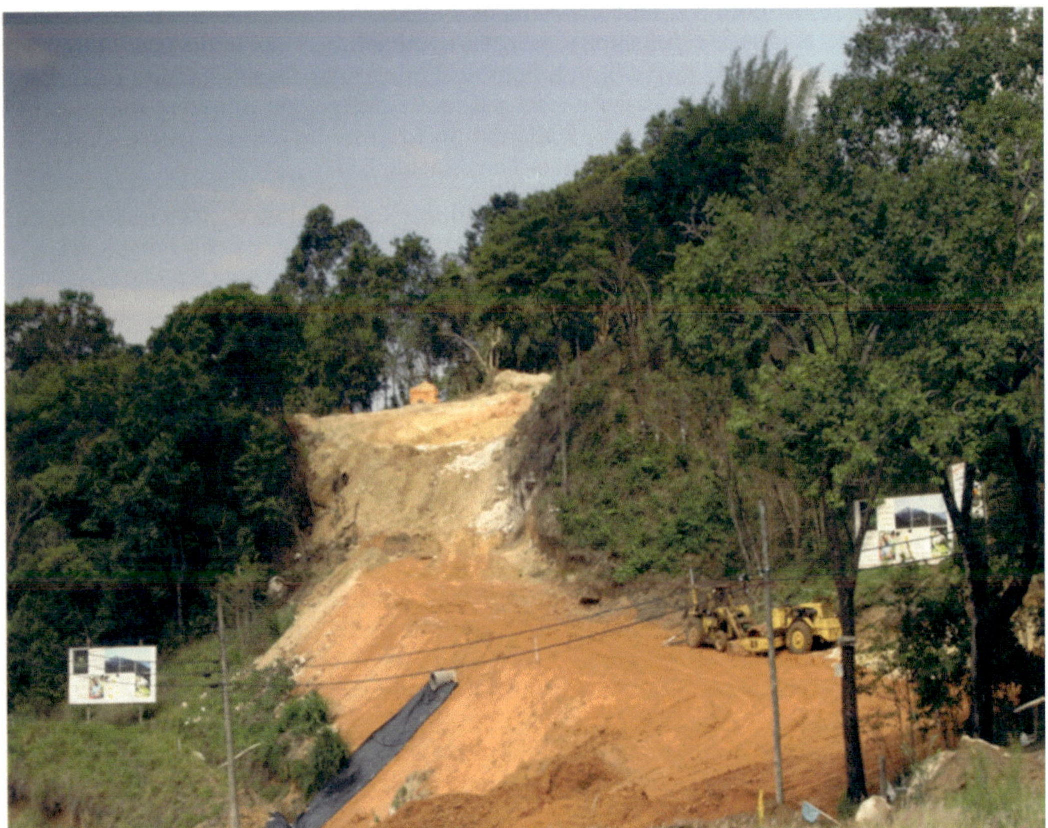

Fig. 1. Environmental damage caused by houses building in Botucatu, Sao Paulo State, Brazil. The human changes in natural areas, the vector adaptation and the high number of possible reservoirs species represent a serious VL transmission risk to human and animals.

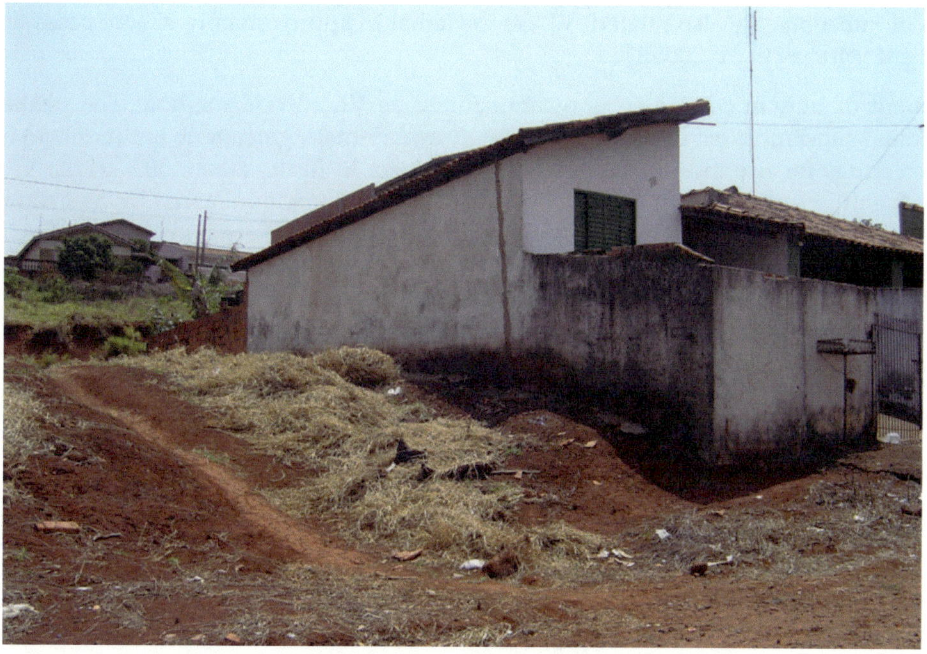

Fig. 2. Organic material accumulation near to a house in Sao Manuel, Sao Paulo State, Brazil. This situation may represent a risk for vector multiplication and VL transmission to both human and animals, especially in tropical countries.

2.7 Susceptibility

People of both sexes and all ages are susceptible to VL. However, the incidence is highlighted in children with nine years of age or less, and in immunossupressed individuals. On the other hand, in recent endemic areas, a new situation regarding VL susceptibility has been observed, and the number of VL cases in children and adults is practically the same. This fact could be related to the protozoa`s pathogeny/pathogenicity variations and also to immunossupressor influences which adult persons are continuously exposed, like stress.

Approximately 12 million of people in the world are infected by *Leishmania* and about 1.5-2 million new cases (25-50% as VL type) are notified by year. However, the official data does not represents the real number of cases, due passive detections, under-diagnosticated cases, asymptomatic cases and low number of countries with obligatory notification (only 32 of 88 endemic countries demand obligatory cases registration). In accordance with the Regional Program of Leishmaniasis, all American countries registered more than 5,000 VL cases in 2006.

3. Clinical signs in human and treatment

The incubation period of VL in human is variable, ranging from 10 days to 24 months, with average of two to six months. Clinical manifestations of the disease in humans are presented gradually, starting with apathy, weight loss, anemia, fever and lymphadenopaty, and liver and spleen enlargement. Pneumonia and other severe manifestations due secondary bacterial infections are also related. VL can be lethal in approximately 95% of cases without treatment (Murray et al., 2005).

Treatment of human cases also is recommended as VL control method. The pentavalent antimonial substances (sodium estibogluconate and N-metil glucamine antimoniate) are the election drugs for use in humans, since 70 years ago. In India, where 50% of the VL cases occur, the miltefosin is being used - since March of 2002 – administered by oral route, also indicated in oncology. This drug presents relatively efficient safety and allows up to 98% of cure. It is indicated in refractory cases to the therapy with conventional antimoniates. However, the patients can develop gastric, intestinal and theratogenic collateral effects. Amphotericin B is another therapeutic option that also determines collateral effects and is considered a high cost drug.

4. HIV-VL co-infection

More than 30 million people in the world are infected by HIV, and at least one third of this population lives in leishmaniasis endemic areas (WHO). The overlapping of geographic areas where leishmaniasis and HIV occur is due to the process of urbanization.

In Europe, 70% of LV cases in adults are associated with HIV, and more than 9% of the individuals with AIDS suffer a just acquired or reactivated leishmaniasis. Users of intravenous drugs are considered of high risk for the co-infection, by sharing needles. From 80's on, this co-infection started to be described in the Europe, particularly in Spain, Italy and South France. In people infected by HIV, leishmaniasis presents severe clinical manifestations and determines lethal immunosuppressive synergism with HIV with stimulation of the viral response. However, the opportunistic behavior of *Leishmania* on HIV-VL co-infection is still not clear.

The HIV-VL co-infection is considered a world priority by WHO. In this context, it was established a worldwide network of further notification of cases.

5. Clinical signs in dogs

Canine Visceral Leishmaniasis (CVL) determines a chronic systemic disease with several clinical manifestations, with difficult diagnosis. CVL incubation period is variable. Clinical signs can be verified in dogs between three months to various years after infection (mean three to seven months) (Brasil, 2006).

Lymphadenopathy; abdominal distension due liver and spleen enlargement; skin lesions and/or alopecia (Fig. 3); emaciation; apathy; ocular lesions (Fig. 4); onicogryphosis; haemorrhages; diarrhoea and pneumonia are the main clinical signs reported. Locomotors and neurological alterations are occasionally related (Slappendel & Ferrer, 1998).

Clinical signs in dogs may have different presentations, depending on the region (Cruz, 2006; Duprey et al., 2006; Albuquerque et al., 2007). In a recent study, the main clinical manifestations observed in 100 examined dogs from an endemic VL area in Brazil were: emaciation (60%); spleen enlargement (57%); alopecia (51%); ocular lesions (46%); skin ulcers (43%); liver enlargement (38%); onicogryphosis (37%) and lymphadenopaty (21%) (Troncarelli et al., 2008).

Symptomatic CVL is frequently reported, but asymptomatic cases represent about 60% of infected dogs. Asymptomatic parasited dogs with or without antibodies have been identified in natural and experimental infections (Farrel, 2002).The infected asymptomatic animals represent a serious problem for public health because they are important unidentified reservoirs. On the other hand, when an infected asymptomatic dog is diagnosed, control measures may be difficult because the euthanasia is usually not authorized by dog's owner.

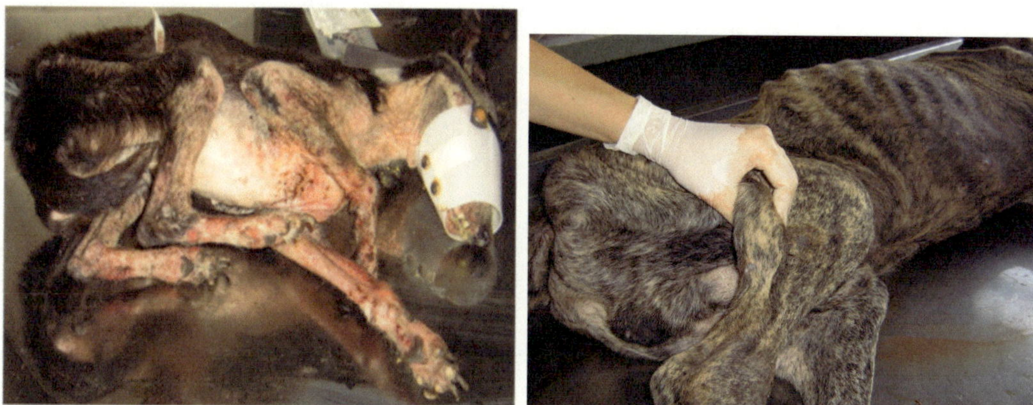

(A) (B)

Fig. 3. Symptomatic VL seropositive dogs in the Zoonosis Control Center (ZCC) in Bauru - an important VL endemic area of Sao Paulo State, Brazil. A: alopecia, emaciation, skin lesions, onicogriphosis and apathy. B: lymphadenopathy (popliteal), emaciation, dehydratation.

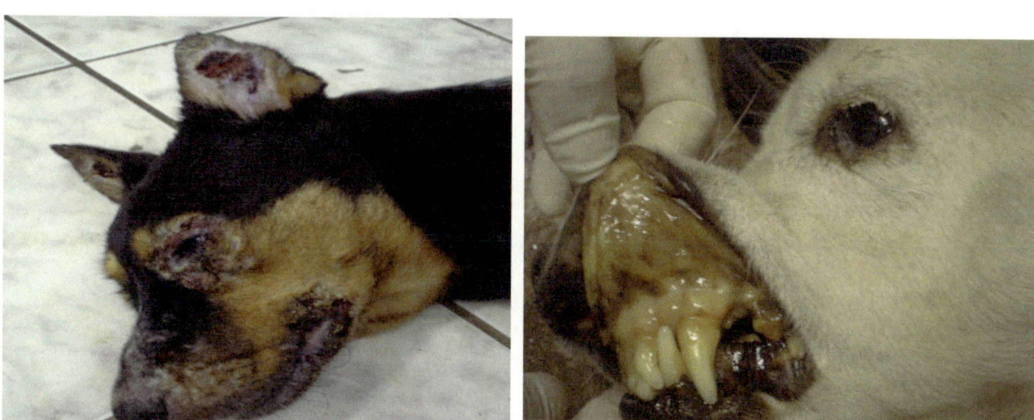

(A) (B)

Fig. 4. Symptomatic VL seropositive dogs from Bauru, Sao Paulo State, Brazil. A: severe periocular, nasal and auricular skin lesions (humid dermatitis, alopecia, crusts and secondary bacterial infection). B: ocular lesions, jaundice.

6. Diagnosis

6.1 Dogs

Considering that VL is a further notification zoonosis and reinforcing the risks to public health represented by *Leishmania* infected dogs, CVL diagnosis must be the more accurate than possible. It is important that the technical groups involved on CVL diagnosis specifically know about the available tests, as its limitations and clinical interpretation (Luz et al., 2001; Gradoni, 2002; Ikeda-Garcia & Marcondes, 2007).

The diagnosis result must not be individually analyzed. There are various dependent factors that must be evaluated, like epidemiological issues, clinical signs, laboratory diagnosis results, etc. A positive result, if punctually analyzed, can condemn a non-infected dog to the euthanasia and a negative result if not correctly evaluated can contribute to the maintenance of an infected dog as a *Leishmania* reservoir (Machado, 2004; Zivicnjak et al., 2005).

6.1.1 Serology

Detection of circulating antibodies anti-*Leishmania* spp. in dogs by serological tests is an essential tool for CVL diagnosis. Serum samples or eluted blood samples can be examined by serological tests (Fig. 5).

Dogs generally present seroconvertion after three months post-infection. Antibodies titles remain high for at least two years after *Leishmania* infection (Ikeda-Garcia & Marcondes, 2007). CVL clinical signs and antibodies titers are not necessarily dependent factors (Reis, 2001; Ferreira et al., 2007).

Available serological tests commonly used for CVL diagnosis are Indirect Haemagglutination (IHA); Agglutination in Latex (AL); Direct Agglutination (DA); Immunoeletrophoresis; Indirect Immunofluoresence Antibody Test (IFAT) (Fig. 5); Enzyme-linked Immunosorbent Assay (ELISA); Complement Fixation; Immunopreccipitation in gel and Western blot. Brazilian Health Ministry (Brasil, 2006) determined that the official labs must apply ELISA as a selection diagnosis and IFAT as a confirmatory test, in CVL surveillances.

IFAT usually shows high sensitivity and specificity values, ranging from 68 to 100% and 74 to 100%, respectively (Grosjean et al., 2003; Alves & Bevilacqua, 2004). ELISA` sensitivity and specificity values range from 71 to 100% and 85 to 100%, respectively. These tests are feasible, fast and inexpensively executed (Ikeda-Garcia & Marcondes, 2006). However, a positive result may not represent an active disease and also infected dogs may have negative results by serological tests. Two tests with 21-30 days interval are recommended.

Due to the phylogenetic similarity between *Leishmania* genus and *Trypanosoma cruzi* (*T. cruzi*), serological cross-reactions (Fig. 6) and false-positive results are quite common (Zanette et al., 2006). There are endemic areas, especially in the Americas, where *Leishmania* spp. and *T.cruzi* incidences are superposed and co-infection with the two parasites may occur both in dogs and in human beings (Savani et al., 2005; Madeira et al., 2006). In fact, the results from serological tests may show *Leishmania* spp. and *T.cruzi* antibodies, signifying the occurrence of infection by the two parasites, rather than cross-reactions (Grosjean et al., 2003; Rosypal et al., 2007). By this way, the improvement of diagnosis methods for the correct identification of canine infection is necessary to better comprehend the disease's status in dogs and also to contribute to its control.

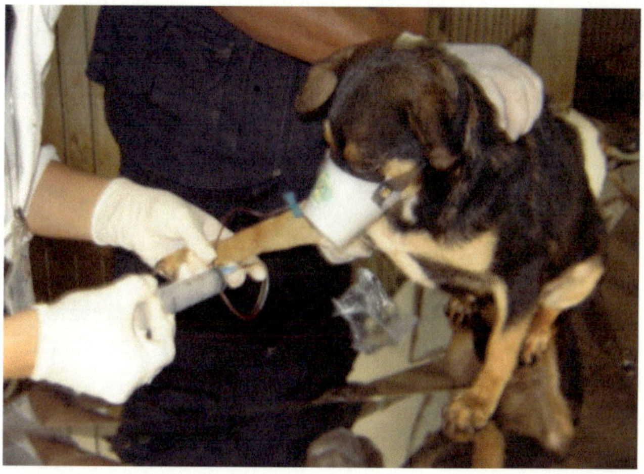

Fig. 5. Blood sampling for CVL serological diagnosis at Zoonosis Control Center (ZCC) of Bauru, Sao Paulo State, Brazil.

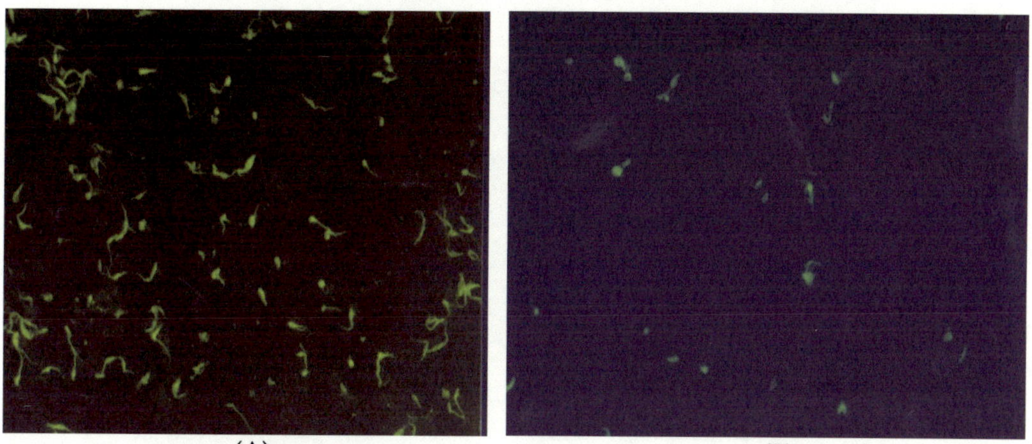

(A) (B)

Fig. 6. Positive results for *Leishmania* spp. and *Trypanosoma cruzi* by indirect immunofluorescence tests in serum samples collected from a dog in an VL endemic area in Brazil. Note the morphologic similarity between the protozoan parasites. A: promastigotes forms of *L. major*. B: trypomastigotes forms of *T. cruzi* "Y"strain. Pictures credits: Zoonosis Research Nucleous (NUPEZO), Univ Estadual Paulista (UNESP), Botucatu, Sao Paulo, Brazil.

A 16.5% (33/200) cross-reaction between *Leishmania* spp. and *T.cruzi* in blood samples collected from dogs in an endemic VL area in Brazil was verified. Twenty-six (78.8%) of 33 dogs that showed anti-*Leishmania* spp. and anti-*T.cruzi* antibodies also tested positive by direct parasitological examination and PCR for *Leishmania* spp., which indicates that these dogs presented leishmaniasis. No liver or spleen sample from the 200 dogs analyzed showed a positive PCR result for *T.cruzi*. These findings support the occurrence of cross-reactions between *Leishmania* spp. and *T.cruzi* in IFAT; they also corroborate the need for simultaneous PCR and/or parasitological examination to establish canine leishmaniasis (CL) diagnosis.

On the other hand, it is important to reinforce that cross-reactions between *Leishmania* and other tripanosomatids or different microorganisms (including *Ehrlichia* canis; *Babesia* canis;, *Toxoplasma gondii* or *Dirofilaria immitis*) can occur, producing false-positive results (Rosario, 2002; Luvizotto, 2003; Alvar et al., 2004). The use of recombinant or purified antigens (like gp63, gp72 and gp70; rK39, rK9 and rK26) improves the sensitivity and specificity of serological tests (Rosário, 2002; Zijlstra et al., 2001).

6.1.2 Culture

Blood samples and lymph node, bone marrow and spleen aspirates can be used for VL diagnosis by culture in special medium like Liver Infusion Tryptosis (LIT); NNN and RPMI-1640 (Sundar & Rai, 2002).

Leishmania amastigotes forms presented in original biological samples collected from vertebrate hosts modify to promastigotes (flagellar) forms in culture medium and can be visualized by optical microscope (Fig. 7).

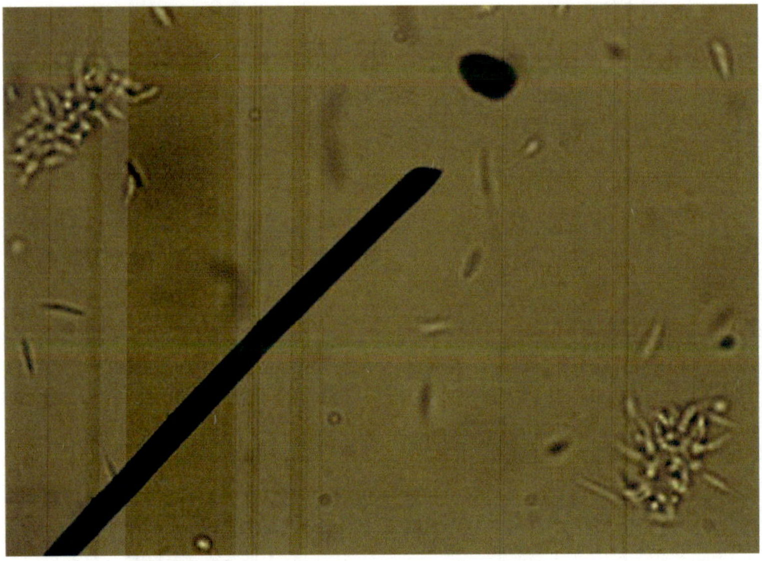

Fig. 7. *Leishmania* promastigotes forms isolated in Liver Infusion Tryptosis (LIT) medium after four weeks incubation at 27ºC. Optical microscopy 1000X.

Culture diagnosis is commonly used for researches purposes because it is a time and material-consuming method. Results are lately obtained because *Leishmania* presents a slow multiplication in culture media. A positive result can be verified until four months post-incubation, especially in case of low parasite load presented in biological collected samples.

6.1.3 Parasitological identification

6.1.3.1 Citology

Leishmania amastigote forms can be visualized in lymph nodes squashes (or aspirate); bone marrow; spleen aspirate; skin biopsy; skin nodules aspirate; liver biopsy and blood squashes. Giemsa, Leishman, Wright and Panotico are the most common dyes used (Sundar & Rai, 2002). Amastigotes forms have 2-5 µm size. For the correct diagnosis, it is necessary to observe three parasites` structures: cytoplasm, nucleous and kinetoplast (Fig. 8).

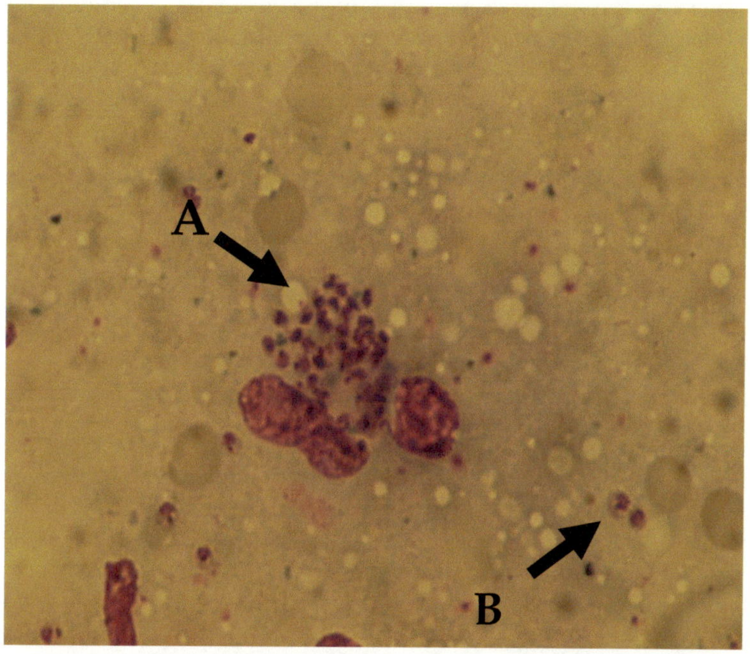

Fig. 8. Dog`s liver *imprint* showing the protozoa`s amastigote structures. Giemsa dye, 1000X. A: amastigotes forms in a macrophage cytoplasm. B: individual protozoa`s amastigote form presenting cytoplasm, nucleus and kinetoplast.

Aspirative cytology is generally used in vet clinics because it is a relatively easy and low invasive procedure. Citology sensitive values are directly related to parasite load, biological material collected, technical experience and time for slide examination (Ikeda-Garcia & Feitosa, 2006). This test presents sensitivity levels of 58%, 70% and 96%, for lymph node, bone marrow and spleen aspirates, respectively (Zijlstra et al., 2001). The 100% specificity allows the indication of cytology as a gold standard method. However, negative results are not uncommon, especially in chronic and/or asymptomatic CVL cases.

6.1.3.2 Immunohistochemistry

Skin, liver and lymphoid tissues are the election materials for VL diagnosis by immunohistochemistry/immunocytochemistry (IHC). Blood squashes; cytological slides; histological and frozen tissues can also be examined (Ikeda-Garcia & Feitosa, 2006). IHC allows retrospective studies and can be indicated for skilful exams.

Immunoglobulins conjugated to enzymes are used to identify *Leishmania* amastigotes forms in tissues. High sensitivity and specificity values of this method allow an accurate and fast diagnosis despite the eventual low parasites load on samples (Ikeda-Garcia & Marcondes, 2007). Amastigotes presents a hazel-brown coloration, easily visible by conventional optical microscopy.

6.1.4 Molecular diagnosis

Polymerase Chain Reaction (PCR) allows the parasite's DNA detection and does not depend on the dog's immunological and/or clinical status (Soares et al., 2005; Reithinger & Dujardin, 2007). PCR can be used in cases of inconclusive reactions, anergy or cross reactions in serological tests, and shows sensitivity and specificity values near 100% (Lachaud et al., 2002; Gomes et al., 2007). Blood samples (Silva et al., 2001a); lymph node aspirates; bone marrow aspirates; biopsy fragments (skin, liver, spleen, etc.) and any kind of biological material can be tested by PCR for Leishmania`s DNA search.

Different PCR protocols have been studied for leishmaniasis diagnosis in animals (Strauss-Ayali et al., 2004), human and vectors (Aransay et al., 2000). Primers used are usually *Leishmania* genus-specific (Fig. 9.) or specie-specific (Solano-Gallego et al., 2001). Detection of more than one *Leishmania* species can be obtained by multiplex PCR (mPCR) protocols (Lachaud et al., 2002a,b). Parasite load can be evaluated by real time PCR (qPCR) techniques (Nicolas et al., 2002). The association of molecular methods with conventional diagnosis tests for VL diagnosis allows an accurate evaluation and also contributes to epidemiological and genetic studies (Singh & Sivakumar, 2003; Moreira et al., 2007).

PCR also contributes with diagnosis elucidation, especially in case of cross reactions results by serological tests. 93.9% sensitivity and 85.8% specificity levels were obtained by PCR for leishmaniasis diagnosis in spleen and liver fragments collected from dogs in Bauru, an endemic CVL area in Brazil (Troncarelli et al., 2009). Using the LINR4 and LIN19 (Ikonomopoulos et al., 2006) primers it was possible to identify 30 of 33 *Leishmania* infected dogs that were both positive for *Leishmania* and *T. cruzi* by IFAT.

720 bp →

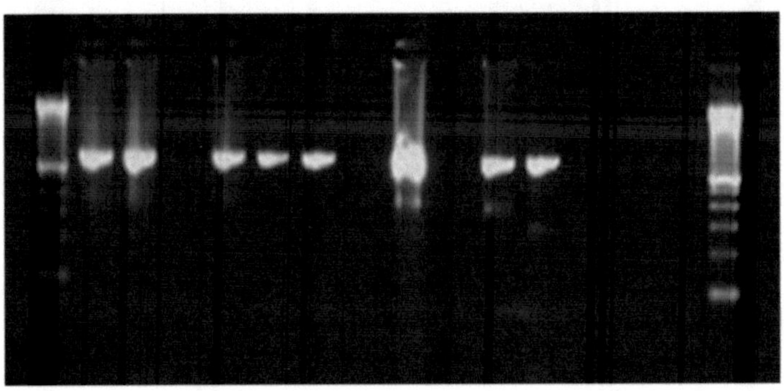

Fig. 9. *Leishmania* spp. kDNA amplification by Polimerase Chain Reaction. Samples: spleen fragments collected from euthanized dogs from Bauru (a Visceral Leishmaniasis endemic area in Sao Paulo State, Brazil). Primers LIN19 and LINR4. Agarosis gel 2%. bp - base pairs; LD - DNA ladder; C+ positive control (*L.major*); 1,3,4,5,9,10 – positive samples; 7 – positive sample with high DNA concentration; 2,6,8,11 – negative samples; 12 – negative control (milliQ water); 13 – PCR negative control (MIX-PCR).

6.2 Human

VL human diagnosis is difficult, because it is generally based on clinical signs that are lately identified. VL is a chronic disease, with a long incubation period with gradual and slow clinical manifestations, in the main number of cases. Infected people just call for a doctor when clinical signs are evident like abdominal distension - due liver and spleen enlargement, hypoproteinemia, anemia - besides progressive emaciation; pain; lymphadenopahty or other severe disorders. In these cases, the diagnosis is done, but the prognostic is reserved to bad, especially in case of young and/or immunossupressed patients (Brasil, 2006).

Serology tests can be done, but results are questionable and normally do not depend on patient infection and/or clinical status. The intra-dermal reaction (Montenegro`s test) is usually negative in VL human cases during disease`s clinical course, but can be positive in asymptomatic individuals or after the clinical cure (Ikeda-Garcia & Marcondes, 2007).

Culture of blood marrow aspirates and direct parasitological exam of blood marrow squashes are the main sensitive tests for human VL diagnosis, but sampling method is invasive and painful. Liver and spleen biopsy are not recommended, especially in chronic cases, due haemorrhages risks due organs enlargement caused by *Leishmania* infection.

7. Epidemiological vigilance, prophylaxis and control

Considering the difficulties of VL control and monitoring, actions are centered on the better definition of risk transmission areas. The new target is to reinforce vigilance measures in States and counties where no LV human or canine cases are related, in order to avoid or to minimize the disease transmission in these non endemic areas. In the VL endemic areas, after the epidemiological stratification, the control measures generally are individually evaluated and implemented. However, it is important that integrated measures are adopted for an effective control.

VL incidence especially in Americas is very high, but control strategies must be improved. Surveillance systems are usually inadequate and there are no sufficient human resources for diagnosis, treatment and control methods implementation. The Regional Program supported by the Global Program on leishmaniasis prevention and control prepared an action plan to be started in 2007. This plan includes a collective work for diagnosis tests standardization; strengthening of human resources; decentralization of public health programs of VL prevention and control; surveillance system improvement; strategic partnerships development and communities` involvement.

7.1 Vector control

The control strategy of this zoonosis includes: the early identification/treatment of human cases, the residual insecticides spraying in domiciles and near-house areas and add physical barriers in doors and windows in order to prevent the exposition to the vector. Photo-stables pyrethroids are usually sprayed in the human houses' walls, and animals' installations, like hen and swine houses, stables, etc; considering that these animals and its organic substances attract phlebotomines. It is important to reinforce the adequate destination of garbage, the removal of rubbish and organic substances in the near-house areas.

7.2 Control in dogs

7.2.1 Euthanasia

The identification of serologically positive dogs, followed by euthanasia (Fig. 10) is one of control measures adopted in endemic areas (Brasil, 2006). VL coexists in dogs and humans but generally the disease in dogs precedes the occurrence of human cases. This reinforces the importance of fast diagnosis in dogs, especially in endemic areas. Dogs are considered competent and abundant reservoirs, and cohabit with humans.

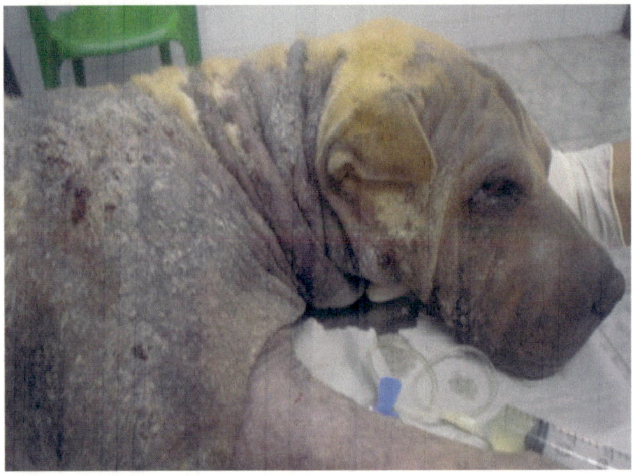

Fig. 10. Euthanasia of a symptomatic VL seropositive dog in Zoonosis Control Center (ZCC) in Bauru, Sao Paulo State, Brazil. Approximately 20-30 dogs are euthanized at the ZCC daily.

The impact of the control by positive dogs' elimination is very conflicting, because it is showing laborious, with doubtful effectiveness and for the veterinarians and owner's point of view. The euthanasia of seropositive dogs is frequently discussed. In recent studies, the evolution of seropositivity levels in humans, in two areas - one with elimination and another one without elimination of the seropositive dogs - were evaluated and there was no significant difference after one year of serological monitoring. However, the risk to the domestic man and to other animals - considering the importance of dog as a reservoir, and the low efficiency of therapeutical protocols for dogs - justifies, until the moment, the recommendation for euthanasia of infected dogs, as complementary method of control and prophylaxis of VL.

7.2.2 Collars with repellent substances

Collars impregnated with deltamethrin or other repellent substance can be associated with other control measures for VL prevention in dogs. This measure avoids dogs to be bitted by the vector.

A study done in Andradina (Camargo Neves, 2005), an endemic VL area in Sao Paulo State, Brazil, demonstrated that both CVL and human VL prevalences had decreased when a prevention program was initiated with deltamethrin collars putting in dogs. It is important to reinforce that collars were replaced each three to four months interval, in order to maintain the residual action of the repellent.

7.2.3 Vaccination

Vaccination is considered another control method of CVL. There are several studies regarding dogs' immunization, and the main researches' objective is to develop a safe, low cost and highly immunogenic vaccine against VL in dogs. In experimental studies, filtered proteins from *Leishmania* promastigotes culture stimulated high immunity in different hosts, and conferred good protection in BALB/c mice infected with *L. major*. In other research, it was demonstrated that the vaccine produced from promastigotes antigens of *L. infantum* allowed 92% of protection in dogs from endemic areas.

The Fucose Manose Ligand (FML) was the first antigenic glycoprotein approved for dogs`s immunization in Brazil. The main question regarding this vaccine was the probable difficulties to differentiate naturally infected from vaccinated animals by conventional serological tests.

A new recombinant vaccine using the A2 *Leishmania* antigen fragment was recently approved by Brazilian Ministry of Agriculture.

National researches institutes in Brazil are also involved on CVL vaccines development. The main effort is to produce a recombinant CVL vaccine associated with Rabies virus, to be used in national vaccination programs.

7.2.4 Treatment

Treatment of dogs with drugs indicated for human application is not recommended in Brazil (Brasil, 2006). Despite several studies have been conducted demonstrating that clinical signals are minimized or eliminated after treatment, there are some controversies about the parasitological cure versus the apparent clinical cure. Some researches reinforce that dogs could remain as *Leishmania* reservoirs representing a public health risk.

On the other hand, CVL treatment is allowed in Spain and in other endemic countries. Glucantime is sold for veterinary use, and the doses volume is adjusted for use in small animals. Moreover, there are some medical pet foods with low protein levels indicated for dogs with leishmaniasis, considering that CVL commonly determines hepatic and renal lesions by immune-complexes deposition.

7.3 Control difficulties

7.3.1 General factors

One of the biggest challenges for the strategies control improvement is the identification of each element of the epidemiological chain and its impact on VL transmission. The high prevalence of VL in endemic areas, especially in tropical countries are due environmental and climatic changes; low financial support on Health and Education programs; discontinuing of control measures; vector's adaptation to environments modified by human; vectors genetic variances; co-infection with immune-suppressor diseases like AIDS, or chemotherapy treatment; urban problems like under-nutrition, house lacking and sanitary deficiencies.

7.3.2 Diagnosis fails

The delay on human and canine VL diagnosis usually determines under-notification of cases and treatment fails. This may be determined by lack of information on VL by population and eventually by some health professionals contributing to VL severity increase, high mortality levels and dissemination risks. The time between sampling, diagnosis and control measures is too long (more than 80 days), determining the maintenance of infected dogs as reservoirs during several months. The strategy of seropositive dogs culling after 80 days blood sampling and diagnosis reduces in 9% the VL prevalence. If the euthanasia of seropositive dogs is done after 7 days of sampling and diagnosis, there is a 27% reduction in seroprevalence.

7.3.4 Vectors`characteristics

Phlebotomines are highly adaptable insects. As they multiply in organic materials, its control is very hard. The use of insecticides must be done by official agents with extremely sense, due the insecticides` residues that can prejudice the ecosystem and the environment.

It is also important to consider the potential of other species of insects and mites as VL transmitters.

7.3.5 Reservoirs` characteristics

Dog is generally considered a family member. Its close contact with human may represent a serious public health risk considering the VL transmission potential in endemic areas. In some situations, when an infected dog is identified by diagnosis methods, it is sent to another place by its owners, in order to avoid the dog`s euthanasia. As there is no control about dogs' transit from endemic to non endemic areas, the risk of introduction and dissemination of VL in different regions is very high.

It is also important to consider the reservoirs potential of wild animals as and the role of some domestic animals like cats on VL transmission.

8. Continued education

Continued education programs on VL are essential for population orientation and to establish directing global actions involving community and public health organs for the disease prevention and control. The educative actions must be implemented in schools and neighbor associations in order to provide information regarding the main VL clinical signs and the prevention methods. Responsible ownership must be emphasized because dogs' replacement levels after infected dogs' removal for euthanasia are extremely high, especially in VL endemic areas.

9. Conclusion

VL represents a serious Public Health challenge in the world. The high disease expansion both in number of cases and in geographic areas reinforces the necessity of effective VL monitoring and control strategies. The complexity of causal agent, the variability of reservoirs species and the vectors adaptability to different ecosystems demand systematic and integrated actions in different points of the epidemiological chain. These factors explain why leishmaniasis is an old disease with continuous impact on public health.

The improvement of diagnosis methods, the surveillance studies, the vaccine immunoprophylaxy, the systematic control of vectors, the researches for effective antimicrobials and therapeutical protocols for dogs and humans, the continued education regarding VL and responsible ownership are some measures for the VL control success.

10. Acknowledgments

We thanks to Zoonosis Control Center (ZCC) of Bauru, Sao Paulo State, Brazil to allow the CVL research studies; to Zoonosis Research Nucleous (NUPEZO) - School of Veterinary Medicine and Animal Science - Univ Estadual Paulista (UNESP) Botucatu, Sao Paulo, Brazil, for lab support; to Fundação de Amparo à Pesquisa do Estado de São Paulo (FAPESP) for the financial support to VL studies; and to all students/researches on VL that contribute with leishmaniasis prevention and control in the world.

11. References

Albuquerque, A.R.; Aragão, F.R.; Faustino, M.A.G.; Gomes, Y.M.; Lira, R.A.; Nakasawa, M. & Alves, L.C. (2007). Aspectos clínicos de cães naturalmente infectados por *Leishmania (Leishmania) chagasi* na região metropolitana do Recife. *Clínica Veterinária*, No.71, pp.78-80, ISSN 1413-571X.

Alves, W.A. & Bevilacqua, P.D. (2004). Reflexões sobre a qualidade do diagnóstico da leishmaniose visceral canina em inquéritos epidemiológicos: o caso da epidemia de Belo Horizonte, Minas Gerais, Brasil, 1993-1997. *Cadernos de Saúde Pública*, Vol.20, No.1, pp.259-265.

Aransay, A.M.; Scoulica, E. & Tselentis, Y. (2000). Detection and Identification of *Leishmania* DNA within Naturally Infected Sand Flies by Seminested PCR on Minicircle Kinetoplastic DNA. *Applied Environmental Microbiology*, Vol.66, pp.1933-1938.

Brasil. Ministério da Saúde. Secretaria de Vigilância em Saúde. Departamento de Vigilância Epidemiológica. (2006). *Manual de vigilância e controle da leishmaniose visceral.* Brasília, Brazil, pp.9-18.

Camargo-Neves, V.L.F. *Leishmaniose visceral americana*: doença emergente no estado de São Paulo. São Paulo: Superintendência de Controle de Endemias - SUCEN, Coordenadoria de Controle de Doenças, Secretaria de Estado de Saúde de São Paulo, 2005. Available in: <http://www.comciencia.br/reportagens/2005/06/17.shtml>. Accessed in September 2007.

Camargo-Neves, V.L.F. Utilização de coleiras impregnadas com deltametrina a 4% para o controle da leishmaniose visceral americana. Resultados preliminares de um estudo conduzido no Estado de São Paulo, Brasil. Consulta de Expertos OPS/OMS sobre Leishmaniasis Visceral en Las Américas Brasilia, 2005 p99.

Cruz, B. (2006). *Cães apresentam alta incidência de leishmaniose em município pernambucano.* Rio de Janeiro: Agência Fiocruz de Notícias. Available in: <http://www.fiocruz.br/ccs/cgi/cgilua.exe/sys/start.htm?infoid=776&sid=9>. Accessed in September 2007.

Dantas-Torres, F.; Simões-Matos, L.; Brito, F.L.C.; Figueiredo, L.A. & Faustino, M.A.G. (2006). Leishmaniose felina: revisão de literatura. *Clínica Veterinária*, ano XI, Vol.61, pp. 32-40, ISSN 1413-571X.

De Lima, H.; Carrero, J.; Rodriguez, A.; De Guglielmo, Z. & Rodriguez, N. (2006). Trypanosomatidae de importância en salud pública en animales silvestres y sinantrópicos en un área rural del município Tovar del estado Mérida. *Venez. Biomédica*, Vol.26, pp.42-50.

Desjeux, P. (2004). Leishmaniasis: current situation and new perspectives. Comparative Immunology. *Microbiologic Infectious Diseases*, Vol.27, pp.305-318.

Duprey, Z.H.; Steurer, F.J.; Rooney, J.A.; Kirchhoff, L.V.; Jackson, J.E.; Rowton, E.D. & Schantz, P.M. (2006). Canine visceral leishmaniasis, United States and Canada, 2000-2003. *Emergent Infectious Diseases,* Vol.12, No.3, p.440-446.

Farrell, J.P. (2002). *Leishmania.* World class Parasites: Vol.4. London: Kluwer Academic Publishers, pp.45-57.

Ferreira, E.C.; Lana, M.; Carneiro, M.; Reis, A.B.; Paes, D.V.; Silva, E.S.; Schallig, H. & Gontijo, C.M.F. (2007). Comparison of serological assays for the diagnosis of canine visceral leishmaniasis in animals presenting different clinical manifestations. *Veterinary Parasitology,* Vol.146, pp.235-241.

Gomes, A.H.S.; Ferreira, I.M.R.; Lima, M.L.S.R.; Cunha, E.A.; Garcia, A.S.; Araújo, M.F.L. & Pereira-Chioccola, V.L. (2007). PCR identification of *Leishmania* in diagnosis and control of canine leishmaniasis *Veterinary Parasitology,* Vol.144, Supl. 3-4, pp.234-241.

Gontijo, C.M.F. & Melo, M.N. (2004). Leishmaniose visceral no Brasil: quadro atual, desafios e perspectivas. *Revista Brasileira de Epidemiologia,* Vol.7, pp.338-349, 1415-790X.

Gradoni, L. (2002). The diagnosis of canine leishmaniasis. Canine Leishmaniasis: moving towards a solution. *Proceedings of International Canine Leishmaniasis Forum,* 2., 2002, Sevilla, Spain. Salamanca: Intervet International bv, pp.7-14.

Grosjean, N.L.; Vrable, R.A.; Murphy, A.J. & Mansfield, L.S. (2003). Seroprevalence of antibodies against *Leishmania* spp. among dogs in the United States. *Journal of American Veterinary Medical Association,* Vol.222, No.5, pp.603-606.

Ikeda-Garcia, F.A. & Feitosa, M.M. (2006). Métodos de diagnóstico da leishmaniose visceral canina. *Clínica Veterinária,* No.62, pp.32-38.

Ikeda-Garcia, F.A. & Marcondes, M. (2007). Métodos de diagnóstico da leishmaniose visceral canina. *Cínica Veterinária.* Ano 12, No.71, pp.34-42, ISSN 1413-571X.

Ikonomopoulos, J.; Kokotas, S.; Gazouli, M.; Zavras, A.; Stoitsiou, M. & Gorgoulis, V.G. (2003). Molecular diagnosis of leishmaniosis in dogs. Comparative application of traditional diagnostic methods and the proposed assay on clinical samples. *Veterinary Parasitology,* Vol.113, pp.99-103.

Lachaud, L.; Machergui-Hammami, S.; Chabbert, E.; Dereure, J.; Dedet, J.P. & Bastien P. (2002a). Comparison of Six PCR Methods Using Peripheral Blood for Detection of Canine Visceral Leishmaniasis. *Journal of Clinical Microbiology,* Vol.40, pp.210-215.

Lachaud, L.; Chabbert, E.; Dubessay, P.; Dereure, J.; Lamothe, J. & Dedet, J.P. (2002b). Value of two PCR methods for the diagnosis of canine visceral leishmaniasis and the detection of asymptomatic carriers. *Parasitology,* Vol.125, No.3, pp.197-207.

Lainson, R.; Shaw, J. J.; Silveira , F.T. & Braga, R. (1987). American visceral leishmaniais: on the origin of *Leishmania (Leishmania) chagasi. Transactions Royal Society of Tropical Medicine Hygiene,* Vol. 81, pp. 517.

Lindoso, J.A.L. & Goto, H. (2006). Leishmaniose visceral: situação atual e perspectivas futuras. *Boletim Epidemiológico Paulista,* Vol.3, No.26.

Lukes, J.; Mauricio, I.L.; Schönian, G.; Dujardin, J.C.; Soteriadou, K.; Dedet, J.P.; Kuhls, K.; Tintaya, K.W.Q.; Jirku, M.; Chocholová, E.; Haralambous, C.; Prationg, F.; Obornik, M.; Horák, A.; Ayala, F.J. & Miles, M.A. (2007). Evolutionary and geographical history of the *Leishmania donovani* complex with a revision of current taxonomy. *PNAS,* Vol.104, No.22, pp.9375-9380.

Luvizotto, M.C.R.; Biazzono, L.; Eugenio, F.R.; Andrade, A.L.; Moreira, M.A.B. (1999). Leishmaniose visceral canina autóctone no município de Araçatuba-SP. *Anais do*

Congresso Brasileiro de Clínicos Veterinários de Pequenos Animais, 2., Águas de Lindóia, Sao Paulo, Brazil, p.24.

Luz, Z.M.P.; Pimenta, D.N.; Cabral, A.L.L.V.; Fiúza, V.O.P. & Rabello, A. (2001). A urbanização das leishmanioses e a baixa resolutividade diagnóstica em municípios da região metropolitana de Belo Horizonte. *Revista da Sociedade Brasileira de Medicina Tropical*, Vol.34, No.3, pp.249-254.

Machado, J.G. (2004). *Comparação do diagnóstico sorológico da Leishmaniose visceral Canina entre laboratórios de Belo Horizonte, 2003-2004.* 48f. Dissertação (Mestrado) Universidade Federal de Minas Gerais, Belo Horizonte.

Madeira, M.F.; Schubach, A.; Schubach, T.M.P.; Pacheco, R.S.; Oliveira, F.S.; Pereira, S.A.; Figueiredo, F.B.; Baptista, C. & Marzochi, M.C.A. (2006). Mixed infection with *Leishmania* (*Viannia*) *braziliensis* and *Leishmania* (*Leishmania*) *chagasi* in a naturally infected dog from Rio de Janeiro, Brazil. *Transactions of Royal Society of Tropical Medicine Hygiene*, Vol.100, pp.442-445.

Moreira, M.A.B.; Luvizotto, M.C.R.; Garcia, J.F.; Corbett, C.E. & Laurenti, M.D. (2007). Comparison of parasitological, immunological and molecular methods of the diagnosis of leishmaniasis in dog with different clinical signs. *Journal of Veterinary Parasitology*, Vol.42, pp.65.

Murray, H.W.; Berman, J.D.; Davies, C.R. & Saravia, N.G. (2005). Advances in leishmaniasis. *Lancet*, Vol.366, pp.1561-1577.

Nicolas, L.; Prina, E.; Lang, T. & Milon, G. (2002). Real-time PCR for detection and quantitation of *Leishmania* in mouse tissues. *Journal of Clinical Microbiology*, Vol.40, No.5, pp.1666-1669.

Nunes, V.L.B.; Galati, E.A.B.; Nunes, D.B.; Zinezzi, R.O.; Savani, E.S.M.M.; Ishikawa, E.; Camargo, M.C.G.O.; D'Áuria, S.R.N.; Cristaldo, G. & Rocha, H.C. (2001). Ocorrência de leishmaniose visceral canina em assentamento agrícola no Estado de Mato Grosso do Sul, Brasil. *Revista da Sociedade Brasileira de Medicina Tropical*, Vol.34, No.3, pp.301-302.

Reis, A.B. (2001). *Avaliação de parâmetros laboratoriais e imunológicos de cães naturalmente infectados com Leishmania (Leishmania) chagasi, portadores de diferentes formas clínicas da infecção.* 176f. Tese (Doutorado) Universidade Federal de Minas Gerais, Belo Horizonte, Brazil.

Reithinger, R. & Dujardin, J.C. (2007). Molecular diagnosis of leishmaniasis: current status and future applications. *Journal of Clinical Microbiology*, Vol.45, No.1, pp.21-25.

Rosário, E.Y. (2002). *Avaliação de testes sorológicos utilizando antígenos brutos e recombinantes para o diagnóstico da leishmaniose visceral canina.* 99f. Dissertação (Mestrado), Universidade Federal de Minas Gerais, Belo Horizonte, Brazil.

Rosypal, A.C.; Cortés-Vecino, J.A.; Gennari, S.M.; Dubey, J.P.; Tidwell, R.R. & Lindsay, D.S. (2007). Serological survey of *Leishmania infantum* and *Trypanosoma cruzi* in dogs from urban areas of Brazil and Colombia. *Veterinary Parasitology*, Vol.149, p.172-177.

Santiago, M.E.B.; Vasconcelos, R.O.; Fattori, K.R.; Munari, D.P.; Michelin, A.F.& Lima, V.M.F. (2007). An investigation of *Leishmania* spp. in *Didelphis* spp. from urban and peri-urban areas in Bauru (Sao Paulo, Brazil). *Veterinary Parasitology*, Vol.150, pp.283-290.

Savani, E.S.M.M.; Nunes, V.L.B.; Galati, E.A.B.; Castilho, T.M., Araujo, F.S.; Ilha, I.M.N.; Camargo, M.C.G.O.; D'Auria, S.R.N. & Floeter-Winter, L.M. (2005). Ocurrence of co-infection by *Leishmania* (*Leishmania*) *chagasi* and *Trypanosoma* (*Trypanozoon*) *evansi* in a dog in the state of Mato Grosso do Sul, Brazil. *Memórias do Instituto Oswaldo Cruz Rio de Janeiro*, Vol.100, No.7, pp.739-741.

Silva, E.S.; Gontijo, C.M.; Pirmez, C.; Fernandez, O.; Brazil, R.P. (2001a). Short report: detection of *Leishmania* DNA by polymerase chain reaction on blood samples from dogs with visceral leishmaniasis. *American Journal of Tropical Medicine Hygiene*, Vol.65, No.6, p.896-898.

Silva, E.S.; Gontijo, C.M.F.; Pacheco, R.S.; Fiuza, V.O.P.; Brazil, R.P. (2001b). Visceral leishmaniasis in the metropolitan region of Belo Horizonte, State of Minas Gerais, Brazil. *Memórias do Instituto Oswaldo Cruz Rio de Janeiro*, Vol.96, No.3, pp.285-291.

Singh, S. & Sivakumar, R. (2003). Recent Advances in the diagnosis of Leishmaniasis. *Journal of Postgraduation Medicine*, Vol.49, pp.55-60.

Slappendel, R.J. & Ferrer, L. (1998). *Leishmaniasis*. Infectious Diseases of the dog and the cat. pp. 450-457, ISBN 0721623395. Philadelphia, Pensilvania, USA.

Soares, M.J.V.; Moraes, J.R.E. & Roselino, A.M.F. (2005). Polymerase chain reaction in detecting *Leishmania* spp. in symptomatic and asymptomatic seropositive dogs. *Journal of Venomous Animals and Toxins including Tropical Diseases*, Vol.11, No.4.

Solano-Gallego, L.; Morell, P.; Arboix, M.; Alberola, J.; Ferrer, L. (2001). Prevalence of *Leishmania infantum* infection in dogs living in an area of canine leishmaniasis endemicity using PCR on several tissues and serology. *Journal of Clinical Microbiology*, Vol.39, pp.560-563.

Strauss-Ayali, D.; Jaffe, C.L.; Burshtain, O.; Gonen, L.; Baneth, G. (2004). Polymerase chain reaction using noninvasively obtained samples, for the detection of *Leishmania infantum* DNA in dogs. *Journal of Infectious Diseases*, Vol.189, pp.1729-1733.

Sundar, S. & Rai, M. (2002). Laboratory diagnosis of visceral leishmaniasis. *Clinical Diagnosis on Laboratory Immunology*, Vol.9, No.5, pp.951-958.

Troncarelli, M.Z.; Machado, J.G.; Camargo, L.B.; Hoffmann, J.L.; Camossi, L.; Greca, H.; Faccioli, P.Y. & Langoni, H. (2008). Associação entre resultados sorológicos no diagnóstico da leishmaniose e da tripanossomíase canina, pela técnica de imunofluorescência indireta. *Veterinária e Zootecnia*, Vol.15, No.1, pp.40-47.

Troncarelli, M.Z.; Camargo J.B.; Machado, J.G.; Lucheis, S.B. & Langoni, H. (2009). *Leishmania* spp. and/or *Trypanosoma cruzi* diagnosis in dogs from endemic and nonendemic areas for canine visceral leishmaniasis. (2009). *Veterinary Parasitology*. Vol.164, No.2-4, pp.118-123. ISSN 0304-4017.

Zanette, M.F.; Feitosa, M.M.; Ikeda, F.A.; Rossi, C.N.; Camacho, A.A. & Souza, A.I. (2006). Ocorrência de reação cruzada entre doença de Chagas e Leishmaniose visceral canina pela técnica de ELISA. *Anais do congresso brasileiro da Anclivepa, 27., Congresso da Fiavac, 3.*, 2006, Vitória - Espírito Santo, Brazil.

Zijlstra, E. E.; Nur, Y.; Desjeux, P.; Khalil, E.A.G.; El-Hassan, A. M. & Groen, J. (2001). Diagnosing visceral leishmaniasis with the recombinant K39 strip test: experience from Sudan. *Tropical Medicine International Health*, Vol.6, pp.108-113.

Zivicnjak, T.; Martinkovic, F.; Marinculic, A.; Mrljak, V.; Kucer, N.; Matijatko, V.; Mihaljevic, Z. & Baric-Rafaj, R. (2005). A seroepidemiologic survey of canine visceral leishmaniasis among apparently healthy dogs in Croatia. *Veterinary Parasitology*, Vol.131, pp.35-43.

Part 4

Zoonotic Nematoda

16

Zoonosis Caused by *Baylisascaris procyonis*

José Piñero, Jacob Lorenzo-Morales, Carmen Martín-Navarro, Atteneri López-Arencibia, María Reyes-Batlle and Basilio Valladares
University Institute of Tropical Diseases and Public Health of the Canary Islands, Departament of Parasitology, Ecology and Genetics, University of La Laguna, Spain

1. Introduction

The raccoon roundworm, *Baylisascaris procyonis,* is classified under the Phylum Nemathelminthes (the roundworms) and Class Nematoda. It is a member of Family Ascaridae and Superfamily Ascaridoidea, which represents intestinal worms with direct life cycles. Other, more familiar ascarids are *Ascaris lumbricoides,Toxocara canis,* and *Toxocara cati,* nematode parasites of humans, dogs, and cats, respectively.

Baylisascaris procyonis was first named as *Ascaris columnaris* and isolated from raccoons in the New York Zoological Park in 1931(McClure, 1933). It was later recognized as a different species (*Ascaris procyonis*) in raccoons in Europe (Stefanski & Zarnowski, 1951). The genus *Baylisascaris* was defined by Sprent in 1968 and included eight recognized and two provisional species previously classified as members of the*Ascaris* or *Toxascaris* genus (Sprent, 1968). The new genus was namedafter H. A. Baylis, formerly member of the British Museum of Natural History, London, United Kingdom.The possibility of human infection was anticipated by Beaver (Beaver, 1969) and later by Kazacos (Kazacos& Boyce, 1989). The marked zoonotic potential of *B. procyonis* has become apparent only in the last 2 decades. The first confirmed cases of NLM in humans were described to have occurred in two young boys, in 1984 and 1985 (Huff et al., 1984; Fox et al., 1985).

This parasite is common in raccoons (*Procyon lotor*) in North America and Europe and also is frequent in racoons kept in zoos or peltry farms. Other members of this genus are found in bears, skunks, badgers and other carnivores. There is also evidence that dogs can acquire patent *B. procyonis* infections after scavenging intermediate, hosts.

Baylisascaris procyonis is considered the most common cause of clinical larva migrans (LM) in animals, in which it is usually associated with fatal or severe neurological disease. In humans, particularly children, has emerged in recent years as one of the most serious causes of zoonotic visceral, ocular, and neural LM (VLM; OLM; NLM) and has been recognized as a source of severe, often fatal, neurologic disease.

2. Morphology and life cycle

B. procyonis biologically and morphologically resembles the intestinal roundwormof dogs *Toxocara canis.* Adult worms measure are tan-white in color, cylindrical and tapered at both ends. The female reaching 20–22 cm long and the male 9–11 cm long (Kazacos, 2001). Cervical alae are vestigial and inconspicuous, the vulva is located one-fourth to one-third the body length fromthe anterior end, and males possess pericloacal roughened áreas. The egg itself is a typical ascarid egg, although smaller than a *Toxocara canis* egg, with a thick pitted shell and a large, dark zygote that almost completely fills the shell.The eggs of *B. procyonis* are ellipsoidal in shape, brown in color, and have a thickshell with a finely granular surface; theyrange in size from 63–88 x 50—70 μm, with most averaging 68–76 x 55–61 μm.

Adult female worms in the small intestine of raccoons and produce between 115,000 and 179,000 eggs/worm/day. In nature, infected raccoons shed an average of 20,000 to 26,000 eggs per gram of feces, with higher shedding rates in juvenile raccoons than in adults, and can shed in excess of 250,000 eggs per gram of feces. Thus, infected raccoons can shed millions of *B. procyonis* eggs daily, leading to widespread and heavy environmental contamination. The numbers of eggs produced by infected raccoons combined with their defecation behaviour, ensures that latrine sites will become heavily contaminated. The eggs possess a sticky proteinaceous outer coat that enables them to adhere to objects and facilitates transmission. *B. procyonis* eggs become infective (secondstagelarva) in ~2–4 weeks, depending on environmental temperature and moisture. *B. procyonis* eggs are very resistant to environmental conditions, especially in moist soil. Although they can be killed eventually by extreme heat and dryness, the eggs survive harsh winters, and under appropriate conditions, they can remain viable for years, contributing to the long-term danger posed by latrines.

Young raccoons become infected by ingesting infective eggs, whereas older raccoons become infected byingesting third-stage larvae (L3's) in paratecnic hosts, usually rodents. Young raccoons become infected at an early age by ingesting eggs fromtheir mother's contaminated teats or fur, from the contaminated den, or from raccoon latrines near their den.

In young raccoons, larvae hatching from eggs enter themucosa of the small intestine and develop there several weeks before reentering the intestinal lumen to mature, the worms reaching patency in 50–76 days. In older raccoons, larvae from intermediate hosts develop to adults in the intestinal lumen, reaching patency in 32–38 days.

The higherparasite burden of juvenile raccoons (mean burden, 48 to 62 worms) than in adults (mean burden, 12 to 22 worms) likely reflects differences in mechanisms of infection.

Like other parasite (*Toxocara* spp.) *B. procyonis* can be borne by intermediate hosts when eggs are swallowed by a different vertebrate. Most commonly the intermediate host is a rodent, birds or lagomorph. In these animals, parasite eggs hatch in the small intestine, penetrate the intestinal wall and are get to the bloodstream through the liver to the lungs, where they are eventually distributed via the blood to various organs. Larvae eventually become encapsulated within eosinophilic granulomas, where they remain viable until they are ingested by raccoonsor for the lifetime of the host (Kazacos& Boyce, 1989).

B. procyonis larvae often invading the central nevous system (CNS). Invasion of the brain seems to be particularly common in rodents, rabbits, birds and primates. In mice, approximately 5-7% of *B. procyonis* larvae are estimated to enter the CNS. These larvae can cause considerable damage, both from mechanical damage during migration and from the inflammatory reaction they stimulate. Larvae in the eye can damage the retina and other structures. Eventually the larvae encyst, mainly in the connective tissues and muscles.

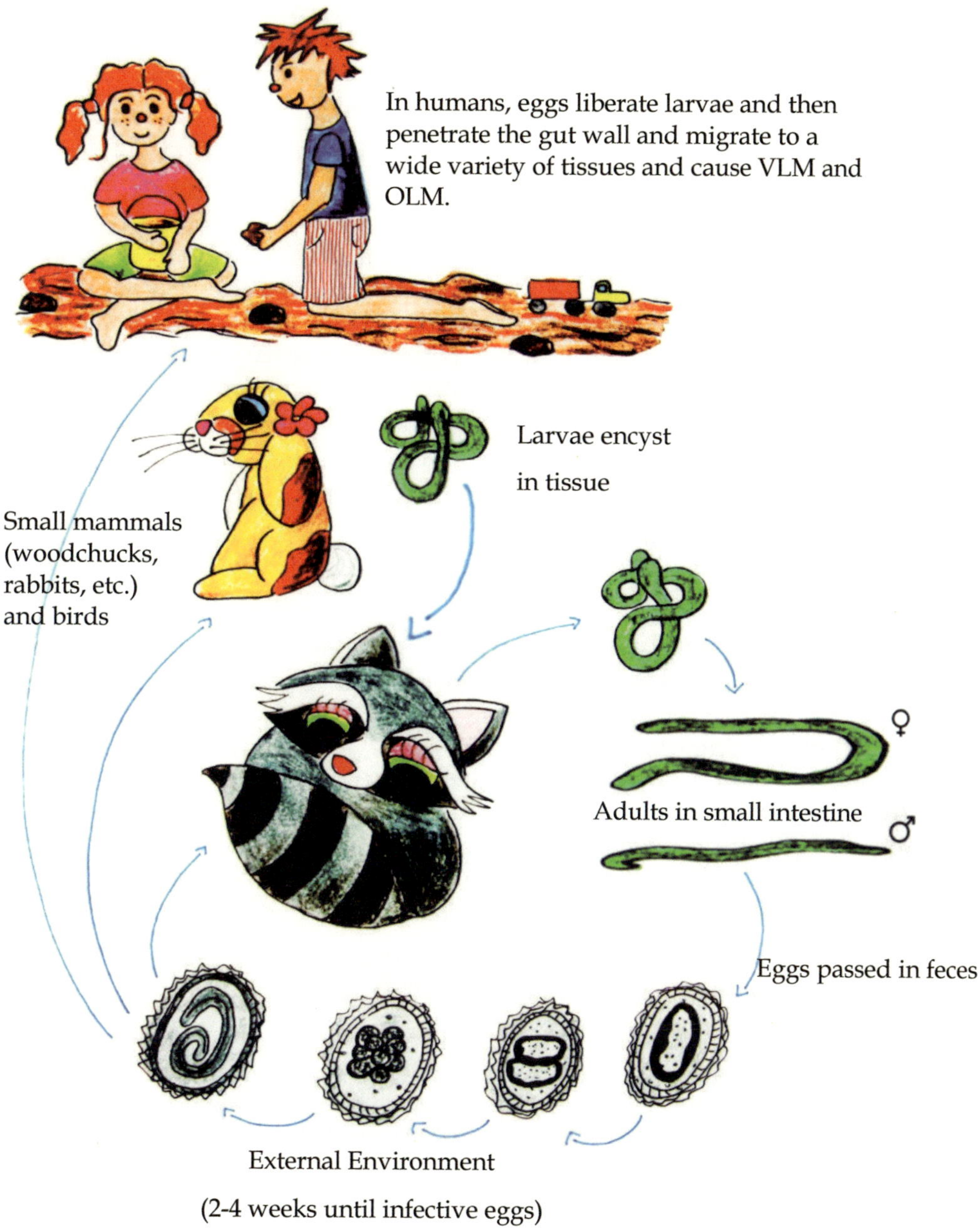

Fig. 1. Life cycle of *Baylisascaris procyonis*.

Humans are accidental intermediate hosts and infection typically occurs in young children with pica or geophagia after ingestion of infective *B. procyonis* eggs from environments or items contaminated with raccoon feces (Kazacos, 2000).

In humans, *B. procyonis* larvae have a tendency to invade the eyes, spinal cord, and brain, causing inflammatory reactions and tissue damage. The result can be blindness, neurological damage, and even death. *B. procyonis* infection typically results in fatal disease or severe sequelae.

3. Epidemiology

Raccoons, which are the definitive hosts for *B. procyonis,* are native to the Americas, where they can be found from Canada to Panama. They were introduced into Europe, the former U.S.S.R. and Asia for the commercial fur trade and into Japan as pets, and have become naturalized in some of these areas. The prevalence of *B. procyonis* infection is high in wild raccoons in Germany and those kept in zoos or as pets in Japan (Baeur &Gey, 2002; Kazacos, 2001; Miyashita,1993; Sato et al., 2001). Although surveys of feral raccoons in Japan have not detected this organism, it is possible that some pets released into the wild were infected.

In areas where *B. procyonis* is common in raccoons, it has much higher prevalence in juvenile raccoons (> 90%) than in adults (37%–55%). Average parasite intensity ranges from 43 to 52 worms, with juvenile raccoons having a higher mean intensity (48–62, range 1–480) than adult raccoons (12–22, range1–257) (Snyder & Fitzgerald 1985; Ermer& Fodge 1986; Kazacos, 2001).

In United State *B. procyonis* roundworms are most prevalent in the midwestern, northeastern, and Pacific western states. Numerous surveillance studies have been conducted in the southeastern United States, and parasite are most common in the mountainous regions of Virginia, Kentucky, and West Virginia (Kazacos, 2001; Souza et al., 2009). Geographic expansion of *B. procyonis* roundwormshas been recently documented in Georgia (Eberhard et al., 2003; Blizzard et al., 2010a) and into northwestern and southeastern of Florida (Blizzard et al., 2010b).Recently, and study about the prevalence of *B. procyonis* in raccoons in Portland, Oregon, showed that 58% of sampled raccoons were found to be infected with parasite (Yeitz et al., 2009).

In Canada, the prevalence of *B. procyonis* was estimated in 37.1% of the urban raccoon population of Winnipeg (Manitoba) (Sexsmith et al., 2009).

In most areas where raccoons occur, there should be no environmental limitationson the presence of *B. procyonis,* although conditions for optimal egg development and survival willvary based on temperature and humidity. *Baylisascaris procyonis* eggs become infective in 11–14 days at 22°C–25° C and 100% humidity (Sakla et al. 1989), similar to eggs of *B. columnaris* (11–16 d) (Berry, 1985). Under natural conditions, with cooler and/or fluctuating temperatures, egg development will beslower and will take several weeks to months.

Under sufficiently warm but fluctuating temperaturas (e.g., cooler nights), most eggs should reach infectivity in 3–4+ weeks. Embryonated *B. procyonis* eggs stored 9–12 years at4° C retained their infectivity and central nervous system pathogenicity for mice (Kazacos, 2001). Given adequate moisture, embryonated eggs will last years in the soil, including through harsh winters(Kazacos 1986, 1991; Kazacos & Boyce 1989).Conditions of extreme heat and dryness, as occur inbarn lofts and attics in summer months, will kill *B. procyonis*eggs by desiccation, probably in a few weeks ormonths (Kazacos & Boyce 1989).

The epidemiology of *Baylisascaris* infection is linked to the defecation habits of raccoons. Presumably for communication or territorial reasons, individuals and groups of raccoons habitually defecate in focal areas called "latrines", where large amounts of feces and *B. procyonis* eggs accumulate (Kazacos, 2001; Roussere et al., 2003; Page et al., 1998; Page et al., 1999). Raccoon latrines are found directly on the ground, particularly at the base of trees; along and on the tops of fences; on roofs, decks, and stored firewood; and in outbuildings, attics, and various other locations (Kazacos, 2001; Roussere et al., 2003; Page et al., 1998). Homeowners are often unaware that there are latrines on roofs or hidden elsewhere on their property, thus increasing the risk of exposure to raccoon feces. Moreover, decomposition of the feces can occur rapidly under outdoor conditions, making it less obvious that these areas are contaminated.

The primary risk factors for human *B. procyonis* infection include contact with raccoon latrines, pica/geophagia, young age (<4 years), and male sex. Older persons who have pica or exhibit geophagia are alsoat risk for significant infection. People are commonly exposed to the eggsof this parasite in peridomestic areas where infected raccoons are common.

4. Pathology

4.1 Infections in humans

Baylisascaris procyonis causes neurologic disease in wild, zoo, and domestic animals as well as human beings. The full clinical spectrum of human baylisascariasis is unknown but includes VLM, NLM, and OLM. In addition, preliminary evidence suggests that asymptomatic infection also occurs.

The severity of CNS disease is related to the number of eggs ingested, the extent and location of larval migration, and the severity of ensuing inflammation and necrosis (Kazacos 2000, 2001).When infective *B. procyonis* eggs are ingested, infective larvae emerge from the eggs, penetrate the gut, and after migrating through the liver and lungs, become distributed via the bloodstream to various somatic tissues, including skeletal muscles, the viscera, brain, and eyes; here, they continue to migrate and eventually become encapsulated in granulomas (Kazacos, 1997, 2001). The pathogenicity of the larvae is related to their aggressive migratory behavior in the tissues and the fact that they molt and grow considerably during migration (Kazacos, 1997, 2000, 2001; Goldberg et al., 1993). Only 5%–7% of ingested larvae enter the CNS (Kazacos, 2000, 2001); thus, although theyare not neurotropic per se, their large size, aggressive migration, and stimulation of intense eosinophilic inflammatory reactions cause extensive damage to nervous (and ocular) tissues (Kazacos, 1997). Baylisascaris larvae entering the brain migrate there for extended periods before becoming walled off by host reactions.In heavy infections, the brain undergoes postinflammatory atrophy, leading to the progressive neurologic impairment and severe incapacitation seen in surviving patients with neural LM (Gavin et al., 2002a; Rowley et al., 2000a). Pathologic changes are further exacerbated by diagnostic and treatment delays.

The incubation period in humans is uncertain, but NLM may occur as soon as 2 to 4 weeks after ingestion of the eggs.

NLM occurs when the parasites migrate through the CNS, and the symptoms vary with the location and number of the migrating larvae. The initial signs may be mild, with subtle behavioral changes, lethargy, somnolence or irritability, weakness, speech defects and/or mild changes in vision, but they can rapidly become severe. A variety of symptoms including ataxia, paresis or paralysis, developmental regression, tremors, torticollis, nystagmus and coma have been reported. Seizures are common and can be severe. Ocular signs, including blindness, also occur in many cases.

NLM is associated with eosinophilic meningoencephalitis, an elevated peripheral cerebrospinal fluid eosinophilia can be detected in cases of meningoencephalitis.

Some cases of NLM are fatal, almost all surviving patients have been left with serious neurological defects despite treatment. It has been reported only a one case of a child who developed relatively mild symptoms (headache, right arm pain, vomiting, mild upper extremity tremors and dysmetria, progressing to ataxia) and appeared to recover completely.

OLM has been reported more frequently than neural larva migrans, and can occur without neurological signs. Inflammatory and degenerative changes are mainly seen in the retina and optic disk, usually only in one eye. The clinical signs may include transient obscuration of the vision, photophobia, other signs of diffuse unilateral subacute neuroretinitis (DUSN) and loss of vision. Some visual defects can be permanent.

VLM by *B. procyonis* showed non-specific signs such as low-grade fever, nausea and lethargy. Invasion of the liver can result in hepatomegaly, and migration through the lung may cause symptoms of pneumonitis. A macular rash, seen mainly on the face and trunk, has also been reported. VLM is associated with eosinophilic cardiac pseudotumors (cardiac myofibroblastic tumors with high percentage of eosinophils). Subclinical cases might also occur in infection with *B. procyonis.*

Human infections with *B. procyonis* have been documented most often in the U.S., but suspected cases have been reported from Europe, and a patient with neural larva migrans was reported in Canada in 2009. One case of ocular larva migrans in Brazil was reported as a probable *B. procyonis* infection, but the identification was not definitive. No exposure to raccoons was documented in the latter case, although the patient had been exposed to skunks.

Other *Baylisascaris* species have been less well studied, but probably occur in most areas where their definitive hosts are found.

Year of published report	Location	Age	Sex	Clinical	Risk factor	Diagnostic method	Treatment	Outcome
1975	Missouri	18 mo	Female	Eosinophilic meningo-encephalitis	Geophagia	Serologic (cross-reacting)		Persistent weakness and spastic right arm and leg
1984	Pennsylvania	10 mo	Male	Eosinophilic meningo-encephalitis	Pica	Autopsy, serologic	None	Death

Year of published report	Location	Age	Sex	Clinical	Risk factor	Diagnostic method	Treatment	Outcome
1985	Illinois	18 mo	Male	Eosinophilic meningo-encephalitis	Down syndrome and pica	Autopsy, serologic	Thiabendazole	Death
1991	Germany	48 y	Female	Diffuse unilateral subacute neuroretinitis				Ocular sequelae
1992	California	29y	Male	Diffuse unilateral subacute neuroretinitis	Exposure to raccoons	Serologic	None	Ocular sequelae
1993	Michigan	9 mo	Male		Pica	Serologic	Not recorded	Neurologic deficits, cortical blindness
1994	Oregon	21 y	Male	Encephalopthy	Developmental delay, pica/geophagia		Not recorded	Persistent residual deficits
1994	New York	13 mo	Male	Eosinophilic meningo-encephalitis	Pica	Serologic	Thiabendazole, ivermectin, and prednisone	Neurologic deficits, cortical blindness, brain atrophy
1995	Massachusetts	10 y	Male	Eosinophilic cardiac pseudotumor	Not date	Not date	None	Death
2000	California	11 mo	Male	Eosinophilic encephalitis	Pica	Serologic	Albendazole and Methyl-prednisolone	Neurologic deficits, seizures, profound visual impairment
2000	California	13 mo	Male	Eosinophilic meningo-encephalitis	Pica/ geophagia	Brain biopsy, serologic	Solumedrol and prednisolone	Neurologic deficits, blindness, seizures, brain atrophy
2001	Minnesota	13 mo	Male	Eosinophilic meningo-encephalitis	Unknown	Serologic	Methyl-prednisolone, vincristine, and thioguanine	Death
2001	Minnesota	19 mo	Male	Eosinophilic meningo-encephalitis	Klinefelter síndrome	Serologic	Prednisone, vincristine, and thioguanine	Death
2002	California	17 y	Male	Eosinophilic meningo-encephalitis	Developmental delay and geophagia	Brain biopsy, serologic	Albendazole and antiinflammatories	Death
2002	California	11 mo	Male	Eosinophilic meningo-encephalitis	Pica/ geophagia	Serologic	Albendazole and antiinflammatories	Neurologic deficits, cortical blindness, seizures

Year of published report	Location	Age	Sex	Clinical	Risk factor	Diagnostic method	Treatment	Outcome
2002	Illinois	2.5 y	Male	Progressive encephalo-pathy	Pica/ geophagia	Serologic	Albendazole and solumedrol	Neurologic deficits, blindness, generalized spasticity
2002	Illinois	6 y	Male	Progressive encephalopathy, diffuse unilateral subacute neuroretinitis	Developmental delay,pica/ geophagia	Serologic	Albendazole and prednisone	Neurologic deficits, seizures
2003	Michigan	6 y	Male	Diffuse unilateral subacute neuroretinitis, neurologic deficits	Pica	Serologic		Severe neurologic sequelae
2003	Michigan	2 y	Male	Eosinophilic meningo-encephalitis, chorioretinitis	Pica	Serologic		Severe neurologic sequelae
2004	Louisiana	4 y	Male	Eosinophilic meningitis	Raccoons in neighborhood	Serologic	Dexamethasone albendazole	Full recovery
2009	Oregon	17 y	Male	Eosinophilic meningo-encephalitis	Geophagia and substance abuse	Serologic	Methyl-prednisolone	Aphasia and memory deficits
2009	Toronto	7 y	Male	Eosinophilic meningo-encephailitis	Autism, raccoons in backyard	Serologic	Albendazole, methyl-prednisone, prednisone	No longer used speech to communicate, cortical visual impairment, seizure disorder
2010	New York	12 mo	Male	Eosinophilic encephalo-myelitis	Geophagia	Serologic	Albendazole, prednisone and methyl-prednisolone	Neurologic deficits

Table 1. Reported human cases caused by *Baylisascaris procyonis*.

4.2 Infections in animals

Susceptibility to *Baylisascaris* larva migrans varies among animal groups and species (Wirtz 1982; Sheppard & Kazacos 1997). Animal groups particularly susceptible to parasite NLM include rodents, rabbits, primates, and birds, based on the number of cases and species affected. For example, in 2007 a *Baylisascaris procyonis* infection in a Moluccan cockatoo (*Cacatua moluccensis*), was reported. An adult female Moluccan cockatoo was evaluated for a 10-day history of progressive ataxia and weakness. The bird had been exposed intermittently over a 3-day period to a cage that had previously housed juvenile raccoons. Results of diagnostic tests were inconclusive and, despite supportive care, the bird died 7 days after the initial presentation. Histopathologic examination revealed a single nematode larva in the midbrain that was consistent with *Baylisascaris* species and multifocal granulomas in the left ventricle of the heart (Wolf et al., 2007).

Some animal groups and species are only marginally susceptible, with limited migration occurring in the intestinal wall or viscera; others appear to be resistant. For example, no cases of *B. procyonis* NLM have been documented in opossums, which are commonly exposed through foraging at raccoon latrines(Page et al., 1998, 1999), or in adult domestic livestockor zoo hoofstock, which are commonly exposed through contaminated hay. Very limited or no migration was seen in sheep, goats, and swine experimentally infected with *B. procyonis* (Dubey, 1982; Snyder, 1983; Kazacos & Kazacos 1984). No cases have been documented in cats or raptors, which eat rodents possibly contaminated with eggs and/or containing L3's. (Kazacos, 2001). The apparent species limitations to *Baylisascaris* infection should be regarded with caution.

Except in very heavy infections with intestinal obstruction, raccoons infected with *B. procyonis* appear clinically normal with no outward signs of infection. Similarly, other species with *Baylisascaris* larva migrans usually are asymptomatic if no larvae enter the brain. The severity and progression of central nervous system disease in NLM depends on the number of eggs ingested, the number of larvae entering the brain, the location and extent of migration damage and inflammation in the brain, and the size of the brain.Thus, clinical disease will vary from mild, insidious, slowly progressive central nervous system disease with subtle clinical signs to acute, fulminating, rapidly progressive central nervous system disease with marked clinical signs. Although larvae enter the somatic tissues, eyes, and brain of some species as early as 3 days postinfection, clinical central nervous system disease is not usually apparent before 9–10 days postinfection, and in many cases not until 2–4+ weeks postinfection, due to the lag time in causing central nervous system damage and inflammation (Kazacos, 1997; Sheppard& Kazacos, 1997).

5. Diagnostic

The diagnosis of baylisascariasis is difficult in live patients; there is no widely available, non-invasive definitive test. The combination of encephalopathy with cerebrospinal fluid (CSF) and peripheral eosinophilia and diffuse white matter disease on neuroimaging, with or without eye disease, in a patient from North America or Europe should strongly suggest the diagnosis of *Baylisascaris* NLM, and a history of exposure to raccoons or their feces should be sought.

Unless a brain biopsy is done and a larva is found, antemortem diagnosis usually depends on serology, with supportive evidence from other tests.

5.1 Serology

In neural larva migrans, antibodies to *Baylisascaris* can be found in serum and CSF; a rising titer is usually seen. An enzyme linked immunosorbent assay (ELISA), indirect immunofluorescence and immunoblotting (Western blotting) have been developed to detect anti-*Baylisascaris* antibodies. These serological assays are not commercially available, but they may be provided by university research laboratories. In the U.S., an ELISA is available from the Department of Comparative Pathobiology at Purdue University, West Lafayette, IN. Indirect immunofluorescence tests use frozen sections of *B. procyonis* third-stage larvae as an antigen. Enzyme-linked immunosorbent assay and Western blotting use excretory-secretory products from *in vitro* cultures of *B. procyonis* larvae as the antigen (Boyce et al., 1989). Larval excretory-secretory antigens have been characterized as complex glycoproteins, with molecular masses of 10 kDa to 200 kDa, that contain several different sugar residues(Boyce et al, 1989). Protein epitopes of 33-kDa to 45-kDa antigens appear to be recognized selectively by antibodies from *B. procyonis*-infected humans and animals but not by normal human or *T. canis* antibody-positive sera (Boyce et al, 1989). In addition, children with clinical *B. procyonis* NLM are strongly positive for anti-*Baylisascaris* antibodies in CSF and serum and have consistently been negative for anti-*Toxocara* antibodies (Cunningham et al., 1994; Fox et al., 1985; Gavin et al., 2002; Kazacos, 2001; Moertel et al., 2001; Murray, 2002; Park et al., 2000; Rowley et al., 2000). In several of these cases, positive *B. procyonis* serology was confirmed by brain biopsy or at autopsy (CDC, 2002; Fox et al., 1985; Huff et al., 1984; Rowley et al., 2000). Acute and convalescent-phase titers characteristically demonstrate several fold increases in both serum and CSF anti-Baylisascaris antibody levels (Gavin et al., 2002; Moertel et al., 2001).

Although *B. procyonis* excretory-secretory (BPES) antigen-based ELISA and Western blot assays are useful in the immunodiagnosis of this infection, cross-reactivity remains a major problem. Recently, a recombinant *B. procyonis* antigen, BpRAG1, was reported for use in development of improved serological assays for the diagnosis of *Baylisascaris* larva migrans (Dangoudoubiyam et al., 2010). In a recent study, authors tested a total of 384 human patient serum samples in a BpRAG1 ELISA, including 20 patients with clinical *Baylisascaris* larva migrans, 137 patients with other parasitic infections (8 helminth and 4 protozoan), and 227 with unknown/suspected parasitic infections. A sensitivity of 85% and specificity of 86.9% was observed with the BpRAG1 ELISA, compared to only 39.4% specificity with the BPES ELISA. In addition, the BpRAG1 ELISA had a low degree ofcross-reactivity with antibodies to *Toxocara* spp. infection (25%), while the BPES antigen showed 90.6% cross-reactivity. Based on these results, BpRAG1 antigen has a high degree of sensitivity and specificity and should be very useful and reliable in the diagnosis and seroepidemiology of *Baylisascaris* larva migrans by ELISA (Dangoudoubiyam et al., 2011)

5.2 Laboratory tests

Although no routine laboratory test is considered diagnosticof *B. procyonis* NLM by itself, a number of studies provide additional supporting evidence. Most importantly, the presence of eosinophilia, particularly eosinophilic meningitis,

should alert the physician to the possibility of a parasitic etiology(Lo Re& Gluckman, 2003; Rothenberg, 1998; Weller, 1993). Eosinophils are not normally present in CSF; their presence narrows the differential diagnosis of CNS disease and provides an early or theonly etiologic clue. In documented cases of NLM, the peripheral white blood cell count is usually mildly elevated, but eosinophilia may be marked. Cerebrospinal fluid cell counts may be normal at presentation and generally demonstrate only mild leukocytosis, again with eosinophilia. Notably, even in the absence of pleocytosis, demonstrable CSF eosinophilia may be evident. Because eosinophils are easily missed in unstained or Gram-stained CSF, it may be necessary to request Wright's orGiemsa stain of cytocentrifuged CSF specimens. In documented cases of NLM, CSF protein is generally normal or only mildly elevated, while

CSF glucose levels are normal. Although the finding of elevated serum isohemagglutinins, caused by cross-reactions between larval glycoproteins and human blood group antigens, is not specific for baylisascariasis, it does provide an additional clue to the diagnosis (Boyce et al., 1989).

5.3 Other techniques

Imaging techniques and encephalography provide supportive evidence and help rule out other causes. In ocular larva migrans, an ophthalmoscopic examination may occasionally reveal large, motile larvae in the retina, as well as choroidioretinitis and other signs of DUSN. The presence of *Baylisascaris* larvae in the eye is also suggestive in cases with neurological signs. Biopsies of the CNS are occasionally definitive, but larvae are often absent from the sample. A definitive diagnosis can also be made retrospectively from CNS samples taken at autopsy. *Baylisascaris* larvae are much larger (up to 80 µm in diameter and up to 1900 µm long) than *Toxocara* larvae, and can also be distinguished by their morphology. However, parasite larvae can be difficult to identify within tissues, and misidentification is common. In tissues, the third stage larvae of *B. procyonis* cannot be differentiated from *B. columnaris* or *B. melis*. Epidemiological evidence, such as a history of exposure to raccoons but not skunks or badgers, can be suggestive.

6. Treatment

The prognosis for *B. procyonis* NLM is grave with or without treatment; among documented cases,there are no neurologically intact survivors. In this parasite is very important early clinical suspicion of raccoon roundworm meningoencephalitis.

The majority of cases have been treated with anthelmintics and corticosteroids. Empirical anthelmintic treatment with thiabendazole, fenbendazole, tetramisole, or ivermectin has failed to prevent death or unfavorable outcomes. Animal data suggest that albendazole and diethylcarbazinehave the best CSF penetration and larvicidal activity (Kazacos, 2001).

Treatment with albendazole is protective in animal models if eggs have been ingested, but symptoms have not yet developed. In humans, albendazole has been used prophylactically after exposure to raccoon latrines or other sources of eggs. Whether it is helpful in patients with clinical signs is uncertain, because the death of the parasite might worsen the inflammation.

Albendazole appears to have the more favorable pharmacologic profile, with good absorption, high serum concentrations of the active metabolite, good penetration across the blood-brain barrier, and minimal toxicity (de Silva et al., 1997; Jung et al., 1990).

Most clinical cases have been treated concurrently with anthelmintics and corticosteroids; the corticosteroids are used to suppress inflammation caused by the death of the larvae, as well as to dampen the existing inflammatory response. In a recent case a early intervention with both, albendazole and steroids, may have contributed to patient's partial recovery (Hajek et al., 2009) and a mild case of suspected *B procyonis* infection, with apparent early complete response after cerebellar edema, was treated with early corticosteroids and later albendazole (Pai et al., 2007).

Other supportive therapy may also be given. Recently, an acute eosinophilic meningoencephalitis, caused by *Baylisascaris procyonis* in a previously healthy teenager with a history of substance abuse, was treated with methylprednisolone; no antihelmintic drugs were administered (Chun et al., 2009).

Laser photocoagulation, systemic corticosteroids and other therapies have been used in ocular larva migrans (Goldberg et al., 1993; Kazacos et al., 1985).

In many cases, significant damage has already occurred by the time treatment is begun, and improvement is not seen. The best chance of recovery is expected with a very early diagnosis and treatment.

7. Prevention and control

In intermediate hosts, the risk of infection can be decreased by avoiding contact with raccoons, other definitive hosts and their feces. Raccoons can be discouraged from visiting homes and farms with the same measures that are used to prevent disease in humans. Infections are difficult to prevent completely in pets allowed outdoors, as the infective eggs can survive for long periods in the environment. In dogs, monthly heartworm/nematode preventatives appear to decrease the risk of intestinal infection with *B. procyonis*. In high-risk areas, dogs that are not on these preventatives should receive regular fecal examinations to decrease the risk that they will shed eggs.

In zoos and other facilities, the housing for intermediate hosts should be designed to minimize exposure to raccoons, skunks and other definitive hosts. Captive raccoons and skunks should be kept in dedicated cages that can be cleaned, if necessary, with the harsh methods required to destroy *Baylisascaris* eggs. They should be tested regularly and dewormed when necessary, and they should not be fed wild animals that might carry larvae. Newly acquired definitive hosts should be quarantined and dewormed. Once contamination has occurred, it can be difficult to remove completely. Intermediate hosts in exhibits are sometimes treated prophylactically with pyrantel tartrate or ivermectin. Similarly to humans, animals with recent exposure might also be treated with albendazole to prevent the development of clinical signs.

In humans, risk of infection is greatest when infants or toddlers with geophagia or pica come in contact with raccoon latrines or an environment contaminated by infected raccoon feces. Young infants and toddlers, particularly those with pica or geophagia, should be kept away from potentially contaminated areas.

Raccoon latrines in and around homes and play areas shouldbe cleaned up and decontaminated. However, the longevity of *B. procyonis* eggs and their resistance to disinfection or decontamination makes successful environmental cleanup difficult. Recently a publication (Shafir et al., 2011) showed that eggs survived complete desiccation for at least 6 months at room temperature. Total loss of viability was observed after 7 months of desiccation. Eggs frozen at –15°C for 6 months demonstrated no reduction in viability. Freeze–thaw, including exposure to 5 cycles, did not affect survival. Although they did not specifically design experiments to assess the effect of chlorine on inactivation of *B. procyonis* eggs, exposure to undiluted household bleach for 90 min toremove the mammillated layer did not affect viability. In this study (Shafir et al., 2011) *B. procyonis* eggs showed alow thermal death point at <62°C, similar to that reported for other ascarids (Shafir et al., 2007; Feachem et al., 1983).Heat is by far the best method of killing *B. procyonis* eggs (Kazacos, 2001). Boiling water, steam-cleaning, flaming, or fire are highly effective and practical methods for decontamination of large or small areas. The use of direct flames from a propaneflame-gun is a favored method (Kazacos, 2001). For heavily contaminated areas a combination of removal and disposal of the top few inches of surface soil with flaming is most effective.

8. Acknowledgment

Jacob Lorenzo Morales was funded by a "Ramón y Cajal" grant 2011 from the Spanish Ministry of Science and Innovation. Carmen Mª Martín was supported by a Ph.D. grant "Beca de Investigación CajaCanarias para Postgraduados 2010" from the University of La Laguna, Spain. Atteneri López was funded by the grant "Ayudas del Programa de Formación de Personal Investigador para la realización de Tesis Doctorales" from the Agencia Canaria de Investigación, Innovación y Sociedad de la Información from the Canary Islands Government. This work was funded by project RICET (project no. RD06/0021/0005 of the program of Redes Temáticas de Investigación Cooperativa, FIS), Spanish Ministry of Health, Madrid, Spain and the project "Protozoosis emergentes por amebas de vida libre: Aislamiento y caracterización molecular, identificación de cepas transportadas de otros agentes patógenos y búsqueda de quimioterapias" PI10/01298, Spanish Ministry of Science and Innovation, Madrid, Spain. Authors are thankful to Cecilia Arrate for drawing the *Baylisascaris procyonis* life cycle.

9. References

Anderson, D.C.; Greenwood, R.; Fishman, M. & Kagan, I.G. (1975). Acute infantile hemiplegia with cerebrospinal fluid eosinophilic pleocytosis: an unusual case of visceral larva migrans. *The Journal of Pediatrics*, Vol.86, nº2, (February 1975), pp. 247–249.

Baeur, C. & Gey, A. (1995). Efficacy of six anthelmintics against luminal stages of *Baylisascaris procyonis* in naturally infected raccoons (*Procyon lotor*). *Veterinary Parasitology*, Vol.60, nº1-2, (November 1995), pp. 155–159, ISSN 0304-4017

Beaver, P. (1969). The nature of visceral larva migrans. *The Journal of Parasitology*, Vol.55, nº1, (February 1969), pp. 3–12, ISSN 0022-3395

Berry, J.F. (1985). Phylogenetic relationship between *Baylisascaris* spp. Sprent, 1968 (Nematoda: Ascarididae) from skunks, raccoons and groundhogs in southern Ontario. M.S Thesis. University of Guelph, Guelph, Ontario, 99 pp.

Blizzard, E.L.; Davis, C.L.; Henke, S.; Long, D.B.; Hall, C.A. & Yabsley, M.J. (2010a). Distribution, prevalence, and genetic characterization of *Baylisascaris procyonis* in selected areas of Georgia. *The Journal of Parasitology*, Vol.96, nº6, (December 2010), pp. 1128-33, ISSN 0022-3395.

Blizzard, E.L.; Yabsley, M.J.; Beck, M.F. & Harsch, S. (2010b). Geographic expansion of *Baylisascaris procyonis* roundworms, Florida, USA. *Emerging Infectious Diseases*, Vol.16, nº11, (November 2010), pp. 1803-4, ISSN 1080-6059.

Boyce, W.M.; Asai, D.J.; Wilder, J.K. & Kazacos, K.R. (1989). Physiochemical characterization and monoclonal and polyclonal antibody recognition of *Baylisascaris procyonis* larval excretory-secretory antigens. *The Journal of Parasitology*, Vol.75, pp. 540–548.

Centers for Disease Control. 2002. Raccoon roundworm encephalitis—Chicago, Illinois, and Los Angeles, California, 2000. *Morbidity and Mortality Weekly Report*, Vol.50, nº51, (January 2002), pp. 1153–1155, ISSN 0149-2195.

Chun, C.S.; Kazacos, K.R.; Glaser, C.; Bardo, D.; Dangoudoubiyam, S. & Nash, R. (2009). Global neurologic deficits with baylisascaris encephalitis in a previously healthy teenager. *The Pediatric Infectious Diseases Journal*, Vol.28, nº10, (October 2009), pp. 925-7, ISSN 0891-3668.

Cunningham, C.K.; Kazacos, K.R.; Lucas, J.A.; McAuley, J.B.; Wozniak, E.J. & Weiner, L.B. (1994). Diagnosis and management of *Baylisascaris procyonis* infection in an infant with nonfatal meningoencephalitis. *Clinical Infectious Diseases*, Vol.18, nº6, (June 1994), pp. 868–872, ISSN 1058-4838.

Dangoudoubiyam, S.; Vemulapalli, R.; Hancock, K. & Kazacos, KR. (2010). Molecular cloning of an immunogenic protein of *Baylisascaris procyonis* and expression in *Escherichia coli* for use in developing improved serodiagnostic assays. *Clinical and Vaccine Immunology*, Vol17, nº12, (December 2010), pp. 1933-9, ISSN 1556-6811

Dangoudoubiyam, S.; Vemulapalli, R.; Ndao, M. & Kazacos KR. (2011). A recombinant antigen-based enzyme-linked immunosorbent assay for specific diagnosis of *Baylisascaris procyonis* larva migrans. *Clinical and Vaccine Immunology* CVI Accepts, (published online ahead of print on 10 August 2011) doi:10.1128/CVI.00083-11

De Silva, N.; Guyatt, H. & Bundy, D. (1997). Anthelmintics. A comparative review of their clinical pharmacology. *Drugs* Vol.53, nº5, (May 1997), pp. 769–788, ISSN 0012-6667.

Dubey, J.P. (1982). *Baylisascaris procyonis* and eimerian infections in raccoons. *Journal of the American Veterinary Medical Association* Vol.181, nº11, (December 1982), pp. 1292–1294, ISSN 0003-1488.

Eberhard, M.L.; Nace, E.K.; Won, K.Y.; Punkosdy, G.A.; Bishop, H.S. & Johnston, S.P. (2003). *Baylisascaris procyonis* in the metropolitan Atlanta area. *Emerging Infectious Diseases*, Vol9, nº12, (December 2003), pp. 1636–7, ISSN 1080-6059.

Ermer, E.M. & Fodge, J.A. (1986). Occurrence of the raccoon roundworm in raccoons in western New York. *New York Fish and Game Journal*, Vol.33, pp. 58–61, ISSN 0028-7210.

Feachem, R.; Bradley, D.J.; Garelick, H. & Mara, D.D. 1983)Ascaris and ascariasis. In: *Sanitation and disease: health aspects of excreta and wastewater management*, John Wiley & Sons for World Bank Studies in Water Supply and Sanitation, p. 391, Washington.

Fox, A.S.; Kazacos, K.R.; Gould, N.S.; Heydemann, P.T.; Thomas, C. & Boyer, K.M. (1985). Fatal eosinophilic meningoencephalitis and visceral larva migrans caused by the raccoon ascarid *Baylisascaris procyonis*. *The New England Journal of Medicine* Vol.312, nº25, (June 1985), pp. 1619–1623, ISSN 0028-4793.

Gavin, P.J.; Kazacos, K.R.; Tan, T.Q.; Brinkman, W.B.; Byrd, S.E.; Davis, A.T.; Mets, M.B. & Shulman, S.T. (2002). Neural larval migrans caused by the raccoon roundworm *Baylisascaris procyonis*. *The Pediatric Infectious Disease Journal*, Vol.21, nº.10, (October 2002), pp. 971–975, ISSN 0891-3668.

Goldberg, M.A.; Kazacos, K.R.; Boyce, W.M.; Ai, E. & Katz, B. (1993). Diffuse unilateral subacute neuroretinitis: morphometric, serologic, and epidemiologic support for *Baylisascaris* as a causative agent. *Ophthalmology*, Vol.100, nº.11, (November 1993), pp. 1695–701, ISSN 0161-6420.

Hajek, J.; Yau, Y.; Kertes, P.; Soman, T.; Laughlin, S.; Kanani, R.; Kazacos, K.; Dangoudoubiyam, S. & Opavsky, M.A. (2009). A child with raccoon roundworm meningoencephalitis: A pathogen emerging in your own backyard?. *The Canadian Journal of Infectious Diseases & Medical Microbiology*, Vol. 20, nº4, (Winter 2009), pp. 177-80, ISSN 1712-9532.

Hoffmann, C.O. & Gottschang, J.L. (1977). Numbers, distribution and movements of a raccoon population in a suburban residential community. *Journal of Mammalogy*, Vol.58, No.4, (November 1977), pp. 623-36, ISSN 0022-2372.

Huff, D.S.; Neafie, R.C.; Binder, M.J.; Leon, G.A.D.; Brown, L.W. & Kazacos, K.R. (1984). The first fatal *Baylisascaris* infection in humans. *Pediatric Pathology*, Vol.2, nº3, (pp. 345–52, ISSN 0277-0938.

Jung, H.; Hurtado, M.; Sanchez, M.; Medina, M. & Sotelo, J. (1990). Plasma and CSF levels of albendazole and praziquantel in patients with neurocysticercosis. *Clinical Neuropharmacology*, Vol.13, nº6, (December 1990), pp. 559–564, ISSN 0362-5664.

Kazacos, K.R. (1986). Raccoon ascarids as a cause of larva migrans. *Parasitology Today*, Vol.2, nº9, (September 1986), pp. 253–255, ISSN 0169-4758.

Kazacos, KR. (1991). Visceral and ocular larva migrans. *Seminars in Veterinary Medicine and Surgery (Small Animal)*, Vol.6, nº3, (August 1991), pp. 227–235, ISSN 0882-0511.

Kazacos, K.R. (1997). Visceral, ocular, and neural larva migrans. In: *Pathology of infectious diseases, Vol. II*. Connor, D.H.; Chandler, F.W.; Schwartz, D.A.; Manz, H.J. & Lack, E.E., pp. 1459–73, Appleton & Lange, Stamford, CT.

Kazacos, KR. (2000). Protecting children from helminthic zoonoses. *Contemporary Pediatrics*, Vol.95, nº3, (Suppl) pp. 1–24, ISSN 8750-0507.

Kazacos, K.R. (2001). *Baylisascaris procyonis* and related species. In: *Parasitic diseases of wild mammals. 2nd ed.* Samuels, W.M.; Pybus, M.J. & Kocans, A.A., pp. 301–41, Iowa State University Press/Ames, Iowa.

Kazacos, K.R. & Kazacos, E.A. (1984). Experimental infection of domestic swine with *Baylisascaris procyonis* from raccoons. *American Journal of Veterinary Research*, Vol.45, nº6, (June 1984), pp. 1114–1121, ISSN 0002-9645.

Kazacos, K.R.; Raymond, L.A.; Kazacos, E.A. & Vestre, W.A. (1985). The raccoon ascarid. A probable cause of human ocular larva migrans. *Ophthalmology*, Vol.92, nº12, (December 1985), pp. 1735–1743, ISSN 0161-6420.

Kazacos, K.R. & Boyce, W.M. (1989). *Baylisascaris* larva migrans. *Journal of the American Veterinary Medical Association*, Vol.195, nº7, (October 1989), pp. 894-903, ISSN 0003-1488.

Lo Re, V.III & Gluckman, S.J. (2003). Eosinophilic meningitis. *The American Journal of Medicine,* Vol.114, n°3, (February 2003), pp. 217–223, ISSN 0002-9343.

McClure, G. (1933). Nematode parasites of mammals. From specimens collected in the New York Zoological Park, 1931. Zoologica (New York) Vol.15 pp. 29–47.

Mets, M.B.; Noble, A.G.; Basti, S.; Gavin, P.; Davis, A.T.; Shulman, S.T. & Kazacos KR. (2003). Eye findings of diffuse unilateral subacute neuroretinitis and multiple choroidal infiltrates associated with neural larva migrans due to *Baylisascaris procyonis. American Journal of Ophthalmology,*Vol.135, n°6, (June 2003), pp. 888-90, ISSN 0002-9394.

Miyashita, M. (1993). Prevalence of *Baylisascaris procyonis* in raccoons in Japan and experimental infections of the worm to laboratory animals. *Journal Urban Living Health Association,* Vol.37, pp. 137–151. (In Japanese.)

Moertel, C.L.; Kazacos, K.R.; Butterfield, J.H.; Kita, H.; Watterson, J. & Gleich, G.J. (2001). Eosinophil-associated inflammation and elaboration of eosinophil-derived proteins in two children with raccoon roundworm (*Baylisascaris procyonis*) encephalitis. *Pediatrics,* Vol.108, n°5, (November 2001), pp. E93, ISSN 0031-4005.

Murray, W.J. (2002). Human infections caused by the raccoon roundworm, *Baylisascaris procyonis. Clinical Microbiology Newsletter,* Vol.24, n°1, pp. 1-7, ISSN 0196-4399.

Murray, W.J. & Kazacos, K.R. (2004). Raccoon roundworm encephalitis. *Clinical Infectious Diseases,* Vol.39, n°10, (November 2004), pp. 1484-92, ISSN 1058-4838.

Page, L.K.; Swihart, R.K. & Kazacos, K.R. (1998). Raccoon latrine structure and its potential role in transmission of *Baylisascaris procyonis* to vertebrates. *American Midland Naturalist,* Vol.140, n° 1, (July 1998), pp. 180-185, ISSN 0003-0031.

Page, L.K.; Swihart, R.K. & Kazacos, K.R. (1999). Implications of raccoon latrines in the epizootiology of baylisascariasis. *Journal of Wildlife Diseases,* Vol.35, n°3, (July 1999), pp. 474-80, ISSN 0090-3558.

Pai, P.J.; Blackburn, B.G.; Kazacos, K.R.; Warrier, R.P. & Bégué RE. (2007). Full recovery from *Baylisascaris procyonis* eosinophilic meningitis. *Emerging Infectious Diseases,* Vol.13, n°6, (June 2007), pp. 928-30, ISSN 1080-6040.

Park, S.Y.; Glaser, C.; Murray, W.J.; Kazacos, K.R.; Rowley, H.A.; Fredrick, D.R. & Bass, N. (2000). Raccoon roundworm (*Baylisascaris procyonis*) encephalitis: Case report and field investigation. *Pediatrics,* Vol.106, n°4, (October 2000), pp. E56, ISSN 0031-4005.

Perlman, J.E.; Kazacos, K.R.; Imperato, G.H.; Desai, R.U.; Schulman, S.K.; Edwards, J.; Pontrelli, L.R.; Machado, F.S.; Tanowitz, H.B. & Saffra, N.A. (2010). *Baylisascaris procyonis* neural larva migrans in an infant in New York City. *Journal of Neuroparasitology,* Vol.1, (June 2010), pp., ISSN 2090-2344

Rothenberg, M.E. (1998). Eosinophilia. *The New England Journal of Medicine,* Vol.338, n°22, (May 1998), pp. 1592-600, ISSN 0028-4793.

Roussere, G.P.; Murray, W.J.; Raudenbush, C.B.; Kutilek, M.J.; Levee, D.J. & Kazacos, K.R. (2003). Raccoon roundworm eggs near homes and risk for larva migrans disease, California communities. *Emerging Infectious Diseases,* Vol.9, n°12, (December 2003), pp. 1516–22, ISSN 1080-6040.

Rowley, H.A.; Uht, R.M.; Kazacos, K.R.; Sakanari, J.; Wheaton, W.V.; Barkovich, A.J. & Bollen, A.W. (2000). Radiologic-pathologic findings in raccoon roundworm (*Baylisascaris procyonis*) encephalitis. *AJNR. American Journal of Neuroradiology*, Vol.21, n°2, (February 2000), pp. 415–420, ISSN 0195-6108.

Sakla, A.A.; Donnelly, J.J.; Khatami, M. & Rockey, J.H. (1989). *Baylisascaris procyonis* (Stefanski and Zarnowski, 1951) Ascarididae: Nematoda. I. Embryonic development and morphogenesis of second stage larvae. Assiut Veterinary Medical Journal, Vol.21, pp. 68–76.

Sato, H.; Furuoka, H. & Kamiya, H. (2002). First outbreak of *Baylisascaris procyonis* larva migrans in rabbits in Japan. *Parasitology international*,Vol.51, n°1, (March 2002), pp. 105–108, ISSN 1383-5769.

Sexsmith, J.L.; Whiting, T.L.; Gree, C.; Orvis, S.; Berezanski, D.J. & Thompson A.B. (2009). Prevalence and distribution of *Baylisascaris procyonis* in urban raccoons (*Procyon lotor*) in Winnipeg, Manitoba. *The Canadian Veterinary Journal*, Vol.50, n°8, (August 2009), pp. 846-50, ISSN 0008-5286.

Shafir, S.C.; Wang, W.; Sorvillo, F.J.; Wise, M.E.; Moore, L., Sorvilo, T. & Eberhard, M.L: (2007). Thermal death point of *Baylisascaris procyonis* eggs. *Emerging Infectious Diseases*, Vol.13, n°1, (January 2007) pp. 172–3, ISSN 1080-6040.

Shafir, S.C.; Sorvillo, F.J.; Sorvillo, T. & Eberhard, M.L. (2011). Viability of *Baylisascaris procyonis* Eggs. *Emerging Infectious Diseases*, Vol.17, n°7, (July 2011), pp. 1293-5, ISSN 1080-6040.

Sheppard, C.H. & Kazacos, K.R. (1997). Susceptibility of *Peromyscus leucopus* and *Mus musculus* to infection with *Baylisascaris procyonis*. *The Journal of Parasitology*, Vol.83, n°6, (December 1997), pp. 1104–1111, ISSN 0022-3395.

Snyder, D.E. (1983). The prevalence, cross-transmissibility to domestic animals and adult structure of *Baylisascaris procyonis* (Nematoda) from Illinois raccoons (*Procyon lotor*). Ph.D. Thesis, University of Illinois at Urbana-Champaign, Urbana, IL, 233 pp.

Snyder, D.E. & Fitzgerald, P.R. (1985). The relationship of *Baylisascaris procyonis* to Illinois raccoons (*Procyon lotor*). *The Journal of Parasitology*, Vol.71, n°5, (October 1985), pp. 596–598, ISSN 0022-3395.

Souza, M.J.; Ramsay, E.C.; Patton, S. & New, J.C. (2009). *Baylisascaris procyonis* in raccoons (*Procyon lotor*) in eastern Tennessee. *Journal of Wildlife Diseases*, Vol.45, n°4, (October 2009), pp. 1231–4, ISSN 0090-3558.

Sprent, J.F.A. (1968). Notes on *Ascaris* and *Toxascaris*, with a definition of *Baylisascaris* gen. nov. *Parasitology*, Vol.58, n°1, (February 1968), pp. 185–198, ISSN 0031-1820.

Stefanski, W. & Zarnowski, E. (1951). *Ascaris procyonis* n. sp. z jelita szopa (*Procyon lotor* L.) *Ascaris procyonis* n. sp. provenant de l'intestin de *Procyon lotor*. Ann. Mus. Zool. Polonici, Vol.14, pp. 199–202.

Weller, P. F. (1993). Eosinophilic meningitis. *The American Journal of Medicine*, Vol.95, n°3, (September 1993), pp. 250–253, ISSN 0002-9343.

Wirtz, W.L. (1982). Cerebrospinal nematodiasis due to the raccoon ascarid, *Baylisascaris procyonis*. M.S. Thesis, Purdue University, West Lafayette, IN, 90 pp

Wolf, K.N.; Lock, B.; Carpenter, J.W. & Garner, M.M. (2007). *Baylisascaris procyonis* infection in a Moluccan cockatoo (*Cacatua moluccensis*). *Journal of Avian Medicine and Surgery*, Vol.21, nº3, (September 2007), pp. 220-5, ISSN 1082-6742.

Yeitz, J.L.; Gillin, C.M.; Bildfell, R.J. & Debess, E.E. (2009). Prevalence of *Baylisascaris procyonis* in raccoons (*Procyon lotor*) in Portland, Oregon, USA. *Journal of Wildlife Diseases*, Vol.45, nº1, (January 2009), pp. 14-8, ISSN 0090-3558.

17

Angiostrongyliasis in the Americas

Arnaldo Maldonado Jr.[1], Raquel Simões[1,2] and Silvana Thiengo[1]
[1]*Oswaldo Cruz Foundation,*
[2]*Federal Rural University of Rio de Janeiro,*
Brazil

1. Introduction

Abdominal angiostrongyliasis, a parasitic disease originally from the Americas, and eosinophilic meningoencephalitis, from Asia, are caused by two species of angiostrongilids nematodes, belonging to the family Metastrongylidae Leiper, 1908. In both cases, rats are the main definitive hosts and snails are the intermediate hosts (Acha & Szyfres, 2003).

The helminth *Angiostrongylus costaricensis* Morera & Céspedes, 1971 is endemic to the Americas and is responsible for a pathological abdominal syndrome, caused by the presence of the adult helminth in the mesenteric arteries. This is microscopically characterized by eosinophilic infiltration, vascular abnormality and a granulomatous reaction (Graeff-Teixeira et al., 1987). The disease was first reported in humans by Céspedes et al. (1967) and Morera (1967) in Costa Rica. The adult worm was subsequently described from specimens recovered during surgical procedures by Morera & Céspedes (1971). The parasite's current distribution ranges from the southern United States to northern Argentina (Morera, 1988), with human cases having been reported in Costa Rica, Honduras, Colombia, Martinique, Dominican Republic, Puerto Rico, Nicaragua, Mexico, Venezuela, Guadalupe, El Salvador, Panama and Brazil (Kaminsky, 1995).

In turn, *Angiostrongylus cantonensis*, the agent that causes eosinophilic meningoencephalitis, was first described in Canton, China, by Chen (1935), and is now dispersed to various Pacific islands, Australia, Africa, and more recently, the Americas (Foronda et al., 2010). It is believed that the initial dissemination to islands in the Pacific resulted from the introduction of naturally infected rats in containers coming from Asia (Diaz, 2008). The growing flows of global trade and tourism, as well as the spread of habits and customs among countries, have enabled the dispersion of the definitive and intermediate hosts of *A. cantonensis* (Cross, 1987). Currently there are reports of human infection in the United States (New et al., 1995), Cuba (Aguiar et al., 1981), Jamaica (Slom & Johnson, 2003), Ecuador (Dorta-Contreras et al., 2010) and Brazil (Lima et al., 2009.) In particular the introduction of the *Achatina fulica* in Brazil (Thiengo et al., 2007) and *Pomacea canaliculata* (Lamarck, 1822)in China are examples of the importance of exotic snails in the spread of this helminthiasis (Lv et al., 2008).

This chapter focuses on the taxonomy, life cycle, endemic and exotic intermediate hosts, natural vertebrate hosts and geographical distribution of these *Angiostrongylus* species together with diagnosis, treatment and prophylaxis of the diseases borne by them.

2. Systematic and general morphology

The system for classifying the *Angiostrongylus* genus basically relies on the morphological characteristics of the rays of the copulatory bursa, host group specificity and/or place where the adult worms are located in the host.

Dougherty (1946) considered the following genera to be synonyms for the genus *Angiostrongylus* Kamensky, 1905: *Haemostrongylus* Railliet and Henry, 1907; *Parastrongylus* Bayle, 1928; *Rodentocaulus* Shul'ts, Orlov and Kutas, 1933; *Pulmonema* Chen, 1935; and *Cardionema* Yamaguti, 1941. Drozdz (1970) separated species of the genus *Angiostrongylus* into two subgroups based on morphological characteristics of the caudal bursa and systematized them into two subgenera - *Angiostrongylus* and *Parastrongylus* - based on the morphology of the lateral rays of the caudal bursa. *Angiostrongylus* has a ventrolateral ray arising independently from the mediolateral and posterolateral rays, which emerge as a single trunk, and is a parasite of the right heart and pulmonary artery of carnivores. In contrast, the subgenus *Parastrongylus* parasitizes rodents and has as taxonomic characteristics the lateral rays arising in a common trunk and a cleft at the same level. A third subgroup, parasitizing insectivores, was classified as belonging to the genus *Stefanskostrongylus,* comprising species with lateral rays similar to the subgenus *Parastrongylus,* but without the gubernaculum. Anderson (1978) accepted such systematic criteria but did not mention biological aspects such as host specificity or site of infection. Furthermore, Chabaud (1972) proposed eight different genera based on the morphology of the bursal rays, types of hosts and infection site. Ubelaker (1986) reorganized the Angiostrongylidae into six genera, based on bursal morphology and on specific host groups. Nevertheless, the host-specificity criteria need to be studied further since infection has been reported of non-human primates and carnivores by *A. costaricensis* (Miller et al., 2006).

In this chapter we accept the classification of Dougherty (1946). To date, 18 species of *Angiostrongylus* have been reported around the world. Four species have been described infecting carnivores: *Angiostrongylus vasorum* Baillet, 1866; *Angiostrongylus raillieti* Travassos, 1927; *Angiostrongylus gubernaculatus* Dougherty, 1946; and *Angiostrongylus chabaudi* Biocca, 1957. In rodents, 14 species have been described: *Angiostrongylus taterone* Baylis, 1928; *A. cantonensis; Angiostrongylus sciuri* Merdevenci, 1964; *Angiostrongylus mackerrasae* Bhaibulaya, 1968; *Angiostrongylus sandarsae* Alicata, 1968; *Angiostrongylus petrowi* Tarjymanova and Tschertkova, 1969; *Angiostrongylus dujardini* Drozdz and Doby, 1970; *Angiostrongylus schmidti* Kinsella, 1971; *A. costaricensis; Angiostrongylus malaysiensis* Bhaibulay and Cross, 1971; *Angiostrongylus ryjikovi* Jushkov, 1971; *Angiostrongylus siamensis* Ohbayashi, Kamiya, and Bhaibulaya, 1979; *Angiostrongylus morerai* Robles, Navone, and Kinsella, 2008; and *Angiostrongylus lenzii* Souza et al., 2009.

Angiostrongylus costaricensis was described from three female specimens and one male specimen, recovered from a patient during surgery. Chabaud (1972) raised the species to the new genus *Morerastrongylus,* but this proposal was not accepted by Anderson (1978) in revising the classification of nematodes. *A. costaricensis* (Figs. 1-3; 7) is a filiform nematode. The cephalic end is round and the esophagus is club-shaped (Fig. 1). The copulatory bursa is slightly asymmetric and well developed. The dorsal ray is short and bifurcates into arms terminating in sharp tips. On its ventral side, behind its bifurcation, there is a conspicuous papilla. The lateral rays emerge from a common trunk, widely separated from the ventral rays, and the mediolateral and the posterolateral rays are fused in their proximal half. The anterolateral ray is thicker and separates form the common trunk just after its emergence from the trunk. The externodorsal ray arises close the lateral trunk and is well separated from the dorsal ray. Its distal end is knoblike. The ventral rays are fused except at the tips and the ventrolateral ray is slightly longer than the ventrolateral one. A gubernaculum is present with two branches that come together just before they terminate in the cloaca (Fig. 7). Behind the cloacal opening, there are three papillae. The spicules are slender, striated and of equal size. The caudal extremity of the female is roughly conical, with a small projection at the tip (Fig. 3) (Morera, 1973).

Angiostrongylus cantonensis was initially described as *Pulmonema cantonensis* Chen, 1935, a new genus, from specimens recovered from the lungs of naturally infected rats (*Rattus norvegicus* and *Rattus rattus*) collected in Canton, China. The adult worms of *cantonensis* (Figs. 4-6; 8) are characterized by a filiform body in both sexes, tapering at the anterior end. Females are larger and more robust than males. The cephalic vesicle is absent, the oral aperture is simple, circular and surrounded by six papillae (two dorsal, two lateral and two ventral) and two lateral amphids. The esophagus is claviform and the excretory pore is posterior to the esophagus (Fig. 4). The nerve ring is anterior to the middle of the esophagus, the male caudal bursa is small and slightly asymmetric, the ventroventral rays are smaller than the ventrolateral ones, with a common origin, bifurcated at the proximal half and do not reach the bursal margins. The dorsal ray is thick, bifurcating into three branches, with digititoform externodorsal rays separated at the base. The right mediolateral ray is thinner than the left one, with the right mediolateral and posterolateral rays bifurcating at the middle of the trunk and the left mediolateral and laterolateral rays at the distal third. The lateral rays arise from a common trunk, with the ventrolateral ray being cleft-shaped and smaller than the other lateral rays (Fig. 5). The gubernaculum is conspicuous and curved. Uterine tubules spiral around the blood-filled intestine, easily seen through the transparent cuticle. The tail is long and rounded without cuticle expansion and papillae, and is slightly ventrally curved (Fig. 6) (Thiengo et al., 2010).

	Angiostrongylus costaricensis		*Angiostrongylus cantonensis*	
	Male	Female	Male	Female
Body lenght	19.9	32.8	22.82	32.84
Width	0.28-0.31	0.32-0.35	0.35	0.48
Widht at the base of esophagus	0.12-0.14	0.14-0.15	0.04	0.05
Esophagus	0.18-0.23	0.23-0.26	0.31	0.34
Nerve ring	-	-	0.09	0.10
Excretory pore	-	-	0.43	0.40
Spicules	0.32-0.33	-	1.29	-
Gubernaculum	-	-	0.08x0.02	-
Vuva-tail	-	0.24-0.29	-	0.19
Anus-tail	-	0.06-0.07	-	0.06
Eggs	-	-	-	0.06

Table 1. Measurements comparasion of *Angiostrongylus costaricensis* from Costa Rica (Morera, 1973) and *Angiostrongylus cantonensis* from Brazil (Thiengo et al., 2010).

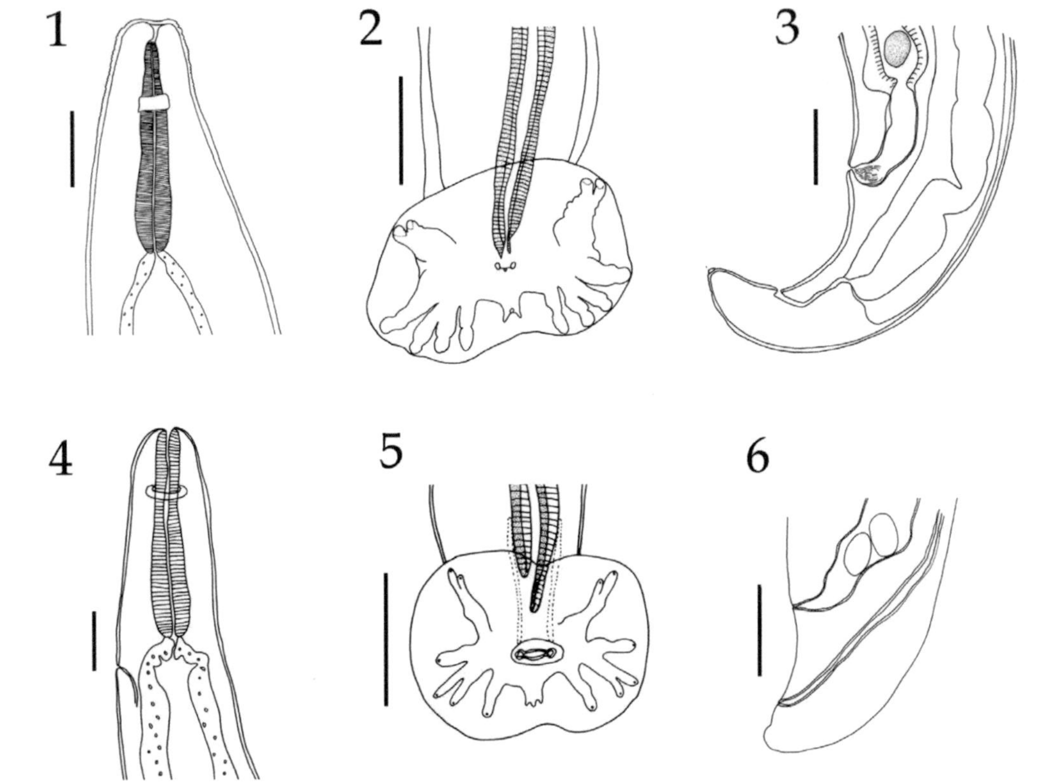

Fig. 1-3. *Angiostrongylus costaricensis;* 1. Anterior extremity, right lateral view, female. Scale bar: 50 µm. 2. Male, caudal bursa, ventral view. Scale bar: 100µm .3. Female, posterior extremity, lateral view. Scale bar: 100µm. 4-6. *Angiostrongylus cantonensis;* 4. Anterior extremity, right lateral view, female. Scale bar: 100 µm. 5. Male, caudal bursa, ventral view. 6. Female, posterior extremity, lateral view. Scale bar: 100 µm.

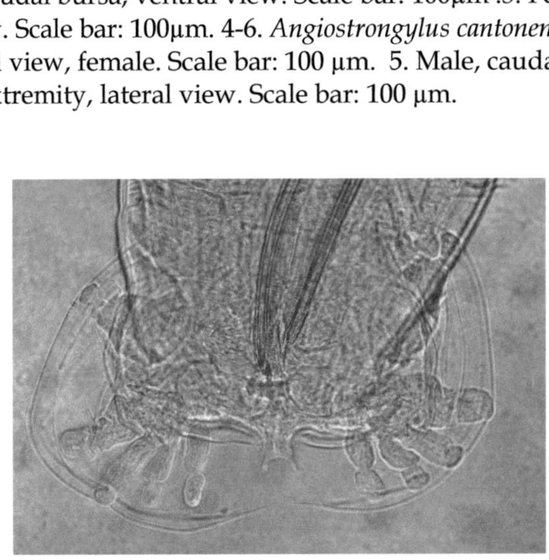

Fig. 7. Light microscopy of *Angiostrongylus costaricensis.* Scale bar: 100 µm.

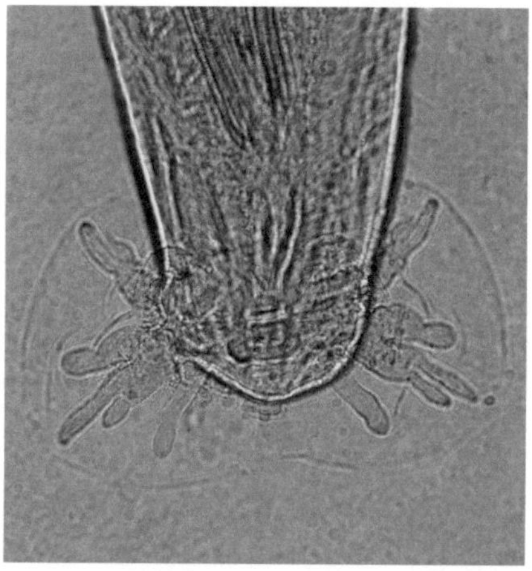

Fig. 8. Light microscopy of *Angiostrongylus cantonensis.* Scale bar: 100 μm.

3. Life cycle of main species of *Angiostrongylus* infecting man

Species of *Angiostrongylus* cause a nematode infection in domestic dogs and wild mammals (Anderson, 1978). Some species can accidentally infect humans, causing characteristic clinical symptoms of the disease: *A. cantonensis* and *A. costaricensis,* which respectively cause eosinophilic meningoencephalitis and abdominal disease in humans (Graeff-Teixeira et al., 1991a; Wang et al., 2008). The biological cycle of these helminths requires an intermediate host, usually a snail, and a definitive host, most often a wild rodent. Humans participate in the biological cycle as accidental hosts, since the cycle does not complete itself in people.

Infection by *A. costaricensis* happens when the definitive host ingests the snail, which can be infected with third stage larvae (L_3), or food contaminated with snail mucus. The larvae migrate to the ileocecal region, penetrating the intestinal wall and entering the lymphatic vessels, where they molt twice before migrating to the mesenteric arteries, where they reach sexual maturity. The females release eggs, which are carried by the bloodstream, causing embolisms in the arterioles and capillaries of the intestinal wall. The eggs hatch when they reach the first larval stage (L_1), penetrating the intestinal lumen, where they are released in the feces. To continue the cycle, the L_1 larvae must be ingested or actively penetrate the tissue of the intermediate host (Thiengo, 1996). After 19 days of the initial infection, the larvae will have molted twice (passing through the L_2 and L_3 stages, the latter of which is the infective stage for the definitive host). The wild rodents become infected by ingesting parasitized snails, mainly the species *Vaginulus* (*Sarasinula*) *plebeius* in Costa Rica (Morera, 1970) or *Phyllocaulis variegatus* (Semper, 1885) in Brazil (Graeff-Teixeira et al., 1989). The main rodent hosts are *Sigmodon hispidus* (Morera et al., 1970) and *Oligoryzomys nigripes* (Graeff-Teixeira et al., 1990) in these two countries, respectively. The worms reach sexual maturity in the mesenteric arterioles of the rodent *S. hispidus,* where they lay their eggs. The L_1 larvae are found in the feces 24 days after experimental infection (Morera, 1973; Motta & Lenzi, 1995).

Humans become infected by eating raw infected snails or food contaminated by snail mucoid secretions containing L_3 larvae. Although the helminth reaches sexual maturity and releases eggs that stimulate a granulomatous reaction in the infected person intestinal wall due to their degeneration, it does not produce L_1 larvae, thus interrupting the biological cycle.

The nematode *A. cantonensis* is commonly known as the lungworm because its niche in the adult phase is in the pulmonary arteries of the definitive host, in general the rodents *R. rattus* and *R. norvegicus*. In experimental infection of *R. norvegicus*, the female worm lays eggs inside the pulmonary arterioles, where they develop into the first-stage larvae (L_1), which then move to the interior of the alveoli. The larvae then migrate to the pharynx and are swallowed, pass through the gastrointestinal tract and are eliminated in the feces (Bhaibulaya, 1975; Yousif & Ibrahim, 1978). Land or freshwater snails are the principal intermediate hosts. They can become infected by ingestion of or penetration by L_1 larvae. The helminths then molt two times and become infective L_3 larvae, generally within 21 days after infection. Rats become infected by ingesting the intermediate hosts infected by L_3 larvae. These larvae then penetrate the intestinal wall and enter the bloodstream a few hours after being ingested. They reach the pulmonary circulation from the heart and are dispersed to various other organs by the arterial circulation. Many reach the brain and molt again, becoming L_4 larvae. The fifth molting into L_5 occurs in the subarachnoid space, from where after developing they migrate to the pulmonary arteries where they are found as of 25 days after infection. The worms then reach sexual maturity at around 35 days and the L_1 larvae can be found in the rodent's feces as of 42 days after the exposure to the previous generation of L_1 larvae (Weinstein et al., 1963; Bhaibulaya, 1975).

Humans become infected by eating raw or undercooked snails and slugs or through paratenic hosts (crabs, freshwater shrimps). In humans, the young larvae reach the brain, where they die rather than migrating further and terminating their development. This causes eosinophilic meningoencephalitis, which has neurological symptoms. Normally the infection is regenerative and does not kill the victim, but the parasitism can be serious enough to kill when there is massive exposure to infective L_3 larvae (Lima et al., 2009) (Fig. 9).

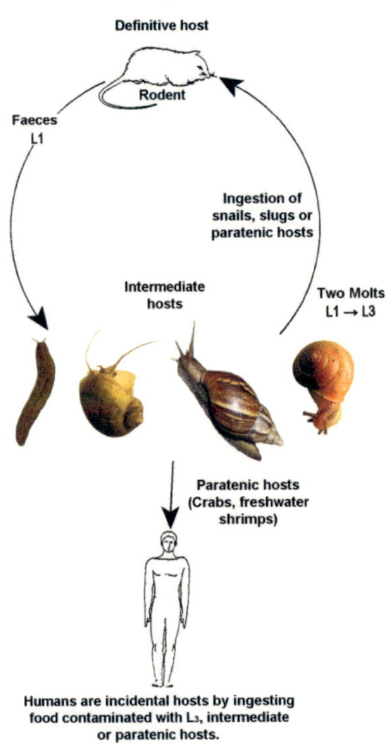

Fig. 9. Life cycle of *Angiostrongylus cantonensis*.

4. Endemic and exotic mollusks as intermediate hosts

The life cycle of *A. cantonensis* (Fig. 9) involves different species of terrestrial and freshwater gastropods as intermediate hosts. Mollusks become infected either by ingestion of L_1 present in the rat feces or by penetration of these larvae through the body wall or respiratory pores. In the mollusk tissues the L_1 molts twice (L_2 and L_3) and the period necessary for the development is around 15 days. Details of the life cycle may be seen in Cheng & Alicata, 1965, Chao et al. 1987 and Graeff-Teixeira et al. 2009.

Because the parasite displays broad nonspecificity for intermediate hosts, various species of terrestrial and freshwater mollusk species had been found naturally infected, such as: *Achatina fulica* Bowdich, 1822, *Bradybaena similaris* (Férussac, 1821), *Subulina octona* (Bruguière, 1792), *Pomacea canaliculata* (Lamarck, 1822), *Pomacea lineata* (Spix in Wagner, 1827); *Deroceras laeve* (Muller, 1774), *Pila* spp. (Wallace and Rosen,1969; Malek and Cheng, 1974; Caldeira et al., 2007; Thiengo et al., 2010).

It is noteworthy in the epidemiology of the transmission of *A. cantonensis* the occurrence of paratenic hosts (or carrier hosts) such as land crabs, freshwater prawns, frogs and planarians. Those are passive hosts where the parasite does not undergo any development. However, they play an important role as they improve parasite opportunities (in time and space) to get the definitive host.

In China where *P. canaliculata* and *A.fulica* are widespread in the south of the country, the number of cases of eosinophilic meningoencephalatis has been increasing, and the transmission is linked to both species (Lv et al., 2008, 2009). In the last years, various outbreaks have been reported and the transmission in most of the cases was directely related to the consumption of *P. canaliculata*, considered currently the main cause of the spread of angiostrongyliasis in China (Lv et al. 2011).

The first cases of eosinophilic meningitis recorded to South America were to Brazil in 2007 and in 2008 and *A. fulica* was considered the vector for three out of the four reported cases. One of the cases reported to Pernambuco, Northeastern region, was attributed to the ingestion of undercooked *P. lineata* specimens (Caldeira et al., 2007; Lima et al., 2009; Thiengo et al., 2010). In fact, specimens of *A. fulica* have been found infected with *A. cantonensis* larvae from two of the main Brazilian regions, South and Southeast, in the last five years (Maldonado et al., 2010). Hence, the emergence of eosinophilic meningitis is a matter of concern in Brazil as it is currently experiencing the explosive phase of the invasion of *A.fulica*, recorded in 24 out the 26 states and the Federal District (Thiengo et al., 2007, Zanol et al., 2010).

The life cycle of *A. costaricensis* is quite similar to that of *A. cantonensis*, although paratenic hosts do not occur.

To continue the cycle, the L_1 larvae must be ingested or actively penetrate the tissue of the intermediate host (Thiengo, 1996). After 19 days of the initial infection, the larvae will have molted twice (passing through the L_2 and L_3 stages, the latter of which is the infective stage for the definitive host). The wild rodents become infected by ingesting parasitized snails, mainly the species *Vaginulus* (*Sarasinula*) *plebeius* in Costa Rica (Morera, 1970) or *Phyllocaulis variegatus* (Semper, 1885) in Brazil (Graeff-Teixeira et al., 1989; Motta & Lenzi, 1995).

5. Parasitism by *Angiostrongylus costaricensis* and *Angiostrongylus cantonensis* in naturally infected rat populations

The nematode *A. costaricensis* has little specificity for its definitive host. The main hosts involved in its life cycle in nature are rodents of the Cricetidae family, although rodents of the Heteromydae and Muridae families have also been found to be infected (Table 2). The rodent *S. hispidus* has been indicated as the principal natural host due to its abundance, parasite prevalence rates in Panama and aspects of its ecology (Rodríguez et al., 2000).

Definitive Host	Family	Country	References
Rodentia			
Sigmodon hispidus	Cricetidae	Costa Rica; Panamá; United States	Morera, 1970; Tesh et al., 1973; Ubelaker & Hall, 1979
Rattus rattus	Muridae	Costa Rica; Panamá; Puerto Rico; Guadoulupe	Morera, 1970; Tesh et al., 1973; Andersen et al., 1986; Juminer et al., 1993;
Rattus norvegicus	Muridae	Guadoulupe; Dominican Republic; Puerto Rico	Juminer et al., 1993; Vargas et al., 1992; Andersen et al., 1986
Liomys adspersus	Heteromyidae	Panamá	Tesh et al., 1973
Zygodontomys microtinus	Cricetidae	Panamá	Tesh et al., 1973
Oryzomys fulvescens	Cricetidae	Panamá	Tesh et al., 1973
Oryzomys caliginosus	Cricetidae	Colombia	Malek, 1981
Oligoryzomys nigripes (=*Oryzomys eliurus*)	Cricetidae	Brazil	Graeff-Texeira et al., 1990
Sooretamys angouya (=*Oryzomys Ratticeps*)	Cricetidae	Brazil	Graeff-Texeira et al., 1990
Proechimys sp.	Echimyudae	Venezuela	Santos, 1985
Didelphimorphia			
Didelphis virginiana	Didelphidae	United States	Miller et.al, 2006
Carnivora			
Nasua narica bullata	Procyinidae	Costa Rica	Morera, 1970
Procyon lotor	Procyinidae	United States	Miller et.al, 2006
Primates			
Hylobates syndactylus	Hylobatidae	United States	Miller et.al, 2006
Aotus nancymaae	Aotidae	United States	Miller et.al, 2006
Saguinus mystax	Cebidae	Peru	Sly et al., 1982

Table 2. Vertebrate hosts infected with *Angiostrongylus costaricensis* in the Americas.

Other mammals have also been found naturally infected, such as the coati *Nasua narica bullata* in Costa Rica, in which parasitism by *A. costaricensis* was confirmed after experimental infection of *S. hispidus* from isolation of L_1 larvae obtained from the host's feces, and in specimens of the marmoset *Saguinus mystax* imported from Peru after histopathological examination, which demonstrated the presence of the adult worm in the lamina propria of the host's mesenteric artery.

Recently, *A. costaricenis* was reported parasitizing siamangs (*Hylobates syndacttylus*), night monkeys (*Aotus nancymaae*), raccoons (*Procyon lotor*) and opossums (*Didelphis virginiana*) in a zoo in the United States (Miller et al., 2006).

In Brazil, only two species of cricetids rodents, *O. nigripes* and *Sooretamys angouya*, are involved in transmission of *A. costaricensis*, in the Southern region of the country (Graeff-Teixeira et al., 1990). Although no evidence has been found of the participation of wild rodents in the Southeastern region (Graeff-Teixeira et al., 2010), there are various reports of abdominal angiostrongyliasis in the Midwestern and Southeastern regions (Pena et al., 1995; Magalhães et al., 1982).

In the Americas in general, the presence of *R. rattus* and *R. norvegicus* infected by *A. cantonensis* confirms the endemism of this zoonosis in Cuba, the United States, Jamaica, Puerto Rico, Dominican Republic, Haiti and Brazil (Table 3). The infection rate of these rodents is highly variable (Wang et al., 2008) and does not suggest specificity among the murids. Some findings of infected rodents in urban areas are associated with epidemiological investigations after the occurrence of cases of eosinophilic meningoencephalitis, such as in Cuba, Jamaica and Brazil (Aguiar et al., 1981; Lindo et al., 2002; Simões et al., 2011).

Definitive Host	Family	Country	References
Rodentia			
Rattus rattus	Muridae	Jamaica; Haiti	Lindo et al., 2002; Raccurt et al., 2003
Rattus norvegicus	Muridae	Cuba; United States; Jamaica; Haiti; Brazil	Aguiar et al., 1981; Campbell & Little, 1988; Lindo et al., 2002; Raccurt et al., 2003; Simões et al., 2011
Neotoma floridanus	Cricetidae	United States	Kim et al., 2002
Didelphimorphia			
Didelphis virginiana	Didelphidae	United States	Kim et al., 2002
Primates			
Varecia variegata rubra	Lemuridae	United States	Kim et al., 2002

Table 3. Vertebrate hosts infected with *Angiostrongylus cantonensis* in the Americas.

Kim et al. (2002) reported *A. cantonensis* infection *in* a lemur (*Varecia variegata rubra*), in a wood rat (*Neotoma floridanus*) and in 4 opossums (*Didelphis virginiana*) in Lousiana, United States.

How *A. cantonensis* arrived and became established in the Americas is not well established, but Diaz (2008) attributed the spread of *A. cantonensis* to the American continents to the introduction of *R. norvegicus* by containers carried by ships. In Brazil, two arrival routes of this parasite have been postulated: in parasitized rats during the country's colonial period, when there was frequent contact with Africa and Asia (Maldonado et al., 2010) and/or by recent invasion of the African snail *A. fulica*, some two decades ago (Thiengo et al., 2007).

6. Geographic distribution of angiostrongyliasis in the Americas

The first report of abdominal angiostrongyliais was in 1952 in children in Costa Rica (Céspedes et al., 1967; Morera, 1967). Nearly 20 years later, in the same country, the parasite was reported naturally infecting *S. hispidus* and *R. rattus* (Cépedes & Morera, 1971). Since the description of this parasite, various cases have been reported in both South and North America, in countries including Honduras (Sierra & Morera, 1972), Venezuela (Zambrano, 1973), Mexico (Zavala et al., 1974), El Salvador (Sauerbrey, 1977), Brazil (Ziliotto et al., 1975), Ecuador (Lasso, 1985), Nicaragua (Duarte et al., 1991) and Guatemala (Kramer et al., 1998).

In the United States (Ubelaker & Hall, 1979; Hulbert et al., 1992), Colombia (Malek, 1981), Panama (Tesh et al., 1973) and Caribbean islands (Juminer et al., 1993; Jeandel et al., 1998), reports of the presence of the parasite in the definitive host preceded the finding of cases of abdominal angiostrongyliais. It is thus possible that the distribution of this zoonosis in the Americas and the world at large is more ample than currently known.

Angiostrongyliais caused by *A. cantonensis* was originally reported in Asia. It has been postulated that this zoonosis spread to the Americas in the twentieth century (Pascual et al., 1981), where there have been reports of sporadic outbreaks. The first report of eosinophilic meningoencephalitis occurred in Cuba (Aguiar et al., 1981), followed by United States (News et al., 1995), Jamaica (Barrow et al., 1996), Brazil (Lima et al., 2009) and more recently Ecuador (Dorta-Contreras et al., 2011). After the reports of parasitism in humans, the naturally infected definitive host was identified, except in Ecuador. In contrast, in Puerto Rico, Dominican Republic and Haiti, only the parasite infecting snails and/or rats has been reported (Andersen et al., 1986; Vargas et al., 1992; Raccurt et al., 2003), with no cases of diseased reported so far.

7. Diagnostic methods for detection of abdominal angiostrongyliasis and eosinophilic meningoencephalitis

Abdominal angiostrongyliasis is caused by the presence of *A. costaricensis* worms in the mesenteric arteries of the ileocecal plexus, where they cause a predominantly eosinophilic granulomatous reaction in the mesentery, intestinal wall and lymph nodes. Although it is not generally a serious disease and frequently clears up spontaneously, its evolution to occlusion or perforation of the intestine can lead to death (Palomino et al., 2008). The main clinical signs include acute eosinophilic abdominal pain and occasionally fever (Morera, 1995). Palpation of the tumoral mass in the lower right abdominal quadrant, vomiting and anorexia suggest parasitism, but definitive diagnosis is only confirmed by observation of the worms inside the arteries after histological examination of biopsy material (Graeff-Teixeira et al, 1991). Laboratory diagnosis includes the serological latex agglutination test (Morera & Amador, 1998), enzyme-linked immunosorbent assay (ELISA) Graeff-Teixeira et al., 1997) and indirect immunofluorescence assay (Abrahams-Sandi et al., 2011). Nevertheless, the choice of the antigen and specificity of the tests need improvement.

Presumptive diagnosis of angiostrongyliasis caused by *A. cantonensis* is mainly based on the clinical signs presented by the patients, which include eosinophilic meningitis, eosinophilic encephalitis and ocular angiostrongyliasis. The symptoms in general are not very specific and can include headache, vomiting, fever, history of paresthesia and neck stiffness (Sawanyawisuth & Sawanyawisuth, 2008). Results of laboratory analysis of the blood and cerebrospinal fluid showing readings of eosinophils above 10%, including serological tests, despite their low sensitivity (Eamsobhana & Yong, 2009), along with diagnosis by cerebral imaging, help to confirm the infection (Kampittaya et al., 2000). The information reported by the patient, such as ingestion of the intermediate host snail or raw or undercooked paratenic hosts, is important to substantiate the diagnosis of eosinophilic meningoencephalitis caused by *A. cantonensis*. Confirmation of the parasitism by observation of the worm in the cerebrospinal fluid is not common (Yii, 1976; Punyagupta et al., 1975). More recently, infection has been confirmed by the presence of the helminth's DNA in the cerebrospinal fluid by real-time polymerase chain reaction (PCR) (Lima et al., 2009). The inflammatory process of the subarachnoid space and meninges is accompanied by intense eosinophilia and associated with an elevation in the number of eosinophils in the peripheral blood and cerebrospinal fluid (Tseng, et al., 2011).

8. Treatment of the infections and prophylaxis

The use of anthelmintics such as diethylcarbamazine, thiabendazole and levamisole to treat abdominal angiostrongyliasis is not recommended, because it can induce erratic migration of the worms and/or worsening of the lesions due to the inflammatory response to the death of the helminths at the infection sites (Morera & Bontempo, 1985). Therefore, any time possible, the treatment of choice is surgery (Cépedes et al., 1967).

The main procedure to treat eosinophilic meningoencephalitis is based on reduction of the symptoms by the use of analgesics and/or corticoids and careful removal of the cerebrospinal fluid (CSF) at frequent intervals (Slom et al., 2003). The combined use of albendazole and prednisolone for two weeks has been shown to be safe and effective (Chotmongkol et al., 2004). Generally, infections caused by *A. cantonensis* are slight or self-limiting and the prognosis is good. In a few weeks most of the symptoms disappear and rarely leave prolonged effects.

Prophylaxis for angiostrongyliasis requires some precautions: (a) consume snails or animals that can be intermediate or paratenic hosts only after adequate cooking; (b) do not consume raw vegetables that have not been hygienized by soaking in a sodium hypochlorite solution; (c) control the populations of snail vectors and synanthropic rats near houses and in planted fields; and (d) provide information to people on the ways *A. costaricensis* and *A. cantonensis* are transmitted as well as the measures to follow to minimize the risk of infection by the parasite.

9. Conclusion

Under public health point of view, the spread of *A. costaricensis* and *A. cantonensis* in the New World and the presence of rats and snails in the peridomestic area poses substancial risk for future outbreaks. Therefore, reinforce the need to awareness the population about the risk of contracting angiostrongyliasis and healthcare providers should consider these parasites in the American continent to detect in time and adequate medical response. Moreover, surveillance and control of intermediate and definitive host as well as health education should be done to avoid human infections.

As for eosinophilic meningitis the epidemiology of its transmission has got importance for travel medicine currently. The increasingly widespread travel of people worldwide has led to the detection of many imported cases of this zoonosis and noteworthy for the differential diagnosis of neurological disease in travel medicine (Graeff-Teixeira et al., 2009).

10. References

Abrahams-Sandi, E., Mesén-Ramírez, P., Suarez-Chacón, D. & Fernández-Quesada, K. (2011). An indirect immunofluorescence antibody test employing whole eggs as the antigen for the diagnosis of abdominal angiostrongyliasis. *Memórias do Instituto Oswaldo Cruz*, Vol.106, No.4, pp. 303-304

Acha, P. & Szyfres, B. (2003). *Zoonoses and Communicable Diseases Man and Animals* (Third edition). Pan American Health Organization, Scientific and Tech. Publications, Washington, DC

Aguiar, P., Morera, P. & Pascual, J. (1981). First record of *Angiostrongylus cantonensis* in Cuba. *American Journal of Tropical Medicine and Hygiene*, Vol. 30, No. 5, pp. 963–965

Alicata, J. & Jindrak, K. (1970). *Angiostrongylosis* in the Pacific and Southeast Asia. Chales C.Thomas, Springfield, Illinois.

Alicata, J. (1965). Biology and distribution of the rat lungworm, *Angiostrongylus cantonensis*, and its relationship to eosinophilic meningoencephalitis and other neurological disorders of man and animals. *Advances in Parasitology*, Vol.3, pp. 223-248

Alicata, J. (1991). The discovery of *Angiostrongylus cantonensis* as a cause of human eosinophilic meningitis. *Parasitology Today*, Vol.7, No. 6,pp.151-153

Andersen, E., Gubler, D., Sorensen, K., Beddard, J. & Ash, L. (1986). First report of *Angiostrongylus cantonensis* in Puerto Rico. *American Journal of TropicalMedicine and Hygiene*, Vol. 35, No.2, pp. 319–322

Anderson, R. C. 1978. Keys to genera of the Superfamily Metastrongyloidea, In *CIH Keys to the nematodes parasites of vertebrates*, R.C. Anderson, A.G. Chabaud & S. Willmott (Eds.), 1-40, Common wealth Agricultural Bureaux, Farnham Royal, Bucks, U. K.

Archer, C. , Appleton, C. Mukaratirwa, S. & Hope, K. (2011). The rat lung-worm Angiostrongylus cantonensis: A first report in South Africa. *South Africa Medical Journal*, Vol.101, No.3, pp. 174-175

Asato, R., Taira, K., Nakamura, M., Kudaka, J., Itokazu, K. & Kawanaka, M. (2004). Changing epidemiology of *Angiostrongylus cantonensis* in Okinawa Prefecture, Japan. *Japanese Journal of Infectious Diseases*, Vol.57, pp.184-186

Ash, L. (1976). Observations on the role of mollusks and planarians in the transmission of*Angiostrongylus cantonensis* infection to man in New Caledonia. *Revista de Biologia Tropical*, Vol.24, No. 1, pp.163-174

Bahaibulaya, M. (1975). Comparative studies on the life history of *Angiostrongylus mackerrasae* Bhaibulaya 1968 and *A. cantonensis* (Chen, 1935). *International Journal of Parasitology*, Vol.5, pp. 7-20

Barrow, K., St Rose, A. & Lindo, J. (1996). Eosinophilic meningitis: is *Angiostrongylus cantonensis* endmic in Jamaica? *West Indian Medical Journal*, Vol. 45, No.2, pp. 70-71

Caldeira, R., Mendonça, C., Gouveia, C., Lenzi, H., Graeff-Teixeira, C., Lima, W., Mota, E., Pecora, I., Medeiros, A. & Carvalho, O. (2007). First Record of molluscs naturally infected with *Angiostrongylus cantonensis* (Chen, 1935) (Nematoda: Mestastrongylidae) in Brazil. *Memórias do Instituto Oswaldo Cruz*, Vol,102, No.7, pp.887-889

Campbell, R. & Little, M. (1988). The finding of *Angiostrongylus cantonensis* en rats in New Orleans. *American Journal of Tropical Medicine and Hygiene*,Vol. 38, pp.568-573

Céspede, R., Salas, J., Mekbel, S.,Troper, L., Mullner, F & Morera, P. (1967). Granulomas entéricos y linfáticos con intensa eosinofilia tisular producidos por um estrongilídeo (Strongylata). *Acta Médica Costarricence*, Vol. 10, pp. 235-255

Chabaud, A. (1972). Description de *Stefanskostrongylus dubosti* n sp. parasite du Potamogale et essai de classification des Nématodes Angiostrongylinae. *Annales de Prasitologie Humaine et Comparée*, Vol. No., pp. 735-744

Chao, D., Lin, C-C. & Chen, Y-A. (1987). Studies on growth and distribution of *Angiostrongylus cantonensis* larvae in *Ampullarium canaliculatus*. *Southeast Asian Journal of Tropical Medicine and Public Health*, Vol.18, No.7, pp. 248-252

Chen, H.T., 1935. Un nouveau nematode pulmonare. *Pulmonema cantonensis*, N. G., N sp. des rats de Canton. *Annales de Parasitologie Humaine et Comparée*,Vol.13, No.4, 312-317

Cheng, T. & Alicata, J. (1965). On the modes of infection of *Achatina fulica* by the larvae of *Angiostrongylus cantonensis*. *Malacologia*, Vol.2, pp.267-274

Chotmongkol, V., Wongjitrat, C., Sawadpanit, K. & Sawanyawisuth, K. (2004). Treatment of eosinophilic meningitis with a combination of albendazole and corticosteroid. *Southeast Asian Journal of Tropical Medicine and Public* Health, Vol. 35, No. 1, pp.172-174

Cross, J. & Chi, C. (1982). ELISA for the detection of *Angiostrongylus cantonensis antibodies* in patients with eosinophilic meningitis. *Southeast Asian Journal of Tropical Medicine and Public Health*, Vol.13, No. 1, pp. 73-76

Cross, J. (1987). Public health importance of Angiostrongylus cantonensis and its relatives. *Parasitology Today*, Vol. 3, No. 12, pp.367-369

Dorta-Contreras, A., Padilla-Docal, B., Moreira, J., Robles, L., Aroca, J., Alarcón, F. & Bu-Coifu-Fanego, F. (2011). *Arquivo de Neuropsiquiatria*, Vol. 69, No.3, pp. 466-469

Diaz, J. (2008). Helminth eosinophilic meningitis: emerging zoonotoc diseases in the South. *Journal of the Louisiana State Medical Society*, Vol.160, No. 6, pp. 333-342

Dougherty, E. (1946). The genus *Aelulostrongylus* Cameron, 1927 (Nematoda : Metastrongylidae) and its relatives withj description of parafilaroides gen. Nov., and *Angiostrongylus gubernaculatus* sp. nov. *Proceedings of the Helminthological Society of Washington*, Vol.13, pp. 16-26

Drozdz, J. (1970). Révision de le systématique du genre *Angiostrongylus* Kamensky, 1905 (Nematoda :Matastronguloidea). *Annales de Parasitologie (Paris)*, Vol.45, No.5, pp. 597-603

Duarte, Z., Moreira, P. &Vuong, P. (1991). Abdominal angiostrongyliasis in Nicaragua: a clinico-pathological study on a series of twelve case reports. *Annales de Parasitologie Humaine et Comparée*, Vol.66, No.6, pp. 259-262

Eamsobhana, P. & Yong, H. (2009). Immunological diagnosis of human angiostrongyliasis due to *Angiostrongylus cantonensis* (Nematoda: Angiostrongylidae). *International Journal of Infectious Diseases*, Vol.13, No.4, pp. 425-31

Foronda, P., López-González, M., Miquel, J., Torres, J., Segovia, M., Abreu-Costa, N., Casanova, J., Valladares, B., Mas-Coma, S., Bargues, M. & Feliu, C. (2010). Finding of *Parastrongylus cantonensis* (Chen, 1935) in *Rattus norvegicus* in Terrife, Canary Island (Spain). *Acta Tropica*, Vol.114, pp. 123-127, 2010

Graeff-Teixeira, C., Camillo-Coura, L. & Lenzi, H. (1987). Abdominal angiostrongyliasis-an underdiagnosed disease. *Memórias do Instituto Oswaldo Cruz*, Vol.82, No.4, pp 353-354

Graeff-Teixeira, C., Thomé, J., Pinto, S., Camillo-Coura, L. & Lenzi, H. (1989). *Phyllocaulis variegatus* - an intermediate host of *Angiostrongylus costaricensis* in South Brazil. *Memórias do Instituto Oswaldo Cruz,* Rio de Janeiro, Vol.84, No.1, pp. 65-68

Graeff-Teixeira, C., Pires, F., Machado, R., Camillo-Coura, L. & Lenzi, L. (1990). Identificação de Roedores Silvestres como hospedeiros do *Angiostrongylus costaricensis* no sul do Brasil. *Revista do Instituto de Medicina Tropical de São Paulo,*Vol.32, No.3, pp. 147-150

Graeff-Teixeira, C., Camillo-Coura, L., Lenzi, H. (1991a). Angiostrongilíase Abdominal - Nova Parasitose no Sul do Brasil. *Revista da Associação Medica do Rio Grande do Sul,* Porto Alegre, Vol.35, No.2, pp. 91-98

Graeff-Teixeira, C., Camillo-Coura, L., Lenzi, H. (1991b). Histopathological criteria for the diagnosis on abdominal angiostrongyliasis. *Parasitology Research,* Vol.77, No.7, pp. 606-611

Graeff-Teixeira, C., Agostini, A., Camillo-Coura, L. & Ferreira-da-Cruz, M. (1997). Seroepidemiology of abdominal angiostrongyliasis: the standardization of an immunoenzymatic assay and prevalence of antibodies in two localities in southern Brazil.*Tropical Medicine & International Health,* Vol.2, No.3, pp. 254-260

Graeff-Teixeira, C., Silva, A. & Yoshimura, K. (2009). Update on Eosinophilic Meningoencephalitis and its Clinical Relevance. *Clinical Microbiology Reviews,* pp.322-348

Jeandel, R., Fortier, G., Pitre-Delaunay, C. & Jouannele, A. (1988). *Angiostrongylus intetsinale à Angiostrongylus costaricensis.* A propôs d`um case em Martinique. *Gastroentérologie Clinique et Biologique,* Vol. 2, No. , pp. 390-393

Juminer, B., Borel., G., Mauleon, H., Durette-Desset, M., Raccurt, C., Roudier, M., Nicolás, M. & Péres, J. (1993). Natural murine infestation by *Angiostrongylus costaricensis* Morera and Céspedes, 1971, in Guadaloupe. *Bulletin de la Societé de Pathologie Exotique,* Vol.86, No.5, pp. 502-505

Kaminsky, R., Caballero, R. & Andrews, K. (1995). Presencia de *Angiostrongylus costaricensis* en Honduras y sus relaciones agro-ecológicas y humanas. *Parasitología al Día,* Vol. 19, No. 1, pp. 81-90

Kanpittaya, J., Jitipmolmard, S., Tiamkao, S. & Mairiang, E. (2000). MR findings of eosinophilic meningoencephalitis attributed to *Angiostrongylus cantonensis. Am. J. Neuroradiol,* Vol.21, No.6, pp. 1090-1094

Kliks, M. & Palumbo, N. (1992). Eosinophilic meningitis beyond the Pacific basin: The global dispersal of a peridomestic zoonosis caused by *Angiostrongylus cantonensis,* the nematode lungworm of rats. *Social Science and Medicine, Vol.34,* No.2,pp.199-212

Kramer, M., Greer, G., Quinonez, J., Padilla, N., Hernandez., Barana, B., Lorenzana, R., Moreira, P., Hightower, A., Eberhard, M. & Herwaldt, B. (1998). First reported outbreak of abdominal angiostrongyliasis. *Clinical Infectious Diseases,* Vol.26, No.2, pp. 365-372

Lasso, R. 1985. Angiostrongyliasis em Ecuador. *Universidad de Guayaquil Comisión de Ciencia y tecnologia Boletín informativo,* No.3

Lima, A., Mesquita, S., Santos, S., Aquino, E., Rosa, L., Duarte, F., Teixeira, A., Costa, Z. & Ferreira, M. (2009) Alicata disease: neuroinfestation by *Angiostrongylus cantonensis* in Recife, Pernambuco, Brazil. *Arquivos de Neuropsiquiatria,* Vol.67, No.4, pp. 1093-1096

Lindo, J., Waugh, C., Hall, J., Cunningham-Myrie, C., Ashley, D., Eberhard, M., Sullivan, J., Bishop, H., Robinson, D., Holtz, T. & Robinson, R. (2002). Enzootic *Angiostrongylus cantonensis* in rats and snails after outbreak of human eosinophilic meningitis Jamaica. *Emerging Infectious Diseases,* Vol.8, No.3, pp. 324-326

Lv S, Zhang Y, Steinmann P. & Zhou XN 2008. Emerging angiostrongyliasis in mainland China. *Emerging Infectious Diseases,* Vol.14, No.1,pp.161-164

Lv, S., Zhang, Y, Liu H., Zhang, C., Steinmann, P., Zhou, X. & Utzinger, J. (2009). *Angiostrongylus cantonensis*: morphological and behavioral investigation within the freshwater snail *Pomacea canaliculata. Parasitology Research,* Vol.3, No.2, 368

Lv, S., Zhang, Y., Steinmann, P., Yang, G-J., Yang, K., Zhou, X-N. & Utzinger, J. (2011). The emergence of angiostrongyliasis in the People's Republic of China: the interplay between invasive snails, climate change and transmission dynamics. *Freshwater Biology,* Vol.56, No.4, pp. 717-734

Magalhães, A., Andrade, G., Koh, L., Soares, M., Alves, E., Tubino, P., Santos, F. & Raick, A. (1982). Novo caso de angiostrongilose abdominal. *Revista do Instituto de Medicina Tropical de São Paulo,* Vol.24, No.4, pp. 252-256

Maldonado Jr., A, Simões, R., Oliveira, A., Motta, E., Fernandez, M., Pereira, Z., Monteiro, S., Torres, E., Thiengo, S. (2010) First report of *Angiostrongylus cantonensis* (Nematoda: Metastrongylidae) in *Achatina fulica* (Mollusca: Gastropoda) from Southeast and South regions of Brazil. *Memórias do Instituto Oswaldo Cruz*Vol.105, No.7, pp. 938-941

Malek, E. & Cheng, T. (1974). *Medical and Economic Malacology.* Academic Press, New York, London

Malek, E. (1981). Presence of *Angiostrongylus costaricensis* Morera and Cépedes, 1971 in Colombia. *The American Journal of Tropical Medicine and Hygiene,* Vol.30, No.1, pp. 81-83

Miller, C., Kinsella, J., Garner, M., Evans, S., Gullet, P. & Schmidt, R. (2006). Endemic infections of *Parastrongylus* (=*Angiostrongylus*) *costaricensis* in two species of non human primates, raccons, and opossum from Miami, Florida. *Journal of Parasitology* Vol.92, No.2, pp. 406-408

Morera, P. (1967). Granulomas entericos y linfaticos con intensa eosinophilia tisular producidos por um estrongilideo (Strongylata; Railliet y Henry, 1913): II. Aspectos parasitológico. *Acta Médica Costarricence,* Vol. 10, pp. 257-265

Morera, P. (1970). Investigación del huésped definitivo de Angiostrongylus costaricensis (Morera y Céspedes, 1971). *Boletin Chileno de Parasitologia,* Santiago, Vol.25, pp.133-134

Morera, P. (1973). Life History and Redescription of *Angiostrongylus costaricensis* Moreira and Céspedes. *The American Journal of Tropical Medicine and Hygiene,* Vol.22, No.5, pp. 613-621

Morera, P. (1988). Angiostrongilosis abdominal: um problema de salud pública? *Revista de la Sociedad Guatemalteca de Parasitología y Medicina Tropical*, Vol.2, No.1, pp. 9-11

Morera, P. (1995). Abdominal angiostrongyliasis, In: *Enteric infection: intestinal helminths*, P. Morera (Ed.), 225-230, Chapman & Hall, London

Morera, P. & Céspede, R. (1971). *Angiostrongylus costaricensis* n. sp. (Nematoda: Metastrongyloidea), a new lungworm occurring in man in Costa Rica. *Revista de Biologia Tropical*, Vol.50, No.2, pp. 377-394

Morera, P. & Bontempo, I. (1985). Accion de lagunos antohelminticos sobre *Angiostrongylus costaricensis*. *Revista Medica del Hospital Nacional de Niños Costa Rica*, Vol.20, pp.165-174

Morera, P. & Amador, J. (1998). Prevalencia de la angiostrongilosis abdominal y la distribución estacional de la precipitación. *Revista Costarricense de Salud Pública*, Vol.7, No.13, pp. 1-14, ISSN 1409-1429

Motta, E. & Lenzi, H. (1995). *Angiostrongylus costaricensis* life cycle: a new proposal. *Memórias do Instituto Oswaldo Cruz*, Vol.90, No.6. PP.707-709

Narain, K., Mahanta, J., Dutta, R. & Dutta, P. (1994). Paddy Field dermatitis in Assam: A cercarial dermatitis. *Journal of Communicable Disease*, Vol.26, No.1,pp.26-30

Narain, K., Mahanta, J., Dutta, R. & Dutta, P. (1994). Paddy Field dermatitis in Assam: A cercarial dermatitis. *Journal of Communicable Disease*, Vol.26, No.1,pp.26-30

New, D., Little, M. & Cross, J. (1995). *Angiostrongylus cantonensis* infection from eating raw snails. *The New England Journal of Medicine*, Vol.332, No.16, pp. 1105-1106

Palominos, P., Gasnier, R., Rodriguez, R., Agostini, A. & Graeff-Teixeira, C. (2008). Individual serological follow-up of patients with suspected or confirmed abdominal angiostrongyliasis. *Memórias do Instituto Oswaldo Cruz*, Vol.103, No.1, pp. 93-97

Pascual, J., Bouli, R. & Aguiar, H. (1981). Eosinophilic meningoencephalitis in Cuba, cusedb by *Angiostrongylus cantonensis*. *The American Journal of Tropical Medicine and Hygiene*, Vol. 30, No. 5, pp. 960-962

Prociv, P., Spratt, D. & Carlisle, M. (2000). Neuro-angiostrongyliasis: unresolved issues. *International Journal of Parasitology, Vol.30*, No.12-13,pp.1295-1303

Punyagupta, S., Juttijudata, P. & Bunnag, T. (1975). Eosinophilic meningitis in Thailand. Clinical studies of 484 typical cases probably caused by *Angiostrongylus cantonensis*. *The American Journal of Tropical Medicine and Hygiene*, Vol.21, No.6, pp. 921-931

Raccurt, C., Blaise, J. & Durette-Desset, M. (2003). Présence d'*Angiostrongylus cantonensis* en Haiti. *Tropical Medicine and International Health*, Vol.8, No.5, pp. 423–426

Rodríguez, B., Gonzáles, R. & Chinchilla, M. (2000). Helmintos parásitos de la rata *Sigmodon hispidus* (Rodentia: Cricetidae) de un hábitat estacional y otro perenne en Costa Rica. *Revista de Biología Tropical*, Vol.48, No. 1, pp. 121-123

Sauerbrey, M. (1977). A precipitin test in the diagnosis of human abdominal angiostrongyliasis. *The American Journal of Tropical Medicine and Hygiene*, Vol. 26, No.6, pp. 1156-1158

Sawanyawisuth, K. & Sawanyawisuth, K. (2008). Treatment of angiostrongyliasis.*Transaction of the Royal Society of Tropical Medicine and Hyiene*, Vol.*102*, No.10, pp. 990-996

Sierra, E. & Morera, P. (1972). Angiostrongilosis abdominal. Primer caso humano encontrado em Honduras (Hospital Evangélico de Siguatepeque). *Acta Médica Costarricense*, Vol.14, pp. 95-99

Simões, R., Monteiro, F., Sánchez, E., Thiengo, S., Garcia, J., Costa-Neto, S., Luque, J. & Maldonado Jr., A. (2011). Endemic Angiostrongyliasis, Rio de Janeiro, Brazil. *Emerging Infectious Diseases*, Vol.17, No.7, pp. 1331-1333

Slom, T. & Johnson, S. (2003). Eosinophilic Meningitis. *Current Infection Disease Reports*, Vol.5, No.4, pp. 322-8

Tesh, R., Ackermann, L., Dietz, W. & Williams, J. (1973). *Angyostrongylus costaricensis* in Panamá. Prevalence and Pathologic Findings in wild rodents infected with this parasite. *The American Journal of Tropical Medicine and Hygiene*,Vol.22, No.3, pp.348-356

Thiengo, S. (1996). Mode of infection of Molluscs with Angiostrongylus costaricensis larvae (Nematoda). *Memórias do Instituto Oswaldo Cruz*, Vol.91, No.3, pp. 277-288

Thiengo, S., Faraco, F., Salgado, N., Cowie, R. & Fernandez, M. (2007). Rapid spread of an invasive snail in Soth America: the giant African snail, *Achatina fulica*, in Brasil. *Biological Invasions*, Vol.9, No.6, pp.693-702

Thiengo, S., Maldonado, A., Mota, E., Torres, E., Caldeira, R., Oliveira, A., Simões, R., Fernandez, M. & Lanfredi, R. (2010). The giant African snail *Achatina fulica* as natural intermediate host of *Angiostrongylus cantonensis* in Pernambuco, northeast Brazil. *Acta Tropica*, Vol.115, No.3, pp. 194-199

Ubelaker, J. & Hall, N. (1979). First report of *Angiostrongylus costaricensis* Morera and Céspede, 1971 i the United States. *Journal of Parasiology*, Vol.65, pp. 307, ISSN 0399-8320

Ubelaker, J. (1986). Systematics of species referred to the genus *Angiostrongylus*. *Journal of Parasitology*, Vol.72, No.2, pp. 237-244

Ubelaker, J., Bullick, G. & Caruso, J. (1980). Emergence of third-stage larvae of *Angiostrongylus costaricencis* Morera and Cespedes 1971 from *Biomphalaria glabrata* (Say). *Journal of Parasitology*, Vol.66,pp.856-857

Vargas, M., Gomez Perez, J. & Malek, E. (1992). First record of *Angiostrongylus cantonensis* (Chen 1935) (Nematoda: Metastrongylidae) in the Dominican Republic. *Tropical Medicine and* Parasitology,Vol.43, No.4, pp. 253–255

Wang, Q., Lai, D., Zhu, X., Chen, X. & Lun, Z. (2008). Human angiostrongyliasis. *The Lancet Infectious Diseases*, Vol.8, No.10, pp. 621-30

Wallace, G. & Rosen, L. (1969). Studies on eosinophilic meningitis V- Molluscan hosts of *Angiostrongylus cantonensis* on Pacific Islands. *American Journal of Tropical Medicine and Hygiene*, Vol.18, No.2, pp.206-216

Weinstein, P., Rosen, L., Laqueuer, G. & Sawyer, T. (1963). *Angiostrongylus cantonensis* infection in rats and rhesus monkeys, and observations on the survival of the parasite in vitro. *American Journal of Tropical Medicine and Hygiene*, Vol.12, pp. 358-377

Yii, C. (1976). Clinical observations on eosinophilicmeningitis and meningoencephalitis caused by *Angiostrongylus cantonensis* on Taiwan. *The American Journal of Tropical Medicine and Hygiene*, Vol.25, No.2, pp. 233-249

Yousif, F. & Ibrahim, A. (1978). The first record of *Angiostrongylus cantonensis* from Egypt, Vol.56, pp. 73-80

Zambrano, Z. (1973). Ileocolitis seudotumoral eosinofílica de origen parasitario. *Revista Latinoamerica de Patología*, Vol.12, No., pp.43-50

Zanol, J., Fernandez, M., Oliveira, A., Russo, C. & Thiengo S. (2010). The exotic invasive Snail *Achatina fulica* (Stylommatophora, Mollusca) in the State of Rio de Janeiro (Brazil): current status. *Biota Neotropica,* Vol.10, No.3, pp. 447-451

Zavala, V., Ramírez, B., Reyes, P. & Bates, F. (1974). *Angiostrongylus costaricensis. Primeiros casos MexicanosRevista de investigación clínica (Mexico),* Vol.26, No. ,pp.389-394

Zilioto, A., Kunzle, J., Rus Fernandes, L., Prates-Campos, C. & Britto-Costa, R. (1975). Angiostrongilíase: apresentação de um provável caso. *Revista do Instituto de Medicina Tropical de São Paulo,* Vol.17, No.5, pp. 312-318.

Part 5

Veterinary Zoonosis

18

Echinococcosis

Mesut Akarsu, Funda Ugur Kantar and Aytaç Gülcü
Dokuz Eylul University, Faculty of Medicine, Turkey

1. Introduction

Echinococcosis is a parasitic zoonosis caused by adult or larval stages of cestodes belonging to the genus *Echinococcus* (family Taeniidae). There are two major species of echinococcosis which are *Echinococcus granulosus* and *Echinococcus multilocularis,* which cause cystic echinococcosis (CE) and alveolar echinococcosis (AE), respectively. In endemic areas, the diseases are important for both medical and social aspects. CE and AE are both serious diseases, the latter especially so, with a high fatality rate and poor prognosis if careful clinical management is not carried out (Zhang&McManus,2006).

The annual incidence of CE ranges from <1 to 200 per 100,000 inhabitants, whereas the annual incidence of AE ranges from 0.03 to 1.2 per 100,000. It may be significantly higher in certain endemic areas. The global human burden of CE averages 285,000 diasability-adjusted life years (DALYs) and causes an annual economic loss of US $194,000,000. The mortality is also high, especially in untreated cases. The mortality, which is higher in AE than CE, reaches about %90 in untreated or inadequatelly treated cases of AE (Brunetti, 2010).

In this chapter, we evaluated this complex parazitic disease, which is a challange for the physicians in both diagnostic and theraupetic aspects. We also mentioned about the social and economic burden of the disease and investigated the control and preventive measures.

2. Epidemiology

2.1 Epidemiology of *E. granulosis*

CE has a serious impact on human health and livestock production in endemic areas such as in South and Central America, the Middle East, some sub-Saharan African countries, China, and the former Soviet Union. The overall prevelance of echinococcal infection is not clear because of the lack of systemic population surveys.

In some European countries or regions, the annual incidences of hospital cases of human CE vary between 1 and 8 per 100,000 population. High incidence rates or prevelances have also been recorded from countries in northern and eastern Africa (prevalences of 3%) and South America (for example; an annual incidence of 9.2 per 100,000 population in Uruguay in 1995).(Eckert&Deplazes,2004)

Epidemiological studies in endemic villages of Peru have shown human infection prevalences ranging from 5.5% to 9.1%, with the prevalence of CE in sheep and cattle as high as 77% and 68%, respectively(Moro et al. 2011).

A recent surveyin Spain showed human CE annual incidence rates in the range of 1.1 to 3.4 cases per 10^5 person-years, in combination with ovine or bovine CE prevalence proportions of up to 23%.(Benner et al.2010)

In China where CE is highly endemic, farmers (76%) were the main group of echinococcosis patients, followed by students (12.4%), workers including those self employed (5.2%), cadres (4.8%) and others (2%). Females outnumbered male patients with a ratio of 1.38. For 2000, the population ratio showed a significantly higher morbidity in females for echinococcosis (Yang et al,2010).

Cystic echinococcosis(CE) is an endemic zoonosis in Iran particularly in rural regions. Harandi et al prepared a study to determine the prevalence of CE among rural communities in Kerman using ultrasonography (US) and serology in southeastern Iran. Two hydatid cases (0.2%) were detected by ultrasound. Serological results showed 7.3% seropositivity, and females (8.3%) were significantly more positive than males (2.1%). There were significant difference between CE seropositivity and sex, age and occupation. Dog ownership does not appear to be a significant risk factor for CE in the region. The serological study showed that many people, especially women, had been exposed to Echinococcus eggs and had seroconverted but were not infected (Harandi et al, 2011).

Greece is another cauntry where national surveillance programmes are running for Cystic echinococcosis. The prevelance of human hydatidosis, declined from an annual incidence of 14.8 per 100,000 inhabitants during 1967-1971 to 0.3 in 2008. Late surveys revealed that in Greece the prevalence of echinococcosis was 23-39.2% for sheep, 7.6-14.7% for goats, 0% in cattle and 0.6% in pigs (Sotirakis&Chaligiannis,2010).

The prevelance of CE in sheep reported to European Food Safety Authority (EFSA) in 2008 is 4.3% in Bulgaria, 11.3% in Italy , 6.7% in Poland and 5% in Romania. High levels of sheep CE were also reported in Portugal and Greece in 2007 (9.4% and 3.9%, respectively) (http://www.efsa.europa.eu/en/scdocs/scdoc/1496.htm)

Mastin et al. evaluated the prevalence of canine echinococcosis by using coproantigen in mid/south Wales. The coproantigen prevalence identified in dogs was 10.6% , with 20.6% of farms containing at least one coproantigen-positive dog (Mastin et al, 2011).

2.2 Epidemiology of *E. multilocularis*

Although generally rare, AE deserves public health attention due to the high fatality rate of untreated patients and the high costs of treatment. Echinococcus multilocularis occurs across the Northern Hemisphere, in parts of central Europe, Russia, western China, areas of North America, and Northern Africa. In Europe, the endemic area of Echinococcus multilocularis covers parts of the western continent (France, Benelux States) and all countries of central Europe, including the Baltic States. Furthermore, foci exist in Denmark and on the Norwegian Svalbard Island In Eastern Europe, Russia belongs to the endemic area, and the parasite has also been found in Byelorussia, Ukraine, Moldavia, and Armenia(Jenkins et al,2005).

Ultrasonographic and immunodiagnostic surveys (1991 to 1997) have revealed a very high prevalence within a focus in China, where 135 (4%) of 3,331 people examined had documented AE (Craig et al,2000). A recent study from Western China including the Tibetan Plateau reported total prevalence rate of 8.1% (3.9% for alveolar echinococcosis and 4.2% for cystic echinococcosis) which is the highest level for echinococcosis ever reported in the world (Li et al,2010).

3. Pathogenesis

3.1 Pathogenesis of *E. granulosus*

The hydatid cyst has three layers:

1. The outer pericyst is a dense and fibrous zone and composed of modified host cells. It is the protective layer.
2. The middle is the laminated membrane. It is acellular and allows the passage of nutrients.
3. The inner layer is the germinative layer which gives rise to the hydatid fluid and small secondary cysts (brood capsules) which bud internally from this layer. Fragmentation of the germinative layer and brood capsules gives rise to daughter cysts. These may develop within the original cyst or separately.

The middle laminated membrane and the germinal layer form the true wall of the cyst, usually referred to as the endocyst, although the acellular laminated membrane is occasionally referred to as the ectocyst (Pedrosa et al,2000). Daughter vesicles (brood capsules) are small spheres that contain the protoscolices and are formed from rests of the germinal layer. 10-12 months after infection, protoscolices are produced in broad capsules. Cysts containing protoscolices are fertile and can produce daughter cysts, whereas cysts without protoscolices are sterile. Before becoming daughter cysts, these daughter vesicles are attached by a pedicle to the germinal layer of the mother cyst. At gross examination, the vesicles resemble a bunch of grapes. Daughter cysts may grow through the wall of the mother cyst, particularly in bone disease (Pedrosa et al,2000)

The pattern of *E. granulosus* infection varies in different geographic regions and among different populations. Among patients in Turkana, Kenya, for example, many cysts are large, unilocular and fertile. In contrast, cysts among individual in the northern hemisphere tend to be calcified, small, and infertile. The time between infection and diagnosis, intraspecies variation of the parasite and host differences (immunologic, genetic and/or nutritional) can influence these variations (Eckert&Deplazes,2004).

3.2 Pathogenesis of *E. multilocularis*

E. multilocularis can cause severe infection in humans. The metacestode tissue invades and destroys tissue, extends beyond organ borders into adjacent structures, and can metastasize to distant sites. In macroscopic sections of the human liver, the metacestodes of *E. multilocularis* exhibit an alveolar spongy structure composed of numerous irregular vesicles with diameters between less than 1 and 20 mm. There is no sharp demarcation from surrounding organ tissue. The vesicles are embedded in a very dense and hard fibrous stroma so, fibrosis and in some cases central necrosis are hallmarks of alveolar echinococcosis. The lack of limiting membrane allows exogenous budding, proliferation and infiltration into adjacent tissues, resulting in necrosis of surrounding host tissue. (Ammann& Eckert,1996; Kern 2010).

In the human host, there may be adjacent organ metastases (gall bladder, pancreas, diaphragm,etc.) or spread to distant localizations (lungs, bones, muscles, skin, brain, spine, etc.) by haematogenous or lymphatic route. The morphological structure of the *E. multilocularis* metacestode in other organs is essentially similar to that in the liver.

Microscopically, the cysts are composed of a thin laminated layer with minimal or no germinative layer. Brood capsules and protoscolices form in less than 10 percent of these cysts. The metacestode of *E. multilocularis* proliferate either by exogeneous budding and separation of smaller daughter vesicles from larger old ones, or by endogenous formation of small daughter vesicles originating from the germinal layer of older large vesicles (Hemphil et al 2010). Metacestodes can die spontaneously, followed by degeneration (Rausch et al, 1987).

4. Genetic variation and immunity

E granulosus shows genetic variations which are important for the formation of different strains. There are 10 distinct genetic types of E Granulosis (genotypes G1-10) with different biological properties important for life cycle patterns, host specificity, development rate, antigenicity, transmission dynamics, sensitivity to chemotherapeutic agents and pathology with important implications for the design and development of vaccines, diagnostic reagents and drugs (Zhang&McManus,2006).On the other hand, E multilocularis lacks this property and exhibit limited genetic variation.

Echinococcosis is mostly asymptomatic for a long period after infection but hosts' immune responce is continuous.

4.1 Immune responce against Cystic Echinococcosis (CE)

The immune responce against early *E. granulosus* infection begins after the oncosphere locates a target organ and forms hydatid cyst that causes infiltration of macrophages and eosinophil cells, and low-level polarized Th1 responses (Zhang&McManus,2006). This generally does not result in a severe inflammatory response and aged cysts tend to become surrounded by a fibrous layer that separates the laminated layer from host tissue. Antibody responses are also weak and are, normally, undetectable in the early two to three weeks following infection (Zhang et al, 2003).

As the parasite grows, it produces significant quantities of antigens that modulate the immune responses which include polarized Th2 responses, balanced with Th1 responses. Elevation of IL-4, IL-5, IL-6 and IL-10 also has been recorded in most hydatid patients where cytokine levels have been measured. In addition, IgG, especially IgG1 and IgG4, IgE and IgM are elevated as the cyst grows and becomes established. When a cyst dies naturally, is killed by chemotherapy treatment or is removed by surgery, Th2 responses drop rapidly, and Th1 responses become dominant. This can be interpreted as Th1 lymphocytes contribute significantly to the inactive stage of hydatid disease, with Th2 lymphocytes being more important in the active and transitional stages. IgG levels can be maintained in humans for several years after the cyst has been removed. In case of relaps, the Th2 responses regenerate very quickly. (Zhang&McManus,2006). These patients have high levels of IgE and IgG4, increased levels of IL-5, IL4, and IL-10, and low levels of IFN-γ compared to patients with a primary infection (Rigano et al,1995a; Rigano et al,1996). Patients with a primary infection have higher levels of IL-2, IFN-γ, and IL-5. The high level of IL-5 is in agreement with the high levels of IgG4 and IgE observed (Rigano et al,1996). There is a significant correlation between IgE and IgG4 production in sera from patients with hydatid disease and a trend toward increased IL-4 and IL-10 levels in patients who are high producers of IgE and IgG4 (Rigano,1995b; Zang et al, 2003) Serum IL-4 may be a useful marker for the follow up of patients with CE (Rigano et al, 1999).

Eosinophilis and high levels of IgE are the common consequences of infection by helminths (Bell,1996; Capron,1992). They may be important as a defense against the tissue stages of parasites that are too large to be phagocytosed (Haynes,1990). IgE-dependent mast cell reaction can be involved both in localization of eosinophils near the parasite and enhancing their antiparasitic functions (Bell,1996). Eosinophils are less phagocytic than neutrophils, but, like neutrophils, they can kill larval stages of parasites such as Echinococcus. Their activities are also enhanced by cytokines (Rainbird et al,1998; Meeusen&Balic, 2000).

4.2 Immune responce against Alveolar Echinococcosis (AE)

Human AE is a chronic and often fatal disease which is characterized by slowly developing cysts, mainly in the liver. It destroys the liver parenchyma, bile ducts and blood vessels forming necrotic cavities, causes biliary obstruction and portal hypertension. Like CE infection, Th1 responses predominate in the early stages of AE infection, with the immune response switching to a Th2 polarized profile in later progression (Zhang &McManus ,2006; Wei et al, 2004). Pathological examination of AE infection shows large granulomatous infiltrate surrounding the parasitic lesions (Vuitton et al., 1989; Ricard-Blum et al., 1996; Grenard et al., 2001).The cells involved in the formation of the periparasitic granuloma are mainly macrophages, myofibroblasts and T lymphocytes. In patients with abortive or dead lesions, a large number of CD4 T lymphocytes are present, whereas patients with active metacestodes display a significant increase in activation of predominantly CD8 T cells (Manfras et al., 2002), indicating that CD4 T cells play a role in the killing mechanism. In the absence of T cells, the cellular immune response to infection decreases that will disturb the hepatic granuloma formation. Today it is known that CD4 T cells play in limiting *E. multilocularis* proliferation, while CD8 T and B cells appeared to play a minor role in the control of parasite growth. (Dai et al 2004)

Significantly higher levels of IL-10 and IL-5 have been found in AE patients than in controls (Wellinghausen et al,1999; Sturn et al,1995; Riley et al,1985) . In contrast, IL-4 was measurable in only a minority of patients and controls. IL-12 levels were comparable between AE patients and controls and showed a similar distribution pattern to IL-10 with regard to disease progression (Zang et al,2003) AE patients experiencing a relapse of the disease have a tendency to increased production of IL-5 but lower IFN-γ_ production accompanied by significantly higher levels of IgE and IgG4 compared to patients with a primary infection (Godot et al,1997).

One of the most important issue about *E. multilocularis* is the interplay between the immunity of the host and the parasite. The disease spectrum is clearly dependent on the genetic background of the host as well as on acquired disturbances of Th1-related immunity. The laminated layer of the metacestode, and especially its carbohydrate components, plays a major role in tolerance induction. Th2-type and anti-inflammatory cytokines, IL-10 and TGF-beta, as well as nitric oxide, are involved in the maintenance of tolerance and partial inhibition of cytotoxic mechanisms. The production of nitric oxide by intraperitoneal macrophages of mice during secondary infection with Echinococcus multilocularis mediates immunosuppression at early and late stages of infection. Results of these studies in the experimental mouse model and in patients suggest that immune modulation with cytokines, such as interferon-alpha, or with specific antigens could be used in the future to treat patients with alveolar echinococcosis and/or to prevent this very severe parasitic disease (Dai et al,2003; Vuitton&Gottstein,2010)

5. Life cycle and transmission

The life cycle of Echinococcus includes a definitive host (usually dogs or related species) and an intermediate host (herbivores such as sheep, horses, cattle, pigs, goats and camels,etc). Humans are incidental hosts; they do not play a role in the transmission cycle. *E. granulosus* adult tapeworms are usually found in dogs or other canids. *E. multilocularis* adult tapeworms are usually found in foxes, other canids, or occasionally cats.

The tapeworm of *E. granulosus* in definitive host is composed of at least three proglottid segments which have both male and female sexual organs, which are about 2-7 mm long. They can produce thousands of parasite eggs 30 to 40 µm in size containing embryos (oncospheres). Gravid proglottids or released eggs are shed in the faeces and, following their ingestion by a human or ungulate host, an oncosphere larva is released that penetrates the intestinal epithelium into the lamina propria. This is then transported passively through blood or lymph to the target organs where it develops into a hydatid cyst. About 5 days after ingestion of eggs of *E. granulosus*, the metacestode forms. It is a small vesicle which is about 60 to70 mm in diameter consisting of an internal cellular layer (germinal layer) and an outer acellular, laminated layer. Endocyst gradually expands and induces a granulomatous host reaction, followed by a fibrous tissue reaction and the formation of a connective tissue layer (pericyst). *E. granulosus* cysts in the human body is highly variable in size and usually ranges between 1 and 15 cm but much larger cysts (20 cm in diameter) may also ocur (Ammann&Eckert,1996; Eckert&Plazes ,2004).

E. multilocularis worms are up to 4 mm long with two to six proglottic segments. The metacestode stage of *E. multilocularis* is a tumor-like multivesicular, infiltrating structure consisting of numerous small vesicles embedded in stroma of connective tissue; the larval mass usually contains a semisolid matrix rather than fluid (Eckert & Plazes, 2004). This exogenous tumour-like proliferation, which leads to infiltration of the affected organs and, in progressive cases, to severe disease and even death. The single vesicle has a wall structure similar to that of the metacestode of *E. granulosus* (germinal and laminated layer).

E. granulosus eggs can survive under humid conditions for several weeks or months in areas of warm and cold climates,but they are sensitive to desiccation (Eckert et al,2001). Eggs of *E. multilocularis* remain infective for approximately 1 year in a suitable, moist environment at lower temperatures, but they are sensitive to desiccation and high temperatures (Veit et al,1995). These eggs can survive at(-) 50°C for 24 h but are killed at (-) 70°C within 96 h and at (-)80 to (-)83°C within 48 h. Deep-freezing at (-)70°C for at least 4 days or at (-)80°C for at least 2 days is recommended for inactivating *E. multilocularis* eggs in carcasses or intestines of final hosts or in fecal material before examination in the laboratory.

Humans acquire primary CE by oral uptake of *E. granulosus* eggs excreted by infected carnivores. The infection may be acquired by handling infected definitive hosts, egg-containing feces, or egg-contaminated plants or soil followed by direct hand-to-mouth transfer . Transmission frequently occurs in settings where dogs eat the viscera of slaughtered animals. The dogs then excrete infectious eggs in their feces, which are passed on to other animals or humans via fecal-oral transmission. This may occur via environmental contamination of water and cultivated vegetables, or contact between infected domestic dogs and humans (often in children). It has been shown that Echinococcus eggs adhere to the coat of dogs, particularly to the hairs around the anus and on the thighs, muzzles, and paws. It is generally assumed that humans can become exposed to the eggs of *E. multilocularis* by handling infected definitive hosts or by ingesting food or water contaminated with eggs. Direct transmission of echinococcosis from human to human does not occur since two mammalian species are required for completion of the life cycle. Prenatal transfer of *E. granulosus* does not play a role (Conn,1994; Eckert et al, 2001).

The identification of risk factors of transmission is also an important issue. In a case-control study in Argentina, spending the first years of life surrounded by a large number of dogs was found to be an important risk factor (Larrieu et al,2002). In Tibetan aeras of China (Sichuan), increased risks for CE were associated with nomadic life, age, playing with dogs, not protecting food from flies, and raising yaks or sheep (Wang et al,2001). In another study, risk factors for human cystic echinococcosis were found to be pastoral occupation, history of dog ownership, poor education, age, sex, and drinking water source (McManus,2003).

Domestic dogs and cats can also be infected with *E. multilocularis*. In a previous study in France, 5.6% of 36 dogs were identified as carriers of *E. multilocularis*, and in a further five studies in Germany and France, 0.5 to 3.7% of cats (58 of 498) were identified (by necropsy) as carriers (Eckert et al,2000). In an area of endemic infection in eastern Switzerland with an average prevalence of *E. multilocularis* in foxes of approximately 33%, only 0.30% of 660 dogs and 0.38% of 265 cats from "normal" populations were parasite carriers (Deplazes,1999). Dogs are highly susceptible to *E. multilocularis*, but cats appear to have a lower and a more variable degree of susceptibility, as observed both in several older and in more recent experimental studies (Jenkins&roming,2000). However, naturally infected cats can harbor small numbers of *E. multilocularis* worms containing fully developed eggs and are therefore potential sources of infection.

6. Clinical aspects of Echinococcus disease

6.1 Clinics in *Echinococcus granulosus*

CE can be seen in all age groups. In endemic areas, most hospital cases are recorded in the age groups between 21 and 40 years. Many infections are acquired in childhood but do not cause clinical manifestations until adulthood. The initial phase of primary infection is always asymptomatic. Latent periods may be very long such as 50 years. An analysis of 8,596 individuals in areas of endemic infection in Uruguay has revealed a significant age dependent increase of hepatic cysts detectable by ultrasonography from 0.33% in the age group from 0 to 9 years to 3.80% in the age group from 70 to 79 years. Similar observations were made in other areas of endemic infection. Morbidity is higher in younger individuals aged between 6 and 20 years (Eckert&Deplazes,2003)

The cysts of E granulosis may grow at a rate of 1-5 cm yearly or may persist without changes for years (Brunetti et al,2010). Hydatid cysts can be found in any part of the body, but liver is the most affected organ (Figure 1). Lung, brain, muscle, kidney, bone, heart and pancreas can be involved also. Up to 80% of patients infected with E granulosus have single organ involvement and a solitary cyst located in the liver (Yang et al,2006;) or lung (Brunetti&Junghanss,2009). The clinical presentation of *E. granulosus* infection depends upon the site of the cysts and their size. Small and/or calcified cysts may remain asymptomatic indefinitely. In larger cysts, there may be symptoms due to compression or rupture into neighbouring structures. (Brunetti et al,2010).

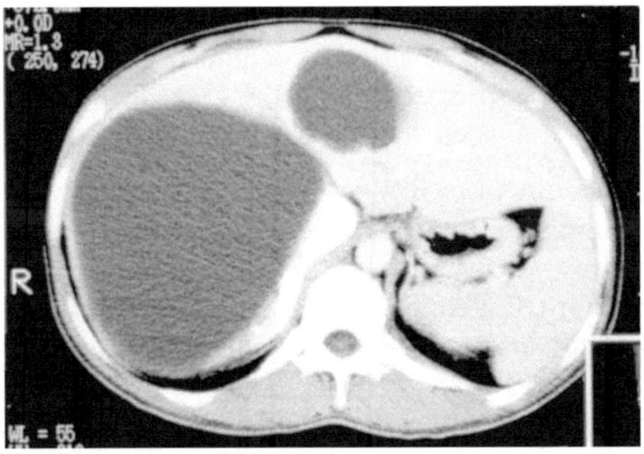

Fig. 1. CT examination shows two hypodense cystic liver lesions. Well defined fluid collections, consistent with cyst hydatid.

6.1.1 Liver involvement

E. granulosus infection of the liver frequently produces no symptoms. The right lobe is affected in 60 to 85 percent of cases. Significant symptoms are unusual before the cyst has reached at least 10 cm in diameter. The rate of growth of cysts is variable depending on the strain differences and the organ involved. Typical measurements state that the average cyst growth is 1 cm to 1.5 cm/year. Moreover, small, well-encapsulated, or calcified cysts typically do not elicit major pathology. Hydatid hepatic cyst symptoms include pain in the upper abdominal region, hepatomegaly, cholestasis, biliary cirrhosis, portal hypertension, and ascites. Serious complications include cyst rupture either into the peritoneal cavity resulting in anaphylaxis or secondary cystic Echinococcosis, cyst rupture into the biliary tree resulting in cholangitis and cholestasis. Secondary bacterial infection of the cysts can result in liver abscesses.(Scherer et al,2009)

In a study of Avgerinos et al. where they shared their 20 year experience with liver hydatidosis, the presenting symptoms or findings leading to the diagnosis of liver echinococcosis were jaundice (six cases, 17%), abdominal pain (five cases, 14%), gastrointestinal discomfort of the upper abdomen (e.g. nausea, vomiting, distention, anorexia) (two cases, 6%), acute pancreatitis (one case, 3%) and portal hypertension (one case, 3%). The rest of the cases were diagnosed incidentally (20 cases, 57%). (Avgerinos et al,2006)

6.1.2 Lung involvement

The ratio of lung:liver involvement is higher in children than in adults. Most pulmonary cases are discovered incidentally on routine radiograph evaluation; also most infected individuals remain asymptomatic until the cyst enlarges sufficiently to cause symptoms(Santivanez &Garcia,2010). Approximately 60 percent of pulmonary hydatid disease affects the right lung and 50 to 60 percent involve the lower lobes. Multiple cysts are common. Approximately 20 percent of patients with lung cysts also have liver cysts. Symptoms are usually caused by mass effect from the cyst. Complications such as cyst rupture and aggregated infection change the clinical presentation, producing cough, chest pain, hemoptysis, or vomiting. If cysts rupture into the pleural space, a pleural effusion or empyema may develop. Diagnosis is obtained by chest radiographs or computed tomography, and supported by serology. (Baden&Elliot,2003; Santivanez &Garcia,2010)

6.1.3 Other organs

Involvement of heart, central nervous system, kidneys, bone and eye have been reported in the literature. Echinococcal infections of these organs are rare but can lead to significant morbidity and mortality.Cardiac involvement is a rare, but potentially a very serious complication of the hydatid disease. The diagnosis of cardiac cyst hydatid may be difficult due to the nonspecific symptoms and varying clinical presentations. The most common localizations within the heart are left ventricle, interventricular septum, right ventricle, pericardium and right or left atrium. Infection of the heart can result in mechanical rupture with widespread dissemination or pericardial tamponade (Demircan et al,2010)

Cerebral hydatid cysts are usually supratentorial, whereas infratentorial lesions are quite rare. Clinically the disease presents as intracranial space occupying lesion and is more common in children. It can produce symptoms such as seizures and stroke(Ali et al,2009).

Cysts in the kidney can cause hematuria or flank pain, immune complex-mediated disease, glomerulonephritis leading to the nephrotic syndrome, and secondary amyloidosis (Gogus et al,2003; Gelman et al,2000) (Figure 2).

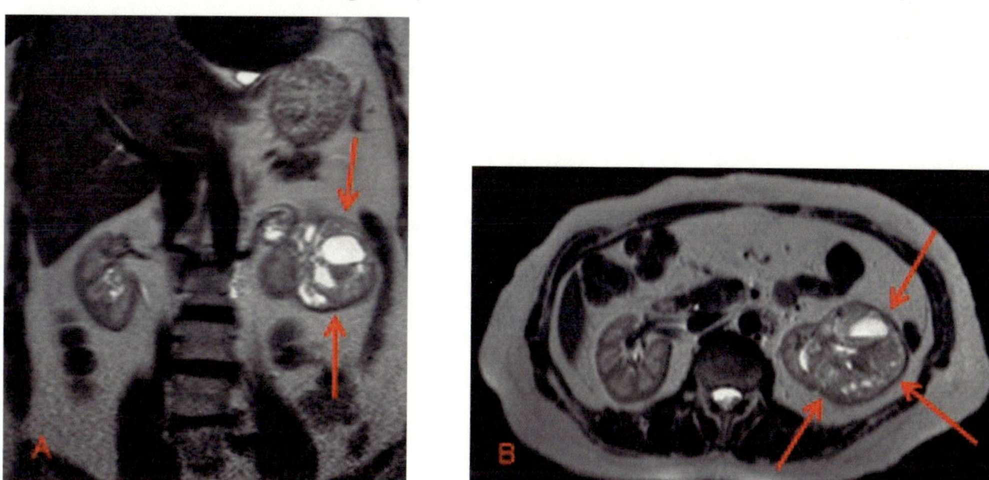

Fig. 2. A,B: MRI T2W coronal and axial images show a heterogenous semisolid cyst hydatid lesion (Gharbi type 4, WHO CE4) with hyperintense cystic areas located at the left kidney.

Bone involvement is rare (0.2-4%), affecting the spine in almost half of the cases. The other localizations are pelvis and long bones. The disease is usually silent until a complication such as paraplegia or pathologic fracture occurs. Many cases are diagnosed intraoperatively. Pre-operative diagnosis is based on radiological findings and serological assays (Papanikolaou,2008).

Ocular cysts also occur(Schallenberg et al,2007).

Cyst rupture is another severe complication of cyctic echinococosis. Acute hypersensitivity reactions including anaphylaxis, may be the principal manifestations of cyst rupture. Fever can be seen. Hypersensitivity reactions are related to the release of antigenic material and secondary immunologic reactions

Calcification occurs mostly with hepatic cyst but can also be seen in pulmonary or bone cysts. It usually requires five to 10 years to develop. Total calcification of the cyst wall suggests that that the cyst may be nonviable.

6.2 Clinics in *Echinococcus multilocularis*

Alveolar echinococcosis is characterized by an initial asymptomatic incubation period of 5–15 years and a subsequent chronic course. The infection may persist for years within an initial phase and might be detected by chance or during screening programmes. The most common presenting complaints include malaise, weight loss and right upper quadrant discomfort due to hepatomegaly. Later, severe hepatic dysfunction occurs and is often associated with portal hypertension. Cholestatic jaundice, cholangitis and the Budd-Chiari syndrome can also occur(Kern,2010).

Alveolar echinococcosis is a rare chronic and progressive disease, which can involve mostly liver and in rare cases lung and brain. It devolops predominantly in the right lobe, from foci of a few millimetres to areas of 15–20 cm in diameter, sometimes with central necrosis. Giant lesions are reported occasionally (Yapici et al,2011).

Rarely, parasitic cysts may cause compression and thrombosis of the hepatic venous outflow tract. It may present as portal hypertension and variceal upper gastrointestinal bleeding (Dulger et al,2010).

Extrahepatic primary disease is very rare (1 percent of cases). Thirteen percent of cases present as multiorgan disease where metacestodes involve the lungs, spleen,bone or brain in addition to the liver. In patients with cerebral alveolar echinococcosis, neurological symptoms prevailed, such as headache, seizures, vomiting, blindness, left face numbness, aphasia, or ataxia(Kern,2010).

Immunodeficiency, such as HIV or transplantation, may accelerate the manifestations of alveolar echinococcosis. If left untreated, mortalitiy is high(more than 90 percent of patients will die within 10 years of the onset of clinical symptoms, and virtually 100 percent by 15 years). Since treatment with albendazole has been introduced, the prognosis has improved considerably

In a recent study from France, where 362 patients with AE were evaluated. 83%of the patients were presented with clinical patterns evocative either of a digestive or a hepatic disorder. Other symptomatic patients presented with clinical pictures, generally due to metastasis or extra-hepatic location of the parasite. Except for a few patients with particularly severe AE who died shortly after the diagnosis, most patients were treated using benzimidazoles and their mortality tends to merge with that of the general French population, matched by sex, age, and calendar year (Piarroux et al,2011).

7. Diagnosis

7.1 Diagnosis of *Echinococcus granulosus*

7.1.1 Routine laboratory tests

Nonspecific leukopenia or thrombocytopenia, mild eosinophilia, and nonspecific liver function abnormalities may be detected, but are not diagnostic. Eosinophilia is seen in 15% of cases and generally occurs only if there is leakage of antigenic material.

7.1.2 Imaging

Computed tomography (CT) scanning, magnetic resonance imaging (MRI), and ultrasound are used to detect hydatid cysts and to evaluate their characteristics. Ultrasound is employed most widely because it is easy to perform and less expensive.

Plain radiography may reveal calcification within a cyst, but cannot detect uncalcified cysts and is not the imaging technique of choice.

7.1.2.1 Ultrasound

US examination is the basis of CE diagnosis in abdominal locations, at both the individual and population levels (Macpherson and Milner, 2003). It has a sensitivity of approximately 90 to 95 percennt. US may visualize cysts in liver or in other organs, including lung when cysts are peripherally located (El Fortia et al.2006). The most common appearance on ultrasound is an anechoic smooth, round cyst, which can be difficult to distinguish from a benign cyst. When the liver cyst contains membranes, mixed echoes will appear that can be confused with an abscess or neoplasm. Internal septations are due to daughter cysts. Pulmonary lesions may be single or multiple, usually do not calcify, rarely lead to daughter cyst formation, and may contain air if the cyst has ruptured.

The ultrasonographic (US) appearance of hydatid cysts may vary. The cyst wall usually manifests as double echogenic lines separated by a hypoechogenic layer. Simple cysts do not demonstrate internal structures, although multiple echogenic foci due to hydatid sand may be seen within the lesion by repositioning the patient. The term "hydatid sand," reflects a complex image which consists predominantly of hooklets and scolexes from the protoscolices. This finding may be visible when shifting the patient's position during imaging. The echogenic foci quickly fall to the most dependent portion of the cavity without forming visible strata. This finding has been referred to as the snowstorm sign (Pedrosa et al,2000).

US is the most sensitive modality for the detection of membranes, septa, and hydatid sand within the cyst. US also allows for the classification of the cyst(s) by biologic activity. Cyst may be active, transitional, or inactive. An inactive lesion include a collapsing, flattened elliptical cyst which means low pressure within the cyst, detachment of the germinal layer from the cyst wall, coarse echoes within the cyst, and calcification of the cyst Wall (Salama et al,1995; Suwan,1995). Detachment of the endocyst from the pericyst is probably related to decreasing intracystic pressure, degeneration, host response, trauma, or response to therapy. Complete detachment of the membranes inside the cyst has been referred to as the US water lily sign because of its resemblance to the radiographic water lily sign in pulmonary cysts. Cysts with a calcified rim may have an "eggshell" appearance.

Multivesicular cysts manifest as well-defined fluid collections in a honeycomb pattern with multiple septa representing the walls of the daughter cysts. Daughter cysts appear as cysts within a cyst. The matrix represents hydatid fluid containing membranes of broken daughter vesicles, scolices, and hydatid sand. Membranes within the matrix can be seen as serpentine linear structures and this finding is highly specific for hydatid disease.

When the matrix fills the cyst completely, a mixed echogenic pattern is created that mimics a solid mass. Daughter vesicles or membranes are very important images for differential diagnosis of the lesion. Cyst calcification usually occurs in the cyst wall, although internal calcification in the matrix may also be seen. When the cyst wall is heavily calcified, only the anterior portion of the wall is visualized and appears as a thick arch with a posterior concavity. Partial calcification of the cyst can not be assumed as the death of the parasite but densely calcified cysts are mostly inactive.

There are some classification systems based upon ultrasound appearance: One is the Gharbi classification, which divides cysts into five types (Gharbi,1981). Type I cysts consist of pure fluid (Figure 3); type II have a fluid collection with a split wall; type III cysts contain daughter cysts (with or without degenerated solid material); type IV have a heterogeneous echo pattern (Figure 4); and type V have a calcified wall.

In 1995, the WHO-IWGE developed a standardised classification that could be applied in all settings allowing grouping of the cysts into three relevant groups: active (CE1 and 2), transitional (CE3) and inactive (CE4 and 5) (WHO and Echinococcosis, 2003).

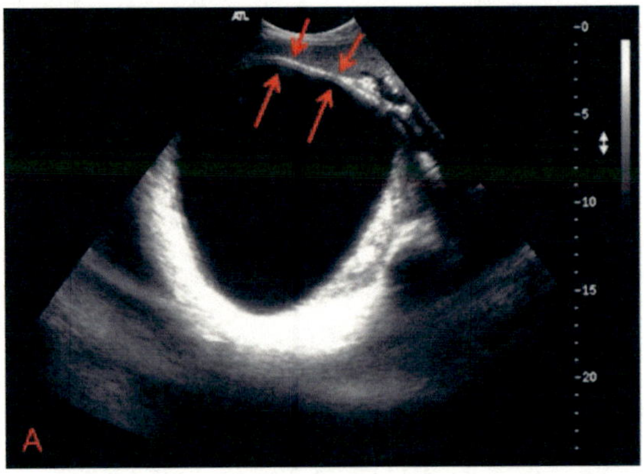

Fig. 3. A: B-mode ultrasonography demonstrating an anechoic, smooth cyst located at the right lobe of the liver: Cyst Hydatid (Gharbi type 1, WHO; CE 1). The cyst wall manifests as double echogenic lines separated by a hypoechogenic layer *(arrows)*.

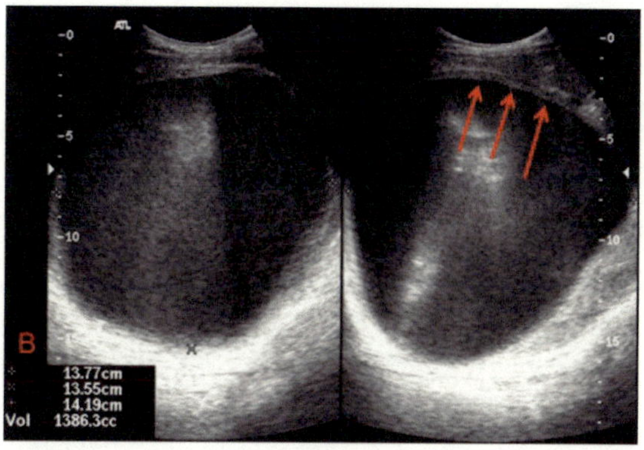

Fig. 3. B: Cyst volume: 1386 cc. Arrows indicating cyst wall.

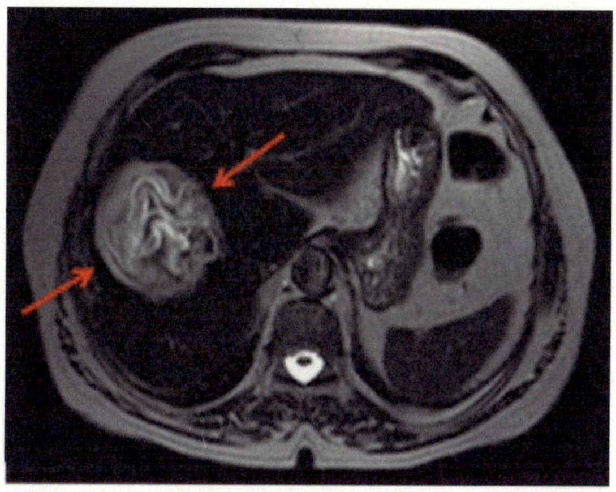

Fig. 4. MRI T2W image shows a hyperintense heterogenous cyst hydatid (Gharbi Type 4, WHO CE 4) (arrows) located at right liver lobe.

Gharbi	I	II	III	IV	V
	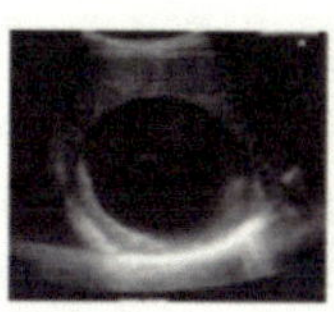	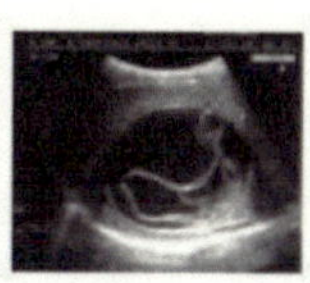	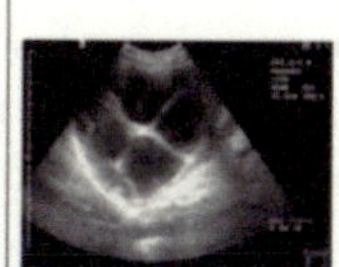	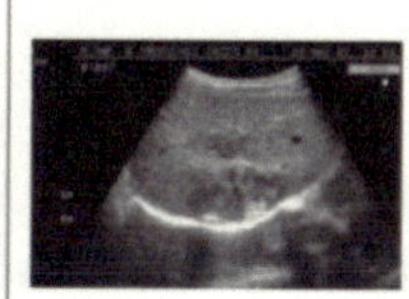	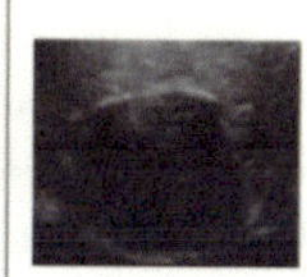
WHO	CE1	CE3a	CE2	CE4	CE5
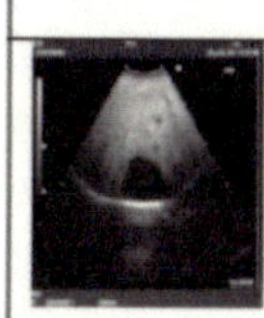			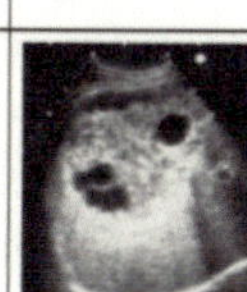		
CL			CE3b		

Table 1. Comparison of Gharbi's and WHO-IWGE ultrasound classification. (Brunetti,2010)

WHOIWGE classification differs from Gharbi's classification introduced in 1981 by adding a "cystic lesion" (CL) stage (undifferentiated), and by reversing the order of CE Types 2 and 3 . CE3 transitional cysts may be differentiated into CE3a (with detached endocyst) and CE3b (predominantly solid with daughter vesicles) (Junghanss et al et al. 2008). CE1 and CE3a are early stages and CE4 andCE5 late stages.

7.1.2.2 Computed tomography

CT is indicated in cases in where US could not be used due to patient-related difficulties such as obesity, excessive intestinal gas, abdominal wall deformities, previous surgery or disease complications. It has a high sensitivity and specificity for hepatic hydatid disease (Figure 5). Intravenous administration of contrast material is not necessary unless complications are suspected, especially infection and communication with the biliary tree. CT is best in showing cyst wall calcification, cyst infection and peritoneal seeding(Ilica et al,2007).

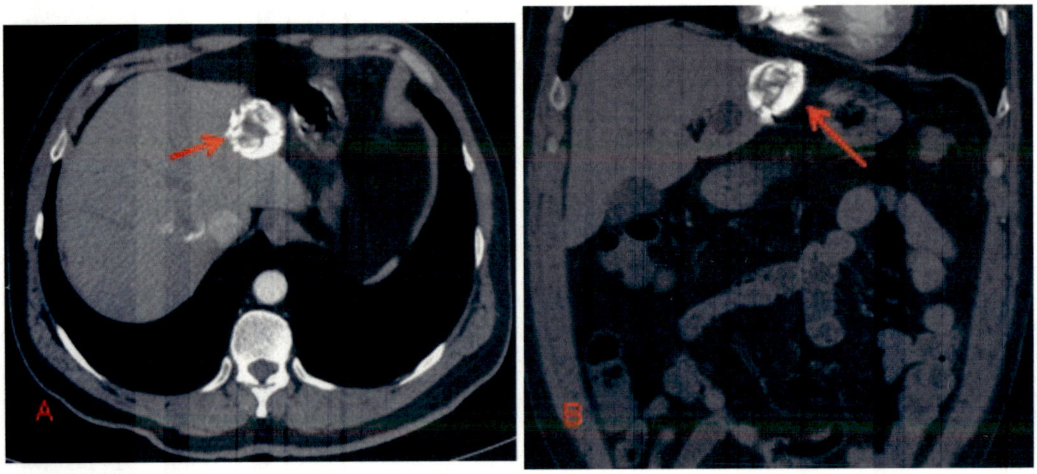

Fig. 5. A, B: CT axial (A) and coronal (B) images show hyperdense calcified cyst hydatid (arrows) (Gharbi type 5, WHO CE 5) located at the left liver lobe. Another smaller hypodense cyst hydatid lesion (arrowhead) can be seen on the coronal plane.

CT may show hepatic cystic lesion which includes many small round shaped cystic lesions that have a lower density of inner substance than the density of the inner substance of the mother cystic lesion. The presence of daughter cysts is a pathognomonic sign of the cystic hydatid nature, and these CT findings are thought to be specific for cystic echinococcosis in spite of the low appearance rate of 30%. (Ohnishi et al,2008)

In one study, ultrasound performed better than CT in the investigation of the cyst wall, hydatid sand, daughter cysts, and splitting of the cyst wall, while CT was superior in detecting gas and minute calcifications within the cysts, in attenuation measurement, and in anatomic mapping. Detachment of the laminated membrane from the pericyst can be visualized as linear areas of increased attenuation within the cyst. Daughter vesicles manifest as round structures located peripherally within the mother cyst.

Extrahepatic abdominal hydatid lesions have nearly identical imaging features, including the presence of cyst wall calcification, daughter cysts, and membrane detachment. The combinations of radiologic and serologic tests especially in patients living in the endemic areas contribute to the diagnosis(Ohnishi et al,2008; Ilica et al,2007).

7.1.2.3 Magnetic Resonance Imaging (MRI)

MRI shows the characteristic low-signal-intensity rim of the hydatid cyst on T2-weighted images(Reiterova,2005). It probably represents the outer layer of the hydatid cyst (pericyst), which is rich in collagen and is generated by the host. Although cyst wall calcification is more clearly depicted at CT, MR imaging is superior in demonstrating irregularities of the rim. These irregularities probably represent incipient detachment of the membranes (Davilo et al,1990) (Figure 6).

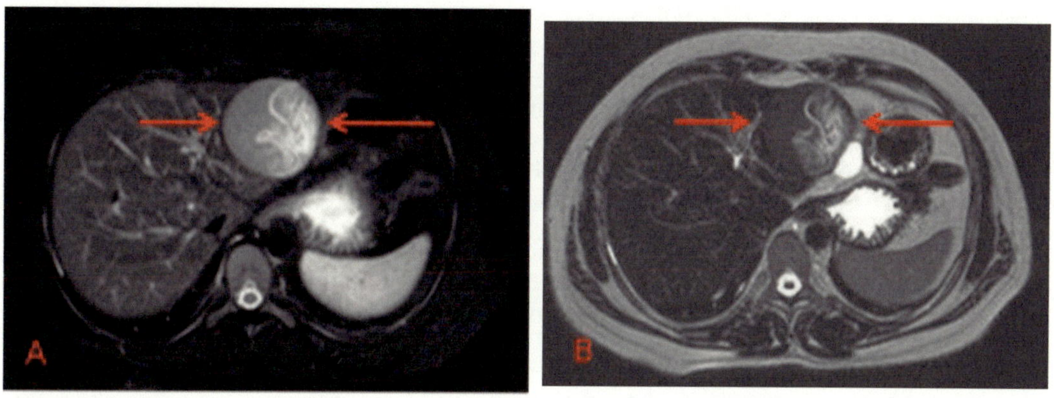

Fig. 6. A,B: MRI T2W (A) and Heavy T2W (B) images show hypointense cyst hydatid lesion with a hyperintense split wall located at the left liver lobe (Gharbi Type 2, WHO C3a).

According to WHO, computed tomography and magnetic resonance imaging, and if possible cholangiopancreatography (MRCP) are indicated in

1. Subdiaphragmatic location,
2. Disseminated disease,
3. Extraabdominal location,
4. In complicated cysts (abscess, cysto-biliary fistulae) and
5. Pre-surgical evaluation.

Whenever possible, MR imaging should be preferred to CT due to better visualization of liquid areas within the matrix (Hosch et al, 2008).

Other imaging techniques such as cholangiography may be indicated to diagnose biliary involvement, particularly in patients with cholestatic jaundice. ERCP can be performed in patients with liver cysts prior to intervention.

7.1.3 Serology

Sensitivity of serum antibody detection using indirect hemagglutination, enzyme-linked immunosorbent assay (ELISA), or latex agglutination, with hydatid cyst fluid antigens, ranges between 85 and 98% for liver cysts, 50–60% for lung cysts and 90–100% for multiple organ cysts (Siracusano and Bruschi, 2006; Ito and Craig, 2003; Siles-Lucas and Gottstein, 2001). Detection of circulating *E. granulosus* antigens in serum is less sensitive than antibody detection, which remains the method of choice. Neverthless, due to the cross-reactions with other cestode infections (*E. multilocularis* and Taenia solium), some other helminth diseases, malignancies, liver cirrhosis and presence of anti-P1 antibodies, the specificity of all tests are limited and confirmatory tests must be used (arc-5 test; Antigen B (AgB) 8 kDa/12 kDa subunits or EgAgB8/1 immunoblotting) in dubious cases (Siracusano and Bruschi, 2006; Ito and Craig, 2003.

Detection of parasite-specific IgE or IgG4 has no significant diagnostic advantage since these antibodies remain in serum for long periods following surgical removal or effective drug treatment of cysts, or even if the infection self-cures. Bulut et al showed that after surgical treatment of the disease, total IgE levels in the sera of the patients decreased to normal six months after surgery. Specific IgE against echinococcal antigens decreased one year after operation, but serum levels were still significantly high. There were no changes in the levels of anti-*Echinococcus* IgG and total IgG in follow-up period. Additionally, other parameters, such as IgA, IgM, C3 and C4, were not affected (Bulut et al, 2001). There may be also false negative results with varying frequency depending upon the site of the lesion and the cyst's integrity and viability. Antigen-antibody complexes that remove all antibodies may lead to false negative reactions. Thus, a negative serologic test generally does not rule out echinococcosis.

In fact ELISA using crude hydatid cyst fluid has a high sensitivity (over 95%) but its specificity is often unsatisfactory. If purified antigens like antigen B or other techniques such as immunoblot analysis, detection of immunoglobulin G4 (IgG4) antibodies and immunoelectropheresis are used, specificity is improved but average sensitivity is much lower. Furthermore, it should be remembered that approximately 10 to 20% of patients with hepatic cysts and about 40% with pulmonary cysts do not produce detectable specific serum antibodies (IgG) and therefore give false-negative results. Cysts in the brain, bone, or eye and calcified cysts often induce no or low antibody responses. Children and pregnant women more frequently have negative serology than other patient populations. Neverthless, immunoblotting may be used as a first-line test and is best for differential diagnosis (Akisu et al,2006; Eckert &dePlazes,2004)

7.1.4 Cyst aspiration or biopsy

Microscope examination of protoscoleces after cyst fluid aspiration using vital staining gives evidence for the parasitic nature and viability of a cyst (WHO/OIE, 2001). Detection of parasitic antigens gives no indication of viability. Presence of calcification is not reliable as an indicator of non-viability: more frequent in CE4 and CE5, it may be observed at all stages (Hosch et al, 2007).

MRS may be used to examine cyst fluid ex vivo and prepare detailed quantitative metabolite profiles, enabling a multivariate metabolomics approach to cyst staging. (Hosch et al., 2008). In vivo evaluation of cyst viability has already been performed using MR spectroscopy in cysts that do not move with respiration such as brain cysts. In a patient with hydatid disease of the brain and on albendazole treatment, Seckin et al. performed MRS before the medical therapy was begun, which revealed the typical findings of a hydatid cyst with resonance of alanine, acetate, and succinate that were specific for hydatid disease, and additional nonspecific lactate peaks with an additional small peak of choline. Two sequential MRS imaging revealed a prominent decrease of the succinate and acetate resonance, accompanied by a smaller decline of the alanine resonance progressively, correlated with the conventional MRI findings of the cyst, which had a smaller size with blurred margins in the meantime.

After 5 months of medical treatment, the cyst had completely disappeared. The patient has been monitored for 5 years and remains well without recurrence. The author concluded that changes in the metabolic profile of the cyst, especially those regarding succinate and acetate may represent the efficacy of the medical treatment.(Seckin et al, 2008) and might become possible for other locations in the future (Hosch et al, 2008).

Percutaneous aspiration of an active cysts reveal clear watery fluid containing scolices and have elevated pressure, whereas inactive cysts exhibit cloudy fluid without detectable scolices and do not have elevated pressure (Salama et al,1995). Percutaneous aspiration of liver cyst contents is associated with very low rates of complications, but this method of diagnosis is generally reserved for situations when other diagnostic methods are inconclusive because of the potential for anaphylaxis and secondary spread of the infection (Gargouri et al,1990; Khuroo et al,1993; Filice et al,1990; Giorgio et al,1992).To prevent secondary echinococcosis if a hydatid cyst is punctured, chemotherapy with albendazole is recommended for 4 days before the procedure. Chemotherapy should be continued for at least 1 month a fter puncturing a lesion that was diagnosed as an *E. granulosus* cyst even after its immediate surgical removal Increasingly, cyst puncture also is performed as a therapeutic measure.

According to WHO, the diagnostic criterias for cystic echinococcus are:

1. Typical organ lesion(s) detected by imaging techniques (e.g. US, CT-scan, plain film radiography, MR imaging
2. Specific serum antibodies assessed by high-sensitivity serological tests, confirmed by a separate high specificity serological test.
3. Histopathology or parasitology compatible with cystic echinococcosis (e.g. direct visualization of the protoscolex hooklets in cyst fluid).
4. Detection of pathognomonic macroscopic morphology of cyst(s) in surgical specimens.

WHO defines the possible versus probable versus confirmed cases as follows:

Possible case: Any patient with a clinical or epidemiological history, and imaging findings or serology positive for CE.

Probabale case: Any patient with the combination of clinical history, epidemiological history, imaging findings and serology positive for CE on two tests

Confirmed case: The above, plus either

1. Demonstration of proto scoleces or their components, using direct microscopy or molecular biology, in the cyst contents aspirated by percutaneous puncture or at surgery, or
2. Changes in US appearance, e. g. Detachment of the endocyst in a CE1 cyst, thus moving to a CE3a stage, or solidification of a CE2 or CE3b, thus changing to a CE4 stage, after administration of ABZ (at least 3 months) or spontaneous

7.2 Diagnosis of *Echinococcus multilocularis*

7.2.1 Routine laboratory tests

Nonspecific leukopenia or thrombocytopenia, mild eosinophilia, and nonspecific liver function abnormalities may be detected, but are not diagnostic. Hypergammaglobulinemia and elevated serum IgE levels are present in more than 50 percent of cases. In a recent study, absence of eosinophils in the peritoneal cavity and a low number of such cells in the blood of infected animals was observed and this was related to metacestode antigens (in vitro generated vesicle fluid and E/S products) that were able to proteolytically digest eotaxin. Proteolysis of eotaxin was, thus, dose-dependent and proportional to the time of incubation with the metacestode antigens. Absent eosinophils, thus, may be a part of a series of events that maintain a low level of inflammation displayed within the peritoneal cavity of experimentally infected mice (Mejri&Gottstein, 2009).

7.2.2 Imaging

7.2.2.1 Ultrasound

US examination is the basis of AE diagnosis in abdominal locations, at the individual and population levels, but needs an experienced examiner (Bartholomot et al., 2002; Romig et al.,1999). The lesion resembles a tumor, but the patient's overall condition is usually better than would be expected for a malignancy.

Typical findings (70% of cases) include

1. Juxtaposition of hyper- and hypoechogenic areas in a pseudo-tumour with irregular limits and scattered calcification and
2. Pseudo-cystic appearances due to a large area of central necrosis surrounded by an irregular hyperechogenic ring.

Less typical features (30% of cases) include

1. 1- Hamangioma-like hyperechogenic nodules as the initial lesion and
2. 2- A small calcified lesion due either to a dead or a smallsized developing parasite (Bresson-Hadni et al., 2000, 2006).

US with colour Doppler provides information on biliary and vascular involvement.

7.2.2.2 CT and MRI

CT gives an anatomical and morphological characterization of lesions and best depicts the characteristic pattern of calcification (WHO/OIE, 2001). In cases of diagnostic uncertainty, MR imaging may show the multivesicular morphology of the lesions, thereby supporting the diagnosis (Bresson-Hadni et al., 2006) It is the best technique to show invasions to adjacent structures. For pre-operative evaluation, MRCP has replaced percutaneous cholangiography to study the relationship between the AE lesion and the biliary tree (Bresson-Hadni et al., 2006). Initial radiological examination to exclude pulmonary and cerebral AE is recommended.

Common CT and MR imaging findings of cerebral lesion seen with *E. multilocularis* is a well-defined multiseptated mass consisting of solid and cystic components with calcification in the solid portion (Bukte et al,2004).

The characteristic radiological findings of pulmonary alveolar hydatid disease include intersegmental distribution involving the segmental veins. Alveolar hydatid disease probably spreads via emboli, in a manner similar to that of metastatic neoplasms.The absence of marked retraction of adjacent organs such as pleura, bronchus and pulmonary vessels seems to be characteristic of pulmonary alveolar hydatid disease caused by *E. multilocularis* (Ohsaki et al,2007).

7.2.3 Serology

Serology can also be helpful in the diagnosis of *E. multilocularis* infection. Immunodiagnostic tests for primary diagnosis or confirmation of imaging results are more reliable in the diagnosis of AE than of CE since more specific antigens are available. For example, the Em2plus-ELISA, using a mixture of affinity-purified *E. multilocularis* metacestode antigens (Em2-antigen) and a recombinant antigen (EmII/3-10), exhibited a diagnostic sensitivity of 97% in patients with confirmed AE and an overall specificity of 99% for infections due to other helminths. The use of purified and/or recombinant, or in vitro-produced *E. multilocularis* antigens (Em2, Em2+, Em18, etc) has a high diagnostic sensitivity of 90–100%, with a specificity of 95–100%. Most of the purified antigens allow discrimination between AE and CE in 80–95% of cases. Immunoblotting tests may be used for confirmation or as a firstline investigation if easily available. Serology usually remains positive indefinitely in patients receiving chemotherapy, yet may become negative within a few years following complete surgical resection. Clinical recurrence is often associated with rising serologic titers. IgG1 and IgG4 antibodies are the most sensitive isotypes for monitoring the success of therapy (Schantz et al,1983; Ito et al,1995; Brunetti et al,2010)

For AE screening, a combined approach using US and serology discriminates different infection status among seropositive individuals:

1. Patients with active hepatic lesions,
2. Individuals presenting with fully calcified lesions and
3. Individuals presenting with no detectable lesion at all.

The latter two variants refer to persons exposed to infection but in whom the parasite has not become established or does not progress (Vuitton et al., 2006).

According to WHO, the diagnostic criteria for alveolar echinococcus are:

1. Typical organ lesions detected by imaging techniques (e.g.abdominal US, CT, MR).
2. Detection of Echinococcus spp. specific serum antibodies by highsensitivity serological tests and confirmed by a high specificity serological test.
3. Histopathology compatible with AE.
4. Detection of *E. multilocularis* nucleic acid sequence(s) in a clinical specimen.

WHO defines the possible versus probable versus confirmed cases as follows:

Possible case: Any patient with clinical and epidemiological history and imaging findings or serology positive for AE.

Probable case: Any patient with clinical and epidemiological history, and imaging findings and serology positive for AE with two tests.

Confirmed test: The above, plus (1) histopathology compatible with AE and/or (2) detection of *E. multilocularis* nucleic acid sequence(s) in a clinical specimen

8. Treatment

8.1 Treatment of *Echinococcus granulosus*

A number of surgical and non-surgical options exist to treat cystic echinococcosis of the liver. Pre- and post-intervention chemotherapy with albendazole or mebendazole reduces the risk of disease recurrence and intraperitoneal seeding of infection that may develop by cyst rupture and spillage occurring spontaneously or during surgery or needle drainage. PAIR appears to be more effective treatment method with lower rates of major and minor complications, mortality, and disease recurrence. Hospitalization period is also shorter compared to patients treated surgically. PAIR is a safe and effective procedure of choice for patients with hepatic echinococcosis, and perhaps other anatomic sites of infection such as lung, peritoneum, kidney, and other viscera when the medication are ineffective. Surgery should be reserved for patients with hydatid cysts refractory to PAIR because of secondary bacterial infection or for those with difficult-to-manage cyst-biliary communication or obstruction(Smego et al,2005).

8.1.1 Open surgery

Indications for surgery should be evaluated carefully before making decision. Open surgery is the first treatment choice for complicated cysts, and it is also an option for complete removal of the parasite in patients who can tolerate surgery and who have cysts in amenable locations. According to WHO-IWGE experts, the indications for surgery are:

1. Removal of large CE2-CE3b cysts with multiple daughter vesicles,
2. Single liver cysts, situated superficially, that may rupture spontaneously or as a result of trauma when PTs are not available,
3. Infected cysts, again, when PTs are not available,
4. Cysts communicating with the biliary tree (as alternative to PT) and
5. Cysts exerting pressure on adjacent vital organs(Brunetti et al, 2010).

Surgery is also preferred for large liver cysts (diameter >10 cm, especially if associated with multiple daughter cysts); superficially located single liver cysts; complicated cysts such as those accompanied by infection, compression, or obstruction; or cysts in the lung, kidney, bone, brain, or other organs (Dervenis et al,2005; Safioleas et al,2006; Junghanss et al,2008).

Contraindications of surgery are (Brunetti et al, 2010):

1. Patients to whom general contraindication for surgery apply,
2. Inactive asymptomatic cyst
3. Difficult to Access cyst
4. Very small cyst

8.1.1.1 Surgical techniques

Total removal of the cyst is usually described as "pericystectomy." "Closed total pericystectomy" removes the cyst without opening it, and "open total pericystectomy" sterilizes the metacestode with protoscolicidal agents, evacuates the contents of the cyst, then removes the pericystic tissue. There is a cleavage plane between the inner layer of the host's reaction facing towards the parasite and the outer layer, or adventitia which limits the damage to liver parenchyma when dissecting around the cyst and allows safer removal of the cyst (Peng et al. 2002). All these operations can be named as total cystectomy. Partial cystectomy, in which the cyst content is sterilized and removed after opening, with the pericyst partially resected, is especially suited for endemic areas where the operations are performed by general surgeons. But the risk of secondary echinococcosis from protoscolex dissemination is higher than with total pericystectomy or total cystectomy(Brunetti et al, 2010) .

The main goals of surgical therapy include:

1. Evacuation of the cyst while avoiding spillage of its contents,
2. Neutralization of the cyst, and
3. Obliteration of the residual cavity (Safioleas et al,2006).

Adequate drainage and obliteration of the remaining cavity is a necessary procedure to minimize the possibility of serum or blood accumulation or liver abscess formation. Although conservative surgical procedures are considered simpler and safer to perform, the rate of postoperative complications such as biliary fistula, residual cavity and recurrence, and cavity suppuration has been reported to be about 35%. On the other hand, radical surgery can be performed with low risk of recurrence (3.2%).(Aydin et al. 2008).

The treatment modalities for liver cysts include total pericystectomy, partial hepatic resection and more conservative procedures including simple-closure tube drainage and cavity management via capitonnage (obliteration of residual cavity after cyst extrusion using deep purse-string suturing). Marsupialization (now rarely done), omentoplasty, introflexion or internal drainage are not commonly performed.

The surgical options for lung cysts include lobectomy, wedge resection, pericystectomy, intact endocystectomy, and capitonnage. In a large study of 842 patients followed for 3 to 20 years, a recurrence rate of 1.9 percent was noted after intact endocystectomies(Qian,1998).

Any effort made to avoid fluid spillage is recommended, including protection of peritoneal tissues and organs with protoscolicide-soaked surgical drapes and injection of protoscolicide into the cyst before opening(Brunetti et al, 2010). Twenty percent hypertonic saline is recommended, and should be in contact with the germinal layer for at least 15 minutes. (WHO/OIE, 2001). In order to reduce the risk of chemically-induced sclerosing cholangitis, its use should be avoided when communication between the cyst and the bile ducts is found. Formalin, which frequently was used for this purpose in the past, is no longer recommended because of an increased risk of sclerosing cholangitis.

Ivermectin, praziquantel (PZQ) and BMZ solutions have been used as protoscolicodal agents however, they should be further studied in humans for efficacy and safety (Bygott and Chiodini, 2009; Dziri et al., 2009). Peri-operative BMZ may reduce cyst pressure and decrease the risk of secondary CE. The length of administration usually ranges between 1 day before and 1 month after surgery but has never been formally evaluated.

8.1.1.2 Cysto-Biliary fistulas

In clinically asymptomatic patients, cyst diameter can be a clue for the presence of cysto-biliary fistulas. With a cyst diameter of 7.5cm as a cut-off point, a 79%, likelihood to find a cysto-biliary fistula was calculated (Aydin et al. 2008). When this complication is detected, sphincterotomy alone is not an adequate treatment. Most communications can be managed with suture during surgery. However, biliary-intestinal anastomosis or liver resection are sometimes necessary. It is also advisable to do an ERCP pre-PAIR and to perform postaspiration imaging of the cyst using contrast to rule out possible communication with the biliary tree.

8.1.1.3 Outcome

Complications of surgery include infection of the residual cavity, intraabdominal abscesses, anaphylactic reactions, spillage of parasite material leading to secondary echinococcosis, biliary fistulation, and sclerosing cholangitis. Surgical mortality is usually 0.5 to 4 percent for the first intervention, but increases with repeated interventions and with inadequate experience or operative facilities. Surgery is not the optimal treatment for complicated liver CE and disseminated CE (Dziri et al., 2004).

8.1.2 Laparoscopy

Laparoscopic treatment of liver echinococcosis has become increasingly popular, most suitable treatment option for the cases with anteriorly located hepatic cysts; have high success, low complication and low recurrence rates(Bickel et al,1998). Laparoscopic treatment includes partial or total pericystectomy and cyst drainage with omentoplasty. Disadvantage of laparoscopy is the lack of precautionary measures to prevent spillage under the high intraabdominal pressures caused by pneumoperitoneum(Dervenis et al,2005). Allergic reactions are more common in laparoscopic interventions due to peritoneal spillage, although length of stay is generally shorter and morbidity rates lower than for open procedures. Laparoscopic treatment is not suitable for deep intraparenchymal cysts or posterior cysts situated close to the vena cava, more than three cysts with thick and calcified walls (Chowbey et al,2003; Ertem et al,2002; Seven et al,2000).

8.1.3 Percutaneous treatments

Percutaneous treatments can broadly be divided into:

1. Those aiming at the destruction of the germinal layer (puncture, aspiration, injection and reaspiration, or PAIR) and
2. Those aiming at the evacuation of the entire endocyst (also known as Modified Catheterization Techniques). (Brunetti et al,2010)

8.1.3.1 PAIR procedure

Puncture, aspiration, injection and reaspiration (PAIR) is a percutaneous cyst puncture procedure performed under ultrasound or CT guidance followed by aspiration of substantial amounts of cyst fluid and injection of a protoscolicidal agent into the cyst cavity. PAIR confirms the diagnosis and removes parasitic material. It is minimally invasive, less risky and usually less expensive than surgery (Smego et al., 2003).

Protoscolicides used in PAIR are mainly 20% NaCl and 95% ethanol. Transhepatic cyst puncture prevents peritoneal protoscolex spillage. The cyst is then reaspirated after a period of at least 15 minutes. Prophylaxis with ABZ 4 h before and 1 month after PAIR is mandatory (WHO-IWGE, 2003a,b).

PAIR is a minimally invasive technique used in the treatment of cysts in the liver and other abdominal locations (WHO-IWGE, 2003a,b). It is indicated for inoperable patients and those who refuse surgery, in cases of relapse after surgery or failure to respond to BMZ alone. Best results with PAIR + BMZ are achieved in >5cm CE1 and CE3a cysts and suggested as first-line treatment (Khuroo et al., 1993). PAIR is contraindicated for CE2 and CE3b, for CE4 and CE5, and for lung cysts. The presence of biliary fistulae is also a contraindication for PAIR because of protoscolicide use. It should not be used in patients with inaccessible cysts, superficially located liver cysts where there is a risk of spillage into the abdominal cavity, cysts with nondrainable solid material or echogenic foci and inactive or calcified cysts.

The potential risks of this procedure include anaphylaxis, secondary echinococcosis, hemorrhage, infection, chemical sclerosing cholangitis, and biliary fistulas. PAIR should only be performed by experienced physicians with drugs and resuscitation equipment to manage anaphylactic shock at hand and a surgical back-up team. The WHO panel concluded that the use of PAIR is widespread and increasing in all areas where cystic hydatid disease is a problem and PAIR appears to be a safe and effective therapeutic tool.

In a study from Bulgaria, PAIR was performed in 230 patients with 348 echinococcal cysts. At 12-month follow-up, 77.6% of the cysts, all cystic echinococcosis (CE) 1 and CE3a cysts according to the World Health Organization Informal Working Group classification, showed various degrees of obliteration. In 11.5% of cysts, all of which were > 10 cm-type CE1, a significant amount of fluid persisted, and they were punctured again. Of those, 16 (4.6%) contained protoscolices and were treated by a second PAIR. The remaining 24 (6.9%) cysts were treated by simple aspiration or drainage. No significant reduction in size and no changes in the structure were observed in 10.9% of cysts, all of which were classified as CE2 or CE3b. Complications developed in 25.2% of patients, including severe anaphylactic reaction in two (0.9%) patients(Golemanov et al,2011).

Percutanous treatment of hydatid cysts in pregnancy is also an efficient and safe procedure in cases where percutaneous treatment is indicated (Ustunsoz et al,2008).

Ustunsoz has reported six pregnant patients (age range 19-28 years; mean age 23 years) with six hepatic hydatid cysts who underwent percutaneous treatment without albendazole prophylaxis. PAIR technique was used to treat the cysts. They used hypertonic saline solution as cytotoxic agent and followed-up patients mainly by sonography every 2 weeks during pregnancy, every third month post-partum for the first year, every 6 months for the second year, and once a year thereafter. Average hydatid cyst volume which was 2,145 ml before treatment was reduced to 145 ml post-treatment at the time of delivery. A cystobiliary fistula was found in one patient and a percutaneous catheter was placed into the postresidual cavity and a nasobiliary catheter was placed into the common bile duct after syphincterotomy. The fistula was closed in 2 weeks. This patient has a follow-up time of 1 year so far without any problem. No mortality, morbidity, fetal loss, abdominal dissemination, or tract seeding was observed among these cases.

Another paper from Turkey reported a single-center experience comparing surgery, laparoscopic surgery, and percutaneous treatments in 355 patients with 510 hydatid cysts of the liver over a period of 10 years. There were two postoperative deaths (1.08%) in the open surgery group. Biliary leakage was observed in 28 patients treated with open surgery, in 10 patients after PT, and in 2 after laparoscopic treatment. Recurrence rates were 16.2%, 3.3%, and 3.5% after open surgery, laparoscopic surgery, and percutaneous treatment, respectively. They stated that characteristics of the cyst, presence of cystobiliary communications, and the availability of a multidisciplinary team are the factors affecting the results and concluded that PAIR is effective and safe (Yagcı et al,2005).

Gabal et al. performed a modified PAIR techique for percutaneous high risk hydatid cysts. In this method, they used a coaxial catheter system to achieve concomitant evacuation of cyst contents while infusing scolicidal agent. Hypertonic saline was used to wash out cyst contents and to kill protoscolices which was followed by injection of a sclerosant (ethyl alcohol 95%) into the residual cyst cavity to prevent formation of a cyst collection after the procedure. 17 cysts in 14 patients were successfully aspirated. They found gradual decrease in cyst size (17 cysts, 100%), thickening and irregularity of the cyst wall due to separation of endocyst from pericyst (7 cysts, 41%), development of a heterogeneous appearance of the cyst components (8 cysts, 47%) and development of pseudotumor (2 cysts, 12%). They concluded that modified PAIR technique is a reliable method for percutaneous treatment of risky and symptomatic hydatid cysts (Gabal et al, 2005).

8.1.3.2 Other percutaneous treatments

Modified Catheterization Techniques are reserved for cysts that are difficult to drain or for cysts that tend to relapse after PAIR. These procedures aim to remove the entire endocyst and daughter cysts from the cyst cavity using large-bore catheters and cutting devices together with an aspiration apparatus. Among more than 1000 patients, rates of short- and medium-term success are satisfactory with minimal complications. These techniques have also been successfully employed for CE2 cysts located outside the abdomen (Akhan et al., 2007). However, long-term follow-up of patients is unavailable, and the procedure should be done with caution. (Brunetti et al,2010)

8.1.4 Antiparasitic drug treatment

Benzimidazoles (BMZ) inhibit the assembly of tubulin into microtubules, thus impairing glucose absorption through the wall of the hydatid parasite. This causes glycogen depletion and degeneration of the endoplasmic reticulum and mitochondria of the germinal layer of the metacestode, and results in an increase in lysosomes and subsequent cellular death.

WHO recommendations state that medical therapy should be used for (Brunetti et al,2010):

1. 1-Inoperable patients with liver or lung CE,
2. 2-Patients with multiple cysts in two or more organs,
3. 3-Peritoneal cysts,
4. 4-Small (<5 cm) CE1 and CE3a cysts in the liver and lung
5. 5-Prevention of recurrence following surgery or PAIR

According to WHO-IWGE experts, the contraindications for benzimidazoles are:

1. 1-Cysts at risk of rupture
2. 2-In early pregnancy

Adverse effects of benzimidazoles include hepatotoxicity, leucopenia, thrombocytopenia and alopecia, so benzimidazoles must be used with caution in patients with chronic hepatic disease and should be avoided in those with bone-marrow depression. Inactive or calcified asymptomatic cysts should not be treated unless they are complicated. BMZ alone are not effective in large cysts (over 10 cm), as their effect is extremely slow in cysts with large volumes of fluid .

BMZ can be used in patients of any age. However, there is little experience with children under-6 years old; it is less limited by the patient's status than surgery. The cure rate after a treatment period of 3-6 months with standart doses is 30%. Stojkovic et al. collected and analysed data from 711 treated patients with 1,308 cysts from six centres (five countries). Analysis was restricted to 1,159 liver and peritoneal cysts. They evaluated the importance of cyst stage and size in determining response to treatment They found that 1-2 y after initiation of benzimidazole treatment 50%-75% of active C1 cysts were classified as inactive/disappeared compared to 30%-55% of CE2 and CE3 cysts. They showed that 50%-60% of cysts <6 cm responded to treatment after 1-2 y compared to 25%-50% of cysts >6 cm. However, 25% of cysts reverted to active status within 1.5 to 2 y after having initially responded and multiple relapses were observed; after the second and third treatment 60% of cysts relapsed within 2 years. (Stojkovic et al., 2009).

8.1.4.1 Mebendazole

It is the first benzimidazole agent tested against Echinococcus. The usual dosage is 40 to 50 mg/kg per day, given in three divided doses with fat-rich meals. Maximal daily dose that can be given is 6 g. Therapy is usually indicated for at least three to six months. It is used if albendazole is not available or not tolerated.

8.1.4.2 Albendazole

Albendazole is currently the drug of choice to treat CE, either alone or together with PT. Given orally, at a dosage of 10–15 mg/kg/day, in two divided doses, with a fat-rich meal to increase its bioavailability. The hepatic metabolite of albendazole, albendazole sulfoxide, is also active against the parasite. Because of safety concern, albendazole was administered intermittently in four week courses, followed by an interval of two drug-free weeks but today it is recognised that continuous therapy does not increase the risk of side effects, and efficacy may be improved.

In cases of preoperative treatment with albendazole, the results were in favor of the 3-month treatment while even the 1-month treatment was associated with improved effectiveness compared to no treatment.(Gil-Grande et al,1993) Wen H et al and Aktan et al also performed prospective controlled trials that showed that 4-month cyclic (30 days on-therapy and 10 days off-therapy) and 3-week continuous preoperative treatment with albendazole, respectively, resulted to fewer viable cysts at the time of operation compared to no treatment. In a recent study, Stankovic et al reported statistically fewer viable protoscolices at the time of surgery for patients that received 3 weeks preoperative treatment with albendazole compared to those that received no preoperative treatment.(Wen et al,1994; Aktan et al,1996; Stankovic et al,2005)

8.1.4.3 Flubendazole

Flubendazole is another benzimidazole drug, which has been evaluated for CE treatment in both mice and men. Flubendazole has shown poor in vivo efficacy against CE in humans and mice. However, flubendazole causes marked in vitro damage on *E. granulosus* protoscoleces (Ceballos et al,2010). In a study by Ceballos et al, pharmacological performance of the benzimidazole compounds flubendazole (FLBZ) and albendazole (ABZ) were evaluated. And they stated that flubendazole offers a great potential to become a drug of choice in the treatment of cystic echinococcosis(Ceballos et al,2011)

8.1.4.4 Praziquantel

This isoquinoline has been shown to have effective protoscolicidal activity, and may be more effective than albendazole in vitro. It can be used alone or in combination with albendazole. The dose of praziquantel is 40 mg/kg once a week or 25 mg/kg orally each day. Praziquantel increases serum concentrations of albendazole sulfoxide fourfold so combination of the two drugs seems more effective in killing protoscoleces than any alone(McManus et al,2003). It usually is well tolerated but occasionally causes headache, nausea or abdominal discomfort. However, the efficacy of praziquantel has varied in clinical studies, and its role in primary chemotherapy has not been clearly defined(Wen et al,1993). In a study of Mohamed et al. 41 patients with hepatic hydatid cysts were treated with either albendazole alone or in combination with praziquantel. Albendazole alone resulted in the complete disappearance of the cyst in 36 percent of subjects with treatment periods ranging from six months to two years, while the combination led to the complete disappearance of cysts in 47 percent after only two to six months of drug therapy (Mohamed et al,1998). In another study Cobo showed that in a patient cohort with intraabdominal hydatidosis, significantly greater number of patients treated preoperatively with albendazole and praziquantel had nonviable protoscolices at the time of surgery compared to patients receiving albendazole alone, at doses of both 10 mg/kg/day and 20 mg/kg/day. (Cobo et al,1998; Smego et al, 2005)

8.1.4.5 Problems with chemotherapy

Low penetrate of the drugs through the tissue barriers to reach inner compartments of the metacestode is an important problem in clinical practice. Manterola et al. studied the plasmatic and intracystal concentrations of albendazole sulfoxide (AS) and correlated them with the viability of the scolices in patients surgically treated for hepatic hydatid cysts that received albendazole preoperatively, as an indirect way of evaluating the scolicide efficacy of the drug. The patients were given 10 mg/kg/day of albendazole for 4 days prior to the surgery. Intraoperative samples of venous blood and hydatid fluid were taken, in which the plasmatic concentration and intracystal concentration of AS were measured by means of high-performance liquid chromatography. They found that there was no association between intracystal levels of AS and the viability of the scolices and concluded that albendazole is ineffective as a scolicidal agent administered preoperatively for 4 days (Manterola et al,2005).

Since the intracystic concentration of albendazole is not correlated with the efficacy of the drug, duration of therapy may be an important issue.

8.1.4.6 Outcome

Albendazole is the drug of choice fo the treatment of CE. Studies that have directly compared mebendazole and albendazole have shown that mebendazole leads to an improvement in radiologic appearance in approximately 50 to 60 percent of patients, while 75 to 85 percent of patients show a response to albendazole (Horton,1997; Teggi et al,1993; Todorov et al,1992). The duration of treatment is shorter than mebendazole with a better response rate. The results of chemotherapy are affected by cyst characteristics such as size, age and location, as well as by host characteristics (El-On,2003).

8.1.5 Management of cysts in extra-hepatic sites

The frequency of CE in extra-hepatic site is very low, and WHO recommendations for treatment is as follows:

8.1.5.1 Lung

The presentation of pulmonary CE varies widely, making a uniform treatment recommendation impossible. BMZ used alone showed good efficacy on small, uncomplicated lung cysts but should be avoided pre-operatively in larger lung cysts. Surgery aims at removing the parasite and treating associated pathology. It should be as conservative as possible. Radical procedures are required for extended parenchymal involvement, severe pulmonary suppuration, and complications (Isitmangil et al. 2002).

8.1.5.2 Bone

Bone involvement accounts for 0.5–2% of the total number of cases and is potentially the most debilitating form of CE. The most effective treatment is radical resection of the affected bone (Zlitni et al., 2001). Surgical procedures can be repeated because of the recurrences, and some serious complications such as spinal involvement, fistulae, acute and chronic osteomyelitis, have an extremely poor prognosis. When the hip is involved, broad resections should be carried out, with the implantation of a prosthetic hip absolutely contraindicated. CE in bone is less sensitive to ABZ than cysts at other sites and high dosage and long-term administration (years) are indicated(Brunetti et al,2010).

8.1.5.3 Heart

Cardiac involvement accounts for 0.5–2% of total cases with 10% of cases showing various symptoms. Surgery is the treatment of choice (Thameur et al., 2001). Venous filters are used to prevent dissemination. If complete removal of the cysts is possible, the prognosis is good, with a low rate of recurrence.

8.1.5.4 Disseminated disease

When cysts are widespread, usually after cyst rupture, spontaneously or during surgery, a surgical approach is often impractical. If the cysts are very large or located in or near vital organs the treatment should be combined surgery and ABZ, despite its palliative nature. However, medical treatment alone with ABZ, maintained for an indefinite length of time, is the only option available in most cases, with an acceptable response (reduction in the number and/or size of lesions) (Chawla et al., 2003). Discontinuation is often associated with recurrence.

8.1.6 Watch and wait

The idea of leaving certain cyst types untreated and just monitoring them over time is a logical consequence because of two main findings:

1. A good proportion of cysts are consolidating and calcifying and becoming completely inactive without any treatment and

2. Cysts that have arrived at this stage, not compromising organ functions or causing discomfort seem to remain like this or stabilize even further(Junghanss et al,2008).

CE4 and CE5 cysts do not require any treatment if uncomplicated, CL cysts should not be treated, until their parasitic nature has been proven. Long-term follow-up of with US imaging has increased clinicians' confidence that in selected cases, i.e. when inactive cysts are not complicated, treatment can be put on hold. This decision must, however, be accompanied and verified by long-term ultrasonographic follow- up. Ten years seem to be an adequate time frame ((Junghanss et al. 2008).

8.1.7 Comparisons of therapy for *E. granulosus*

There have been few studies that have directly compared the various forms of therapy for cystic echinococcosis.

A number of surgical and non-surgical options exist to treat cystic echinococcosis of the liver. Pre- and post-intervention chemotherapy with albendazole or mebendazole reduces the risk of disease recurrence and intraperitoneal seeding of infection that may develop by cyst rupture and spillage occurring spontaneously or during surgery or needle drainage. PAIR appears to be more effective treatment method with lower rates of major and minor complications, mortality, and disease recurrence. Hospitalization period is also shorter compared to patients treated surgically. PAIR is a safe and effective procedure of choice for patients with hepatic echinococcosis, and perhaps other anatomic sites of infection such as lung, peritoneum, kidney, and other viscera when the medication are ineffective. Surgery should be reserved for patients with hydatid cysts refractory to PAIR because of secondary bacterial infection or for those with difficult-to-manage cyst-biliary communication or obstruction(Smego,2005)

8.1.8 Monitoring the response to therapy

Follow-up visits, including US examination should be done every 3–6 months initially and every year once the situation is stable. Leukocyte counts and aminotransferase measurements are necessary at monthly intervals to detect adverse reactions. Serum levels of the drugs can be measured but only few laboratories have the capacity to determine plasma drug levels (Brunetti et al,2010).

8.1.8.1 Ultrasound

Radiologic changes are not entirely reliable in assessing response to therapy. However, changes seen on ultrasound that seem to correlate with effective therapy include (Khuroo et al,1993; Sciarrino et al, 1991):

1. Reduction in cyst size and volume
2. Separation of the endocyst from the pericyst and detachment or collapse of membranes leading to a split wall (water lily sign)
3. Decrease in size or number of daughter cysts and/or rupture of vesicles in multivesicular cysts
4. Decrease in fluid within the cyst and increase of the solid component, leading first to development of internal echoes within the cyst (heterogeneous echo pattern) and then to obliteration of the cyst cavity by echogenic material (pseudotumor echo pattern)

5. Thickening and irregularity of the cyst wall
6. Complete disappearance of the cyst (Figure 7, 8).

Development of new cysts, increase in its volume or its liquid component and disappearance of visibly detaching membrane can be interpreted as relaps.(Echinonet,2005)

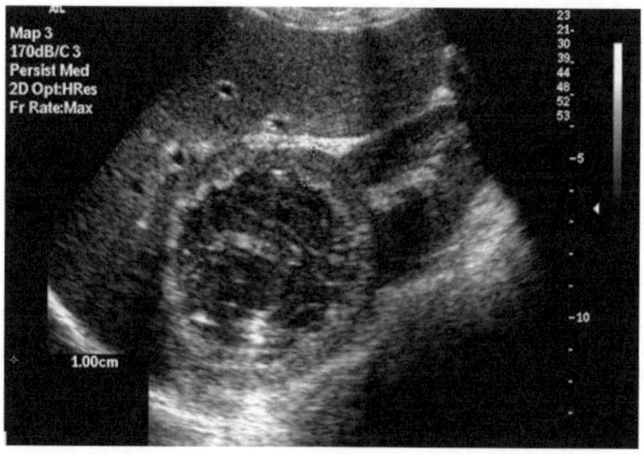

Fig. 7. Post percutaneous treatment. B-mod US shows inactive cyst containing membranes and coarse echoes. Cyst wall is markedly thickened.

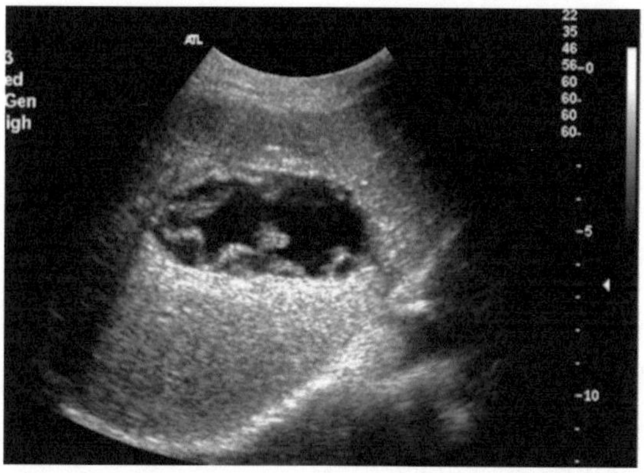

Fig. 8. Post percutaneous treatment. B-mode US shows collapsed flattened elliptical cyst (low pressure within the cyst), germinal layer detached from the cyst wall.

8.1.8.2 Serology

Serologic titers usually fall 1-2 years after successful surgery but it is not a rule. Antibodies may remain elevated even many years after cyst removal (Rigano et al,2002; Galitza et al,2006). Specific IgE antibody titers, IgG4 antibody and arc 5-based tests have been shown to be more sensitive than other tests (Baldelli et al,1992; Guisantes et al,1994; Shambesh et al,1997; Rigano et al,2002; Galitza et al,2006). There are also some new antigens which can be important in post-treatment monitoring. Nouir et al. synthesized recombinant *Echinococcus granulosus* protoscolex recP29 antigen to be preliminarily assessed by ELISA and immunoblotting and carried out on 54 young patients with cystic echinococcosis (CE). RecP29 ELISA showed a gradual decrease of antibody concentrations in all cured-CE cases that were initially (before treatment) seropositive to this antigen or that seroconverted following treatment. A complete seronegativity was reached within 3 years post-surgery in all of these cases. They showed that recombinant P29 protein appears prognostically useful for monitoring those post-surgical CE cases with an initial seropositivity to this marker (Ben Nouir ,2009). In a recent study of the same author, *Echinococcus granulosus* protoscolex soluble somatic antigens (PSSAs) were assessed for their prognostic value in the serological follow-up of young patients treated for cystic echinococcosis (CE), compared to conventional hydatid fluid (HF) antigen. They stated that PSSA represents a useful candidate to carry out a serologic follow-up of CE (Ben Nouir et al,2008).

One of the major problems of CE is the assesment of serological markers to diagnose relapses. Galitza et al. followed six cystic echinococcosis patients who underwent surgery for the removal of echinococcal cysts. All were treated with albendazole prior to and following treatment. After surgery, no cysts were detected in five of the six patients examined. Both ELISA and immunoblot analysis have been used to determine specific IgG, IgG4 and IgE activities. Total elimination of IgG and IgG4 was not achieved in any of the patients studied. Prior to the first surgery/treatment, specific IgG, IgG4 and IgE antibodies were demonstrated in all patients, except one who did not show any IgE activity. The first treatment was followed by highly elevated IgE in two patients; in one of them it was further combined with an apparent decrease in IgG activity. Repeated treatment with albendazole given 0.8-8.5 years after the first treatment/surgery was followed by either moderate or highly reduced IgE activity in two patients, respectively, and a slight increase in IgG4 in another patient. A third course of treatment, given 2-2.5 years after the second treatment, barely affected the antibody activities. The study suggests that anti-echinoccocal antibody activity may remain high many years after successful cyst removal. The presence of anti-echinococcal antibodies after surgery with no cyst detection does not necessarily indicate an active echinococcal infection (Galitza et al., 2006).

8.2 Treatment for *Echinococcus multilocularis*

The following principles should be followed for treatment for alveolar echinococcus:

1. BMZ are mandatory in all patients, temporarily after complete resection of the lesions, and for life in all other cases,
2. Interventional procedures should be preferred to palliative surgery whenever possible,
3. Radical surgery is the first choice in all cases suitable for total resection of the lesion(s) (Brunetti et al,2010).

8.2.1 Antiparasitic drug treatment

Long-term BMZ treatment for several years is mandatory in all inoperable AE patients and following surgical resection of the parasite lesions. Since residual parasite tissue may remain undetected at radical surgery, including liver transplantation(LT), BMZ should be given for at least 2 years and these patients monitored for a minimum of 10 years for possible recurrence. Pre-surgical BMZ administration is not recommended except in the case of LT. The contrandications for medical treatment consist of only the life-threatening side effects of the drugs. In cases of pregnancy, the drug should be used with cautions (Brunetti et al,2010).

The dose of albendazole is 10-15mg/kg/day given in 2 divided doses with a fat-rich meal. Continuous treatment with albendazole is preferred instead of intermittent treatment and it is well tolerated for more than 20 years. If ABZ is not available or not well tolerated, mabendazole may be given at daily doses of 40–50 mg/kg/day divided into three doses with fat-rich meals. Based on experimental data, PZQ has no place in the treatment of human AE (Marchiondo et al., 1994). Nitazoxanide has no efficacy for treatment of AE. (Kern et al., 2008). Conventional and liposomal amphothericin B have been used as a salvage treatment in a few patients who did not tolerate BMZ (Reuter et al., 2003).

During treatment, the clinican must control liver function tests initially every 2 weeks (first 3 months), then monthly (first year), then every 3 months. BMZ administration is crucial in all cases of AE, but if an increase above 5 times the upper limit of normal (ULN) of aminotransferases is observed, the following steps are recommended:

1. Check for other causes of the increase (other medication, viral hepatitis, AE-related biliary obstruction or liver abscess),
2. Monitor drug levels,
3. If ABZ sulfoxide plasma levels are higher than the recommended range of concentrations (1–3 mol/L, 4 h after morning drug intake), decrease ABZ dosage and shift to the alternative BMZ (MBZ if ABZ and vice versa) and
4. If an increase over 5×ULN persists, consult a reference centre.

Decrease of leukocyte count under 1.0×10^{9}/L indicates BMZ toxicity and warrants treatment withdrawal (Brunetti et al,2010).

Medical therapy can improve the quality and length of survival, even though benzimidazoles are only parasitostatic and not curative. Approximately one-half the patients respond with regression or at least stabilization of their lesion. Survival rates of 53 to 80 percent at 15 years have been observed with chemotherapy alone compared to 100 percent mortality at 15 years without treatment(Ammann et al,1990; Wilson et al,1992; Wilson et al,1995).

8.2.2 Surgery

Radical resection is the primary goal. Whenever possible complete resection of AE lesions should be performed. In principle, radical surgery should be avoided when R0- resection is not achievable. Excision of the entire parasitic lesion should follow the rules of tumour surgery, with a 2cm safety margin classified according to the quality of resection: (R0: no residue; R1: microscopic residue; R2: macroscopic residue). Lesions not confined to the liver are not a contraindication to surgery per se, but curative procedures have to meet the criteria for R0- resections as well. Lesions in other organs (e.g. brain) should be managed either by surgery or by alternative measures. Irrespective of the type of procedure, concomitant BMZ treatment is mandatory for at least 2 years. LT is contraindicated in the presence of extra-hepatic locations and if immunosuppressive drugs and/or BMZ are contraindicated.

Li et al published their experiences in treatment of human multiorgan alveolar echinococcis by surgery and drugs. Among 17 cases, 8 cases achieved an excellent effect after taking liposomal albendazole, 3 cases received radical hepatectomy and 1 case pneumonectomy with a better effect, 1 case of palliative liver transplantation had lung metastasis and stayed on a long-term therapy of liposomal albendazole. Another case of liver transplantation received a long-term postoperative chemotherapy. And the metastases of lung and brain were found. Three operative cases suffered serious complications in liver and brain and received a long-term chemotherapy. One of them died of serious brain complications after a 6-month follow-up. And one advanced AE patient died at home due to a refusal of any further treatment. They concluded that multi-organ AE patients may have a prolonged survival and an improved clinical outcome (Li et al,2010)

8.2.3 Liver transplantation

The indications for liver transplantation are:

1. Severe liver insufficiency (secondary biliary cirrhosis or Budd-Chiari syndrome) or recurrent life-threatening cholangitis,
2. Inability to perform radical liver resection
3. Absence of extra-hepatic AE locations: cases with residual AE in lung or abdominal cavity should be regarded as exceptional indications, (Scheuring et al., 2003).

Liver transplantation can be performed in cases with nonresectable lesions and severe liver compromise, but residual parasite tissue may be prone to more rapid growth because of the immunosuppression that is required following transplantation. In order to minimize the risk, post-transplant adjuvant chemotherapy with a benzimidazole is advised (Bresson-Hadni,1999). Moray et al. reported 2 patients with advanced alveolar echinococcal disease that invaded both lobes of the liver and neighboring vital structures including the inferior vena cava. Despite the technical difficulty of the surgery, both patients were successfully treated with living donor liver transplantation. The author concludes that liver transplantation should be accepted as a life-saving treatment of choice in patients with alveolar echinococcosis for whom there is no other medical or surgical treatment options (Moray et al,2009).

Liver transplantation is currently contraindicated in patients with residual or metastatic alveolar echinococcosis lesions. Hadni et al. evaluated the long-term course of such patients who underwent LT and were subsequently treated with benzimidazoles. They found that high doses of immunosuppressive drugs, the late introduction of therapy with benzimidazoles, its withdrawal due to side effects, and nonadherence to this therapy adversely affected the prognosis. They stated that potential recurrence of disease, especially in patients with residual or metastatic AE lesions, should not be regarded as a contraindication to LT when AE is considered to be lethal in the short term (Bresson-Hadni et al,2011).

8.2.4 Endoscopic and Percutaneous Interventions (EPI)

EPIs are indicated for complications if surgery is felt to be too high a risk and total resection of the lesions cannot be safely performed. Main indications include liver abscess due to bacterial infection of necrotic lesions, jaundice due to bile duct obstruction with or without acute cholangitis, hepatic or portal vein thrombosis and bleeding of oesophageal varices secondary to portal hypertension. But EPI spread parasite material and should be avoided if postinterventional BMZ is not possible. EPIs together with BMZ avoid palliative surgery and can improve life expectancy and quality of life of AE patients. In addition, radical resection which was not possible initially may become feasible following the shrinkage of a necrotic cavity after percutaneous drainage. Risks of EPIs include haemorrhage (for all procedures) and internal bile leakage or prolonged bile leakage through an external drain for bile duct drainage.

8.2.5 Monitoring treatment

After initiation of any type of treatment, long-term follow-up by US at shorter intervals and CT and/or MRI at intervals of 2–3 years, should be planned. Progression is documented by enlargement of lesions over time. Determination of ABZ sulfoxide blood levels, 4 h after the morning dose, is recommended 1, 4 and 12 weeks after starting treatment, and 2–4 weeks after each dose adjustment with an estimated therapeutic range of 0.65–3 mol/L. ABZ dosage should be reduced if 2 sequential measurements are above 10 mol/L. Monitoring of MBZ plasma level is possible; plasma levels should be over 250 nmol/L (WHO-IWGE, 1996).

Scheuring et al. reported a case of advanced alveolar echinococcosis which was diagnosed histologically from a subcutaneous nodule with skin inflammation on the right leg. The patient showed bone metastases in the lower thoracic spine and the left third toe by hematogenic spread. The patient was treated with albendazole and remained stable for 6 years. When progression of AE occurred the therapy was changed to mebendazole, resulting in a stable condition for further 4 years. The author showed that serum levels of Anti-Em2 and anti-Em18 antibodies decreases rapidly after complete surgical removal of the lesions. (Scheuring et al., 2003). Interpretation of serological results in patients treated with BMZ without radical resection is more complex (Tappe et al., 2009).

Ammann et al showed that in patients with curative surgery, the profiles of specific antibodies against EmII/3-10 antigen normalized within 3 years but remained above the cut-off value in 40% of non-resectable group. This lack of normalization was associated with lower bioavailability of mebendazole. AE-recurrence after 'radical' surgery was associated with high anti-EmII/3-10 concentrations.Presence of anti-II/3-10/Em18-antibodies is more likely to reflect the presence of a viable metacestode with disappearance of such antibodies indicating lesions dying-out (Ammann et al., 2004).

BMZ are only parasitostatic and many studies have demonstrated that they do not kill *E. multilocularis* metacestodes (WHO-IWGE, 1996). Methods to assess early therapeutic efficacy are lacking. Recently, AE liver lesions were reported to exhibit increased F-18-fluorodeoxyglucose (FDG) uptake in positron emission tomography. This may be an important tool when there is a tendency to stop treatment. Although it does not provide direct evidence of *E. multilocularis* viability and recurrence may occur, this technique, together with the follow-up of specific serum antibodies, may support decision making and follow-up after BMZ withdrawal in highly selected patients. (Reuter et al., 2004; Stumpe et al., 2007).

9. Economic burden of Echinococcosis

Echinococcus is an important public health and economic problem in endemic regions of the world. In humans, CE may have various consequences, including direct costs such as diagnosis, hospitalisation, surgical or percutaneous treatments, medical therapy, post-treatment care, travel for both patient and family members as well as indirect costs such as mortality, suffering and social consequences of disability, loss of working days or "production", abandonment of farming or agricultural activities by affected or at-risk persons (Battelli, 2009). In the literature, there are some studies evaluating the overall economic losses due to human and animal disease. The total estimated cost of human CE in Peru is U.S.$2,420,348 per year. Total estimated livestock-associated costs due to CE ranges from U.S.$196,681 if only direct losses (i.e., cattle and sheep liver destruction) are taken into consideration to U.S.$3,846,754 if additional production losses (liver condemnation, decreased carcass weight, wool losses, decreased milk production) are accounted for. An estimated 1,139 (95% CI: 861–1,489) disability adjusted life years (DALYs) are also lost due to surgical cases of CE (Moro et al,2011).

A study from Spain showed that the overall economic loss attributable to CE in humans and animals in 2005 was estimated at 148 964 534 euros. Human-associated losses were estimated at €133 416 601 and animal-associated losses at €15 532 242(Benner et al,2010). Another study from Turkey where the mean prevalence rates of the cystic echinococcosis disease were calculated to be 7.4% in cattle, 46.3% in sheep and 10.9% in goats, the production losses in an infected ruminant were estimated as US$ 139.2 for cattle, US$ 13.7 for sheep, and US$ 13.9 for goats. The nation-wide annual losses due to CE were estimated as US$ 32.4 million (26.2–39.1) for cattle, US$ 54.1 million (43.8–65.5) for sheep and US$ 2.7 million (2.2–3.3) for goats. The nation-wide production losses due to CE in Turkey in 2008 were calculated as US$ 89.2 million (72.2–107.9) (Sarıozkana&Yalcın, 2009).

In a report from China quantifying the economic losses due to Echinococcus multilocularis and *E. granulosus* in Shiqu County, Sichuan; showed that human losses associated with treatment costs and loss of income due to morbidity and mortality, in addition to production losses in livestock due to *E. granulosus* infection was estimated to reach 218,676 U.S. dollars if only liver-related losses in sheep, goats, and yaks are taken into account. This was equal to approximately 3.47 U.S. dollars per person annually or 1.4% of per capita gross domestic product. They stated that total annual losses could be nearly 1,000,000 U.S. dollars if additional livestock production losses were assumed (Budke et al,2005).

A report from Tunisia states that Echinococcosis causes significant direct and indirect losses in both humans and animals of approximately US dollars 10-19 million annually (Majorowski et al,2005).

The awareness of the social and economic burden of the disease accelerated the use of control and prevention programmes.

10. Control of the disease

10.1 Control of *E. granulosus* infection

Prevention of cystic echinococcosis often can be achieved mostly by avoiding close contact with dogs. Careful washing of vegetables and contaminated fresh produce can also reduce infection. Prohibition of home-slaughter of sheep will prevent dogs from consuming infected viscera, thus disrupting the life cycle of the parasite(23).

In some countries where an eradication program has been attempted (eg, Iceland, Australia and New Zealand), a marked decrease in human cases has occurred (Craig et al,2006).

Vaccination of livestock and dogs, special educational programmes, development of better diagnostics for definitive hosts and human beings (including dog coproantigen detection), more effective antiparasitic treatments and the use of mathematical models to simulate best possible cost-eff ective interventions, will improve the hydatid control programmes(Craig et al,2007).

Albendazole (ABZ), along with levamisol and ivermectin, is one of the most used antiparasitic drug in sheep, goats, cattle, horses and pigs. It has been shown that ABZ is not detected in the plasma of treated sheep at any time after administration, but its active metabolites, albendazole sulphoxide and albendazole sulphone are detectable for about 48 hr after administration. Oxfendazole (OXF), another benzimidazole like ABZ, has broad-spectrum activity against larval stages of gastrointestinal roundworms, tapeworms, and lungworms in many animal species(Lanusse et al, 1995).

In a study of Gavidia et al, effects of Oxfendazole alone (an antiparasitic drug used in animals), Oxfendazole plus Praziquantel, and Albendazole plus Praziquantel against hydatid cysts in sheep were evaluated. They demonstrated that over 4 to 6 weeks of treatment, Oxfendazole at 60 mg, combination Oxfendazole/Praziquantel and combination Albendazole/Praziquantel were successful schemas that could be added to control measures in animals. OXF has not yet been approved for human(Gavida et al,2010).

10.2 Control of *E. multilocularis* infection

Currently, there is no reliable and cost-effective method for sustainable control or eradication of *E. multilocularis* in the sylvatic cycle. Large field trials have been conducted since 1995 in Germany for mass treatment of red foxes with baits containing 50 mg of praziquantel. The baits are repeatedly distributed by light aircraft. Although first reports stated that reducing the prevalence of *E. multilocularis* in the fox population was possible, other trials suggest that long-term control of *E. multilocularis*, in the sylvatic cycle in large areas, is extremely difficult and costly(Eckert & De-Plazes ,2004). In another study in Zurich, praziquantel-containing baits were distributed every month for 2 years in six areas of 1 km2 inhabited by foxes. Preliminary results indicate a significant decrease of the environmental contamination with *E. multilocularis* eggs and of parasite prevalences in voles in baited areas compared to those in control areas (Heglin et al,2003). Monthly praziquantel given to dogs in a 10-year field trial in Alaska was effective in reducing egg contamination(Rausch et al,1990).

In areas of endemic infection with low prevalences of *E. multilocularis* infection in dog and cat populations, mass treatment of these animals may currently be neither indicated nor feasible. In these circumstances it may be appropriate to give regular praziquantel treatment every 4 weeks only to dogs and cats having access to infected rodents(Eckert & De-Plazes ,2004).

For persons at especial risk (for example, laboratory personnel working with *E. multilocularis* eggs or handling infected definitive hosts, children after exposure to feces of infected foxes, etc.), repeated serological screening for anti-*E. multilocularis* antibodies by using highly sensitive and specific tests is recommended, with the aim of detecting an infection in an early stage or excluding it with a reasonable degree of probability. Special safety precautions are recommended for laboratory and field workers possibly exposed to infective *E. multilocularis* eggs (Eckert et al,2001).

11. Vaccination

The life-cycles of *E. granulosus* and *E. multilocularis* include two hosts: an intermediate and a definitive host. Prevention of transmission to either host can reduce or even eliminate the infection in human and livestock populations. Vaccination is the most important issue for the control of the disease. Vaccination of humans would provide the most direct means to prevent echinococcosis but the economic burden might be very high. Instead, vaccination of the normal animal hosts of the parasites, indirectly achieves a reduction in human incidence by decreasing or removing the source of infective material for humans. The latter strategy would be considerably less expensive to develop and implement.(Craig et al, 2007)

The sylvatic nature of the lifecycle of *E. multilocularis* makes a vaccination approach impossible.(Zhang &McManus 2006) But a defined recombinant vaccine for ovine cystic echinococcosis (called EG95) was developed in 1996 by the groups of Marshall Lightowlers and David Heath in Australia and New Zealand. The native molecule is 24.5 kDa and cloned as a 16.5 cDNA fusion peptide of 155 aminoacids with a fibronectin-like motif under the control of seven closely related genes. EG95 vaccine, contains a purified recombinant protein of the parasite oncosphere as well as an adjuvant. Echinococcus vaccines would ideally prevent oncosphere development to hydatid cysts in sheep, and thus stop the development of adult gravid tapeworms in dogs. Two doses of the vaccine are administered initially one month apart, followed by a required annual booster. This vaccine has been studied in animals and appears to afford 95 percent protection to sheep, cattle and goats in preliminary trials(Heath et al,2003; Lightowers et al,1996,2000; Zhang,2003).

The EG95 hydatid vaccine was licensed for application in China in June 2007 and is currently being assessed for registration in Argentina. Field trials are underway in Argentina in the Tehuelche communities of Chubut province and the Mapuche communities of Rio Negro province. Clinical trials are underway in Turkey with a clostridial / EG95 combination vaccine for sheep. It would be better to incorporate EG95 with an existing commercial livestock vaccine such as tetanus, leptospirosis, or sheep orf.(Bethony et al,2011)

Compared with the major advances in vaccinating sheep against *E. granulosus*, there is currently no practical vaccine available for use in canid hosts of *E. granulosus*. However, a vaccine that reduces egg production would potentially be sufficient to limit transmission in areas where the parasite is endemic. In fact, dogs are the major definitive host for *E. granulosus* and plays a very important role in transmission. Interruption of the parasite life cycle in the dog host can provides a very acceptable and cost-effective complementary method for control by vaccination.(Zhang & McManus ,2006) Nevertheless, a series of experiments to induce immunity in dogs through vaccination have been carried out, with some encouraging results.

Zhang et al. used differential-display PCR to isolate three differentially expressed sequences (egM4, egM9 and egM123) belonging to a novel egM family of proteins expressed exclusively by mature adult worms (MAWs) of *E. granulosus* and associated with adult worm maturation and/or egg development(Zhang et al,2003b). Subsequently, the three genes were subcloned into an expression vector that expressed the molecules as soluble glutathione S-transferase (GST) fusion proteins in Escherichia coli. The three fusion proteins were purified for vaccine trials in which the dogs were vaccinated and necropsied 45 days after challenge infection (Zhang et al,2006). Compared with worms in the control dogs that received GST, the three recombinant proteins induced a high level of protection (97-100%) in terms of suppression of worm growth and, especially, of egg development and embryogenesis. This study was the first to demonstrate protection against *E. granulosus* in dogs vaccinated with recombinant proteins derived from MAWs.

Another group isolated a single copy gene (EgA31) from *E. granulosus* encoding a paramyosin-like 66-kDa fibrillar protein present in the muscles and tegument of adult worms(Fu et al, 1999). A recombinant form of EgA31 induced significant cellular immune responses in lymph nodes from dogs after intradermal injection(Fu et al,2000; Saboulard et al, 2003). Subsequently, a polypeptide encoded by the Pst I-Hind III fragment of the complete EgA31 cDNA was shown to be the most potent antigenically during infection in the dog (Saboulard et al,2003). Surprisingly, neither recombinant forms of EgA31 nor the Pst I-Hind III fragment were tested for protective efficacy in dogs challenged with *E. granulosus.*

12. Conclusion

Echinococcosis is a zoonotic parasitic disease distributed widely around the world and is an important cause of human morbidity and mortality, particularly in developing countries. Although imaging and immunological techniques for diagnosing CE and AE are improved, elimination of the disease is still difficult with current treatment modalities. Surveillance programmes and monitoring systems are very important tools in disease control as well as vaccination, although there is still no reliable and cost effective method for sustainable control or eradication of AE. Vaccination is the most reliable method in control of CE. The EG95 vaccine of livestock animals has considerable impact on management of hydatid disease in endemic areas and achieves a reduction in human incidence. Nevertheless, development of EG95 as a human vaccine would provide the most direct way of preventing the disease and be important in reduction of human morbidity and mortality caused by hydatid disease in endemic areas.

13. References

Akhan. O, Gumus, B., Akinci, D., Karcaaltincaba, M., Ozmen, M.. (2007). Diagnosis and percutaneous treatment of soft-tissue hydatid cysts. *Cardiovasc. Intervent. Radiol.* 30, 419–425

Akisu, C., Delibas, S.B., Bicmen, C., Ozkoc, S., Aksoy, U., Turgay, N.,(2006). Comparative evaluation of western blotting in hepatic and pulmonary cystic echinococcosis. *Parasite* 13, 321-326.

Aktan AO, Yalin R.(1996) Preoperative albendazole treatment for liver hydatid disease decreases the viability of the cyst. *Eur J Gastroenterol Hepatol*; 8:877–9.

Ali M, Mahmood K, Khan P.(2009). Hydatid cysts of the brain. *JAyub Med Coll Abbottabad*.21(3):152-4.

Ammann RW, Hirsbrunner R, Cotting J, et al.(1990). Recurrence rate after discontinuation of long-term mebendazole therapy in alveolar echinococcosis (preliminary results). *Am J Trop Med Hyg;* 43:506.

Ammann RW, Eckert J. (1996). Parasitic diseases of the liver and intestine: cestodes, Echinococcus. *Gastroenterol Clin North Am;* 25:655–689

Ammann, R.W., Renner, E.C., Gottstein, B., Grimm, F., Eckert, J., Renner, E.L., (2004). Immunosurveillance of alveolar echinococcosis by specific humoral and cellular immune tests: long-term analysis of the Swiss chemotherapy trial (1976–2001). *J. Hepatol.* 41, 551–559

Avgerinos ED, Pavlakis E, Stathoulopoulos A, Manoukas E, Skarpas G, Tsatsoulis P.(2006). Clinical presentations and surgical management of liver hydatidosis: our 20 year experience. *HPB*, 8: 189-193

Aydin, U., Yazici, P., Onen, Z., Ozsoy, M., Zeytunlu, M., Kilic, M., Coker, A., (2008). The optimal treatment of hydatid cyst of the liver: radical surgery with a significant reduced risk of recurrence. *Turk. J. Gastroenterol.* 19, 33–39.

Baden LR, Elliott DD.(2003). Case records of the Massachusetts General Hospital. Weekly Clinicopathological exercises. Case 4-2003. A 42-year-old woman with cough, fever, and abnormalities on thoracoabdominal computed tomography. *N Engl J Med*, 348:447.

Baldelli F, Papili R, Francisci D, et al. (1992).Post operative surveillance of human hydatidosis: evaluation of immunodiagnostic tests. *Pathology;* 24:75.

Bartholomot, G., Vuitton, D.A., Harraga, S., Shida, Z., Giraudoux, P., Barnish, G., Wang, Y.H., MacPherson, C.N., Craig, P.S., (2002). Combined ultrasound and serologic screening for hepatic alveolar echinococcosis in central China. *Am. J. Trop. Med. Hyg.* 66, 23–29.

Ben Nouir N, Nuñez S, Gianinazzi C, et al(.2008). Assessment of *Echinococcus granulosus* somatic protoscolex antigens for serological follow-up of young patients surgically treated for cystic echinococcosis. *J Clin Microbiol;* 46:1631.

Ben Nouir N, Gianinazzi C, Gorcii M, et al.(2009).Isolation and molecular characterization of recombinant *Echinococcus granulosus* P29 protein (recP29) and its assessment for the post-surgical serological follow-up of human cystic echinococcosis in young patients. *Trans R Soc Trop Med Hyg;* 103:355.

Battelli G. (2009). Echinococcosis: costs, losses and social consequences of a neglected zoonosis.*Vet Res Commun*, 33 (Suppl 1):S47–S52

Bell, R. G. (1996). IgE, allergies and helminth parasites: a new perspective on an old conundrum. *Immunol. Cell Biol.* 74:337–345

Benner C, Carabin H, Sánchez-Serrano LP, Budke CM & Carmena D.(2010). Analysis of the economic impact of cystic echinococcosis in Spain. *Bull World Health Organ;* 88:49–57

Bethony JM, Cole RN, Guo X, Kamhawi S, Lightowlers M, Loukas A, Petri W, Reed S, Valenzuela JG, Hotez PJ. (2011).Vaccines to combat the neglected tropical diseases. *Immunological Reviews*, Vol. 239: 237–270

Bickel A, Daud G, Urbach D, et al.(1998). Laparoscopic approach to hydatid liver cysts. Is it logical? Physical, experimental, and practical aspects. *Surg Endosc;* 12:1073.

Bresson-Hadni S, Koch S, Beurton I, et al.(1999) Primary disease recurrence after liver transplantation for alveolar echinococcosis: long-term evaluation in 15 patients. *Hepatology*; 30:857.

Bresson-Hadni, S., Vuitton, D.A., Bartholomot, B., Heyd, B., Godart, D., Meyer, J.P., Hrusovsky, S., Becker, M.C., Mantion, G., Lenys, D., Miguet, J.P. (2000). A twentyyear history of alveolar echinococcosis: analysis of a series of 117 patients from eastern France. *Eur. J. Gastroenterol. Hepatol.* 12, 327–336.

Bresson-Hadni, S., Delabrousse, E., Blagosklonov, O., Bartholomot, B., Koch, S., Miguet, J.P., Mantion, G., Vuitton, D.A., (2006). Imaging aspects and non-surgical interventional treatment in human alveolar echinococcosis. *Parasitol. Int.* 55 (Suppl.), S267–S272.

Bresson-Hadni S, Blagosklonov O, Knapp J, Grenouillet F, Sako Y, Delabrousse E, Brientini MP, Richou C, Minello A, Antonino AT, Gillet M, Ito A, Mantion GA, Vuitton DA.(2011). Should possible recurrence of disease contraindicate liver transplantation in patients with end-stage alveolar echinococcosis? A 20-year follow-up study. *Liver Transpl.* Jul;17(7):855-65

Brunetti E&Junghanss T(2009). Update on cystic hydatid disease. *Current Opinion in Infectious Diseases*, 22:497–502

Brunetti E, Kern P. Vuitton D.A, Writing Panel for the WHO-IWGE (2010) Expert consensus for the diagnosis and treatment of cystic and alveolar echinococcosis in humans.*J.Acta Tropica*.114,1-16

Budke CM, Jiamin Q, Qian W, Torgerson PR (2005). Economic effects of echinococcosis in a disease-endemic region of the Tibetan Plateau. *Am J Trop Med Hyg*. Jul;73(1):2-10.

Bulut V, Ilhan F, Yucel AY, Onal S, Ilhan Y & Godekmerdan A (2001) Immunological follow-up of hydatid cyst cases. *Mem Inst Oswaldo Cruz* 96: 669–671.

Bükte Y, Kemaloglu S, Nazaroglu H, Ozkan U, Ceviz A, Simsek M. (2004).Cerebral hydatid disease: CT and MR imaging findings. *Swiss Med Wkly*. 7;134(31-32):459-67.

Bygott, J.M., Chiodini, P.L., (2009). Praziquantel: neglected drug? Ineffective treatment? Or therapeutic choice in cystic hydatid disease? *Acta Trop*. 111, 95–101.

Capron, A., and J. P. Dessaint. (1992). Immunologic aspects of schistosomiasis. *Annu. Rev. Med*. 43:209–218.

Ceballos L, Elissondo C, Bruni SS, Confalonieri A , Denegri G, Alvarez L, Lanusse C.(2010). Chemoprophylactic Activity of Flubendazole in Cystic Echinococcosis *Chemotherapy*;56:386–392

Ceballos L, Elissondo C, Sánchez Bruni S, Denegri G, Lanusse C, Alvarez L (2011). Comparative performance of flubendazole and albedazole in cycstic echinococcusis:ex vivo activity, plasma/cysts disposition and efficacy in infected mice.Antimicrob *Agents Chemother*. Sep 19

Chawla, A., Maheshwari, M., Parmar, H., Hira, P., Hanchate, V., (2003). Imaging features of disseminated peritoneal hydatidosis before and after medical treatment. *Clin. Radiol*. 58, 818–820.

Chowbey PK, Shah S, Khullar R, et al.(2003). Minimal access surgery for hydatid cyst disease: laparoscopic, thoracoscopic, and retroperitoneoscopic approach. *J Laparoendosc Adv Surg Tech* A; 13:159.

Cobo F, Yarnoz C, Sesma B, et al.(1998) Albendazole plus praziquantel versus albendazole alone as a pre-operative treatment in intra-abdominal hydatisosis caused by *Echinococcus granulosus*. *Trop Med Int Health*; 3:462.

Conn, D. B. (1994). Cestode infections of mammary glands and female reproductive organs: potential for vertical transmission? *J. Helminthol. Soc. Wash.* 61:162–168.

Craig, P. S.P. Giraudoux, D. Shi, B. Batholomot, G. Barnish, P. Delattre, J. P. Quere, S. Harraga, G. Bao, Y. Wang, F. Lu, A. Ito, and D. A. Vuitton. (2000). An epidemiological and ecological study of human alveolar echinococcosis transmission in south Gansu, China. *Acta Trop.* 77:167–177.

Craig PS, Larrieu E.(2006).Control of cystic echinococcosis/hydatidosis: 1863-2002. *Adv Parasitol*; 61:443

Craig PS, McManus DP, Lightowlers MW, Chabalgoity JA, Garcia HH, Gavidia CM, Gilman RH, Armando E Gonzalez, Myriam Lorca, Cesar Naquira, Alberto Nieto, Peter M Schantz.(2007). Prevention and control of cystic echinococcosis *Lancet Infect Dis*; 7: 385–394

Dai WJ, Waldvogel A, Jungi T, Stettler M, Gottstein B.Immunology. (2003) Inducible nitric oxide synthase deficiency in mice increases resistance to chronic infection with Echinococcus multilocularis. *Immunology Feb*;108(2):238-44.

Dai WJ, Waldvogel A, Siles-Lucas M & Gottstein B (2004) Echinococcus multilocularis proliferation in mice and respective parasite 14-3-3 gene expression is mainly controlled by an alphabeta CD4 T-cell-mediated immune response. *Immunology* 112: 481–488.

Davolio SA, Canossi GC, Nicoli FA, et al. (1990).Hydatid disease: MR imaging study. *Radiology*, 175:701-706.

Demircan A, Keles A, Kahveci FO, Tulmac M, Ozsarac M.(2010). Cardiac tamponade via a fistula to the pericardium from a hydatid cyst: case report and review of the literature *J Emerg Med*.38(5):582-6.

Deplazes, P., P. Alther, I. Tanner, R. C. A. Thompson, and J. Eckert. (1999). Echinococcus multilocularis coproantigen detection by enzyme-linked immunosorbent assay in fox, dog, and cat populations. *J. Parasitol.* 85:115–121.

Dervenis C, Delis S, Avgerinos C, et al.(2005). Changing concepts in the management of liver hydatid disease. *J Gastrointest Surg*; 9:869.

Dziri, C., Haouet, K., Fingerhut, A., (2004). Treatment of hydatid cyst of the liver: where is the evidence? *World J. Surg.* 28, 731–736.

Dziri, C., Haouet, K., Fingerhut, A., Zaouche, A., (2009). Management of cystic echinococcosis complications and dissemination: where is the evidence? *World J. Surg.* 33, 1266–1273

Dülger AC, Küçükoğlu ME, Akdenız H, Avcu S, Kemık O.(2010). Case report: Budd-Chiari syndrome and esophageal variceal bleeding due to alveolar echinococcosis].*Turkiye Parazitol Derg.* 34(3):187-90

Echinonet. Online version of Echinonews: www.medicalweb.it/aumi/echinonet/(Accessed March 8, 2005). WHO; 2000.

Eckert, J., F. J. Conraths, and K. Tackmann.(2000). Echinococcosis: an emerging or reemerging zoonosis? *Int. J. Parasitol.* 30:1283–1294.

Eckert, J.B. Gottstein, D. Heath, and F.-J. Liu. (2001). Prevention of echinococcosis in humans and safety precautions, p. 238–247. *In* J. Eckert, M. A. Gemmell, F.-X. Meslin, and Z. S. Pawlowski (ed.), WHO/OIE manual on echinococcosis in humans and animals: a public health problem of global concern. World Organisation for Animal Health, Paris, France.

Eckert J, De-Plazes P.(2004) Biological, Epidemiological, and Clinical Aspects of Echinococcosis,a Zoonosis of Increasing Concern.*Clin Microbiology Reviews*.17(1),107-135.

El Fortia, M., El Gatit, A., Bendaoud, M.(2006). Ultrasound wall-sign in pulmonary echinococcosis (new application). *Ultraschall Med.* 27, 553–557.

El-On J.(2003). Benzimidazole treatment of cystic echinococcosis. *Acta Trop*; 85:243

Ertem M, Karahasanoglu T, Yavuz N, Erguney S.(2002). Laparoscopically treated liver hydatid cysts. *Arch Surg*; 137:1170

Filice C, Di Perri G, Strosselli M, et al. (1990). Parasitologic findings in percutaneous drainage of human hydatid liver cysts. *J Infect Dis*; 161:1290.

Fu, Y. et al. (1999) A new potent antigen from *Echinococcus granulosus* associated with muscles and tegument. Mol. Biochem. *Parasitol.* 102, 43–52

Fu, Y. et al. (2000) Cellular immune response of lymph nodes from dogs following the intradermal injection of a recombinant antigen corresponding to a 66 kDa protein of *Echinococcus granulosus*. *Vet. Immunol. Immunopathol.* 74, 195–208

Gabal AM, Khawaja FI, Mohammad GA(2005). Modified PAIR technique for percutaneous treatment of high-risk hydatid cysts. *Cardiovasc Intervent Radiol.*;28(2):200-8.

Galitza Z, Bazarsky E, Sneier R, et al.(2006). Repeated treatment of cystic echinococcosis in patients with a long-term immunological response after successful surgical cyst removal. *Trans R Soc Trop Med Hyg*; 100:126.

Gargouri M, Ben Amor N, Ben Chehida F, et al. (1990).Percutaneous treatment of hydatid cysts (*Echinococcus granulosus*). *Cardiovasc Intervent Radiol*, 13:169.

Gavidia CM, Gonzalez AE, Barron EA, Ninaquispe B, Llamosas M,. Verastegui MR, Robinson C, Gilman RH. (2010). Evaluation of Oxfendazole, Praziquantel and Albendazole against Cystic Echinococcosis: A Randomized Clinical Trial in Naturally Infected Sheep. *Neglected tropical disease*.4(2), e616

Gelman R, Brook G, Green J, et al.(2000). Minimal change glomerulonephritis associated with hydatid disease. *Clin Nephrol*; 53:152

Gharbi HA, Hassine W, Brauner MW, Dupuch K.(1981). Ultrasound examination of the hydatic liver. *Radiology*, 139:459.

Gil-Grande LA, Rodriguez-Caabeiro F, Prieto JG, et al. (1993). Randomised controlled trial of efficacy of albendazole in intraabdominalhydatid disease. *Lancet*;342:1269–72.

Giorgio A, Tarantino L, Francica G, et al.(1992). Unilocular hydatid liver cysts: treatment with US-guided, double percutaneous aspiration and alcohol injection. *Radiology*; 184:705

Grenard P, Bresson-Hadni S, El Alaoui S, Chevallier M, Vuitton DA & Ricard-Blum S (2001) Transglutaminase-mediated cross-linking is involved in the stabilization of extracellular matrix in human liver fibrosis. *J Hepatol* 35: 367–375.

Godot, V., S. Harraga, M. Deschaseaux, S. Bresson-Hadni, B. Gottstein, D. Emilie, and D. A. Vuitton (1997). Increased basal production of interleukin- 10 by peripheral blood mononuclear cells in human alveolar echinococcosis. *Eur. Cytokine Netw.* 8:401–408.

Golemanov B, Grigorov N, Mitova R, Genov J, Vuchev D, Tamarozzi F, Brunetti E(2011). Efficacy and safety of PAIR for cystic echinococcosis: experience on a large series of patients from Bulgaria. *Am J Trop Med Hyg.* 2011 Jan;84(1):48-51

Göğüş C, Safak M, Baltaci S, Türkölmez K.(2003).Isolated renal hydatidosis: experience with 20 cases. *J Uro*, 169:186.

Guisantes JA, Vincente-García F, Abril MJ, et al.(1994). Total and specific IgE levels in human hydatid disease determined by enzyme immunoassay: serological follow-up after surgery. *J Investig Allergol Clin Immunol;* 4:301.

Haynes, A. P., and J. Fletcher. 1990. Neutrophil function tests. *Baillieres Clin. Haematol.* 3:871–887.

Harandi MF, Moazezi SS, Saba M, Grimm F, Kamyabi H, Sheikhzadeh F, Sharifi I, Deplazes P.(2011) Sonographical and Serological Survey of Human Cystic Echinococcosis and Analysis of Risk Factors Associated with Seroconversion in Rural Communities of Kerman, Iran. *Zoonoses Public Health.* May 6.1863-2378

Heath DD, Jensen O, Lightowlers MW. (2003).Progress in control of hydatidosis using vaccination--a review of formulation and delivery of the vaccine and recommendations for practical use in control programmes. *Acta Trop;* 85:133

Hegglin, D., P. Ward, and P. Deplazes. (2003). Anthelmintic baiting of foxes against urban contamination with Echinococcus multilocularis. *Emerg. Infect. Dis.* 9:1266–1272

Hemphill A, Stadelmann B, Scholl S, et al.(2010) Echinococcus metacestodes as laboratory models for the screening of drugs against cestodes and trematodes. *Parasitology;* 137:569–587.

Horton RJ.(1997). Albendazole in treatment of human cystic echinococcosis: 12 years of experience. *Acta Trop;* 64:79.

Hosch, W., Stojkovic, M., Janisch, T., Kauffmann, G.W., Junghanss, T.(2007). The role of calcification for staging cystic echinococcosis (CE). *Eur. Radiol.* 17, 2538–2545

Hosch, W., Junghanss, T., Stojkovic, M., Brunetti, E., Heye, T., Kauffmann, G.W., Hull, W.E., (2008). Metabolic viability assessment of cystic echinococcosis using highfield 1H MRS of cyst contents. *NMR Biomed.* 21, 734–754.

Ilıca AT, kocaoglu M, zeybek N, Guven S, Adaletli I, Basgul A, coban H, Bilici A, Bukte Y.(2007). Extrahepatic Abdominal Hydatid Disease Caused by *Echinococcus granulosus*: Imaging Findings. *AJR;* 189:337–343

Isitmangil, T., Sebit, S., Tunc, H., Gorur, R., Erdik, O., Kunter, E., Toker, A., Balkanli, K., Ozturk, O.Y. (2002). Clinical experience of surgical therapy in 207 patients with thoracic hydatidosis over a 12-year-period. *Swiss Med. Wkly.* 132, 548–552.

Ito A, Schantz PM, Wilson JF.(1995).Em18, a new serodiagnostic marker for differentiation of active and inactive cases of alveolar hydatid disease. *Am J Trop Med Hyg;* 52:41.

Ito, A., Craig, P.S.(2003). Immunodiagnostic and molecular approaches for the detection of taeniid cestode infections. *Trends Parasitol.* 19, 377–381.

Jenkins, D. J., and T. Romig. (2000). Efficacy of Droncit Spot-on (praziquantel) 4 % w/v against immature and mature Echinococcus multilocularis in cats. *Int. J. Parasitol.* 30:959–962.

Jenkins DJ, Roming T, Thompson RCA.(2005). Emergence/re-emergence of Echinococcus spp.—a global update. *International Journal for Parasitology* 35, 1205–1219.

Junghanss, T., Menezes da Silva, A., Horton, J., Chiodini, P.L., Brunetti, E., (2008). Clinical management of cystic echinococcosis: state of the art, problems, and perspectives. *Am. J. Trop. Med. Hyg.* 79, 301–311.

Kern, P., Abboud, P., Kern, W., Stich, A., Bresson-Hadni, S., Guerin, B., Buttenschoen, K., Gruener, B., Reuter, S., Hemphill, A., (2008). Critical appraisal of nitazoxanide for the treatment of alveolar echinococcosis. *Am. J. Trop. Med. Hyg.* 79, 119

Kern (2010).Clinical features and treatment of alveolar echinococcosis. *Current Opinion in Infectious Diseases*,23:505–512

Khuroo MS, Dar MY, Yattoo GN, et al.(1993).Percutaneous drainage versus albendazole therapy in hepatic hydatidosis: a prospective, randomized study. *Gastroenterology;* 104:1452.

Lanusse CE, Gascon LH, Prichard RK (1995) Comparative plasma disposition kinetics of albendazole, fenbendazole, oxfendazole and their metabolites in adult sheep. *J Vet Pharmacol Ther* 18: 196–203.

Larrieu, E. J., M. T. Costa, M. Del Carpio, S. Moguillansky, G. Bianchi, and Z. E. Yadon.(2002). A case-control study of the risk factors for cystic echinococcosis among children of Rio Negro province, Argentina. *Ann. Trop. Med. Parasitol.* 96:43–52.

Li HT, Tuerganaili, Ayifuhanahan, Shao YM, Zhao JM, Ran B, Wen H.(2010). Clinical experiences in the treatment of human multi-organ alveolar echinococcosis by surgery and drugs. *Zhonghua Yi Xue Za Zhi.* 2;90(40):2839-42

Lightowlers MW, Lawrence SB, Gauci CG, et al.(1996). Vaccination against hydatidosis using a defined recombinant antigen. *Parasite Immunol;* 18:457

Lightowlers MW, Flisser CG, Gauci CG, Heath DD, Jensen O, Rolfe R. (2000)Vaccination against cysticercosis and hydatid disease. *Parasitol Today;* 16: 191–96.

Li T, Chen X, Zhen R, et al (2010). Widespread co-endemicity of human cystic and alveolar echinococcosis on the eastern Tibetan Plateau, northwest Sichuan/ southeast Qinghai, China. *Acta Trop;* 113:248–256.

Majorowski MM, Carabin H, Kilani M, Bensalah A.(2005). Echinococcosis in Tunisia: a cost analysis. *Trans R Soc Trop Med Hyg.* 2005 Apr;99(4):268-78.

Manfras BJ, Reuter S, Wendland T & Kern P (2002) Increased activation and oligoclonality of peripheral CD8(1) T cells in the chronic human helminth infection alveolar echinococcosis. *Infect Immun* 70: 1168–1174

Manterola C, Mansilla JA, Fonseca F.(2005). Preoperative albendazole and scolices viability in patients with hepatic echinococcosis. *World J Surg.*;29(6):750-3.

Mastin A, Brouwer A, Fox M, Craig P, Guitián J, Li W, Stevens K(2011) Spatial and temporal investigation of *Echinococcus granulosus* coproantigen prevalence in farm dogs in South Powys, Wales. *Vet Parasitol.* 178(1-2):100-7.

Mejri N, Gottstein B.(2009). Echinococcus multilocularis metacestode metabolites contain a cysteine protease that digests eotaxin, a CC pro-inflammatory chemokine. *Parasitol Res.* 105(5):1253-60.

McManus DP, Zhang W, Li J, Bartley PB. (2003)Echinococcosis. *Lancet* ; 362: 1295–304.

Macpherson, C.N., Milner, R. (2003). Performance characteristics and quality controlvof community based ultrasound surveys for cystic and alveolar echinococcosis.*vActa Trop.* 85, 203–209

Marchiondo, A.A., Ming, R., Andersen, F.L., Slusser, J.H., Conder, G.A. (1994). Enhanced larval cyst growth of Echinococcus multilocularis in praziquantel-treated jirds (Meriones unguiculatus). *Am. J. Trop. Med. Hyg.* 50, 120–127.

Meeusen, E. N., and A. Balic. (2000). Do eosinophils have a role in the killing of helminth parasites? *Parasitol. Today* 16:95–101.

Mohamed AE, Yasawy MI, Al Karawi MA. (1998).Combined albendazole and praziquantel versus albendazole alone in the treatment of hydatid disease. *Hepatogastroenterology;* 45:1690.

Moro PL, Budke CM, Schantz PM, Vasquez J, Santivan SJ, Villavicencio J.(2011) Economic Impact of Cystic Echinococcosis in Peru. *Neglected Tropical Disease*.5(5),e1179.

Moray G, Shahbazov R, Sevmis S, Karakayali H, Torgay A, Arslan G, Savas N, Yilmaz U, Haberal M.(2009). Liver transplantation in management of alveolar echinococcosis: two case reports. *Transplant Proc.*;41(7):2936-8.

Ohnishi K 1, Nakamura-Uchiyama F1, Komiya N1,Satoh S2, Ohkubo T, Umekita N.(2008). Hepatic Cystic Echinococcosis with Specific CT Findings. *Inter Med* 47: 803-805.

Ohsaki Y, Sasaki T, Shibukawa K, Takahashi T, Osanaı S.(2007). Radiological findings of alveolar hydatid disease of the lung caused by Echinococcus multilocularis *Respirology* 12, 458–461

Papanikolaou A.2008. Osseous hydatid disease. *Trans R Soc Trop Med Hyg*. 2008 Mar;102(3):233-8.

Pedrosa I, Saiz A, Arrazola J, Ferreiros J, Pedrosa CS.(2000) Hydatid Disease: Radiologic and Pathologic Features and Complications. *RadioGraphics*, 20, 795-817.

Peng, X., Zhang, S., Niu, J.H.(2002). Total subadventitial cystectomy for the treatment of 30 patients with hepatic hydatid cysts. *Chin. J. Gen. Surg*. 17, 529–530.

Piarroux M, Piarroux R, Giorgi R, Knapp J, Bardonnet K, Sudre B, Watelet J, Dumortier J, Gérard A, Beytout J, Abergel A, Mantion G, Vuitton DA, Bresson-Hadni S.(2011). Clinical features and evolution of alveolar echinococcosis in France from 1982 to 2007: Results of a survey in 387 patients. *J Hepatol*.55(5):1025-33

Qian ZX. (1988).Thoracic hydatid cysts: a report of 842 cases treated over a thirty-year period. *Ann Thorac Surg*; 46:342.

Rainbird, M. A., D. Macmillan, and E. N. Meeusen. (1998). Eosinophilmediated killing of Haemonchus contortus larvae: effect of eosinophil activation and role of antibody, complement and interleukin-5. Parasite Immunol. 20:93–103.

Rausch RL, Wilson JF, Schantz PM, McMahon BJ.(1987) Spontaneous death of Echinococcus multilocularis: cases diagnosed serologically (by Em2 ELISA) and clinical significance. *Am J Trop Med Hyg*; 36:576.

Rausch RL, Wilson JF, Schantz PM.(1990). A programme to reduce the risk of infection by Echinococcus multilocularis: the use of praziquantel to control the cestode in a village in the hyperendemic region of Alaska. *Ann Trop Med Parasitol;* 84:239

Reiterova K, Miterpakova M, Turcekova L, Antolova D, Dubinsky P.(2005). Field evaluation of an intravital diagnostic test of Echinococcus multilocularis infection in red foxes. *Vet Parasitol* ,128: 65–71.

Reuter, S., Buck, A., Grebe, O., Nussle-Kugele, K., Kern, P., Manfras, B.J., (2003). Salvage treatment with amphotericin B in progressive human alveolar echinococcosis. Antimicrob. *Agents Chemother.* 47, 3586–3591

Reuter, S., Buck, A., Manfras, B., Kratzer, W., Seitz, H.M., Darge, K., Reske, S.N., Kern, P., (2004). Structured treatment interruption in patients with alveolar echinococcosis. *Hepatology* 39, 509–517.

Ricard-Blum S, Bresson-Hadni S, Guerret S, Grenard P, Volle PJ, Risteli L, Grimaud JA &Vuitton DA (1996) Mechanism of collagen network stabilization in human irreversible granulomatous liver fibrosis. *Gastroenterology* 111: 172–182.

Riley, E. M., J. B. Dixon, D. F. Kelly, and D. A. Cox. (1985). The immune response to *Echinococcus granulosus*: sequential histological observations of lymphoreticular and connective tissues during early murine infection. *J. Comp. Pathol.* 95:93–104.

Rigano, R., E. Profumo, S. Ioppolo, S. Notargiacomo, E. Ortona, A. Teggi,and A. Siracusano. (1995). Immunological markers indicating the effectiveness of pharmacological treatment in human hydatid disease. *Clin. Exp. Immunol.* 102:281–285.

Rigano, R., E. Profumo, G. Di Felice, E. Ortona, A. Teggi, and A. Siracusano. (1995). In vitro production of cytokines by peripheral blood mononuclear cells from hydatid patients. *Clin. Exp. Immunol.* 99:433–439.

Rigano, R., E. Profumo, A. Teggi, and A. Siracusano. (1996). Production of IL-5 and IL-6 by peripheral blood mononuclear cells (PBMC) from patients with *Echinococcus granulosus* infection. *Clin. Exp. Immunol.* 105:456–459.

Rigano R, Profumo E, Ioppolo S, Notargiacomo S, Teggi A & Siracusano A (1999) Serum cytokine detection in the clinical follow up of patients with cystic echinococcosis. *Clin Exp Immunol* 115: 503–507.

Riganò R, Ioppolo S, Ortona E, et al. (2002).Long-term serological evaluation of patients with cystic echinococcosis treated with benzimidazole carbamates. *Clin Exp Immunol;* 129:485.

Romig, T., Kratzer, W., Kimmig, P., Frosch, M., Gaus, W., Flegel, W.A., Gottstein, B., Lucius, R., Beckh, K., Kern, P.(1999). An epidemiologic survey of human alveolar echinococcosis in southwestern Germany. Romerstein Study Group. *Am. J. Trop. Med. Hyg.* 61, 566–573.

Saboulard, D. et al. (2003) The *Echinococcus granulosus* antigen EgA31: localization during development and immunogenic properties. *Parasite Immunol.* 25, 489–501

Safioleas MC, Misiakos EP, Kouvaraki M, et al. (2006).Hydatid disease of the liver: a continuing surgical problem. *Arch Surg;* 141:1101.

Salama H, Farid Abdel-Wahab M, Strickland GT.(1995). Diagnosis and treatment of hepatic hydatid cysts with the aid of echo-guided percutaneous cyst puncture. *Clin Infect Dis,* 21:1372

Santivanez S, Garcia HH.(2010). Pulmonary cystic echinococcosis. *Curr Opin Pulm Med.* 16(3):257-61.

Sarıozkana S, Yalcın C. (2009). Estimating the production losses due to cystic echinococcosis in ruminants in Turkey. *Veterinary Parasitology* , 163, 4, (26) :330-334

Schallenberg M, Gök M, Katsounas A, Mellin KB, Steuhl KP.(2007).Keratitis caused by infection with *Echinococcus granulosus. Klin Monbl Augenheilkd.*;224(3):213-5

Schantz PM, Wilson JF, Wahlquist SP, et al.(1983). Serologic tests for diagnosis and post-treatment evaluation of patients with alveolar hydatid disease (Echinococcus multilocularis). *Am J Trop Med Hyg* 1983; 32:1381

Scherer K, Gupta N, Caine WP, Panda M.(2009). Differential Diagnosis and Management of a Recurrent Hepatic Cyst: A Case Report and Review of Literature. *J Gen Intern Med 24*(10):1161–5

Scheuring, U.J., Seitz, H.M., Wellmann, A., Hartlapp, J.H., Tappe, D., Brehm, K., Spengler, U., Sauerbruch, T., Rockstroh, J.K.(2003). Long-term benzimidazole treatment of alveolar echinococcosis with hematogenic subcutaneous and bone dissemination. *Med. Microbiol. Immunol.* (Berl.) 192, 193–195.

Sciarrino E, Virdone R, Lo Iacono O, et al.(1991) Ultrasound changes in abdominal echinococcosis treated with albendazole. *J Clin Ultrasound*; 19:143.

Seven R, Berber E, Mercan S, et al. (2000).Laparoscopic treatment of hepatic hydatid cysts. *Surgery;* 128:36

Seckin, H., Yagmurlu, B., Yigitkanli, K., Kars, H.Z., (2008). Metabolic changes during successful medical therapy for brain hydatid cyst: case report. *Surg. Neurol.* 70, 186–189.

Shambesh MK, Craig PS, Wen H, et al.(1997). IgG1 and IgG4 serum antibody responses in asymptomatic and clinically expressed cystic echinococcosis patients. *Acta Trop;* 64:53.

Siles-Lucas, M.M., Gottstein, B.B.(2001). Molecular tools for the diagnosis of cystic and alveolar echinococcosis. *Trop. Med. Int. Health* 6, 463–475.

Siracusano, A., Bruschi, F.(2006). Cystic echinococcosis: progress and limits in epidemiology and immunodiagnosis. *Parassitologia* 48, 65–66.

Smego Jr., R.A., Bhatti, S., Khaliq, A.A., Beg, M.A.(2003). Percutaneous aspirationinjection-reaspiration drainage plus albendazole or mebendazole for hepatic cystic echinococcosis: a meta-analysis. *Clin. Infect. Dis.* 37, 1073–1083.

Smego RA Jr, Sebanego P.(2005). Treatment options for hepatic cystic echinococcosis. Int J Infect Dis; 9:69

Sotiraki S, Chaligiannis I.(2010) Cystic echinococcosis in Greece. Past and present. *Parasite.* 17(3):205-10

Stankovic N, Ignjatovic M, Nozic D, et al. (2005). Liver hydatid disease: morphological changes of protoscoleces after albendazole therapy. *Vojnosanit Pregl* 62:175–9.

Stojkovic, M., Zwahlen, M., Teggi, A., Vutova, K., Cretu, C.M., Virdone, R., Nicolaidou, P., Cobanoglu, N., Junghanss, T., (2009). Treatment response of cystic echinococcosis to benzimidazoles: a systematic review. *PLoS Negl. Trop. Dis.3,* e524.

Stumpe, K.D., Renner-Schneiter, E.C., Kuenzle, A.K., Grimm, F., Kadry, Z., Clavien, P.A., Deplazes, P., von Schulthess, G.K., Muellhaupt, B., Ammann, R.W., Renner, E.L.(2007). F-18-fluorodeoxyglucose (FDG) positron-emission tomography of Echinococcus multilocularis liver lesions: prospective evaluation of its value for diagnosis and follow-up during benzimidazole therapy. *Infection* 35, 11–18.

Sturm, D., J. Menzel, B. Gottstein, and P. Kern.(1995). Interleukin-5 is the predominant cytokine produced by peripheral blood mononuclear cells in alveolar echinococcosis. *Infect. Immun.* 63:1688–1697.

Suwan Z. (1995). Sonographic findings in hydatid disease of the liver: comparison with other imaging methods. *Ann Trop Med Parasitol,* 89:261.

Tappe, D., Frosch, M., Sako, Y., Itoh, S., Gruener, B., Reuter, S., Nakao, M., Ito, A., Kern, P.(2009). Close relationship between clinical regression and specific serology in the follow-up of patients with alveolar echinococcosis in different clinical stages. *Am. J. Trop. Med. Hyg.* 80, 792–797.

Teggi A, Lastilla MG, De Rosa F. (1993).Therapy of human hydatid disease with mebendazole and albendazole. *Antimicrob Agents Chemother;* 37:1679.

Thameur, H., Abdelmoula, S., Chenik, S., Bey, M., Ziadi, M., Mestiri, T., Mechmeche, R., Chaouch, H.(2001). Cardiopericardial hydatid cysts. *World J. Surg.* 25, 58–67.

Todorov T, Vutova K, Mechkov G, et al.(1992). Chemotherapy of human cystic echinococcosis: comparative efficacy of mebendazole and albendazole. *Ann Trop Med Parasitol;* 86:59

Ustunsoz B, Ugurel MS, Uzar AI, Duru NK.(2008). Percutaneous treatment of hepatic hydatid cyst in pregnancy: long-term results. *Arch Gynecol Obstet.*277(6):547-50.

Veit, P., B. Bilger, V. Schad, J. Scha¨fer, W. Frank, and R. Lucius. (1995). Influence of environmental factors on the infectivity of Echinococcus multilocularis eggs. *Parasitology* 110:79–86.

Vuitton DA, Bresson-Hadni S, Laroche L, Kaiserlian D, Guerret- Stocker S, Bresson JL & Gillet M (1989) Cellular immune response in Echinococcus multilocularis infection in humans. II. Natural killer cell activity and cell subpopulations in the blood and in the periparasitic granuloma of patients with alveolar echinococcosis. *Clin Exp Immunol* 78: 67–74

Vuitton, D., Zhang, S.L., Yang, Y., Godot, V., Beurton, I., Mantion, G., Bresson-Hadni, S.(2006). Survival strategy of Echinococcus multilocularis in the human host. *Parasitol.* Int. 55(Suppl.), S51–S55

Vuitton DA, Gottstein B (2010) Echinococcus multilocularis and its intermediate host: a model of parasite-host interplay. *J Biomed Biotechnol.* Mar 21.

Wang, Q., J. Qiu, P. Schantz, J. He, A. Ito, and F. Liu. (2001). Investigation of risk factors for development of human hydatidosis among households raising livestock in Tibetan areas of western Sichuan province. *Chin. J. Parasitol. Parasit. Dis.* 19:93–96.

Wei XL, Ding JB, Xu Y, Wen H & Lin RY (2004) Change of cytokines in mice with Echinococcus multilocularis infection. *Zhongguo Ji Sheng Chong Xue Yu Ji Sheng Chong Bing Za* Zhi 22: 361–364.

Wen H, New RR, Craig PS.(1993). Diagnosis and treatment of human hydatidosis. *Br J Clin Pharmacol;* 35:565.

Wen H, Zou PF, Yang WG, et al. (1994).Albendazole chemotherapy for human cystic and alveolar echinococcosis in north-western China. *Trans R Soc Trop Med Hyg;*88:340–3.

Wellinghausen, N., P. Gebert, and P. Kern. (1999). Interleukin (IL)-4, IL-10 and IL-12 profile in serum of patients with alveolar echinococcosis. *Acta Trop.* 73:165–174

WHO-Informal Working Group on Echinococcosis,(1996). Guidelines for treatment of cystic and alveolar echinococcosis in humans. Bull. WHO 74, 231–242.

WHO/OIE Manual on Echinococcosis (2001). Echinococcosis in Humans and Animals: A Public Health Problem of Global Concern. World Organisation for Animal Health (Office International des Epizooties) and World Health Organisation

WHO-Informal Working Group on Echinococcosis, (2003a). PAIR: Puncture, Aspiration, Injection, Re-Aspiration. An Option for the Treatment of Cystic Echinococcosis. WHO, Geneva

WHO-Informal Working Group on Echinococcosis, (2003b). International classification of ultrasound images in cystic echinococcosis for application in clinical and field epidemiological settings. *Acta Trop.* 85, 253–261.

Wilson JF, Rausch RL, McMahon BJ, Schantz PM.(1992). Parasiticidal effect of chemotherapy in alveolar hydatid disease: review of experience with mebendazole and albendazole in Alaskan Eskimos. *Clin Infect Dis;* 15:234.

Wilson JF, Rausch RL, Wilson FR. Alveolar hydatid disease. (1995).Review of the surgical experience in 42 cases of active disease among Alaskan Eskimos. *Ann Surg;* 221:315

Yagci G, Ustunsoz B, Kaymakcioglu N, et al.(2005) Results of surgical, laparoscopic, and percutaneous treatment for hydatid disease of the liver: 10 years experience with 355 patients. *World J Surg;* 29:1670.

Yang YR, Liu XZ, Vuitton DA, et al.(2006). Simultaneous alveolar and cystic echinococcosis of the liver. *Trans R Soc Trop Med Hyg,* 100:597–600.

Yapici O, Erturk SM, Ulusay M, Ozel A, Halefoglu A, Karpat Z, Basak M.(2011). Hepatic alveolar echinococcosis: a diagnostic challenge. *JBR-BTR*. 94(1):21-3.

Yu Rong Yang YR, William GM, Craig PS & McManus DP.(2010) Impact of Increased Economic Burden Due to Human Echinococcosis in an Underdeveloped Rural Community of the People's Republic of China. *Neglected Tropical Disease*,4(9),e801.

Zhang W, Li J & McManus DP (2003) Concepts in immunology and diagnosis of hydatid disease. *Clin Microbiol Rev* 16: 18–36

Zhang, W. et al. (2003b) A gene family from *Echinococcus granulosus* differentially expressed in mature adult worms. *Mol. Biochem.Parasitol*. 126, 25–33

Zhang W, McManus D.P.(2006) Recent advances in the immunology and diagnosis of echinococcosis. *FEMS Immunol Med Microbiol* 47 ,24–41

Zhang, W. et al. (2006) Vaccination of dogs against Echinococcus granulosus, the cause of cystic hydatid disease in humans. *J. Infect. Dis*. 194, 966–974

Zlitni, M., Ezzaouia, K., Lebib, H., Karray, M., Kooli, M.,Mestiri, M.(2001). Hydatid cyst of bone: diagnosis and treatment. *World J. Surg*. 25, 75–82.

19

Zoonotic Abortion in Herds: Etiology, Prevention and Control

Kelvinson F. Viana[1] and Marcos S. Zanini[2]
[1]Federal University of Ouro Preto
[2]Federal University of Espírito Santo
Brazil

1. Introduction

In recent years, an increasing number of zoonotic diseases and outbreaks affecting people around the world and it is estimated that of the emerging infectious diseases of humans, 75% are zoonosis (Merianos, 2007). Clearly, these recent events, a number of issues are involved, a fundamental question to be the livestock production systems, as well as the mismanagement of the health of livestock. In this context it is worth questioning the influence of agruculture genetics of microorganisms and the impact that may result from public health (Rosenthal, 2009). A program of activity in animal health planning is applied regularly veterinary herd management and to maintain good animal health and productivity at optimum levels.

Zoonosis affecting reproductive system animals and potentially humans, are common in herds worldwide, requiring prevent them correctly (Del Fava et al., 2003). This involves education, health and performance of vaccine efficacy in herds. However, although this practice capable of generating results broadly favorable, due to increased herd immunity and reduce the impact of an outbreak, vaccination alone is not able to prevent zoonotic infections and loss (Sanderson & Gnade, 2002). Herds infected with zoonotic agents such as Brucella abortus, Campylobacter spp., Coxiella burnetii, Toxoplasma gondii, among others, are deeply affected both the economic point of view, due to losses in production rates as a whole, they become capable disease transmit to humans. In this context, the susceptibility to infections, mainly farmers and others rural workers who daily with the animals carry zoonosis (Viana & Zanini, 2009b).

This problem is more complex developing countries compared with developed countries, due to a several factors such as lack of intensive programs for control and eradication certain diseases. What is more aggravating the epidemiological situation neglected diseases is underreporting, especially in Latin America, Africa and Asia. Therefore, this chapter provides an approach of some zoonotic agents that cause abortions, as well as attention of farmers in the prophylaxis and control these microorganisms, in view of risks and implications to human health.

2. Brucellosis

Brucellosis is one of the most important worldwide zoonotic diseases affecting livestock and humans (Corbel, 1997). According to Gorvel & Moreno (2002), although the classical definition of *Brucella* species describe these bacteria as facultative intracellular parasites, this definition does not honor their true nature which is better understood as a facultative extracellular intracellular parasite. That means that the *Brucella* preferred niche is the intracellular environment of host cells. This environment sustains extensive replication, allowing bacterial expansion and the subsequent transmission to new host cells, frequently achieved through the heavily infected aborted foetus.

Brucella infection is responsible for the decrease from 20 to 25% in milk production, 10 to 15% in meat production, 15% loss of calves due to abortions, increased 30% in the rate of replacement animals, increased calving interval of 11.5 to 20 months. In addition, every five infected cows abort, one or become permanently infertile (Acha & Szyfres, 2003). Besides the loss of animal productivity, brucellosis is a zoonosis of major importance in health public (Freitas & Oliveira, 2005). The species that may infect man are *B. melitensis*, *B. suis*, *B. abortus*, and *B. canis*. *B. melitensis* colonizes ovine stock and is the frequent cause of brucellosis, globally in humans.

2.1 Important aspects in public health veterinary

The transmission of *Brucella* infection and its prevalence in a region depends upon several factors like food habits, methods of processing milk and milk products, social customs, climatic conditions, socioeconomic status, husbandry practices and environment hygiene. In this context, environmental sanitation is particularly important (Mantur & Amarnath, 2008).

Despite the ongoing demonstrations and disclosures about risk from the consumption of raw inadequately treated by heat, contact with animals without observing safety precautions, handling and manipulations viscera, and by products excretions of animals without the use of equipment individual protection, brucellosis remains an important public health problem world (Freitas et al., 2001). Information relating to the activities of livestock management is fundamental to the generation of animal products high quality. However, often not enough information to small producers, cowboys and others working in rural areas and this lack of information is still an obstacle on the health of livestock (Viana et al., 2009a,b).

Brucellosis in pregnancy has no effect on the incidence of congenital malformations or stillbirths. Preterm delivery and low birth weight can be seen as pregnancy outcomes in brucellosis (Gulsun et al., 2011). It as been shown a remarkably high incidence (43%) of first and second-trimester spontaneous abortions among pregnant women with active brucellosis and the intrauterine fetal death rate in the third trimester was 2% (Khan et al., 2001). Rifampicin is considered the drug of choice for treatment pregnant women because its safety and can be used with or without combination with other antibiotics such as cotrimoxaxole and cephtriaxone (Gulsun et al., 2011; Karcaaltincaba et al., 2010; Pappas et al., 2005; Solera, 2000).

2.1.1 Failures in programs of control and eradication brucellosis

Control and eradication of brucellosis is a measure desired by many countries here the disease is endemic. However, this result is difficult and expensive, taking into account the specific climatic, geographical, socio-economic, technical resources and personnel, prevalence of disease, as well as the strict commitment of farmers in vaccinations programs (Kolar, 1984). In this sense, developing countries have encountered major difficulties both in setting and in achieving success in their programs of control and eradication of animal brucellosis (Blasco & Moryon, 2010; Hegazy et al., 2009; Nateloski et al., 2010). Certainly, some significant flaws can be identified, such as voluntary vaccination and lack of conditions of programs financially afford to economic losses of farmers, the loss of positive animals (Hegazy et al., 2011; Nateloski et al., 2010). Furthermore, cultural issues should also be taken into account, since in India, culling of infected cows is a taboo, affecting effort to eradication disease (Gwida et al., 2010).

The fact that brucellosis be spread herds in several regions has caused concern from the standpoint of public health, especially when it comes to developing countries. The issue is more sensitive in rural areas, where habits of people in eating unpasteurized milk, as well as frequent contact with animal secretions and remains of the placenta (Figure 1) and aborted fetuses are, without doubt, most important risk factors to health human (Almuneef et al., 2004; Makita et al., 2010; Vasconcellos, 3003; Viana et al., 2009). Moreover, risk practices in rural areas such as skinning of stillborn lambs and kids, as well as crushing the umbilical cord of newborn lambs and kids with teeth can also be contributing factors (Hussein et al., 2005). However, situations such as the habit of eating aborted fetuses by populations in Equedor, can be characterized as a risk factors (Mantur & Amarnath, 2008).

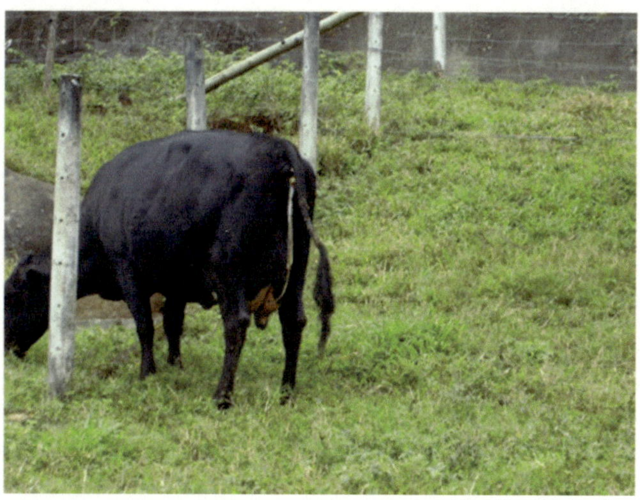

Fig. 1. Cow placenta exposed in the pasture. Situations as shown in this figure are common, characterized as a risk factor for infection by *Brucella abortus* in farmers who deal daily with livestock.

Brucellosis prevalence varies very widely in equine (0.24-37.50%), bovine (0.58-35.90%), caprine (0.40-33.3%), ovine (0.28-16.70%) and camelidae (1.8-7.48%), while humans had the least prevalence (0.89-4.10%) (Gul & Khan, 2007). However, the true incidence of human brucellosis in most countries is still unknown. Really is found in Latin America, Africa, Asia, Middle Eastern and Southern European, certainly due to underreporting (Lucero et al., 2008; Mantur & Amarnath, 2008). In the context, african countries deserve greater attention in the epidemiological scenario, since networks and programmes of surveillance, notification and vaccination are virtually nonexistent. Furthermore, the majority countries are extremely limited economic, in addition, to the habits os people living with their livestock. Besides this, a most aggravating factor is that there is much more morbid endemic infectious diseases such as malaria. Patients presenting with febrile frames are empirically diagnosed with malaria, and only the non-responders are tested for brucellosis (Pappas et al., 2006).

Prevention human brucellosis depends mainly on the control or eradication of the disease in animals. However, few countries were successful in eradication it from their herds, such as Australia, Canada, Denmark, Finland, Netherlands, New Zeland, Norway, Sweden, UK and Japan. Stocks successful these countries are an exemple to those who seek better results in their eradications programs. However, control of infected animals in developing countries requires considerable affort to build solid infrastructure that educates people about the risks of contracting brucellosis (Seleem et al., 2010). Although rural populations, as well as professionals who deal directly with cattle industry are at higher risk situations, it is important to note that urban populations in developing regions are also at risk of acquiring the disease through comsumption products of animal origin in bad (Franco et al., 2007). In the general context, with no interest and mutual effort of all aspects of society, with measures of health education and, above all, political support, the changes success in the eradication brucellosis is almost nonexistent.

3. Campylobacteriosis

Campylobacteriosis it is a zoonotic disease caused by several species of the genus *Campylobacter*. Thermophilic species are important targets of research in veterinary public health due to environmental persistence and a large number of potential hosts (Hannon et al., 2009). *Campylobacter jejuni* (*C. jejuni*) is the leading cause of bacterial gastroenteritis caused food in the world, and interest in this species has increased in recent years as a result of growing appreciation of its importance as a pathogen and the availability of new model systems and technologies genetic and genomic (Young et al., 2007), followed by *Campylobacter coli* (*C. coli*) (Tam et al., 2003).

Often, it is reported that the contamination of poultry meat and eggs is the main cause of infection in man (Friedman et al., 2004). However, it has been reported that the consumption of raw fruits and vegetables is an important risk factor for *Campylobacter* infections, especially for vegetables sold packaged (Verhoeff-Bakken et al., 2011). In addition, water contamination, ingestion of unpasteurized milk and contact with farm animals presenting diarrhea has been associated with outbreaks campylobacteriosis (Butzler et al., 2004; Gilpin et al., 2008; Huang et al., 2009; Pebody et al., 1997).

Infection with *C. jejuni* causes symptoms of diarrhea characterized by often bloody abdominal pain, fever and headache, and the incubation period of 1-10 days. However, not only the infection itself is worrying, but also its consequences, such as Guillain-Barré syndrome, characterized by a subacute polyneuropathy. This syndrome is very severe, mortality rate may reach 2-3% and major neurological sequelae in 20% of cases (Hughes & Rees, 1997; Leonard et al., 2004; Moore et al., 2005). However, patients with *C. jejuni*-related Guillain-Barré syndrome can show transient slowing of nerve conduction, mimicking demyelination, but *C. jejuni* infection does not appear to elicit acute inflammatory demyelinating polyneuropathy (Kuwabara et al., 2004).

3.1 Bovine genital campylobacteriosis

Bovine genital campylobacteriosis (BGC) also known as bovine venereal campylobacteriosis (BVC) is transmitted mainly by *Campylobacter fetus subsp. veneralis* and *Campylobacter fetus subsp. fetus*. The two species cause reproductive problems in cattle; however, the manifestation infection with this subspecies differs in the occurrence and pathogenesis. However, infection with *C. fetus subsp. fetus* is more related to sporadic abortions in cattle, and enzootic infertility in sheep (Stynen et al., 2003). BGC is closely associated with reduced pregnancy rates, low fertility, embryo mortality, abortions and increased calving interval (Mshelia et al., 2010). In males the infection is limited to the preputial cavity, but no clinical abnormalities were absorved in infected animals. However, these animals become asymptomatic carriers and are very important in the transmission of bacteria during intercourse. There may be a decrease in libido for excess service due to high repetition rates of estrus (Jesus, 1999).

The BGC is a difficult disease to control in countries with large cattle herds, were the dominant management system uses natural breeding. Because it is a sexually transmitted disease, initial clinical signs are not always apparent and when the disease is found in the herd, economic losses are already large (Alves et al., 2011).

BGC presents with worldwide distribution, paying attention to countries that the clinical disease has been recently confirmed as Argentina, Australia, Austria, Brasil, Costa Rica, France, Ireland, Jamaica, Namibia, New Zeland, South Africa, United Kingdom, United States and Uruguay (OIE, 2011) (Figure 2). However, understanding the epidemiology BGC not easy to official agencies, since many countries fail to report the incidence and outbreaks of disease. This is clearly visible in the records of the OIE (Fig. 2), mainly in African and Asian countries.

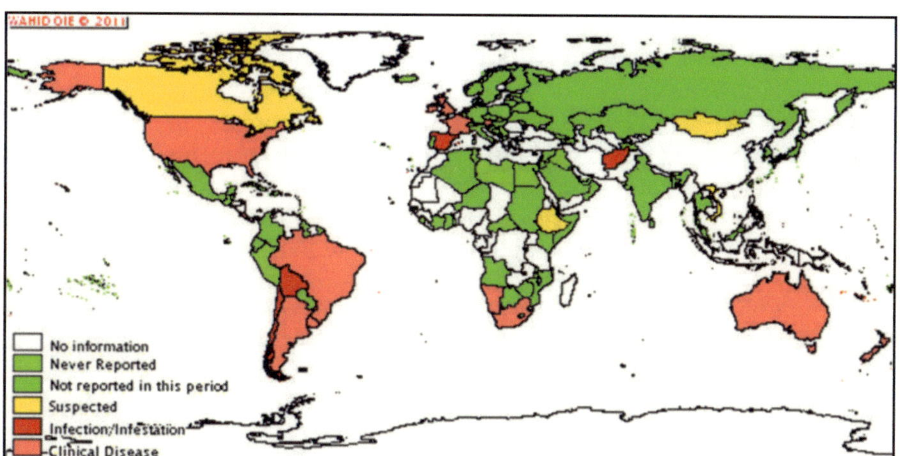

Fig. 2. Global distribution bovine genital campylobacteriosis from July to December 2010. Adapted from OIE (2011)

The establishment control program BGC requires artificial insemination with semen exempt from microorganism (BonDurant, 2005). This factor is paramount to be successful in the program. However, when involved large herds of cattle, where extensive creation system is predominant, and the high cost of litigation, technological difficulties, and properties of human resources, success can be compromised (Alves et al., 2011). Furthermore, detection and identification of the agent are key-factor in control programs, being established in the handbook of the World Organization for Animal Health (OIE) Manual of Diagnostic Tests and Vaccines for Terrestrial Animals. However, a major study showed that, overall, a variety of methods for detection and identification C. fetus subsp. veneralis are in use, these was a lack of harmonization that may have consequences for the description of the health status of countries and may lead to disputes with respect to trade regulations (Van Bergen et al., 2005).

BGC vaccination in herds, despite being a best practice, has not been widely practiced, although it has been quite effective in the prevention of repeated abortions and turnover (BonDurand, 2005). Certainly, the lack of information by farmers is still an obstacle for this practice preventive BGC established in herds. Partly, too, commercial vaccines have not been efficient enough to avoid negative impact of natural infection (Cobo et al., 2003). Furthermore, route vaccine administration can also be correlated with successful prevention, since the vaginal route, compared with subcutaneous route has shown better results compared to commercial vaccines (Cobo et al., 2004) due to generation IgA antibodies are responsible for mucosal immunity. Nevertheless, cost-benefit control of BGC by vaccination is positive because has been shown that return is around 18 times the amount invested in vaccination, and the gain of only a weaned calf equivalent about cost vaccination of 100 animals (Leite, 1977).

4. Q fever

Q fever is a zoonosis of worldwide distribution caused gram-negative intracellular bacteria *Coxiella burnetii*, which can infect arthropods, birds and animals (Cutler et al., 2007). In humans, infection is usually asymptomatic, however, can progress to acute or chronic, with flu-like illness, pneumonia, hepatitis or endocarditis, spontaneous abortion and stillbirths respectively (Arrycau-Bouvery & Rodolakis, 2005). The infection mainly occurs after direct or indirect contact with infected animals, principally mammals, usually as a result of inhalation of contaminated aerosols from amniotic fluid or placenta. Currently it is not possible to accurately estimate the true prevalence infection in domestic ruminants, due to lack of well designed studies. However, there has been detection *C. burnetii* in all five continents (except in New Zealand being only country with a reported apparent prevalence of zero), with a wide range, in whatever kind. The apparent prevalence is slightly higher in cattle (20.0% and 37.7%) than in small ruminants sheep and goats (around 15% to 25%) (Guatteo et al., 2011).

4.1 Reproductive disorders in farm animals

Infections by *C. burnetii* in animal production are mostly asymptomatic, however, may be related reproductive disorders such as abortion, stillbirths, repetition heat, low birth weight animals and metritis. Nevertheless, latter clinical manifestation appears to be unique in cattle (To et al., 1998), occurring during first three weeks after birth, with fetid vaginal discharge and/or increase in body temperature (Sheldon et al., 2006). However, in dutch dairy herds, as been shown infection with *C. Burnetii* is not a major cause of metritis, although apparently microorganism has been circulated in animals (Muskens et al., 2011).

In most cases, abortion occurs late pregnancy; with free that can range from 3 to 80% (Angelakis & Raoult, 2010) with unspecified characteristic clinical signs infection with *C. burnetii*. Aborted fetuses appear normal but infected placentas exhibit intercotyledonary fibrous thickening and discolored exudates, which are not specific to Q fever (Arrycau-Bouvery & Rodolakis, 2005). *C. burnetii* can also be recovered from milk for up to 32 months. Goat shed *C. burnetii* in feces before and after kidding and the mean duration of excretion is 20 days (Angelakis & Raoult, 2010). Furthermore, there may be shedding bacteria in the urine, semen and vaginal discharge mucus. An important factor related to abortion rates in herds is the temperature, since fewer abortions lake place between months November and December. However, this occurrence increases gradually from January to February, decreasing again in March (Cantas et al., 2011).

A relevant issue is infestation of cattle by ticks during months when temperature is higher. Previous studies have shown that ticks seem to play an important role in the dissemination of bacteria in animals, especially wild, believing it to be an important factor in the transmission to domestic animals (Marrie et al., 1986; Psaroulaki et al., 2006). On the other hand, a recent study developed in the Netherlands, after three years of an outbreak Q fever, researchers investigated the role ticks in the transmission *C. burnetii*, showing that actual risk of this infection by ticks is negligible. Moreover, for future risk assessments, it might be relevant to sample more ticks in the vicinity of previously *C. burnetii* infected goat farms and to assess whether *C. burnetii* can be transmitted transovarially and transstadially in *I. ricinus* ticks (Sprong et al., 2011).

4.2 The zoonosis

Certainly, the main rout transmission of *C. burnetii* to humans is through inhalation of contaminated aerosols from placenta, amniotic fluid, wool, clothing contaminated with faces, manure, or transhumance herds infected through a valley (Arrycau-Bouvery & Rodolakis, 2005). In addition, person to person transmission is possible and coughing is associated with some proportion of Q fever cases and emits many particles of respiratory fluid that quickly attain diameters less than 100 μm; these particles can be inspired and, depending on particle aerodynamic diameter, deposit in the alveolar region or upper respiratory tract (Jones et al., 2006). Nevertheless, infected ruminants can shed *C. burnetii* during lactation period, transmission can occur by consumption raw milk (Maurin & Raoult, 1999). This form transmission can be aggravated by increasing the number of farms targeted for rural tourism (Chang et al., 2010).

There are no specific clinical sings for infection by *C. burnetii* in the acute phase, with variation in symptom severity from patient to patient. However, there is often a prolonged fever, usually accompanied by severe headache, pneumonia, which in most cases are clinically asymptomatic or mild, hepatitis, can be found three ways: an infectious hepatitis-like form of hepatitis with hepatomegaly but seldom with jaundice, clinically asymptomatic hepatitis, and prolonged fever of unknown origin with characteristic granulomas on liver biopsy; pericarditis, skin rash, neurological signs such as meningoencephalitis, lymphocytic meningitis and peripheral neuropathy. The clinical care of the chronic phase is mainly characterized by endocarditis, occurring in predisposed patients with vascular changes and the heart valves (Angelakis & Raoult, 2010).

In pregnancy, there is risk of mortality for both the mother and fetus as result of Q fever other serious complications include spontaneous abortion, oligoamnios, stillbirth, and premature delivery. Obstetric complications occur significantly more often as *C. burnetii* infects the patient at an early stage of her pregnancy (Carcopino et al., 2009). Although traditional treatment is with doxycycline, other drugs has also been used in pregnant women, such as azithromycin (Cerar et al., 2009) and cotrimoxazole, allowing the birth healthy babies (Carcopino et al., 2009).

Studies have shown that professional veterinarians and other workers who deal directly with farm animals in slaughterhouses, dairy industry and laboratory workers are at greater risk of infection by *C. burnetii* (Chang et al., 2010; Monno et al., 2009). Moreover, on can speculate that humans can act as reservoirs of the microorganism due to occurrence of spontaneous excretion of *C. burnetii* in faces and milk (Mediannikov et al., 2010). Another relevant issue is the presence bacteria in chicken eggs and mayonnaise, with strong possibility of this zoonotic agent these products to be feasible (Tatsumi et al., 2006). Thus, risk factors for infection can transcend rural people, wounded in urban areas and consequently generate more grievances in public health.

It is essential that certain preventive measures are taken to prevent spread infection by *C. burnetii*. Shares health education farmers to avoid environmental contamination, tick control, handling of placental membranes, fetal fluids and aborted fetus. Only seronegative animals and/or be included vaccinated herds. Furthermore, in herds were infection installed, cows must give birth in isolated locations that should be disinfected as well as the tools used in childbirth. Laboratories should provide necessary information and secure facilities to its employees (Angelakis & Raoult, 2010; Arrycau-Bouvery & Rodolakis, 2005).

5. Toxoplasmosis

Toxoplasmosis is a cosmopolitan disease caused by obligate intracellular protozoan *Toxoplasma gondii*. Certainly one of the most successful parasite in the world and can infect all warm-blooted animals, characterized as an important zoonotic agent (Dubey et al., 2009; Innes et al., 2009). Domestic and wild cat are the only definitive hosts of the parasite. After ingestion of tissue cysts, parasites invade enterocytes; undergo cycles of division and differentiation in microgametocytes and macrogametocytes merging to form an oocyst. This is shed in faces in the environment (Ajioka et al., 2001). Intermediate hosts to be infected with oocysts, two phases allow multiplication of the parasite. The first, rapidly multiplying, stage of the parasite is known as tachyzoite. After 1 to 3 weeks tachyzoites transform into bradyzoites: the slowly replicating form that is contained in tissue cysts (Dubey et al., 1998).

In humans, there is correlation between alterations nervous and infection *T. gondii*, such as car accidents, personality changes and schizophrenia. In addition, it has been suggested to have positive relationship between toxoplasmosis and the etiology of suicide attempt (Yagmur et al., 2010), especially in women of postmenopausal age (Ling et al., 2011). Nevertheless, further researches in this area are needed to confirm this association complex.

5.1 Infection in farm animals

5.1.1 Ruminants

In sheep flocks, toxoplasmosis is a major cause of abortion (Buxton, 1990), and consequently economic losses. Certainly, environmental contamination with *Toxoplasma* oocysts from cat feces is a major source of risk from infection at these farm animals (Buxton et al., 2007). In this context, it is important to note that domestic cats are kept on farms to control presence of rodents in the local feed store. Ingestion of infected aborted foetuses and placentas, and rodents infected birds can lead to the excretion of large amounts of oocysts environment (Zedda et al., 2009). These oocysts are very resistant to environmental conditions. They survive short periods of cold and dehydration, and to remain infectious in moist soil or sand up to 18 months. Moreover, they are highly waterproof and resistant to disinfectants (Tenter et al., 2000).

Although the prevailing view of sheep infected with *T. gondii* is this happens after birth, some studies have suggested that in exceptional circumstances, vertical transmission can occur with greater frequency (Buxton et al., 2006; Rodger et al., 2006). On the other hand, other researchers have suggested that infection via placenta is not that unusual, obtaining high rates of congenital transmission (Duncanson et al., 2001; Morley et al., 2005; Morley et al., 2008). However, there is a severe criticism concerning these recent studies, since authors conclusions were based only on PCR results, no other agents that cause abortions in sheep flocks involved in the studies (Dubey, 2009a).

The cattle is not considered an important reservoir of *T. gondii* (Dubet et al., 2009b), and offer no major risks for transmission of the agent to humans (Kijlstra & Jongert, 2008). On the other hand, has been suggested possible sexual transmission of the parasite among cattle, due to the presence *T. gondii* oocysts and in the forms of thachyzoites in semen samples (Scarpelli et al., 2009). Another interesting question is related to risk factors infection to cattle, since, if the increase in the number of cats on a farm increases possibility infection, presence of chickens is considered protective factor. The protection is provided by chicken presence probable due to the chickweed and other forage plants, seeds, and insects that partially clean environment from contaminating oocysts (Albuquerque et al., 2011).

5.2 Congenital toxoplasmosis in woman

Congenital toxoplasmosis can cause fetal abnormalities, abortion, stillbirth, and can interfere with the quality of life of children who survived the prenatal infection (Tenter et al., 2000). This form of infection is the consequence of a primary contact with the parasite during pregnancy (Cenci-Goga et al., 2011). However, the severity of congenital toxoplasmosis and the risk of intrauterine infection are closely related to the immunocompetence of the mother during parasitemia, the number and virulence of parasites transmitted to the fetus, as well as the age of the fetus at the time of transmission (Tenter et al., 2000). The damage generated in the fetus are more pronounced when they are infected in early pregnancy. Retinochoroiditis, hydrocephalus, microcephaly, and calcification are among the largest endocranial injuries (Goldenberg & Thompson, 2003). However, if fetal infection occurs in the final third pregnancy, damage to the fetus are smaller, asymptomatic newborns (Tenter et al., 2000).

However, if fetal infection occurs in the final third of pregnancy, damage to the fetus are smaller, asymptomatic newborns (Tenter et al., 2000). Pregnant immunocompromised, especially those infected with HIV, are more likely to reactivation of retinochoroiditis (Vogel et al., 1996), and the risk of fetal involvement varies between 2 and 5% (Remington et al., 2006). However, it is not ruled out the possibility of congenital toxoplasmosis in an immunocompetent mother with reactivation of chronic infection Tues eye disease during pregnancy (Andrade et al., 2010).

Serological screening in prenatal and epidemiological surveillance can be critical to reducing the risk of congenital toxoplasmosis (Mioranza et al., 2008). In regions with low prevalence of the disease, this may be an alternative strategy. However, in regions of high prevalence, these two factors are essential. Pregnant women who present with a suspected infection with *T. gondii* acquired during pregnancy should be immediately treated with spiramycin (Thiébaut et al., 2007). If the fetal *T. gondii* infection is confirmed, or in infections acquired in the later stages of pregnancy (when the rate of maternal-fetal transmission is highest), the specific treatment of the mother with pyrimethamine, sulfadiazine and folinic acid should be considered (Montoya et al., 2008). Still, there are still uncertainties related to the effectiveness of treatment of congenital toxoplasmosis. In a meta-analysis study of 2007, researchers found weak evidence for association between early treatment and reduced risk of congenital toxoplasmosis. In 550 liveborn infants infected identified by prenatal or neonatal screening, no evidence that prenatal treatment significantly reduced the risk of clinical manifestations was found (Thiébaut et al., 2007).

5.3 Vaccination against *T. gondii*

Veterinary vaccines against toxoplasmosis may have different purposes, such as the prevention of congenital toxoplasmosis, reduction of tissue cysts or vaccines to reduction oocyst shedding (Innes et al., 2007). There is a vaccine against *T. gondii* licensed for veterinary use in sheep and goats. The vaccine consists of living and a modified strain of the parasite (S48), and commercially known as Toxovax®, suitable for prevention of congenital toxoplasmosis in these ruminants. It is recommended to apply the vaccine three weeks before mating and it is estimated that the application of this immunobiological 2 mL subcutaneously induces protective immunity for at least 18 months (Dubey, 2009). However, this vaccine is not indicated for use in women because it is a parasite living in their composition. It is important that killed vaccines with high immunogenic power are able to stimulate an immune response strong and durable, providing good security for use in women and, thus, preventing congenital infection (Innes, 2010).

From the standpoint public health a vaccine to prevent shedding oocysts by cats is a great alternative (Cenci-Goga et al., 2011) in order to avoid contamination of environments. Nevertheless, as *T. gondii* does not cause clinical disease in cats, the private sector shows no interest in developing an immunobiological for this purpose, even though use a vaccine composed of a mutant strain of T-263 bradyzoites, able to avoid shedding oocysts per cats, has succeeded in reducing exposure the parasite of pigs (Mateus-Pinilla et al., 1999). Just as financial support toward the development of vaccines for neglected diseases such as visceral leishmaniasis and malaria comes from public agencies, the incentive to produce a vaccine for cats that would come from public health agency and cat owners have to be persuaded to purchase and use the vaccine for the public good (Innes, 2010).

6. Perception farmers in control and prevention abortive zoonosis in herds

6.1 Aspects in livestock

Production agriculture is associated with a variety of occupational illnesses and injuries. Agricultural workers are at higher risk of death or disabling injury than most other workers.

Traumatic injury commonly occurs from working with machinery or animals. Respiratory illness and health problems from exposures to farm chemicals are major concerns, and dermatosis, hearing loss, certain cancers, and zoonotic infections are important problems (Von Essen & McCurdy, 1998). In relation to animal production, the current situation of dairy farming, which also coincides with trends observed in other agricultural activities, is reducing the number of units production (dairy cows) and increased productivity (volume of milk per lactation) (Hayirli et al., 2002). However, productivity growth has been associated with increased incidence of diseases that can lead to economic losses for the producer, the greatest risk of antibiotic residues in milk, as well as increased frequency of antimicrobial resistant microorganisms isolated from the milk of dairy herds (Bal et al., 2010; Call et al., 2008; Nam et al., 2010), and negative perception of the population by the dairy industry (Grummer, 1995). In this context, an animal health program should consist veterinary activities in planning regularly applied and good management to maintain the herd health animal and productivity at optimum levels.

The profitability of any livestock production system basically depends on production efficiency, product quality, and especially reproductive efficiency, since the raw material needed to carry out productive characteristics is dependent on the reproductive process and the animal health status a herd. Infectious diseases, bacterial, viral or parasitic origin are important in this context, since they affect the reproductive system of males and females, preventing fertilization, causing abortions, repetition of heat, and the birth of animals with below average size. In addition, many of these organisms have zoonotic, such as bacteria and protozoa discussed in this chapter. Thus, the preventive control of males and females is crucial to get as many animals healthy at birth and hence more profitable production system (Viana & Zanini, 2009b).

Currently, the increasingly globalized world, is no longer possible to treat individual countries as the requirements for marketing for both domestic consumption and for import and export of food is becoming increasingly stringent, homogeneous, the norms established by the bodies international. Any country which has a large potential to double its food production, increasing its share in the international market of products of animal origin, should urgently develop a Strategic Security Program Food (SSPF). These measures are correlated with trends in the global market. Today there is greater concern in producing good quality products with social responsibility. In this sense, is charged to the farmer greater commitment on the quality of products, processes, and animal welfare as well as environmental responsibility and human resource availability (Jakobsen & Kristensen, 2011a). Moreover, in recent decades there has been a drastic change on the view that prevention could bring more satisfactory results rather than curative treatment. Furthermore, studies in veterinary medicine sought to identify and limit reproductive disorders at an early stage. In this sense, the concept of prevention of zoonotic diseases in livestock can be raised through an analysis of environmental or ecosystems health, linking cattle and people (LeBlanc et al., 2006).

6.2 Farmers and health education

6.2.1 Inside farm

The lack of knowledge and awareness of farmers on the importance of prevention and control of zoonosis in the farm, is not limited to developing countries. The same problem related to health education has been observed in developed countries. The decisions taken by farmers in the farm can generate great impact on society, especially in public health (Ellis-Iversen et al., 2010). Unlike the European Union (EU) that has a law that transferred responsibility to the farmers to implement animal disease control programs within the farm EU Zoonosis Directive (EC) No. 2003/99 and the Zoonosis Regulation (EC) No. 2160/2003, in many countries there are not well-established plans, mainly in South America, Africa and Asia. However, even in European countries, the attempt to implement the hazard analysis critical control points (HACCP), so that guide to good hygiene practices is adopted on farms, it is not feasible (Cavirani, 2008).

Surveys have shown that smallholder, although knowing that zoonotic agents can be transmitted through milk, do not you name them, and lacking basic information about the spread of pathogens in a herd. However, brucellosis is usually the most remembered among the zoonosis that cause reproductive disorders. This is due in part to the economic losses generated by *Brucella abortus* due to reproductive failure. Moreover, in many countries established compulsory vaccination against this disease (John et al. 2008; Mosalagae et al., 2011, Viana & Zanini, 2009a).

Another important issue is related biosecurity, which provides for the adoption of a set of measures and their benefits have been proven not only to achieve eradication, but also to keep the property free of disease infectious diseases in animal populations. A recent study showed that to implement biosecurity measures on farms, it is necessary motivation for farmers, since results are more likely to benefit society than individual farmer. However, farmers and policy-makers are faced with important questions about biosecurity at farm-level related to the sanctioning system within the contextual framework of social dilemmas. Therefore, the authors proposed the development of a market-mediated system to (1) reduce the risk of free-riders, and (2) provide farmers with incentives to improve biosecurity at farm-level (Kristensen & Jakobsen, 2011). Researchers of South-East Asia suggest that in lieu of a widespread public awareness program to deliver mass education of smallholder in disease prevention and biosecurity, livestock development projects in region, should be encouraged to include training in disease risk management as an important intervention if the current momentum for trade in large ruminant livestock and large ruminant meat is to continue to progress and contribute to addressing global food security concerns (Nampanya et al., 2011). Another study conducted in Sweden, 50% of livestock farmers living in herds with no previous isolation (Noremark et al., 2010). This decision making is crucial in the dissemination of zoonotic pathogens into a herd.

6.2.2 Attention to vaccination and veterinarian as advisor

Vaccination against infectious abortion can be an effective part in a program of animal health and biosecurity. However, although this practice capable of generating results broadly favorable, due to increased herd immunity and reduce the impact of an outbreak, vaccination alone is not able to prevent zoonotic infections and loss (Sanderson & Gnade, 2002). In the practical context of vaccination livestock, it is important to highlight a sensitive issue: smallholders in regions most in need of infrastructure and government support have greater difficulties in joining such practices. Farmers have limited resources more difficult to observe the benefits of vaccination a herd with no imminent risk of certain disease (Rogers, 2003). On the other hand, an important study developed with poor farmers in Bolivia, revealed that, contrary to recent literature, the behavior of livestock vaccination is strongly linked to social and cultural characteristics, rather than economic. Furthermore, uptake of livestock vaccination was unlikely to improve without knowledge transfer that acknowledges local epistemologies for livestock disease (Heffernan et al., 2008).

The veterinarian is an important tool management process. However, to exercise its role of advisor, you need confidence to the farmers. Is a suggested veterinarian undergo training on communication and reflection. For the farmer recognizes his work as trusted advisor in order to herd health, the veterinarian must go through a personal learning (Kristensen & Jakobsen, 2011b). The veterinarian's role in this matter may go further. Under study developed Ohio, 92 physicians were interviewed about self-assessment of knowledge of zoonosis. The survey demonstrated that over 50% of physicians were either mostly uncomfortable or strongly uncomfortable with their knowledge of zoonosis, and in their ability to diagnose and make recommendations on how to prevent zoonotic infections. Furthermore, fifty-three percent felt a collaborative relationship with a veterinarian who possessed specialty training in zoonosis would be valuable to their practice. A gap may exist in the delivery of zoonosis information and patient care, requiring better communication between health care providers, veterinarians, and public health officials serving farmers (Kersting et al., 2009).

7. Conclusion

The issues addressed in this chapter on zoonotic agents responsible for reproductive disorders in herds, extend beyond the economic losses generated by consequent loss of production (milk and meat) and reproductive (abortion, stillbirth, repetition of heat). Much has been emphasized on the generation of livestock products of excellent quality, free of virulent zoonotic pathogens, and this is not a recent warning. Unfortunately, no easy task control infections discussed in this work, especially in countries located below the Equator, as previously discussed. Recent studies have demonstrated how unprepared the farmer with simple sanitary and health education, either by socioeconomic and / or cultural. In this regard, the authors recommend the approach between three factors: (1) Universities, (2) society and (3) political authorities in generation knowledge and awareness of workers from rural areas about the importance of their work public health. The practice of extension becomes a great teaching resource, and associated with a language accessible to farmers, can be very effective, and generate human resources. In this context comes the veterinarian as a key element in mediation. Nevertheless, it is essential commitment of public health policy, is well established in the design of surveillance programs, control and eradication of certain zoonosis, is in direct support to farmers. That is, without mutual collaboration these three factors is practically impossible to obtain satisfactory results after a specific zoonosis.

8. References

Acha, P. N. & Szyfres, B. (2003). *Zoonosis y enfermedades transmisibles comunes al hombre y a los animales*, Organización Panamericana de la Salud/Oficina Sanitária Panamericana, ISBN 92-75-31991-X, 3th ed. Washington

Ajioka, J. W.; Fitzpatrick, J. M. & Reitter, C. P. (2001). *Toxoplasma gondii* genomics: shedding light on pathogenesis and chemotherapy. *Expert Review Molecular Medicine*, Vol.6, No.1, (January 2001), pp. 1-19, ISSN 1462-3994

Albuquerque, G. E.; Munhoz, A. D.; Teixeira, M.; Flausino, W.; Medeiros, S. M. & Lopes, C. W. G. (2011). Risk factors associated with *Toxoplasma gondii* infection in dairy cattle, State of Rio de Janeiro. *Pesquisa Veterinária Brasileira,* Vol.31, No.4, (Abril 2011), pp. 287-290, ISSN 0100-736X

Almuneef, M. A.; Memish, Z. A.; Balkhy, H. H,; Alotaibi, B.; Algoda, S.;Abbas, M. & Alsubaie, S. (2004). Importance of screening household members of acute brucellosis cases in endemic areas. *Epidemiology and Infectious.* Vol.132, No.3, (June 2004), pp. 533-540, ISSN 0950-2688

Alves, T. M., Stynem, A. P. R.; Miranda, K. L. & Lage, A. P. (2011). Campilobacteriose genital bovina e tricomonose genital bovina: epidemiologia, diagnóstico e controle. *Pesquisa veterinária Brasileira,* Vol.31, No.4, (Abril 2011), pp. 336-344, ISSN 1678-5150

Andrade, G. M. Q.; Vasconcelos-Santos, D. V.; Carellos, E. V. M.; Romanelli, R. M. C.; Vitor, R. W. A.; Carneiro, A. C. A. V. & Januario, J. N. (2010). Congenital toxoplasmosis from a chronically infected woman with reactivation of retinochoroiditis during pregnancy. *Jornal de Pediatriai,* Vol.86, No.1, (January 2010), pp. 85-88, ISSN 0021-7557

Angelakis, E. & Raoult, D. (2010). Q fever. *Veterinary microbiology,* Vol.140, No.4, (January 2010), pp. 297-309, ISSN 0378-1135

Arricau-Bouvery, N. & Rodolakis, A. (2005). Is Q fever an emerging or reemerging zoonosis? *Veterinary Research,* Vol.36, No.3, (June 2005), pp. 327-349, ISSN 1297-9716

Bal, E. B. B.; Bayar, S. & Bal, M. A. (2010). Antimicrobial susceptibilities of Coagulase-Negative *Staphylococci* (CNS) and *Streptococci*from bovine subclinical mastitis cases. *The Journal of Microbiologyi,* Vol.48, No.3, (June 2010), pp. 267-274, ISSN 1976-3794

Blasco, J. M. & Moryon, I. (2010) Eradication of bovine brucellosis in the Azores, Portugal-Outcome of a 5-year programme (2002-2007) based on test-and-slaughter and RB51 vaccination. *Preventive Veterinary Medicine,* Vol.94, No.2, (April 2010), pp. 154-157, ISSN 0167-5877

BonDurant, R. H. (2005). Venereal diseases of cattle: natural history, diagnosis, and the role of vaccines in their control. *Veterinary Clinics of North America: Food Animal Practice,* Vol.21, No.2, (July 2005), pp. 383-408, ISSN 0749-0720

Butzler, J. P. (2004). *Campylobacter,* from obscurity to celebrity. *Clinical Microbiology and Infection,* Vol.10, No.10, (October 2004), pp. 868-876, ISSN 1198743X

Buxton, D. (1990). Ovine toxoplasmosis: a review. *Journal of the Royal Society of Medicine,* Vol.83, No.8, (August 1990), pp. 509-511, ISSN 1758-1095

Buxton, D.; Rodger, S. M.; Maley, S. W. & Wright, S. E. (2006). Toxoplasmosis: the possibility of vertical transmission. *Small Ruminant Research,* Vol.62, No.2, (March 2006), pp. 43-46, ISSN 0921-4488

Buxton, D.; Maley, S. W.; Wright, S. E.; Rodger, S.; Bartley, P. & Innes, E. A. (2007). *Toxoplasma gondii* and ovine toxoplasmosis: New aspects of an old story. *Veterinary Parasitology,* Vol.149, No.2, (October 2007), pp. 25-28, ISSN 0304-4017

Call, D. R.; Davis, M. A. & Sawant, A. A. (2008). Antimicrobial resistence in Beef and dairy cattle production. *Animal Health Research Reviews,* Vol.9, No.2, (December 2008), pp. 159-167, ISSN 1475-2654

Cantas, H.; Muwonge, A.; Sareyyupoglu, BYardimci, H. & Skjerve, E. (2011). Q fever abortions in ruminants and associated on-farm risk factors in northern Cyprus. *Veterinary Research,* vol.17, No.1, (March 2011), pp. 7-13, ISSN 1746-6148

Carcopino, X.; Raoult, D.; Bretelle, F.; Boubli, L. & Stein, A. (2009). Q fever during pregnancy A cause of poor fetal and maternal outcome. *Annals of The New York Academy of Sciences*, Vol.1166, No.1, (May 2009), pp. 79-89, ISSN 0077-8923

Cavirani, S. (2008). Cattle industry and zoonotic risk. *Veterinary Research Communications*, Vol.32, No.1, (August 2008), pp. 19-24, ISSN 1573-7446

Cenci-Goga, B. T.; Rossitto, P. V.; Sechi, P.; McCrindle, C. M. E. & Cuçços, J. S. (2011). Toxoplasma in animals, food, and humans: an old parasite of new concern. *Foodborne Pathogens and Disease*, Vol.8, No.7, (July 2011), pp. 751-762, ISSN 1556-7125

Cerar, D.; Karner, P.; Avsic-Zupanc, T. & Strle, F. (2009). Azithromycin for acute Q fever in pregnancy. *Wiener Klinische Wochenschrift*, Vol.121, No.14, (July 2009), pp. 469-472, ISSN 1563-248X

Chang, C. C.; Lin, P. S.; Hou, M. Y.; Lin, C. C.; Hung, M. N.; Wu, T. M.; Shu, P. Y.; Shih, W. Y.; Lin, J. H. Y.; Chen, W. C.; Wu, H. S. & Lin, L. J. (2010). Identification of risk factors of *Coxiella burnetii* (Q fever) infection in veterinary-associated populations in Southern Taiwan. *Zoonoses and Public health*, Vol.57, No.8, (December 2010), pp. 95-101, ISSN 1863-2378

Cobo, E. R.; Cipolla, A.; Morsella, C.; Cano, D. & Campero, C. (2004). Immunization in heifers with dual vaccines containing *Tritrichomonas foetus* and *Campylobacter fetus* antigens using systemic and mucosal routes. *Theriogenology*, Vol.62, No.8, (November 2004), pp. 1367-1382, ISSN 0093-601X

Cobo, E. R.; Cipolla, A.; Morsella, C.; Cano, D. & Campero, C. (2003). Effect of two commercial vaccines to *Campylobacter fetus subspecies* on heifers naturally challenged. *Journal of Veterinary Medicine*, Vol.50, No.2, (March 2003), pp. 75-80, ISSN 0931-1793

Corbel, M. J. (1997). Brucellosis : an overview. *Emergengy Infectious Diseases*, Vol.3, No.2, (June 1997), pp. 213-221, ISSN 1080-6059

Cutler, S. J. ; Bouzid, M. & Cutler, R. R. (2007). Q fever. *Journal of Infection*, Vol.54, No.4, (April 2007), pp. 313-318, ISSN 0163-4453

Del fava, C.; Arcaro, J. R. P.; Pozzi, C. R.; Arcaro Junior, H.; Fagundes, E. M.; Pituco, E.; De Stefano, L. H.; Okuda, S. & Vasconcellos, A. (2003). Manejo sanitário para o controle de doenças da reprodução em um sistema leiteiro de produção semi-intensivo. *Arquivos do Instituto Biológico*, Vol.70, No.1, (Março 2003), pp.25-33, ISSN 0020-3653

Dubey, J. P.; Linday, D. S. & Speer, C. A. (1998). Structures of *Toxoplasma gondii* Tachyzoites, Bradyzoites, and Sporozoites and biology and Development of Tssue Cysts. *Clinical Microbiology Reviews*, Vol.11, No.2, (April 1998), pp. 267-299, ISSN 0893-8512

Dubey, J. P. (2009a). Toxoplasmosis in sheep - The last 20 years. *Veterinary Parasitology*, Vol.163, No.2, (July 2009), pp.1-14, ISSN 0304-4017

Dubey, J. P. (November 2009b). *Toxoplasmosis in Animals and Humans* (2th Edition), USDA/ARS, ISBN 9781420092363, Maryland, USA

Duncanson, P.; Terry, R. S.; Smith, J. E. & Hide, G. (2001). High levels of congenital transmission of *Toxoplasma gondii* in a commercial sheep flock. *International Journal for Parasitology*, Vol.31, No.14, (December 2001), pp. 1699-1703, ISSN 0020-7519

Ellis-Iversen, J.; Cook, A. J. C.; Watson, E.; Nielen, M.; Larkin, L.; Wooldridge, M. & Hogeveen, H. (2010). Perceptions, circumstances and motivators that influence implementation of zoonotic control programs on cattle farms. *Preventive Veterinary Medicinei*, Vol.93, No.4, (March 2010), pp. 276-285, ISSN 0167-5877

Franco, M. P.; Mulder, M.; Gilman, R. & Smits, H. L. (2007) Human brucellosis. *The Lancet Infectious Diseases*, Vol.7, No.12, (December 2007), pp. 775-786, ISSN 1473-3099

Freitas, J. A. & Oliveira, J. P. (2005). Pesquisa de infecção brucélica em bovídeos abatidos portadores de bursite. *Arquivos do Instituto Biológico*, Vol.72, No.4, (December 2005), pp. 427-433, ISSN 1808-1657

Friedman, C. R.;Hoekstra, R. M.; Samuel, M.; Marcus, R.; Bender, J.; Shiferaw, B.; Reddy, S.; Ahuja, S. D.; Helfrick, D. L.; Hardnett, F.; Carter, M.;Anderson, B. & Tauxe, R. V. (2004). Risk factors for sporadic *Campylobacter* infection in the United States: a case-control study in FoodNet sites. *Clinical Infectious Diseases*, Vol.38, No.3, (April 2004), pp. 285–296, ISSN 1537-6591

Gilpin, B. J.; Scholes, P.; Robson, B. & Savill, M. G. (2008). The transmission of thermotolerant *Campylobacter* spp. to people livingor working on dairy farms in New Zeland. *Zoonoses and Public Health*, Vol.55, No.7, (September 2008), pp. 352-360, ISSN 1863-2378

Goldenberg, R. L. & Thompson, C. (2003). The infectious origins of stillbirth. *American Journal of Obstetrical & Gynecology*, Vol.189, No.3, (September 2003), pp. 861-873, ISSN 0002-9378

Gorvel, P. J. & Moreno, E. (2002). Brucella intracellular life: from invasion to intracellular replication. *Veterinary Microbiology*, Vol.90, No.4, (December 2002), pp. 281-297, ISSN 0378-1135

Grummer, R. R. (1995). Impact of changes in organic nutrient metabolism on feeding the transition dairy cow. *Journal of Animal Science*, Vol.73, No.9, (September 1995), pp. 2820-2833, ISSN 1525-3163

Guatteo, R.; Seegers, H.; Taurel, A. F.; Joly, A. & Beaudeau, F. (2011). Prevalence of *Coxiella burnetii* in domestic ruminants: A critical review. *Veterinary Microbiology*, Vol.149, No.2, (April 2011), pp. 1-16, ISSN 0378-1135

Gul, S. T. & Khan, A. (2007). Epidemiology and epizootology of brucellosis: a review. *Pakistan Veterinary Journal*, Vol. 27, No.3, (September 2007), pp. 145-151, ISSN 0253-8318

Gulsun, S.; Aslan, S.; Satici, O. & Gul, T. (2011). Brucellosis in pregnancy. *Tropical Doctor*, Vol.41, No.2, (April 2011), pp. 82-84, ISSN 1758-1133

Gwida, M.; Al Dahouk, S.; Melzer, F.; Rosler, U.; Neubauer, H. & Tomaso, H. (2010). Brucellosis - Regionally Emerging Zoonotic Disease? *Croatian medical Journal*, Vol.51, No.4, (December 2010), pp. 289-295, ISSN 1332-8166

Hannon, S. J.; Allan, B.; Waldner, C.; Rusell, M. L.; Potter, A.; Babiuk, L. A. & Townsend, H. G. (2009). Prevalence and risk factor investigation of *Campylobacter* species in beef cattle faces from seven large commercial feedlots in Alberta, Canada. *Canadian Journal of Veterinary Research*, Vol.73, No.4, (October 2009), pp. 275-282, ISSN 0830-9000

Hayirli, A.; Grummer, R. R.; Nordheim, E. V. Crump, P. M. (2002). Animal and dietary factors affecting feed intake during the prefresh transition period in Holsteins. *Journal Dairy Science*, Vol.85, No.12, (December 2002), pp. 3430-3443, ISSN 1525-3198

Heffernan, C.; Thomson, K. & Nielsen, L. (2008). Livestock vaccine adoption among poor farmers in Bolivia: Remembering innovation diffusion theory. *Vaccine*, Vol.26, No.19, (May 2008), pp. 2433-2442, ISSN 0264-410X

Hegazy, Y. M.; Ridler, A. L. & Guitian, F. J. (2009). Assessment and simulation of the implementation of brucellosis control programme in an endemic area of the Middle East. *Epidemiology and Infection*, Vol.137, No.10, (October 2009), pp. 1436-1448, ISSN 1469-4409

Hegazy, Y. M.; Molina-Flores, B.; Shafik, H.; Ridler, A. L. & Guitian, F. J. (2011). Ruminant brucellosis in Upper Egypt (2005-2008). *Preventive Veterinary Medicine*, Vol.101, No.4, (September 2011), pp. 173-181, ISSN 0167-5877

Huang, J. L.; Xu, H. I.; Bao, G. Y.; Zhou, X. H.; Ji, D. J.; Zhang, G.; Liu, P. H.; Jiang, F.; Pan, Z. M.; Liu, X. F. &Jiao, X. A. (2009). Epidemiological surveillance of *Campylobacter jejuni* in chicken, dairy cattle and diarrhoea patients. *Epidemiology and Infection*, Vol.137, No.8, (August 2009), pp. 1111-1120, ISSN 1469-4409

Hughes, R. A. & Rees, J. H. (1997). Clinical and epidemiologic features of Guillain-Barré syndrome. *The Journal of Infectious Diseases*, Vol.176, No.2, (December 1997), pp. 92-98, ISSN 0022-1899

Innes, E. A.; Bartley, P. M.; Maley, S.; Katzer, F. & Buxton, D. (2009). Veterinary vaccines against *Toxoplasma gondii*. *Memórias do Instituto Oswaldo Cruz*, Vol.104, No.2, (March 2009), pp. 246-251, ISSN 0074-0276

Innes, E. A. (2010). Vaccination against *Toxoplasma gondii*: as increasing priority for collaborative research? *Expert Review Vaccines*, Vol.9, No.10, (October 2010), pp.1117-1119, ISSN 1476-0584

Jesus, V. L. T.; Trés, J. E.; Jacob, J. C. F.; Latorre, L. B. L. M. & Santos Junior, J. C. B. (1999). Campilobacteriose genital bovina: ocorrência nos estados do Rio de janeiro e Minas Gerais. *Revista Brasileira de medicina Veterinária*, Vol.6. No.3, (Dezembro 1999), pp. 133-136, ISSN 1412-0130

John, K.; Kazwala, R. & Mfinanga, G. S. (2008). Knowledge of causes, clinical features and diagnosis of common zoonoses among medical practitioners in Tanzania. *BMC Infectious Diseases*, Vol.8, No.4, (December 2008), pp. 162-170, ISSN 1471-2334

Jones, R. M.; Nicas, M.; Hubbard, A. E. & Reingold, A. L. (2006). The infectious dose of *Coxiella burnetii* (Q fever). *Applied Biosafety*, Vol.11, No.1, (March 2006), pp. 32-41, ISSN 1535-6760

Karcaaltincaba, D.; Sencan, I.; Kandemir, O.; Guvendag-Guven, E. S. & Yalvac, S. (2010). Does brucellosis in human pregnancy increase abortion rosk? Presentation of two cases and review os literature. *Journal of Obstetries and Ginaecology Research*, Vol.36, No.2, (April 2010), pp. 418-423, ISSN 1447-0756

Kersting, A. L.; Medeiros, L. C. & LeJeune, J. T. (2009). Zoonoses and the physicians role in educating farming patients. *Journal of Agromedicine*, Vol.14, No.3, (August 2009), pp. 306-311, ISSN 1059-924X

Khan, M. Y.; Mah, M. W. & Memish, Z. A. (2001). Brucellosis in pregnant women. *Clinical infectious Diseases*, Vol.32, No.8, (April 2001), pp. 1172-1177, ISSN 1537-6591

Kijlstra, A. & Jongert, E. (2008). Control os the risk of human toxoplasmosis transmitted by meat. *International Journal for parasitology*, Vol.38, No.12, (October 2008), pp. 1359-1370, ISSN 0020-7519

Kolar, J. Diagnosis and control of brucellosis in small ruminants. *Preventive Veterinary Medicine*, Vol.2, No.4, (March 1984), pp. 215-225, ISSN 0167-5877

Kristensen, E. & Jakobsen, E. B. (2011). Danish dairy farmers perception of biosecurity. *Preventive Veterinary Medicine*, Vol.99, No.4, (May 2011), pp. 122-129, ISSN 0167-5877

Kristensen, E. & Jakobsen, E. B. (2011). Challenging the myth of the irrational dairy farmer; understanding decision-making related to herd health. *New Zealand Veterinary Journal*, Vol.59, No.1, (July 2011), pp. 1-7, ISSN 1176-0710

Kuwabara, S.; Oqawara, K.; Misawa, S.; Koqa, M.; Mori, M. Hiraqa, A.; Kanesaka.; Hattori, T. & Yuki, N. (2004). Does *Campylobacter jejuni* infection elicit demyelinating Guallain-Barre syndrome?. *Neurology*, Vol.63. No.3, (August 2004), pp. 529-533, ISSN 0028-3878

Lago, E. G.; Carvalho, R. L.; Jungblut, R.; Da Silva, V. B. & Fiori, R. M. (2009). Screening for *Toxoplasma gondii* antibodies in 2,513 consecutive parturient women and evaluation of newborn infants at risk for congenital toxoplasmosis. *Scientia Medica*, Vol.9, No.1, (March 2009), pp. 27-34, ISSN 1980-6108

LeBlanc, S. J.; Lissemore, K. D.; Kelton, D. F.; Duffield, T. F. & Leslie, K. E. (2006). Major advances in disease prevention in dairy cattle. *Journal Dairy Science*, Vol.89, No.4, (April 2006), pp. 1267-1279, ISSN 1525-3198

Leite, R. C. (1977). Avaliação de alguns métodos de diagnóstico e análise custo/benefício do controle da campilobacteriose bovina. Dissertação de Mestrado em Medicina Veterinária Preventiva, Escola de Veterinária, Universidade Federal de Minas Gerais, Belo Horizonte, MG. 38p

Leonard, E. E.; Tompkins, L. S.; Falkow, S. & Nachamkin, I. (2004). Comparison of *Campylobacter jejuni* isolates implicated in Guillain-Barre syndrome and strains that cause enteritis by a DNA microarray. *Infection and Immunity*, Vol.72, No.2, (February 2004), pp. 1199–1203, ISSN 1098-5522

Ling, V. J.; Lester, D.; Mortensen, P. B.; Langenberg, P. W. & Postolache, T. T. (2011). *Toxoplasma gondii* seropositivity and suicide rates in women. *The Journals of Nervous and mental Disease*, Vol.199, No.7, (July 2011), pp. 440-444, ISSN 1539-736X

Lucero, N. E.; Ayala, S. M.; Escobar, G. I. & Jacob, N. R. (2008). *Brucella* isolated in humans and animals in Latin America From 1968 to 2006. *Epidemiology and Infection*, Vol.136, No.4, (April 2008), pp. 496-503, ISSN 1469-4409

Makita, K.; Fevre, E. M.; Waiswa, C.; Kaboyo, W.; Del Clare Bronsvoort, B. M. & Welburn, S. C. (2008). Human brucellosis in urban and peri-urban areas of kampala, Uganda. *Annals of the New york Academy of Sciences*, Vol.1149, (December 2008), pp. 309-311, ISSN 1749-6632

Marrie, T. J.; Schlech, W. F.; Williams, J. C. & Yates, L. (1986). Q fever pneumonia associated with exposure to wild rabbits. *The lancet*, Vol.22. No.1, (February 1986), pp. 427-429, ISSN 0140-6736

Maurin, M. & Raoult, D. (1999). Q fever. *Clinicam Microbiology Reviews*, Vol.12, No.4, (October 1999), pp. 518-552, ISSN 1098-6618

Mediannikov, O.; Fenolar, F.;Socolovschi, C.; Diatta, G.; Bassene, H.; Molez, J. F.; Sokhana, C.; Trape, J. F. & Raoult, D. (2010). *Coxiella burnetii* in humans and ticks in rural Senegal. *Plos Neglected Tropical Disease*, Vol.4, No.4, (April 2010), pp. e654, ISSN 1935-2735

Merianos, A. (2007). Surveillance and responde to disease emergence. *Current Topics in Microbiology and Immunology*, Vol.315, pp. 477-509, ISSN 0070-217X

Mioranza, S. L.; Meireles, L. R.; Mioranza, E. L. & Andrade Júnior, H. F. (2008). Evidência sorológica da infecção aguda pelo *Toxoplasma gondii* em gestantes de Cascavel, Paraná. *Revista da Sociedade Brasileira de Medicina Tropical*, Vol.41, No.6, (December 2008), pp. 628-634, ISSN 0037-8682

Monno, R.; Fumarola, L.; Trerotoli, P.; Cavone, D.; Giannelli, G.; Rizzo, C.; Cireroni, L. & Musti, M. (2009). Seroprevalence of Q fever, brucellosis and leptospirosis in farmers and agricultural workers in Bali, Southern italy. *Annals of Agricultural and Envoronmental Medicine*, Vol.16, No.2, (December 2009), pp. 205-209, ISSN 1232-1966

Montoya, J. G.; Remington, J. S. (2008). Management of *Toxoplasma gondii* infection during pregnancy. *Clinical Infectious Diseases*, Vol.47, No.4, (July 2008), pp. 554-66, ISSN 1537-6591

Moore, J. E.; Corcoran, D.; Dooley, J. S. G.; Fanning, S.; Lucey, B.; Matsuda, M.; MacDowell, D. A.; Mégraud, F.; Cherie Millar, B.; Mahony, R. O.; Riordan, L. O.; Rourke, M. O.; Rao, R. O.; Rooney, P. J.; Sails, A. & Whyte, P. (2005). *Campylobacter*. *Veterinary research*, Vol.36, No.3, (June 2005), pp. 351-382, ISSN 1297-9716

Morley, E. K.; Williams, R. H.; Hughes, J. M.; Terry, R. S.; Duncanson, P.; Smith, J. E. & Hide, H. (2005). Significant familial differences in the frequency of abortion and *Toxoplasma gondii* infection within a flock of Charollais. *Parasitology*, Vol.131, No.2, (August 2005), pp. 181-185, ISSN 0031-1820

Morley, E. K.; Williams, R. H.; Hughes, J. M.; Tomasson, D.; Terry, R. S.; Duncanson, P.; Smith, J. E. & Hide, H. (2008). Evidence that primary infection of Charollais sheep with *Toxoplasma gondii* may not prevent foetal infection and abortion in subsequent lambings. *Parasitology*, Vol.135, No.2, (February 2008), pp. 169-173, ISSN 0031-1820

Mosalagae, D.; Pfukenyi, D. M. & Matope, G. (2011). Milk producers awareness of milk-borne zoonoses in selected smallholder and commercial dairy farms of Zimbabwe. *Tropical Animal Health and Production*, Vol.43, No.3, (march 2011), pp. 733-739, ISSN 1573-7438

Muskens, J.; van Maanen, C. & Mars, M. H. (2011). Dairy cows with metritis: *Coxiella burnetii* test results in uterine, blood and bulk milk samples. *Veterinary Microbiology*, Vol.147, No.2, (January 2011), pp. 186-189, ISSN 0378-1135

Mshelia, G. D.; Amin, J. D.; Woldehilwet, Z.; Murray, R. D. & Eqwu, G. O. (2010). Epidemiology and bovine venereal campylovacteriosis: geographic distribuition and recent advances in molecular diagnostic techniques. *Reproduction in Domestic Animals*, Vol.45, No.5, (October 2010), pp. 221-230, ISSN 0936-6768

Naletoski, I.; Kirandziski, T.; Mitrov, D.; Krstevski, K.; Dzadzovski, I. & Acevski, S. (2010). Gaps in brucellosis campaing in sheep and goats in Republic of Macedonia: lessons learned. *Croatian Medical Journal*, Vol. 51, No.4, (August 2010), pp. 351-356, ISSN 1332-8166

Nam, H. M.; Lim, S. K.; Kim, J. M.; Kang, H. M.; Moon, J. S.; Jang, G. C.; Kim, J. M.; Wee, S. H.; Joo, Y. S. & Jung, S. C. (2010). Antimicrobial susceptibility of coagulase negative *Staphylococci* isolated from bovine mastitis between 2003 and 2008 in Korea. *Journal of Microbiology and Biotechnology*, Vol.20, No.10, (July 2010), pp. 1446-1449, ISSN 1738-8872

Nampanya, S.; Suon, S.; Rast, L. & Windsor, P. A. (2011). Improvement in smallholder farmer knowledge of cattle production, health and biosecurity in Southern Cambodia between 2008 and 2010. *Transboundary and Emerging Disease*, Vol.58, No.3, (July 2011), pp. 1-11, ISSN 1865-1682

Noremark, M.; Frossling, J. & Lewerin, S. S. (2010). Application of routines that contribute to on-farm biosecurity as reported by Swedish livestock farmers. *Trandboundary and Emerging Diseases*, Vol.57, No.4, (August 2010), pp. 225-236, ISSN 1865-1682

OIE. (August 2011). Bovine genital campylobacteriosis. World Organization for Animal Health,14.08.2011,Availablefromhttp://web.oie.int/wahis/public.php?page=disease_status_map&disease_type=Terrestrial&disease_id=31&disease_category_terrestrial=0&empty=999999&disease_category_aquatic=0&disease_serotype=0&sta_method=semesterly&selected_start_year=2010&selected_report_period=2&selected_start_month=1&page=disease_status_map&date_submit=OK

Pappas, G.; Akritidis, N.; Bosilkovski, M. & Tsianos, E. (2005). Brucellosis. *The New England Journal of Medicine*, Vol.352, No.22, (June 2005), pp. 2325-2336, ISSN 0028-4793

Pebody, R. G.; Ryan, M. J. & Wall, P. G. (1997). Outbreaks of *Campylobacter* infection: rate events for a common pathogen. *Communicable Disease Report CDR Review*, Vol.7. No.3, (March 1997), pp. 33-37, ISSN 1350-9349

Psaroulaki, A.; Hadjichristoudoulou, C.; Loukaides, F.; Soteriades, E.; Konstantinidis, A.; papastergiou, P.; ioannidou, M. C. & Tselentis, Y. (2006). Epidemiological study of Q fever in humans, ruminant animals, and ticks in Cyprus using a geographical information system. *European Journal of Clinical microbiology & Infectious Diseasesi*, Vol.25, No.9, (September 2006), pp. 576-586, ISSN 0934-9723

Remington, J. S.; McLeod, R.; Thulliez, P. & Desmonts, G. (2006). Toxoplasmosis, In: *Infectious Diseases of the Fetus and Newborn Infant*, Remington, J. S.; Klein, J. O.; Wilson, C. B. & Baker, C. J., pp. 947-1091, Elsevier Saunders, ISBN 0721605370, Philadelphia, EUA

Rodger, S. M.; Maley, S. W.; Wright, S. E.; Mackellar, A.; Wesley, F.; Sales, J. & Buxton, D. (2006). Roleof endogenous transplacental transmission in toxoplasmosis in sheep. *Veterinary Record*, Vol.159, no.23, (December 2006), pp. 768-772, ISSN 0042-4900

Rogers, E. M. (2003). *Diffusion of Innovations*. Rogers, E. M, ISBN 0743222091, New York

Rosenthal, B. M. (2009). How has agriculture influenced the geography and genetics of animal parasites? *Trends in Parasitology*, Vol.25, No.2, (February 2009), pp. 67-70, ISSN 1471-4922

Scarpelli, L.; Lopes, W. D. Z.; Migani, M.; Bresciani, K. D. S. & Costa, A. J. (2009). *Toxoplasma gondii* in experimentally infected *Bos Taurus* and *Bos indicus* semen and tssues. *Pesquisa Veterinária Brasileira*, Vol.29, No.1, (January 2009), pp. 59-64, ISSN 0100-736X

Sanderson, M. W. & Gnad, D. P. (2002). Biosecurity for reproductive disease. *Veterinary clinics of North America: Food Animal Practice*, Vol.18, No.1, (March 2002), pp. 79-98, ISSN 0749-0720

Seleem, M. N.; Boyle, S. M. & Sriranganathan, N. (2010). Brucellosis: A re-emerging zoonosis. *Veterinary Microbiology*, Vol.140, No.4, (January 2010), pp. 392-398, ISSN 0378-1135

Sheldon, I. M.; Lewis, G. S.; LeBlanc, S. & Gilbert, R. O. (2006). Defining postpartum uterine disease in cattle. *Theriogenology*, Vol.65, No.8, (May 2006), pp. 1516-1530, ISSN 0093-691X

Solera, J. (2000). Treatment of human brucellosis. *Journal Medical Libanais*, Vol.48, No.4, (August 2000), pp. 255-263, ISSN 0023-9852

Sprong, H.; Tijsse-Klasen, E.; Langelaar, M.; De Bruin, A.; Fonville, M.; Gassner, F.; Takken, W.; Van Wieren, S.; Nijhof, A.; Jongejan, F.; Maassen, c. B.; Scholt, E. J.; Hovius, J. W.; Hemil Hovius, K.; Spiltalská, E. & van Duynhoven, Y. T. (2011). Prevalence of *Coxiella burnetii* in ticks after a large outbreak of Q fever. *Zoonoses and Public Health*, Vol.58, No.4, (June 2011), pp. 1-7, ISSN 1863-2378

Stynen, A. P. R.; Pellegrin, A. O.; Fóscolo, C. B.; Figueiredo, J. F.; Canela Filho, C.; Leite, R. C. & Lage, A. P. (2003). Campilobacteriose genital bovina em rebanhos leiteiros com problemas reprodutivos da microrregião de Varginha-Minas Gerais. *Arquivo Brasileiro de medicina Veterinária e Zootecnia*, Vol.55, No.6, (Dezembro 2003), pp. 766-769, ISSN 0102-0935

Tam, C. C.; O`Brien, S. J.; Adak, G. K.; Meakins, S. M. & Frost, J. A. (2003). *Campylobacter coli* - an important foodborne pathogen. *The Journal of Infection*, Vol.47, No.1, (July 2003), pp. 28-32, ISSN 0163-4453

Tatsumi, N.; Baumgartner, A.; Qiao, Y.; Yamamoto, I. & Yamaguchi, K. (2006). Detection of *Coxiella burnetii* in market chicken eggs and mayonnaise. *Annals of The New York Academy of Sciences*, Vol.1078, No.1, (October 2006), pp. 502-505, ISSN 0077-8923

Tenter, A. M.; Heckeroth, A. R. & Weiss, L. M. (2000). *Toxoplasma gondii*: from animals to humans. *International Journal For Parasitology*, Vol.30, No.13, (November 2000), pp.1217-1258, ISSN 0020-7519

Thiébaut, R.; Leproust, S.; Chêne, G. & Gilbert, R. (2007). Effectiveness of prenatal treatment for congenital toxoplasmosis: a meta-analysis of individual patients' data. *Lancet*, Vol.369, No.9556, (January 2007), pp. 115-122, ISSN 0140-6736

To, H.; Htwe, K. K.; Kako, N.; Kim, H. J.; Yamaguchi, T.; Fukushi, H. & Hirai, K. (1998). Prevalence of *Coxiella burnetii* infection in dairy cattle with reproductive disorders. *Journal of veterinary medical science*, Vol.60, No.7, (July 1998), pp. 359-361, ISSN 1347-7439

Van Bergem, M. A.; Linnane, S.; Van Putten, J. P. & Wagenaar, J. A. (2005). Global detection and identification of *Campylivacter fetus subsp. veneralis. Revue Scientifique et Technique*, Vol.24, No.3, (December 2005), pp. 1017-1023, ISSN 0253-1933

Verhoeff-Bakken, L.; Jansen, H. A.; Veld, P. H.; Breumer, R. R.; Zwietering, M. H. & Van Leusden, F. M. (2011). Consumption of raw vegetables and fruits: a risk factor for *Campylobacter* infections. *International Journal of Food Microbiology*, Vol.144, No.3, (January 2011), pp. 406-412, ISSN 0168-1605

Viana, K. F.; Moraes, G. C. & Zanini, M. S. (2009a). Frequency of anti-*Brucella abortus* antibodies in cattle for Alegre municipality, Espírito Santo State, Brazil. *Acta Veterinaria Brasilica*, Vol.3, No.1, (March 2009), pp. 13-15, ISSN 1981-5484

Viana, K. F. & Zanini, M. S. (2009b). Profile of producers faces vaccination against infectious diseases that abortion in cattle municipality Alegre/ES, Brazil. *Archives of Veterinary Science*, Vol.14, No.2, (June 2009b), pp. 103-108, ISSN 1517-784X

Vogel, N.; Kirisits, M.; Michael, E.; Bach, H.; Hostetter, M.; Bover, K.; Simpson, R.; Holfels, E.; Hopkins, J.; Mach, D.; Mets, M. B.; Swisher, C. N.; Patel, D.; Rolzen, N.; Stein, L.;

Stein, M.; Withers, S.; Mui, E.; Eqwuaqu, C.; Remington, J.; Dorfman, R. & McLeod, R. (1996). Congenital toxoplasmosis transmitted from an immunologically competent mother infected before conception. *Clinical Infectious Diseases*, Vol.23, No.5, (November 1996), pp. 1055-1060, ISSN 1537-6591

Von Essen, S. G. & McCurdy, S. A. (1998). Health and safety risks in production agriculture. *Western Journal of Medicine*, Vol.169, No.4, (October 1998), pp. 214-220, ISSN 1476-2978

Yagmur, F.; Yazar, S.; Temel, H. O. & Cavusoglo, M. (2010). May *Toxoplasma gondii* increase suicide attenpt-preliminary results in Turkish subjects? *Forensic Science International*, Vol.199, No.3, (June 2010), pp. 15-17, ISSN 0379=0738

Young, K. T.; Davis, L. M. & Dirita, V. J. (2007). *Campylobacter jejuni*: molecular biology and pathogenesis. *Nature Reviews Microbiology*, Vol.5, No.9, (September 2007), pp. 665-679, ISSN 1740-1526

Zedda, M. T.; Rolesu, S.; Pau, S.; Rosati, I.; Ledda, S.; Satta, G.; Patta, C. & Masala, G. (2009). Epidemiological study of *Toxoplasma gondii* infection in ovine breeding. *Zoonoses and Public Health*, Vol.57, No.2, (January 2009), pp. 102-108, ISSN 1863-2378

20

Endoparasites with Zoonotic Potential in Domesticated Dogs

Katia Denise Saraiva Bresciani,
Willian Marinho Dourado Coelho, Jancarlo Ferreira Gomes,
Juliana de Carvalho Apolinário, Natalia Marinho Dourado Coelho,
Milena Araúz Viol and Alvimar José da Costa
University of Estadual Paulista, UNESP, Sao Paolo, Brazil

1. Introduction

Dogs play a relevant role as definitive hosts of a large number of parasites, shedding gastrointestinal helminth eggs and protozoan cysts and oocysts in their feces, which favors environmental contamination and possible spread of diseases (Santarém et al., 2004).

Considering the close proximity between men and dogs and the zoonotic potential of these diseases, determining the occurrence of endoparasites in pets has become increasingly relevant. These diseases are frequently diagnosed in spite of the existent therapeutic and prophylactic measures.

Contact with the soil, fomites or hands contaminated with the animals' feces favors accidental human infection either through ingestion of *Toxocara canis* embryonic eggs, resulting in Visceral Larva Migrans (VLM) syndrome (Coelho et al., 2001), or through percutaneous penetration of *Ancylostoma caninum* and *Ancylostoma braziliense* infective larvae, causing Cutaneous Larva Migrans (CLM) Syndrome (Diba et al., 2004).

Studies of animal toxoplasmosis are essential in view of its transmission to men and its pathogenicity in production animals and pets (Garcia et al., 1999a; 1999b, 1999c). Although the dog is not a definitive host, it has contributed to the mechanical dissemination of this protozoal disease (Frenkel & Parker, 1996; Lindsay et al., 1997; Schares et al., 2005).

The risk of acquiring this disease is higher in the postnatal life (Escuissato et al., 2004), when severe behavioral changes such as attention deficit and schizophrenia may occur (Lafferty, 2005), reducing the life quality of individuals (McAllister, 2005). Attention should be drawn to the risk factors for acquiring this prenatal infection, considering its pathogenesis and sequelae (Bachmeyer et al., 2006; Hung et al., 2007). There is strong association of reactivation of this disease in cases of acquired immunodeficiency syndrome - AIDS (Bachmeyer et al., 2006; Hung et al., 2007), commonly leading to secondary infection of the central nervous system in immunocompromised people and severe encephalitis (PASSOS et al., 2000; Mamidi et al., 2002; Collazos, 2003; Yadav et al., 2004; Pradhan et al., 2007). Educational programs directed at reducing environmental contamination by *T. gondii* would eventually decrease the cost of treating humans with clinical toxoplasmosis (Santos et al., 2010).

The dog is considered the main domestic reservoir for *Leishmania* spp. and the Brazilian Ministry of Health has recommended euthanasia for animals affected by this disease (BRASIL, 2006). Visceral leishmaniasis (VL) is a zoonosis worldwide distributed in tropical and subtropical regions, and 90% human cases have been reported for countries like India, Sudan, Bangladesh , Nepal and Brazil (Lindoso & Goto, 2006). Immunodepressed or chemotherapy patients are most susceptible, resulting in lethality of most cases (BRASIL, 2006). The World Health Organization classified leishmaniasis as the second most important current protozoal disease (Troncarelli, 2008).

As to Chagas Disease, millions of people are infected and suffer every year due to this illness (Rosypal, et al., 2007). In São Paulo State (SP), Brazil, infection by *Trypanosoma cruzi* has been detected in dogs (Lucheis et al. 2005; Troncarelli et al. 2009).

Molecular studies have indicated that dogs can transmit the bovine genotype of *Cryptosporidium parvum*, which is known to be pathogenic to humans (Abe et al., 2002). *Cryptosporidium* oocysts are highly resistant under environmental conditions and to the action of chemical products (Plutzer & Karanis, 2009). The protozoan *Cryptosporidium* is included in the Neglected Diseases Initiative of the World Health Organization due to their close relationship with deficient sanitation and low income of the population; thus, it is considered responsible for malnutrition and death in children (Thompson et al., 2008; Bowman & Lucio-Forster, 2010). These evolutionary forms have been detected in foods such as vegetables, seafood, unpasteurized milk, citron and mineral water in several countries. A large number of cryptosporidiosis outbreaks, waterborne, are cited in the literature (Thompson et al., 2008, Smith & Nichols, 2010).

2. Parasitic agents

2.1 Infections by *Ancylostoma* spp. and *Toxocara canis*

2.1.1 Epidemiology

An epidemiological survey carried out by our research group detected *Ancylostoma* spp. in 213 dogs (53.12%), followed by *T. canis* in 83 (20.70%). The high frequency of *Ancylostoma* spp. and *T. canis* justifies the concern about this worldwide problem, emphasizing its relevance from an epidemic-sanitary point of view (Táparo et al., 2006).

Some *Ancylostoma* species present zoonotic potential (Broker et al, 2004), such as *Ancylostoma braziliense* and *A. caninum*, who are the etiologic agents of diseases known as eosinophilic enteritis (Landmann & Prociv, 2003) and cutaneous larva migrans (Caumes, 2006).

Serosurveys have proven that *T. canis* infection is disseminated among the human population (Chieffi & Müller, 1976). Contact with the soil, fomites or hands contaminated with the feces of animals infected by these agents may favor accidental transmission to people (Guimarães et al., 2005; Blazius, 2006).

Our study indicated high occurrence of *T. canis* (67.3%) among young dogs ($P<0.0001$). Helminth and protozoal infections are more prevalent among dogs younger than one year (Gennari et al., 2001), especially when the above-mentioned helminth is involved (Fischer, 2003). There are reports in the literature about the tendency of adult dogs for presenting an effective immune response against nematodes. However, females in the postpartum were noted to shed eggs of *Toxocara* spp. in their feces (Urquhart et al. 1991). Ancylostomatidae were identified in all age ranges of dogs in our studies (Boag et al, 2003; Blazius et al 2005, Táparo et al., 2006).

In our routine laboratory services, we commonly observe dogs in their first month showing a large quantity of *T. canis* eggs in their fecal content. These evolutionary forms of ascarids, known to have thick skin, are characterized by their resistance to environmental adversities, remaining viable for many years, depending on the soil type and the climate conditions (Glickman & Schantz, 1981, Fortes, 1994).

Contributions from Oliveira et al. (1990), Gennari et al. (1999, 2001), Oliveira-Sequeira et al. (2002), Ragozo et al., 2002 and Táparo et al. (2006), in Brazil, have designed the epidemiological aspects of these parasitic disease in the canine species.

Larvae and eggs of helminths shed in the fecal content of dogs lead to great environmental contamination, representing a public health problem (Brener et al., 2005, Pfukenyi et al., 2010) in parks (Moro et al., 2008), affecting children who are in contact with sand tanks in these places, where larvae of *Ancylostoma* spp. are present (Santarém et al., 2004).

In Poland (Borecka, 2005), Venezuela (Ramírez-Barrios et al., 2004), the United States (Bridger &Whitney, 2009) and other regions of Brazil (Sousa-Dantas et al, 2007), the percentages of *Ancylostoma* in dogs were lower than that obtained in our studies, which evidenced 64.2% (27/42) positivity for samples collected from the environment. Of this sampling, 10.86% (5/46) were from child day care centers/parks, 41.30% (19/46) from streets/sidewalks and 47.82% (22/46) from squares/gardens. The genus *Ancylostoma* was present in 65.21% (30/46) samples, *Toxocara* spp. in 15.21% (7/46), *Cryptosporidium* spp. in 4.34% (2/46) and *Giardia* spp. in 10.86% (5/46) (Coelho et al., 2011).

Using parasitological necropsy, Yacob et al. (2007) in Ethiopia and Klimpel et al. (2010) in Brazil reported the occurrence of *A. caninum* in 70% (14/20) and 95.6% (44/46) examined dogs, respectively. These values are lower and higher, respectively, when compared with that obtained in the present study for *Ancylostoma* species. Our group determined the frequency and intensity of *Ancylostoma* spp. in 33 dogs by means of coproparasitological examinations and parasitological necropsy. Willis-Mollay and Sedimentation methods indicated eggs of *Ancylostoma* spp. in 87.8% (29/33) dogs. The species *A. caninum* and *A. braziliense* were found in 63.6% (21/33) and 30.3% (10/33) dogs, respectively (Coelho et al., 2011).

2.1.2 Physiopathogenesis

In dogs, the pathogenic lesions caused by gastrointestinal parasites must be considered for cutaneous, pulmonary (due to pulmonary migration of the larva during its development) and intestinal changes due to the final location of the worm in its adult stage (Fortes, 2004).

Toxocariasis in humans leads to variable clinical signs and symptoms due to the mechanical migration of larvae and the consequent immunological responses inherent in this process (Chieffi & Müller, 1976).

2.1.3 Biology

In the biological cycle of this helminth, T. canis eggs are shed in the feces and become infective under ideal conditions of temperature and humidity after two to six weeks (Scjantz & Glickman, 1983, Overgaauw, 1997).

In terms of biology, the enterohepatic pneumoenteral form is considered the most common infection form in dogs aged up to three months. Above this age range, this migration type has occurred at a lower frequency.. In pregnant bitch,parental infection occurs when larvae becoming mobilized at approximately, three week prior to parturition, and migrate to the lungs of the foetus where they molt into L 3 just prior to birth. In pregnant dogs, migrating larvae mobilize at approximately three weeks before parturition and migrate to the fetal lungs, molting into third-instar larvae before birth. In the newborn pup, the cycle is completed when the larva migrates through the trachea and into the intestinal lumen , where the final molts take placIn the newborn pup, the cycle completes when the larva migrates through the trachea and to the intestinal lumen, where molting into adult worm finally occurs (Urquart, 1991). Once infected, a bitch will usually harbor sufficient larvae to subsequently infect all of her litters, even if she never again encounters an infe

2.1.4 Clinical signs

Percutaneous penetration of *A. can*inum and A. braziliense infective larvae or ingestion of T. canis embryonic eggs leads to Cutaneous Larva Migrans Syndrome (Lee, 1874) or Visceral Larva Migrans Syndrome (Beaver et al., 1952), respectively.

In humans, the evidenced signs of toxocariasis are asymptomatic conditions, fever, hypereosinophilia, hepatomegaly, ocular, pulmonary or cardiac manifestations, nephrosis and cerebral lesion (Overgaauw, 1997).

In dogs, these helminth diseases can lead to organic imbalance such as anemia, changes in appetite, intestinal obstruction or perforation, limited nutrient assimilation, diarrhea, apathy and sometimes death (Fortes, 2004).

2.1.5 Diagnosis

In our laboratory, the following methods have been frequently employed for routine diagnosis of helminth infections: Willis-Mollay floating technique, using saturated sodium chloride solution of 1.182 density (Willis, 1921); Spontaneous Sedimentation in water (Lutz, 1919; Hoffmann et al., 1934); and Direct Examination. The first technique has as basic principle the fecal floating of nematode and protozoan eggs which are less dense, whereas sedimentation is more indicated to recover heavy eggs like those of trematodes and some cestodes; Direct Examination, however, is only recommended to verify barely floating structures since its sensitivity is low (Sloss et. al., 1999).

We carried out a study aimed at analyzing the efficiency of four coproparasitological techniques used in the laboratorial routine to diagnose helminth eggs and protozoan cysts or oocysts in dogs. Association of the methods Willis-Mollay and Sedimentation is considered superior, compared to the Direct method and zinc sulfate flotation centrifugation, to detect these evolutionary and parasitic forms (Táparo et al., 2006).

To elucidate clinical suspicions, either in tests of anthelmintic efficacy or in comparisons between diagnosis techniques for helminth infections, parasitological necropsy is considered the gold standard test, in which the stomach and small and large intestine content is washed in running water, sieved, fixed in 10% buffered formalin and stored in properly labeled flasks. Helminths are obtained by using a stereoscope microscope and the species are identified after clarifying the parasites with 80% acetic acid (Ogassawara et al., 1986).

As a future study, our group intends to standardize the *TF-Test®* kit (Three FecalTest) as the automated standard method to diagnose enteroparasites in dogs (*Canis familiaris*). A data bank will be prepared with images of eggs, cysts, oocysts and trophozoites of the main enteroparasites found and their structures. The parasitological technique *TF-Test®* will be restandardized and associated with a device containing optical microscope, digital camera and motorized platinum to obtain images. Computational techniques of image segmentation and classification of patterns will be employed with the aim of detecting and classifying the parasites found, determining the genus and species of helminths and protozoa, according to their signature or constant identification in the software. The results obtained with the coproparasitological techniques will be compared through statistical analysis, assessing the positivity of animals as to occurrence of enteroparasites and efficiency of techniques. This method will allow the automation of parasitological diagnosis in fecal samples from pets in a rapid and practical way with high efficacy, reducing pre-analytical, analytical and post-analytical errors.

2.1.6 Control

Important therapeutic and control measures to be adopted are addressed in the study of Heukelbach & Feldmeier. Based on the high occurrence of hookworm in dogs and cats in our studies, treatment with anthelmintics is needed, even for animals with negative stool tests, besides adopting a control of the number of animals in public places in order to decrease the likelihood of environmental contamination, since this parasite represents a potential hazard to human and animal health.

2.2 *Leishmania* spp.

2.2.1 Epidemiology

Leishmaniases are enzootic and zoonotic diseases caused by protozoa, morphologically similar, of the genus *Leishmania* (Monteiro et al., 2005). The visceral form has in its etiology *Leishmanias* of the *donovani* complex, including *Leishmania (Leishmania) donovani* in Asia and Africa, *Leishmania (Leishmania) infantum* in Asia, Europe and Africa, and *Leishmania (Leishmania) chagasi* in the Americas (Laison & Shaw, 1987).

This disease is predominantly of places showing low socioeconomic level and promiscuity, and environmental changes have led to its urbanization (Brasil, 2006). In dogs, as well as in humans, prevalence rates are high, reaching 1 to 36%, which varies according to the region of the country (Silva et al., 2001). Among mammals, the fox is the main reservoir in wild and rural environments while the dog is the reservoir in urban sites (São Paulo, 2006).

In Brazil, insects like *Lutzomia longipalpis* and *Lutzomyia cruzi* are identified as vectors related to leishmaniasis transmission (Brasil, 2006).

Araçatuba Municipality, SP, Brazil, our study site, is in an endemic region for canine visceral leishmaniasis, and the data obtained by the Superintendence for Endemic Disease Control (SUCEN) at that locality indicated that 3227 animals were infected from 2006 to 2010. At the Secretariat of Health of that State, a total of 1512 human cases and 138 deaths were recorded from 1999 to 2009, and in 2008, 291 people were diagnosed to have this disease, of which 23 died (Bepa, 2010).

2.2.2 Biology

In studies carried out by Lainson & Shaw, 1987, the vector became infected by ingesting, during the blood meal, amastigote forms of the parasite present in the cells of the monocyte phagocytic system in the dermis of the infected host. In the digestive tube of the insect, amastigotes are transformed into promastigotes, which multiply after three to four days of the first meal. During a new meal, the female phlebotomine inoculates these infective forms into the definitive host and they are phagocytized by macrophages, returning to the amastigote form, when they multiply causing cell rupture. Thus, there is hematogenic dissemination to tissues such as liver, spleen, lymph nodes and bone marrow (Laison & Shaw, 1987).

2.2.3 Diagnosis

The Brazilian Ministry of Health recommends ELISA as the serological screening technique and IFA as the confirmatory test for this disease, as well as euthanasia for seropositive animals, with or without symptoms (BRASIL, 2006).

ELISA (Enzyme Linked Immunosorbent Assay) represents a simple and rapid method for the survey of this canine infection (Lima et al., 2005), allowing the processing of a considerable number of samples in a short time interval (Maia & Campino, 2008).

To diagnose these diseases, serological assays of high sensitivity and specificity are used; however, infected dogs may be seronegative, and seropositive animals may not have the disease. This occurs due to the phylogenetic proximity between *Leishmania* spp. and other hematozoa, especially *Trypanosoma cruzi* (*T. cruzi*), classified into the same family Tripanosomatidae, which favors the occurrence of cross reactions in serology. In Latin countries in particular, we commonly find areas where there was the overlap of leishmaniasis and trypanosomiasis both in humans and in dogs (Troncarelli, 2008). In cases of evident cross reactions, we must consider the serological result, as well as the clinical and epidemiological factors, and carry out another diagnosis method to confirm the disease (Luciano et al., 2009).

With the development of PCR (polymerase chain reaction), a more specific and sensitive methodology, the parasite kinetoplast DNA can be identified and selectively amplified (Alves; Bevilacqua, 2004).

Considering the known phylogenetic similarity between *Leishmania* spp. and *Trypanosoma* spp. (Sundar and Rai, 2002), the consequent risk of false-positive results for these parasites (Zanette, 2006), the high occurrence of euthanized dogs due to visceral leishmaniasis in that endemic area (Nunes et al. 2008), and the absence of epidemiological surveys on canine trypanosomiasis in that region, our study was designed with the aim of detecting cross infections by these two protozoa in Araçatuba Municipality, SP. The obtained results evidence cross reactions by both protozoa in the animals analyzed in this study (Viol, 2011).

2.2.4 Clinical signs

In men, the incubation period varies from ten days to 24 months, and the average is from two to six months. In dogs, the range is wider, between three months and several years, but generally between three and seven months (Brasil, 2006).

Some dogs show few symptoms, rare cutaneous lesions and nodules, while others manifest cachexia, cutaneous changes, peeling, nodules and ulcers, especially in the ear edges or spread all over the body. Cases of conjunctivitis, blepharitis, muzzle swelling, onychogryphosis and paresis of the hind feet have been reported, including splenomegaly, lymphadenopathy, diarrhea and intestinal hemorrhage in advanced stages of the disease (Silva et al., 2001).

2.2.5 Control

Therapeutic protocols based on antimonials, diamidines, aminoglycoside antibiotics, imidazole byproducts and purine analogues are available in the studied literature.

The treatment of canine visceral leishmaniasis, for unknown reasons, is more complicated than that of humans and no medicine is totally efficient in eliminating this parasitic infection, remaining the risk of recurrence after therapy. In endemic regions, a drug protocol consists in the association between allopurinol and pentavalent antimonial like meglumine. Cases of parasite resistance and side effects have been described (Lindsay et al, 2002).

The drugs employed in the treatment of CVL are of uncertain efficacy, and the development of a vaccine has been one of WHO's main strategic alternatives (Da Silva et al., 2001).

Several immunogens have been tested, including live or inactivated vaccines, purified fractions of *Leishmania*, recombinant antigens, antigen expression and *Leishmania* plasmid DNA through the recombinant bacterium (Lima et al., 2010).

Thus, researchers are aware of the need of conducting studies aimed at standardizing, comparing and improving diagnosis methods for both zoonoses in order to facilitate the control in reservoirs and consequently in humans. For leishmaniasis in particular, surveillance programs should recommend a highly sensitive and specific method for the early diagnosis of dogs, preventing mistakes and euthanasia of healthy dogs or the maintenance of positive animals as a source of infection for humans (Troncarelli, 2008).

2.3 Infections by *Trypanosoma* spp.

2.3.1 Epidemiology

Chagas Disease is caused by the flagellate protozoan *Trypanosoma cruzi (T. cruzi)*. Several other trypanosomes parasitize animals and men, including *T. congolensis, T. vivax, T. equiperdum, T. brucei, T. evansi* and *T. rangeli* (Herrera, et al., 2005).

This disease, both in humans and in dogs, is concentrated in rural zones and poor areas of large urban centers, where the transmitting vector proliferates at a higher frequency due to the low social condition and consequently precarious living conditions (Dias et al., 2002).

Several mammals are considered important *T. cruzi* reservoirs; in the domestic environment, however, the dog is highlighted due to the vector's feeding preference for this species (Crisante et al., 2006) and due to its close contact with men, showing great epidemiological and public health importance (Eloy & Lucheis, 2009).

2.3.2 Biology

Vectors, in any stage of their life, become infected by ingesting trypomastigote forms present in the bloodstream of the infected vertebrate host during blood feeding. These forms, which multiply in the intestine of the "barber", are eliminated in their feces during or soon after blood meal (Wanderley, 1994).

2.3.3 Clinical signs

Infected dogs develop the acute or chronic form of the disease. The acute phase, symptomatic or not, lasts about two months, evolving to a chronic phase for the rest of the patient's life. The acute phase affects young dogs aged between five and six months, where generalized infections develop, with lesions in the myocardium and central nervous system, besides anorexia, lymphadenopathy, diarrhea, myocarditis and finally death from cardiac arrhythmia. The chronic phase, after eight to 36 months of the initial infection, is characterized by ventricular arrhythmia and myocardial dilatation. Signs of cardiac failure appear first in the right side of the heart, progressing to biventricular failure (Ettinger & Feldman, 1997).

2.3.4 Diagnosis

The diagnosis of trypanosomiasis has been made by the parasite survey in blood smear, xenodiagnosis, blood culture, samples from bone marrow puncture and lymph nodes (Lucheis, et al., 2005), besides indirect assays with antibody survey. The employed serological methods are ELISA, HAI, and IFA. Cross reaction between *T. cruzi* and *Leishmania* spp. in serological tests has been frequent due to the phylogenetic proximity between these parasites (Troncarelli, 2008, Viol et al., 2011).

Thus, a more accurate diagnosis requires the use of complementary techniques like direct parasitological test and polymerase chain reaction (PCR). The latter allows amplifying DNA sequences of the parasite, consisting in a highly reliable diagnosis method with sensitivity and specificity of almost 100% (Ashford et al., 1995).

2.3.5 Control

Currently, there is no available medicine capable of eliminating *T. cruzi* infection and promoting definitive healing of all treated patients. In addition, there are regional differences due to different parasite strains. Chemotherapy of Chagas Disease remains a challenge. Only two nitroheterocyclic drugs are currently used, Nifurtimox and Benzonidazole, which are active against the blood forms of the parasite, as well as against the tissue forms once administered continuously for an ideal period of 60 days (DIAS et al., 2009).

Treatment of Chagas infection in dogs and cats is still complex since most studies aim to evaluate the canine species as experimental model for therapy in humans. Furthermore, the available drugs do not promote definitive parasitological healing and the side effects are still controversial since therapy is prolonged.

Thus, prevention of Chagas Disease is needed and prophylactic measures include covering cracks, using screens on doors and windows, avoiding the permanence of animals and birds inside the house, avoiding debris, removing the nest of birds from the house eaves, and sending suspect "barbers" to the health service (São Paulo, 2011).

2.4 Infections by *Cryptosporidium*

2.4.1 Epidemiology

The genus *Cryptosporidium* is classified into the Phylum Apicomplexa and the Family Cryptosporidiidae. Genetic analyses allowed the description, according to the host, of 20 *Cryptosporidium* species, of which 12 were in mammals; in addition, 61 *Cryptosporidium* genotypes were determined (Plutzer & Karanis, 2009; Fayer, 2010).

Although there is a report of *C. muris* in dogs (Lupo et al, 2008), the latter are generally infected by *C. canis* (Abe et al., 2002; Thomaz et al., 2007) and *C. parvum* (Xiao et al., 1999). Humans are more frequently infected by *C. parvum* and *C. hominis*. Although *C. felis*, *C. canis*, *C. meleagridis* and *C. muris* were isolated from people, the risk of human infection by direct or indirect contact with pets has not been determined yet (Fayer et al., 2001; Smith et al., 2009).

The occurrence of *Cryptosporidium* in dogs was low in our study (Bresciani et al., 2008), which corroborates other epidemiological surveys in Brazil (Mundim et al, 2007; Huber et al, 2005; Lallo & Bondan, 2006). In the world, there are reports from absence (Fayer et al., 2001) to rates of 44.1% (Hammes et al., 2007). Most authors indicate higher occurrence in pups, which is associated with weaning, nutritional deficits and overcrowding conditions in kennels and/or catteries (Thompson et al., 2008).

Oocysts shed by dogs may represent a source of human infection. According to some authors, however, this animal species does not constitute important risk in terms of public health (Thompson et al., 2008; Tzipori & Griffths, 1998, Smith et al., 2009).

In an attempt to elucidate this issue, our current study included a total of 188 children from different villages of Andradina Municipality, SP, aged between zero and twelve years, as well as their respective pets, a total of 134 dogs and 54 cats, which were examined by using Enzyme-Linked Immunosorbent Assay (ELISA) with the *Cryptosporidium* test Kit TechLab®. To assess the degree of contact between the child and the respective pet, a questionnaire was applied to the 188 interviewees responsible for the children. Thus, 55.9% (104/186) parents confirmed that the animals lick the face of their children, 73.6% (137/186) are used to entering the bedroom, 11.2% (21/186) jump and/or sleep on the bed with the children, only 7.5% (14/186) children wash their hands after having played with the animal, 16.6% (9/54) cats jump onto the kitchen sink and 54.8% children (102/186) play with sand at home. Of the four children positive for *Cryptosporidium* spp. according to ELISA, three had their animals reactive (Coelho, 2009). The next step is to perform the molecular characterization of positive samples through ELISA for children and their respective pets.

2.4.2 Physiopathogenesis

Infection by *Cryptosporidium* causes atrophy, fusion and inflammation on the surface of intestinal microvilli, which result in absorptive surface loss and unbalanced nutrient transport. Diarrhea due to poor absorption is caused by epithelial barrier rupture and immunological and inflammatory responses by the host (Thompson et al., 2008).

2.4.3 Biology

Similarly to other parasites of vertebrates, *Cryptosporidium* spp. has a monoxenic life cycle, which is completed mainly in the gastrointestinal tract of the host. This protozoan, however, has peculiar features that differentiate it from other coccidia, including intracellular but extracytoplasmic location on the cell membrane surface of the infected host since it has a feeding organelle responsible for nutrition; in addition, it is included in a parasitophorous vacuole and has auto-infection capacity (Tzipori & Griffths, 1998).

As to its biology, sporulated oocysts of Cryptosporidium are ingested by the host and, following exposure to the gastric juice and pancreatic enzymes, excystation occurs in the duodenum releasing four sporozoites. The latter are covered by microvilli located in a parasitophorous vacuole and start the asexual reproduction. They develop successive merogony generations, releasing eight and four sporozoites, respectively. The four merozoites released from the second merogony originate the sexual stages, microgametes and macrogametes, which unite to originate the zygote that, after two asexual divisions, forms the oocyst. Sporulation occurs inside the oocyst, developing four sporozoites. Thus, oocysts of thin (capable of starting a new cycle inside the same host) and thick wall (highly resistant under environmental conditions and released in the feces) develop. The infection generally remains in the gastrointestinal tract (Tzipori & Griffths, 1998; Thompson et al., 2008).

2.4.4 Clinical manifestations

Absence of symptoms and release of few fecal oocysts can be more frequently found in dogs. In humans, infection by *Cryptosporidium* is generally subclinical in communities from endemic areas or causes auto-limiting diarrhea with abdominal pain and vomits (Thompson et al., 2008).

2.4.5 Diagnosis

The microscopic diagnosis of cryptosporidiosis requires time and experience of the observer since oocysts are hardly visualized, have small dimensions and do not contain sporocysts. In our laboratorial diagnosis routine, these evolutionary forms can be observed mainly by means of techniques that stain the oocysts, such as Malachite green, Ziehl-Nielsen and Kinyoun.

Intermittent excretion of *Cryptosporidium* oocysts is proven in small animals; thus, repeating the coproparasitological test is indicated, including new sample collection, even after a negative result (Huber et al, 2005).

In a study performed by our team, the parasitological tests of Kinyoun and Sheather were compared with ELISA and the latter was more sensitive in detecting infection by *Cryptosporidium* spp. in dogs (Bresciani et al., 2008).

The distinction between *Cryptoporidium* species and genotypes has been conclusive only by molecular characterization. Thus, continuing our study, Polymerase chain reaction (PCR) will be performed, including genotypic identification, which can be followed by genetic characterization with restriction fragment length polymorphism (RFLP), using the restriction enzyme R*sa*I of a DNA fragment amplified from the gene that codifies *Cryptosporidium* oocyst wall protein (COWP) and/or the sequencing involving the genes codifying 18S rRNA, actin, HSP-70 and GP-60. The latter has shown a high degree of polymorphisms between isolates from *Cryptosporidium* species with identification of several subgenotypes and subtypes. In spite of scientific advances, these cytogenetic analyses are costly and thus maintain the interest in searching for diagnostic methods that can be performed by veterinarians to confirm the clinical suspect and to adopt immediate therapeutic measures (Plutzer & Karanis, 2009).

2.4.6 Treatment

The indicated therapy was rehydration and electrolyte replacement during the initial stages of the infection, before the expression of the host immune response (Thompson et al., 2008). The first drug approved for the treatment of cryptosporidiosis in immunodefficient children and adults, nitazoxanide and its two metabolites, minimized diarrhea and oocyst release (Rossignol., 2010).

2.5 Infections by *Toxoplasma gondii*

2.5.1 Epidemiology

Toxoplasma gondii is a coccidian protozoan, obligate intracellular parasite, which affects almost all warm-blooded animal species (Dubey & Beattie, 1988).

Our research group verified association between dogs positive for *T. gondii* and raised on the ground or lawn ($p < 0.001$), compared to those kept in cemented environment (Bresciani et al., 2007).

As a disease of high seroprevalence, toxoplasmosis has higher incidence with age and is more common among stray dogs (Souza et al., 2003, Cánon-Franco et al., 2004).

Two important data obtained in our studies must be highlighted, with special emphasis on their zoonotic aspect: 1) after infection, we isolated the parasite by means of bioassay from saliva, milk and urine from the animals (Bresciani et al., 2001); 2) we noted that pups from those mothers were born serologically positive, infected, with antibody titers from 1:64 to 1:256, but apparently healthy (Bresciani et al., 2009).

Ingestion of tissue cysts, ingestion of oocysts from the feces of infected cats and congenital infection are the three main forms of *T. gondii* transmission. Other less important forms include ingestion of contaminated milk, transference of organic fluids and organ transplantation (Dubey, 1986; Dubey et al., 1990; Powell et al., 2001; Miró et al., 2004).

Our research group noted that *T. gondii* oocysts are widely distributed on the soil of elementary public schools in our region, likely constituting the main contamination source for these children (Santos et al., 2010).

Silva et al., 2010, showed that toxoplasmosis is related to problems of sanitary education, mainly concerning the appropriate cooking of foods, and was considered a public health problem.

2.5.2 Biology

In its cycle, the protozoan shows as two evolutionary forms in the intermediate host: tachyzoites, structures of rapid multiplication present in organic fluids in the acute phase, and bradyzoites, confined in tissue cysts, especially in the central nervous system and muscles, in the chronic infection. Oocysts, the final product of sexual reproduction, are formed only in the digestive tract of felids, definitive hosts which shed the oocysts with their feces, where by means of sporogony they become infective and extremely resistant to environmental conditions (Miller & Frenkel, 1972).

In more detail, the cycle starts with felids ingesting cysts present in the meat. The cyst wall is dissolved by proteolytic enzymes of the stomach and small intestine, the parasite is released from the cyst and penetrates into the enterocytes (intestinal mucosa cells) of the animal, asexually replicating and originating several generations of *Toxoplasma* through asexual reproduction. After five days of this infection, the sexual reproduction process starts and the merozoites formed in the asexual reproduction originate the gametes. The male (microgamete) and female (macrogamete) gametes, originated from one same or two different parasites, join to form the egg or zygote which, after segregating the cyst wall, originates the oocyst.

2.5.3 Clinical signs

In experimental inoculations, some animals keep asymptomatic, few become ill and deaths are rare (Dubey, 1985). However, there are reports of pulmonary and digestive disorders (Oppermann, 1971), hyperthermia, lymphadenopathy (Bresciani et al., 2001), ocular lesions (Abreu et al., 2002), and loss of consciousness and movement (Brito et al., 2002).

2.5.4 Pathogenesis

The multiplication of tachyzoites will lead the host cell to death, in addition to coagulation necrosis (cream to yellow, in the form of necrosis points of 1 to 2mm diameter) in organs like spleen, liver and lungs of the intermediate host.

2.5.5 Diagnosis

Detection of antibodies against *T. gondii* by indirect immunofluorescence reaction, as well as by modified agglutination test, hemagglutination test and ELISA, is recommended for the epidemiological survey of this zoonosis; however, serology is not always the best form to prove this disease (Zhang et al., 2001) since the bioassay represents an ideal tool to detect this parasite (Abreu et al., 2002). The histopathological test associated with the immunohistochemistry technique, and both in association with PCR, have been widely used in the diagnosis of this infection (Schatzberg et al., 2003, Bresciani et al., 2009).

Studies of the genetic diversity of a parasite have contributed to the evaluation of biological features such as virulence, resistance to drugs and immunological diversity, which can be correlated to the epidemiological tracing of the agent in order to identify infection sources or transmission routes. At the same time, they can generate knowledge to improve diagnosis, treatment and control, besides valuable information to investigate genotypes from infections in animals (Tenter et al., 2000).

Molecular and isoenzymatic studies have shown that *T. gondii* has a highly clonal population structure, although it has the opportunity to genetically recombine in a highly defined sexual cycle in definitive hosts. A consequence of this clonality would be the presence of features related to pathogenicity (Sibley et al., 1995). *T. gondii* would consist thus in three predominant clonal strains, named types I, II and III, globally occurring in animals and men (Dardé et al., 1992; Howe, Siblei, 1995).

The mouse (*Mus musculus*) has been preferably used as experimental model of toxoplasmosis. Most virulent samples for mice are known to belong to type I, while almost all non-virulent isolates are included in type II or III (Howe, Sibley, 1995). Type-II genotype is associated with the reactivation of chronic infections in AIDS patients. These researchers also noted that type-I samples were more related to congenital toxoplasmosis in people and genotype III was preponderant in animals (Howe & Sibley, 1995). Nevertheless, this correspondence between virulence and the sample molecular standard may not be necessarily observed in all hosts (Grigg & Suzuki, 2003).

2.5.6 Control

Other drugs such as pyrimethamine, trimethoprim + sulfonamide and doxycycline (Quadro 2), doxycycline, azithromycin, minocycline and clarithromycin can be employed (Lappin, 2004). Clindamycin hydrochloride can be used at the dosage of 3 to 20 mg / Kg (Quadro 2) and also at 12.5 to 25 mg / Kg, orally, at every 12h for one to two weeks to shorten the oocyst elimination time. The clinical signs of toxoplasmosis resolve within two to four days with the administration of this drug (Greene, 1990; Lppin, 2004). *T. gondii* enteroepithelial stage does not occur in dogs, which become infected by ingesting sporulated oocysts or tissue cysts. Thus, coprophagy must be prevented, while the supply of cooked meat products or commercial food is recommended.

Paratenic hosts such as flies and cockroaches must be eliminated, and the contact with soil or sand possibly contaminated with cat feces must be avoided, paying special attention to the daily cleaning of the feline sandbox in order to reduce environmental contamination (Greene, 1990, Navarro, 2001; Lappin, 2004); in addition, in this context, the birth of stray animals must be controlled, which may contribute to reducing the occurrence of this important zoonosis (Jittapalapong et al., 2007).

3. Final considerations

Considering the importance of the instruction and information level of teachers from municipal early childhood education centers (EMEI.S), the high occurrence of endoparasites in humans and the endemic situation of canine visceral leishmaniasis in Araçatuba Region, we investigated the knowledge degree of those teachers concerning parasitic zoonoses. Thirty EMEI.S from Araçatuba were visited and 85 teachers were interviewed. Descriptive statistical analysis indicated that 96.47% (82 out of 85) teachers answered that walking barefoot may interfere in helminth infection, while 85.88% (73/85) answered that nail biting may interfere in it. We verified that 44.71% (38/85) of them did not know the pathogenesis of helminth diseases and 63.53% (54/85) did not administer anthelmintics to small animals. The participation of cats in toxoplasmosis transmission was known by 92.94% (79/85), of which 82.35% (70/85) did not know the transmission routes. The dog was considered the disseminator of this disease by 80.00% (68/85) interviewees, and only 4.71% (4/85) cited ingestion of meat products as a route of *Toxoplasma gondii* transmission, while 67.06% (57/85) did not know about this issue. As to leishmaniasis, 91.76% (78/85) stated that dogs are the transmitters, but 58.82% (50/85) did not know how and 60.00% (51/85) recommended environmental cleaning as exclusive preventive measure. Based on the obtained data, we can infer that there is the need of implanting a community education program directed to the improvement of basic concepts of control and prevention of parasitic zoonoses (Tome et al., 2005).

Our team interviewed people in the Third Age about basic concepts related to parasitoses. The obtained results proved the need of promoting elucidation campaigns directed to the aged, addressing the control of these diseases (Lima et al. 2008).

More recently, we have carried out a study with the aim of guiding owners about concepts related to the responsible ownership of their pets in an endemic area for canine visceral leishmaniasis. Questionnaires about responsible ownership and control of this disease were applied to the owners of dogs and cats living in Araçatuba Municipality, SP, initially to assess the knowledge degree of these people. Then, based on the deficits verified in their responses, the authors of this study individually instructed the owners of these animals at their houses about the critical points to be reformulated in order to correct erroneous concepts concerning these issues. Thus, 25% (22/88) individuals had already had dogs seropositive for Canine Visceral leishmaniasis in their houses and of these, 54.55% (12/22) sent their animal to veterinarian clinics for euthanasia, 22.73% (5/22) used the services of the Municipal Zoonosis Control Center and 18.18% (4/22) paid for private treatment. However, 35.63% (31/87) dogs were never subjected to exams for the diagnosis of infection by *Leishmania* spp. (MATOS et al., 2011).

These studies indicated misinformation of owners regarding the control of canine endoparasitoses, evidencing the need of continuous implantation of campaigns for community concern.

4. References

Abe N, Sawano Y, Yamada K, Kimata I, Isemi M. *Cryptosporidium* infection in dogs in Osaka, Japan. *Veterinary Parasitology*. Vol. 108, N°3, *September* 2002; pp. 185-93, 545-8585

Abreu, C. B.; Navarro, I. T.; Reis, A. C. F.; Souza, M. S. B.; Machado, R.; Marana, E. R. M.; Prudêncio, L. B.; Mattos, M. R.; Tsutsui, V. S. Toxoplasmose ocular em cães jovens inoculados com *Toxoplasma gondii*. *Ciência Rural*. Vol. 32, N°. 5, Set- Out 2002, pp. 807-812, 0103-8478

Alves, W. A.; Bevilacqua, P. D. Reflexões sobre a qualidade do diagnóstico da leishmaniose visceral canina em inquéritos epidemiológicos: o caso da epidemia de Belo Horizonte, Mina Gerais, Brasil, 1993-1997. *Cadernos de Saúde Pública*, Vol. 20, N°. 1, 2004, pp. 259-265, 0102-311X

Ashford, D. A.; Bozza, M.; Freire, M.; Miranda, J. C.; Sherlock, I.; Eulálio, C.; Lopes, U.; Fernandes, O.; Degrave, W.; Barker Jr, R. H.; Badaró, R.; David, J. R. Comparison of the polimerase chain reaction and serology for the detection of canine visceral leishmaniasis. American Journalof Tropical Medicine and Hygiene. Vol. 53, N°. 3, Setember 1995, pp. 251-255, 0002-9637

Bachmeyer, C.; Mouchnino, G.; Thulliez, P.; Blum, L. Congenital toxoplasmosis from an HIV-infected woman as a result of reactivation. The Journal of Infection, London, February 2006, Vol. 52, N°. 2, pp. e55–e57,

Beaver, P.C., Syndrer, C.H., Carrera, G.M., Dent, J.H., Lafferty, J.W. Chronic eosinophilia due to visceral larva migrans: report of three cases. Pediatrics, Vol. 9, N°. 1, January 1952, p.7-9,

Bepa Comitê de leishmaniose visceral americana (2010) Classificação epidemiológica dos municípios segundo o programa de vigilância e controle da leishmaniose visceral americana no estado de São Paulo, atualizado em maio de 2010 *Bol Epidemiol Paul* 7:21-40

Blazius, R.D.; Emerick. S.; Prophiro, J.S.; Romão, P. R. T.; Silva, O.S. Ocorrência de protozoários e helmintos em amostras de fezes de cães errantes da cidade de Itapema, Santa Catarina. *Revista da Sociedade Brasileira de Medicina Tropical,* Vol. 38, N°. 1, Jan./Feb. 2005, pp. 73-74, 0037-8682

Bowman, DD., & Lucio-Forster, A. 2010. Cryptosporidiosis and giardiasis in dogs and cats: Veterinary and public health importance. *Experimental Parasitology.* Vol. 124, No. 1, january 2010, pp. 121-127, 0014-4894

Boag P.R.; Parsons, J.C.; Presidente, P.J.; Spithill, T.W.; Sexton, J.L. Characterization of humoral immune responses in dogs vaccinated with irradiated Ancylostoma caninum. Veterinary Immunology and Immunopathology, March 2003, Vol. 92, N°. 1-2, pp. 87-94,

Borecka, A. Prevalence of intestinal nematodes of dogs in Warsaw area, Poland. *Helminthologia.* 2005, Vol. 42, N°1, pp.35-9.

Brasil. Ministério da Saúde. Secretaria de Vigilância em Saúde. Departamento de Vigilância Epidemiológica. Manual de Vigilância e controle da leishmaniose visceral. Brasília, 2006. pp. 9-18.

Bradley, C.A., Altizer, S. Urbanization and the ecology of wildlife diseases. *Trends in Ecology & Evolution* . February 2007; Vol. 22, N°2, pp. 95-102,

Brener, B., Lisboa, L., Mattos, DPBG., Arashiro, EKN., Millar, PR., Sudré, AP., & Duque, V. Frequência de enteroparasitas em amostras fecais de cães e gatos dos municípios do Rio de Janeiro e Niterói. *Revista Brasileira de Ciência Veterinária.* Vol. 12, No.1, janeiro-dezembro 2005, pp. 102-105, 1413-0130.

Bresciani, K. D. S.; Toniollo, G. H.; Costa, A. J.; Sabatini, G. A.; Moraes, F. R. Clinical, parasitological and obstetric observations in pregnant bitches with experimental toxoplasmosis. *Ciência Rural,* Vol. 31, N°.6, Dec. 2001, pp. 1039-1043, 0103-8478

Bresciani, KDS., Amarante, AFT., Lima, VFM., Feitosa, MM., Feitosa, FLF., Serrano, ACM., Ishizaki, MN., Tome, RO., Táparo, CV., Perri, SHV., & Meireles., MV. 2008. Infection by Cryptosporidium spp. in dogs from Araçatuba, SP, Brazil: Comparison between diagnostic methods and clinical and epidemiological analysis. *Veterinária e Zootecnia.* Vol. 15, No. 3, Dec. 2008, p.466-468, 0102-5716.

Bresciani, K. D. S., Bridger, K.E., Whitney, H. Gastrointestinal parasites in dogs from the Island of St. Pierre off the south coast of Newfoundland. *Veterinary Parasitology.* May 2009, Vol. 162, N°. 1-2, pp. 167-70.

Bresciani, K. D. S, Costa, A. J. G., Toniollo, H., Luvizzoto, M. C. R., Kanamura, C. T., Moraes, F. R., Perri, S. H. V & S. M. Gennari. Transplacental transmission of Toxoplasma gondii in reinfected pregnant female canines. *Parasitolology Research*, 2009, Vol. 104 pp. 1213–1217

Brooker, S., Bethony, J., Hotez, P.J. Human hookworm infection in the 21st Century. Adv. Parasitol. 2004; 58: 197-288.

Bresciani, K. D. S., Costa, A. J., Nunes, C. M., Serrano, A. C. M., Moura, A. B., Stobbe, N. S., Perri, S. H. V., Dias, R. A., Genari, S. M. Ocorrência de anticorpos contra *Neospora caninum e Toxoplasma gondii* e estudo de fatores de risco em cães de Araçatuba - SP. *Ars Veterinária*, Vol. 23, Nº. 1, 2007, pp. 40-46, 0102-6380

Brito, A. F.; Souza, L. C.; Silva, A. V.; Langoni, H. Epidemiological and serological aspects in canine toxoplasmosis in animals with nervous symptoms. *Memórias do Instituto Oswaldo Cruz*, Vol. 97, Nº. 1, Jan 2002, pp.31-35, 0074-0276

Caumes, E. 2006. It's time to distinguish the sign "creeping eruption" from the syndrome "cutaneous larva migrans". *Dermatology*. Vol. 213, No. 3, 2006, pp. 179-81, 1018-8665

Cañon-Franco, W. A.; Bergamaschi, D. P.; Labruna, M. B.; Camargo, L. M.; Silva, J. C.; Pinter, A.; Gennari, S. M. Ocurrence of anti-Toxoplasma gondii antibodies in dogs in the urban area of Monte Negro, Rondônia, Brazil. *Veterinary Research Communications*, Vol. 28, Nº.2, 2004 pp.113-118,

Chieffi, P. P.; Müller, E. E. Prevalência de parasitismo por Toxocara canis em cães e presença de ovos de Toxocara sp no solo de localidades públicas da zona urbana do município de Londrina, estado do Paraná, Brasil. *Revista de Saúde Pública*, Vol. 10, Nº. 10, 1976, pp. 367-372,

Coelho, LMPS., Dini, CY., Milman, MHSA., & Oliveira, SM. 2001. Toxocara spp. eggs in public squares of Sorocaba, São Paulo State, Brazil. *Revista do Instituto de Medicina Tropical de São Paulo*. Vol. 43, No. 4, july-august 2001, pp. 189-191, 0036-4665.

Coelho, NMD. 2009. *Ocorrência de Cryptosporidium* spp. *em crianças e seus respectivos cães e gatos de estimação no Município de Andradina, SP*. Dissertação (Mestrado em Ciência Animal - Medicina Veterinária Preventiva e Produção Animal), Universidade Estadual Paulista. Araçatuba, SP.

Coelho, W. M. D.; Amarante, A. F. T.; Apolinario, J.C.; Coelho, N. M. D.; & Bresciani, K. D. S. Prevalence of Ancylostoma among dogs, cats and public places from Andradina city, São Paulo State,Brazil. *Revista do Instituto de Medicina Tropical de São Paulo* (in press), 2011.

Crisante, G.; Rojas, A.; Teixeira, M. M.; Añez, N. Infected dogs as a risk factor in the transmission of human Trypanosoma cruzi infection in western Venezuela. *Acta Tropica.*, Vol 98, Nº. 3, July 2006, pp. 247-54,

Da Silva, Vo; Borja-Cabrera, Gp; Correia Pontes, Nn; Paraguai De Souza, E; Luz, Kg; Palatnik, M; Palatnik-De-Sousa, Cb. A Phase III trial of Efficacy of the FML-vaccine against canine kala-azar in an endemic area of Brazil (São Gonçalo do Amarante, RN). Vaccine, Vol. 19, Nº. , , 2001 pp.1082–92.

Dias, E. D. Leishmaniose visceral: estudo de flebotomíneos e infecção canina em Montes Claros, Minas Gerais. *Rev. Soc. Bras. Med. Trop.*, v. 38, n. 2, p.147-152, 2005.

Dias, L.C., Dessoy, M.A. Quimioterapia da doença de Chagas: estado da arte e perspectivas no desenvolvimento de novos fármacos. Quim. Nova, v.32, n.9, p. 2444-2457, 2009

Diba, VC., Whitty, CJM., & Green, T. Cutaneous larva migrans acquired in Britain. *Clinical and experimental dermatology*. Vol. 29, No. 5, september 2004, pp. 555–556, 0307-6938.

Dubey, J. P. Toxoplasmosis in dogs. *Canine Practice*, Vol. 28, pp.7-28, 1985.

Dubey, J. P.; BEATTIE, C. P. *Toxoplasmosis of animals and man*. Boca Raton: CRC, 1988

Ettinger, S. J., Feldman, E. C. In: *Tratado de Medicina Veterinária Interna – Moléstias do cão e do gato*. 4.ed. São Paulo: Manole, 1997, pp. 1185-1217.

Eloy, L.J.; Lucheis, S.B. Canine trypanosomiasis: etiology of infection and implications for public health. *Journal of Venomous Animal and Toxins including Trop. Diseases*, Vol. 4, N°15, 2009, pp. 589-611

Escuissato, D. L.; Aguiar R. O.; Gasparetto, E. L.; Müller, N. L. Disseminated toxoplasmosis after boné marrow transplantation: high-resolution CT appearance. *Journal of Thoracic Imaging*, Philadelphia, Vol. 19, N°.3, 2004, pp.207-209,

Fayer R, Trout JM, Xiao L, Morgan UM, Lal AA, Dubey JP. *Cryptosporidium canis* n.sp. from domestic dogs. Journal Parasitology 2001; 87:1415-22.

Fayer R. 2010. Taxonomy and species delimitation in Cryptosporidium. *Experimental Parasitology*. Vol. 124, No. 1, january 2010; pp. 90-97, 0014-4894

Frenkel, J. K.; Parker, B. B. An apparent role of dogs in the transmission of Toxoplasma gondii . The probable importance of xenosmophilia. Annals of the New York Academy of Sciences, New York, v.791, p.402-407, 1996.

Garcia, J. L.; Navarro, I. T.; Ogawa, L.; OliveirA, R. C. Soroepidemiologia da toxoplasmose em gatos e cães de propriedades rurais do Município de Jaguapitã, Estado do Paraná, Brasil. *Ciência Rural, Santa Maria*, Vol.29, N°.1, 1999[a], pp.99-104,.

Garcia, J. L.; Navarro, I. T.; Ogawa, L.; Oliveira, R. C. Soroprevalência do Toxoplasma gondii em suínos, bovinos, ovinos e eqüinos e sua correlação com humanos, felinos e caninos, oriundos de propriedades rurais do Norte do Paraná- Brasil. *Ciência Rural, Santa Maria*, Vol.29, N°.1, 1999b, pp.91-97,

Garcia, J. L.; Navarro, I. T.; Ogawa, L.; Oliveira, R. C.; Kobilka, E. Seroprevalence, epidemiology and ocular evaluation of human toxoplasmosis in a rural area in Jaguapitã (Parana), Brazil. *Revista Panamericana de Salud Publica*, Washington, Vol.6, N°.3, 1999c, pp.157-163.

Gennari, S. M.; Pena, H. F. J.; Blasques, L. S. Freqüência de ocorrência de parasitos gastrintestinais em amostras de fezes de cães e gatos da cidade de São Paulo. *Veterinary News*, v. 8, n. 52, p. 10-12, 2001.

Gennari, S. M.; Kasai, N.; Pena, H. F. J.; Cortez, A. Ocorrência de protozoários e helmintos em amostras de fezes de cães e gatos da cidade de São Paulo. *Brazilian Journal of Veterinary Research and Animal Science*, Vol. 36, N°.2, 1999, pp. 87-91.

Glickman, L. T.; Schantz, P. M. Epidemiology and pathogenesis of zoonotic toxocariasis. *Epidemiologic Reviews*, Vol. 3, 1981, pp. 230-250.

Greene, C. E. *Infectious diseases of the dog and cat*. Philadelphia: W. B. Saunders, 1990, pp.819-829

Grigg, M. E.; Suzuki, Y. Sexual recombination and clonal evolution of virulence in *Toxoplasma gondii*. *Microbes and Infection*, Paris, Vol.5, N°.7, 2003, pp.685-690,.

Fortes, E. Parasitologia veterinária. 4 ed. rev.amp. Porto Alegre: Ícone, 2004. pp.607

Hammes IS, Gjerde BJ, Robertson LJ. A longitudinal study on the occurrence of *Cryptosporidium* and *Giardia* in dogs during their first year of life. *Acta Veterinari Scandinavica* 2007; Vol.49, pp 1-10.

Herrera, H. M.; Norek, A.; Freitas, T. P. T.; Rademaker, V.; Fernandes, O.; Jansen, A. M. Domestic and wild mammals infection by *Trypanosoma evansi* in a pristine area of Brazilian Pantanal region. *Parasitoogyl. Research.*, Vol. 96, 2005, pp. 121-126,

Hoffman, W.A.; Pons, J.A.; Janer, J.L. The sedimentation-concentration method in schistosomiasis mansoni. *Puerto Rico Journal Public Health*, v.9, p. 281-298, 1934.

Huber F, Bomfim TCB, Gomes RS. Comparison between natural infection by *Cryptosporidium* sp., *Giardia* sp. in dogs in two living situations in the West Zone of the municipality of Rio de Janeiro. *Veterinary Parasitology*; Vol. 130, 2005, pp. 69-72.

Hung, C.C.; Fan, C.K.; Su, K.E.; Sung, F.C.; Chiou, H.Y.; Gil. V.; Ferreira, M.D.A. C.; Carvalho, J.M.; Cruz, C.; Lin, Y.K.; Tseng, L. F.; Sao, K.Y.; Chang, W. C.; Lan; H.S.; Chou, S.H. Serological screening and toxoplasmosis exposure factors among pregnant women in the Democratic Republic of Sao Tome and Principe.Transactions of the *Royal Society of Tropical Medicine and Hygiene*, Vol. 101, N°.2, 2007, pp. 134-139.

Hutchison, W. M.; Dunachie, J. F.; Work, K. The faecal transmission of Toxoplasma gondii. *Acta Pathologica et Microbioloica Scandinavica*, Copenhagen, Vol.74, N°.3, 1968, pp.462-464,.

Hutchison, W. M.; Dunachie, J. F.; Work, K.; Siim, J. C. The life cycle of the coccidian parasite, Toxoplasma gondii in the domestic cat. Transactions of the *Royal Society of Tropical Medicine and Hygiene*, London, Vol.65, N°.3, 1971, pp.380-399.

Jittapalapong, S.; Nimsupan, B.; Pinyopanuwat, N.; Chimnoi, W.; Kabeya, H.; Maruyama, S. Seroprevalence of *Toxoplasma gondii* antibodies in stray cats and dogs in the Bangkok metropolitan area, Thailand . *Veterinary Parasitology*, Amsterdam, Vol.145, N.1-2, pp.138-141, 2007.

Laison, R.; Shaw, J. J.; Silveira, F. T.; Braga, R. American visceral leishmaniasis: on the origin of Leishmania (Leishmania) chagasi. *Transactions of the Royal. Society of Tropical. Medicine and Hyieneg.*, Vol. 81, pp. 517, 1987.

Lafferty, K. D. Look what the cat dragged in: do parasites contribute to human cultural diversity? *Behavioural Processes*, Amsterdam, Vol.68, N°.3, , 2005, pp.279-282.

Landmann, J.K., Prociv, P. Experimental human infection with the dog hookworm, *Ancylostoma caninum*. MJA. 2003; 178: 69-71.

Lappin, M. R. Doenças causadas por protozoários. In: ETTINGER, S. J.; FELDMAN, E. C. (Ed.). *Tratado de medicina interna veterinária*: doenças do cão e do gato. 5.ed. Rio de Janeiro: Guanabara Koogan, 2004. pp. 430-435

Lallo MA, Bondan EF. Prevalência de *Criptosporidium* em cães de instituições da cidade de São Paulo. Rev Saúde Pub 2006; Vol 40, pp. 120-5.

Lee, R.J. Case of creeping eruption. Transactions of the Clinical Society, v. 8, p. 44-45, 1874.

Lima, F.F.; Koivisto, M.B.; Perri, S.H.V.; Amarante, A.F.T.; Bresciani, K.D.S. O conhecimento de idosos sobre parasitoses em instituições não governamentais do município de Araçatuba, SP. 3o Congresso de Extensão Universitária, 2007.

Lima, V.M.F., Ikeda, F.A., Rossi, CN., Feitosa, M.M., Vasconcelos, R.O., Nunes, C.M., Goto, H. Diminished CD4+/CD25+ T cell and increased IFN-γ levels occur in dogs vaccinated with Leishmune® in an endemic area for visceral leishmaniasis. *Veterinary Immunology and Immunopathology* , Vol. 135, pp. 296–302, 2010.

Lima, V. M. F.,Biazzono, L., Silva, A. C., Correa, A. P. F. L., Luvizotto, M. C. R. Serological diagnosis of visceral leishmaniasis by an enzyme immunoassay using protein A in naturally infected dogs. *Pesquisa Veterinaria Brasileira.* Vol. 25, N°. 4, 2005, pp. 215-218,

Lindsay, D. S.; Dubey, J. P.; Butler, J. M.; Blagburn, B. L. Mechanical transmission of *oxoplasma gondii* oocysts by dogs. *Veterinary Parasitology,* v.73, n.1/2, p.27-33, 1997.

Lindsay DS, Zajac AM, Barr SC: Leishmaniasis in American Foxhounds: An Emerging Zoonosis? Compend Cont Educ Pract Vet , Vol. 24, pp. 304-312, 2002

Lindoso, J. A. L. & Goto, H. Leishmaniose Visceral: situação atual e perspectivas futuras. *Boletim Epidemiológico Paulista,* v. 3, n. 26, 2006.

Lucheis, S. B.; Da Silva, A. V.; Araujo Junior, J. P.; Langoni, H.; Meira, D. A.; Marcondes-Machado, J. Trypanosomatids in dogs belonging to individuals with chronic Chagas' disease living in Botucatu town and surrounding region. São Paulo State, Brazil. *Journal. of Venomous Animals and Toxins including. Tropical Diseases,* Vol. 11, N°. 4, p. 492-509, 2005.

Luciano, R.M.; Lucheis, S.B.; Troncarelli, M.Z.; Luciano, D.M.; Langoni, H. Avaliação da reatividade cruzada entre antígenos de *Leishmania* spp e *Trypanosoma cruzi* na resposta sorológica de cães pela técnica de imunofluorescência indireta (RIFI). *Brazilian Journal* of *Veterinary Research* and *Animal Science* - Vol. 46, N°. 3, pp. 181-187, 2009.

Lupo PJ, Langer-Curry RC, Robinson M, Okhuysen PC, Chappell CL. *Cryptosporidium muris* in a Texas canine population. *American Journal Tropical Medicine and Hygiene;* Vol. 78, pp 917-21, 2008

Lutz, A. O Schistosomum mansoni e a schistosomatose segundo observações feitas no Brasil. *Memórias do Instituto Oswaldo Cruz,* Vol. 11, N°. 1, pp. 121-155, 1919

Maia, C. & Campino, L. Methods for diagnosis of canine leishmaniasis and immune response to infection. *Veterinary. Parasitology.* N°158, pp. 274-287, 2008.

McALLISTER, M. M. A decade of discoveries in veterinary protozoology changes our concept of "subclinical" toxoplasmosis. *Veterinary Parasitology,* Amsterdam, v.132, n.3/4, p.241-247, 2005.

Mamidi, A.; DeSimone, J. A., Pomerantz, R. J. Central nervous system infectious in individuals with HIV-1 infection. *Journal of Neurovirology,* Philadelphia, v.8, n.3, p.158-167, 2002.

Miller, N. L.; Frenkel, J. K.; Dubey, J. P. Oral infections with Toxoplasma cysts and oocysts in felines, other mammals and birds. *Journal of Parasitology,* Vol.58, N°.5, pp.928-937, 1972.

Monteiro, E. M.; Silva, J. C. F.; Costa, R. T.; Costa, D. C.; Barata, R. A.; Paula, E. V.; Machado-Coelho, G. L. L.; Rocha, M. F.; Fortes-Dias, C. L.; Dias, E. D. Leishmaniose visceral: estudo de flebotomíneos e infecção canina em Montes Claros, Minas Gerais. *Revista da Sociedade Brasileira de Medicina Tropical. Vol.* 38, N° 2, pp.147-152, 2005.

Moro, F. C. B., Pradebon, J. B., Santos, H. T., Querol, E. Ocorrência de *Ancylostoma* spp. e *Toxocara* spp. em praças e parques públicos dos municípios de Itaqui e Uruguaiana Fronteira oeste do Rio Grande do Sul. Biodivers Pampeana. 2008; Vol.6: pp.25-9.

Mundim MJS, Rosa LAG, Hortêncio SM, Faria ESM, Rodrigues RM, Curi MC. Prevalence of *Giardia duodenalis* and *Cryptosporidium* spp. in dogs from different living conditions in Uberlândia, Brazil. *Veterinary Parasitology* 2007; Vol. 144: pp. 356-9.

Navarro, I T. Toxoplasmose . In: Congresso Da Associação Brasileira De Veterinários Especialistas Em Suinos, 2001, Porto Alegre. *Anais...* Porto Alegre: 2001. (on line)

Nunes CM, Lima VMF Paula HB, Perri SHV, Andrade AM, Dias FEF, Burattini MN (2008) Dog culling and replacement in na área endemic for visceral leishmaniasis in Brazil. *Veterinary Parasitology*, Vol. 153, pp.19-23

Ogassawara, S., Benassi, S., Larsson, C.E.,Leme, P.T.Z., Hagiwara, M.K. Prevalência de infecções helmínticas em gatos na cidade de São Paulo. *Revista da Faculdade de Medicina Veterinária e Zootecnia da Universidade de São Paulo,* Vol.23,pp.145-149, 1986

Oliveira, P.R., Silva, P.L., Parreira, V.F.,Ribeiro, S.C.A., Gomes, J.B. Prevalência de endoparasitos em cães da região de Uberlândia, Minas Gerais. *Brazilian Journal of Veterinary Research and Animal Science,* Vol..27, pp.193-197, 1990.

Oliveira-Sequeira, T.C.G., Amarante, A.F.T., Ferrari, T.B., Nunes, L.C. Prevalence of intestinal parasites in dogs from São Paulo State, Brazil. *Veterinary Parasitology,* Vol. l, N°. 103, pp.19-27, 2002.

Oppermann, W. H. *Versuche zum experimentellen infection des hundes mit Toxoplasma - oozysten.* 1971. Dissertation (Mestrado) - Institute fur Parasitologie dês Fachbereiches Veterinarmedizin, Universität Berlin, Berlin.

Overgaauw, P. A. M. Aspects of Toxocara epidemiology: human toxocarosis. *Critical Reviews in Microbiology,* Vol. 23, N°. 3, pp. 215-231, 1997.

Pfukenyi, D. M. Chipunga, S. L., Dinginya, L., Matenga, E. A survey of pet ownership, wareness, and public knowledge of pet zoonoses with particular reference to roundworms and hookworms in Harare, Zimbabwe. Trop. Anim. Health Prod. 2010; 42: 247-52.

Plutzer J, & Karanis, P. 2009. Genetic polymorphism in *Cryptosporidium* species: in update. *Veterinary Parasitology.* Vol. 165, No. 3-4, pp. 187-199, 0304-4017.

Pradhan, S.; Yadav, R.; Mishra, V. N. *Toxoplasma* meningoencephalitis in HIV-seronegative patients: clinical patterns, imaging features and treatment outcome. *Transactions of the Royal Society of Tropical Medicine and Hygiene,* London, v.101, n.1, p.25-33, 2007.

Ragozo, A.M.A., Muradian, V., Silva, J.C.R.,Caraviere, R., Amajoner, V.R., Magnabosco, C., Gennari, S.M. Ocorrência de parasitos gastrintestinais em fezes de gatos das cidades de São Paulo e Guarulhos. *Brazilian Journal of Veterinary Research and Animal Science,* Vol. 39, pp.244-246, 2002.

Ramírez-Barrios, R. A., Barboza-Mena, G., Muñoz, J., Angulo-Cubillán, F., Hernández, E., González, F., Escalona, F. Prevalence of intestinal parasites in dogs under veterinary care in Maracaibo, Venezuela. *Veterinary Parasitology.* 2004, Vol. 121, pp. 11-20.

Rodrigo Costa da Silva, Vanessa Yuri de Lima, Erika Maemi Tanaka, Aristeu Vieira da Silva, Luiz Carlos de Souza and Hélio Langoni. Risk factors and presence of antibodies to *Toxoplasma gondii* in dogs from the coast of São Paulo State, Brazil. *Pesquisa Veterinaria Brasileira,* Vol. 30, N°2, Fevereiro 2010, pp.161-166.

Rossignol JF. *Cryptosporidium* and *Giardia*: treatment options and prospects for new drugs. Exp Parasitology, 2010; 124: 45-53.

Rosypal, A. C., Corte´S-Vecino, J. A., Gennari, S. M., Dubey, J. P., Tidwell, R. R., Lindsay, D. S. Serological survey of Leishmania infantum and Trypanosoma cruzi in dogs from urban areas of Brazil and Colombia. *Veterinary Parasitology,* Vol. 149, pp. 172-177, 2007.

Santarém, V.A.; Giuffrida, R.; & Zanin, A.Z. 2004. Larva migrans cutânea: ocorrência de casos humanos e identificação de larvas de *Ancylostoma* spp. em parque público do município de Taciba, São Paulo. *Revista da Sociedade Brasileira de Medicina Tropical.* Vol. 37, No. 2, march-april 2004, pp. 179-181, 0037-8682.

São Paulo (Estado). Secretaria de Estado da Saúde. Superintendência de Controle de Endemias - SUCEN e Coordenadoria de Controle de Doenças - CCD. Manual de Vigilância e Controle da Leishmaniose Visceral Americana do Estado de São Paulo. São Paulo, 2006. 158p.

São Paulo (Estado). Secretaria de Estado da Sáude, Superintendência de Controle de Endemias - SUCEN e Coodenadoria de controle de Doenças - CCD. Vetores e Doenças - Doença de Chagas. Capturado: 28 de julho de 2011. Disponível em: <http://www.sucen.sp.gov.br/atuac/chagas.html#ind7>

Schantz, P. M.; Glickman, L. T. Ascarideos de perros y gatos: un problema de salud publica y de Medicina Veterinaria. *Boletin de La Oficina Sanitaria Panamericana,* Vol. 94, pp. 571-586, 1983.

Schares, G.; Pantchev, N.; Barutzki, D.; Heydorn, A. O.; Bauer, C; Conraths, F. J. Oocysts of *Neospora caninum, Hammondia heydorni, Toxoplasma gondii* and *Hammondia hammondi* in faeces collected from dogs in Germany. *International Jounal for Parasitology,* Oxford, Vol .35, N°.14, pp.1525-1537, 2005

Schatzberg, S. J.; Haley, N. J.; Barr, S. C.; Lahunta, A.; Olby, N.; Munana, K.; Sharp, N. J. H. Use of a multiplex polymerase chain reaction assay in the antemortem diagnosis of toxoplasmosis and neosporosis in the central nervous system of cats and dogs. *American Journal of Veterinary Research,* v.64, n.12, p.1507-1513, 2003.

Siblei, L.D; Howe, D.K.; Wan, K.L; Khan, S.; Aslett, M.A.; Ajioka, ,J.W.; *Toxoplasma* as a model genetic system. In: SMITH, D.F.; PARSONS, M. *Molecular biology of parasitic protozoa.* Oxford: *Oxford University Press,* 1995. pp.55-74.

Silva, E. S.; Gontijo, C. M.; Pirmez, C.; Fernandes, O.; Brazil, R. P. Short report: detection of *Leishmania* DNA by polymerase chain reaction on blood samples from dogs with visceral leishmaniasis. *American Journal of Tropical. Medicine and. Hygiene,* Vol. 65, N° 6, pp. 896-898, 2001.

Sloss, W.M.; Zajac, M. A.; Kemp, R. L. Parasitologia Clínica Veterinária. São Paulo: Manole, 1999. p.198

Smith, HV., & Nichols, RAB. 2010. Cryptosporidium: detection in water and food. *Experimental Parasitology.* Vol. 124, No. 1, january 2010, pp. 61-79, 0014-4894.

Smith, RP., Chalmers, KE., Elwin, K., Clifton-Hadley, A., Mueller-Doblies, D., Watkins, J., Paiba, GA., Giles, M. 2009. Investigation the role of companion animals in the zoonotic transmission of cryptosporidiosis. *Zoonoses and Public Health.* Vol. 56, No. 1, february 2009, pp. 24-33, 1863-1959.

Souza, S. L. P.; Gennari, S. M.; Yai, L. E. O.; D'auria, S. R. N.; Cardoso, S. M. S.; Guimarães Junior, J. S.; Dubey, J. P. Ocurrence of *Toxoplasma gondii* antibodies in sera from dogs of the urban and rural areas from Brazil. *Revista Brasileira de Parasitologia Veterinária,* Vol.12, N°.1, p.1-3, 2003.

Sousa-Dantas, L. M., Bastos, O. P. M., Brener, B., Salomão, M., Guerrero, J., Labarthe, N. V. Técnica de centrífugo flutuação com sulfato de zinco no diagnóstico de helmintos gastrintestinais de gatos domésticos. *Ciência Rural.* 2007; 37: 904-6

Sundar S, Rai M (2002) Laboratory diagnosis of visceral leishmaniasis. *Clinical Diagnosis Laboratory Immunology,* Vol.9, pp. 951-958

Táparo, C.V., Amarante, A.F.T, Perri, S. H.V., Serrano, A.C.M., Ishizaki, M.N., Costa, T. P., Bresciani, K. D.S. Ocorrência de endoparasitas em cães da cidade de Araçatuba, SP. *Revista Brasileira de Parasitologia Veterinária*, Vol.15, pp. 1-5, 2006.

Thais Rabelo dos Santos, Caris Maroni Nunes, Maria Cecilia Rui Luvizotto, Anderson Barbosa de Moura, Welber Daniel Zanetti Lopes, Alvimar Jose da Costa, Katia Denise Saraiva Bresciani. Detection of Toxoplasma gondii oocysts in environmental samples from public schools. *Veterinary Parasitology*, Vol. 171, pp. 53–57, 2010

Tome, R.O.; Serrano, A.C.M.; Nunes, C.M.; Perri, S.H.V.; Bresciani, K.D.S. Inquérito epidemiológico sobre conceitos de zoonoses parasitárias para professores de escolas municipais do ensino infantil de Araçatuba-SP. *Revista Científica em Extensão*, Vol. 2, N°.1, pp.38-46, 2005.

Thomaz A, Meireles MV, Soares RM, Pena HFJ, Gennari SM. Molecular identification of *Cryptosporidium* spp. from fecal samples of felines, canines and bovines in the state of São Paulo, Brazil. *Veterinary Parasitology* 2007; Vol. 150, pp. 291-6.

Thompson, RCA., Palmer, CS., & O´Handley, R. 2008. The public health and clinical significance of Giardia and Cryptosporidium in domestic animals. *The Veterinary Journal*. Vol. 177, No. 1., july 2008, pp. 18-25, 1090-0233.

Troncarelli, M. Z.; Machado, J. G.; Camargo, L. B.; Hoffmann, J. L.; Camossi, L.; Greca, H.; Faccioli, P. Y.; Langoni, H. Associação entre resultados sorológicos no diagnóstico da leishmaniose e da tripanossomíase canina, pela técnica de imunofluorescência indireta. *Veterinária e Zootecnia*, Vol. 15, N°. 1, pp. 40-47, 2008.

Troncarelli MZ, Camargo JB, Machado JG, Lucheis SB, Langoni H (2009) *Leishmania* spp. and/or *Trypanosoma cruzi* diagnosis in dogs from endemic and nonendemic áreas for canine visceral leishmaniasis. *Veterinary Parasitology* 164:118-123

Tzipori S, Griffths. Natural History and Biology of *Cryptosporidium parvum*. Adv Parasitol 1998; 40: 4-36

URQUHART, G.M.; ARMOUR, J.; DUNCAN, J.L.; DUNN, A.M.; JENNINGS, F.W. Parasitologia Veterinária. Rio de Janeiro : Guanabara Koogan, 1991. p. 306

Wanderley, D. M. V. Epidemiologia da Doença de Chagas. Rev. Soc. Cardiol. Estado de São Paulo, Vol. 4, N°.2, pp.77-84, 1994.

Willis, H.H. A simple levitation method for the detection of hookworm ova. *The Medical Journal of Australia*,v. 8, p. 375-376, 1921.

Xiao L, Morgan UM, Josef L, Escalante A, Michael A, William S, Thompson RCA, Ronald F, Lal AA. Genetic Diversity within *Cryptosporidium parvum* and related *Cryptosporidium* Species. *Appied and Microbiology Environmental*, 1999; Vol. 65: pp.3386-91.

Zanette MF (2006) Comparação entre métodos de ELISA, imunofluorescência indireta e imunocromatografia para o diagnóstico da leishmaniose visceral canina. Tese de mestrado em ciência animal Universidade Estadual Paulista

Zhang, S.; Wei, M. X.; Wang, L. Y.; Ding, Z. Y.; Xu, X. P. Comparison a modified agglutination test (MAT), IHAT and ELISA for detecting antibodies to *Toxoplasma gondii*. *Acta Parasitologica Medica Entomologica Sinica*, Vol..8, N°.4, pp.199-203, 2001.

21

Gastrointestinal Parasites in Domestic Cats

Willian Marinho Dourado Coelho, Juliana de Carvalho Apolinário, Jancarlo Ferreira Gomes, Alessandro Franscisco Talamini do Amarante and Katia Denise Saraiva Bresciani
Universidade Estadual Paulista - UNESP – Araçatuba, SP, Brazil

1. Introduction

With the domestication of animals, the contact between the latter and humans has intensified, favoring the occurrence of parasitic zoonoses (Brooker et al., 2004; Landmann et al., 2003; Katagiri et al., 2007; Thompson et al., 2008; Araújo et al., 2008). This is more evident in places where hygienic-sanitary conditions are poor (Ederli et al., 2008) and human or animal feces are present in the environment (Gatei et al., 2008; Smith et al., 2010; Sousa et al., 2010; Yoder et al., 2010).

Thus, large human conglomerates and environmental changes made by men have favored the occurrence of several emerging and re-emerging parasitic diseases (Prociv & Croese, 1996; MacCarthy & Moore et al., 2000).

Some parasites show low specificity to their host and may infect a great variety of animals (Tzipori, 1980; Xiao, 2010), causing even more severe infection in immunosuppressed individuals (Gatei et al., 2008; Alves et al., 2010).

Several etiological agents of zoonotic potential have been reported in domestic cats, constituting a severe public health problem (Robertson et al., 2002; Coelho et al., 2010; 2011a; 2011b; 2011c). Although several countries have adopted prophylactic and therapeutic measures, gastrointestinal parasites like helminths (Lima et al., 2006) and protozoa (Palmer et al., 2008) are commonly detected by means of different coproparasitological techniques in fecal samples from felines (Tzanes et al., 2008; Coelho et al., 2009).

Felines play an essential role in the epidemiology of parasites causing zoonoses, including *Ancylostoma caninum*, *Ancylostoma braziliense* (Coelho et al. 2011a), *Toxocara* spp., *Dipylidium caninum* (Abu-Madi et al., 2010; Mircean et al., 2010), and protozoa such as *Cryptosporidium* spp. and *Giardia* spp. (Apelbee et al., 2005; Bresciani et al., 2008).

Toxoplasma gondii is a protozoan capable of infecting a large number of animals and has felines as its definitive host. This parasite represents a great risk to the human population, causing diverse infection and mortality levels, especially among immunosuppressed people and pregnant women (Barbosa et al., 2007; Dubey, 2010).

Although the dog is considered the main urban reservoir for visceral leishmaniasis, the constant reports of this infection in felines have suggested that the latter play an important role in the cycle of this protozoan (Dantas-Torres, 2006; Coelho et al., 2011c).

2. Agents

Ancylostoma spp., *Toxocara* spp., *Dipylidium caninum.*

3. Epidemiology

Occurrence of gastrointestinal helminths in felines have been detected by means of parasitological necropsy in South Africa (Baker et al., 1989), Spain (Calvete et al., 1998), Egypt (Kalafalla, 2011) and Brazil (Ogassawara et al., 1986; Souza et al., 1982; Coelho et al., 2011a).

Analysis of fecal samples has been employed in epidemiological surveys in Iran (Sharif et al., 2010), the Netherlands (Overgaauw, 1997, Overgaauw & Boersena, 1998) and Brazil (Gennari et al., 2001; Labarthe et al., 2004; Coelho et al., 2009).

Ancylostoma was the most prevalent genus among the studied animals, which corroborates data in the literature (Serra et al., 2003, Funada et al., 2007). A large number of studies, however, have shown that the genus *Toxocara* sp. occurs at a higher frequency (Calvete et al., 1998, Ragozo et al., 2002), except for the study carried out by Bittencourt et al., 1996, in Espírito Santo do Pinhal, Brazil, where the proportion of these two helminths was the same (20%).

In a previous study, our team performed parasitological necropsy in 60 cats domiciled in Araçatuba Municipality, São Paulo State, Brazil, and sent to the Zoonosis Control Center of that municipality. The genus *Ancylostoma* spp. was most frequently detected. It must be highlighted that of all animals analyzed, 40 (86.96%) had *A. braziliense* and 11 (23.91%) had the species *A. tubaeforme*, and mixed infection by *A. braziliense* and *A. tubaeforme* occurred in 10 (21.74%) animals (Ishizaki et al., 2006).

Researchers like Campos et al. (1974), Ogassawara et al. (1986), Baker et al. (1989), Calvete et al. (1998) and Overgaauw & Boersema (1998) did not detect the genus *Toxocara* in a survey of the helminth fauna.

Predominance of the genus *Ancylostoma* over the remaining gastrointestinal parasites could be verified by our research group since 96% (49/51), 43.1% (22/51) and 19.6% (10/51) analyzed cats had eggs of *Ancylostoma* spp, *Toxocara* spp. and ovigerous capsules of *D. caninum*, respectively (Coelho et al., 2009).

We must emphasize the low positivity for *D. caninum*; the presence of this parasite is generally underestimated in surveys using coproparasitological tests since its diagnosis is made based on the presence of proglottids in fresh feces or adult forms in necropsy but rarely on the presence of ovigerous capsules in feces (Gennari et al., 1999). The percentages of infection by *D. caninum* are different according to the place of origin of animals. Souza et al. (1982) found prevalence of 51.42% in Rio Grande do Sul, whereas Blazius et al. (2005) obtained prevalence of 1.9% in Santa Catarina State, Brazil.

In São Paulo State, Brazil, Silva et al. (2001) observed that 100% (11/11) cats were positive for *Ancylostoma caninum*. In Minas Gerais State, Brazil, Mundim et al. (2004) verified that 90% (45/50) analyzed cats had eggs of *Ancylostoma* spp.

Environmental contamination by this helminth has been reported in several studies in Brazil (Côrtes et al., 1988; Santarém et al., 1998) and in the world (Shimizu, 1993; Uga, 1993; Şengür et al., 2005).

4. Physiopathogenesis

Parasite migration and spoliation of larvae of *A. braziliense* and *A. caninum* lead to a disease named cutaneous larva migrans (CLM) (Hunter & Worth 1945; Hanslik et al.,, 1998; Kwon et al., 2003; Caumes et al., 2004). High levels of intestinal lesions and is mainly related to the number of worms present in the intestinal lumen, as well as to the age of animals (Rey, 2001; Fortes, 2004).

5. Biology

Except for *D. caninum* which needs fleas as intermediate host, parasites belonging to the genera *Ancylostoma* and *Toxocara* areoelomic cavity of these insects and, when ingested by a mammal biologically defined as host, the parasite is released in the small intestine, where it establishes (Rey, 2001; Fortes, 2004).

6. Clinical signs

The number of adult parasites in the animals is a determinant for the infection severity and the manifestation of clinical signs. Dermatitis, eczema, itch, hypersensitivity and anemia are some of the diverse clinical manifestations shown by animals parasitized by *Ancylostoma* (Rey, 2001; Fortes, 2004).

Human toxocariasis may be associated with the formation of pyogenic abscesses (Rayes & Lambertucci, 1999), asthma (Tonelli, 2005), and several forms of ocular, hepatic and renal disorders (Jacob et al., 1994). These clinical signs are similar to those observed in domestic cats, especially in pups (Fortes, 2004).

Although *D. caninum* is considered slightly pathogenic, hypersensitivity, diarrhea, abdominal pain, as well as nervous manifestations and intussusceptions, may occur (Rey, 2001; Fortes, 2004).

7. Diagnosis

Diagnosis must be based on the animal history, including detailed anamnesis with special attention to the clinical manifestations that may be easily confused with those of other diseases. Thus, skin biopsy can also be performed to detect *Ancylostoma* (Acha & Szyfres, 2003), as well as serological tests to detect anti-*Toxocara* antibodies (Marchioro et al., 2011). In addition, coproparasitological tests have been shown highly effective in detecting these parasites (Hoffmann, 1987; Coelho, 2009).

Different prevalence levels can be found for these parasites according to the adopted diagnosis technique. In our study, parasitological necropsy was the "gold standard" test, while the techniques of flotation in saturated sodium chloride solution of 1.182 density (Willis, 1921) and spontaneous sedimentation in water showed different sensitivity and specificity levels (Coelho et al., 2011a).

This same difference was observed by our group in another study, in which fecal samples from 51 cats were analyzed, indicating the presence of eggs of *Ancylostoma* spp. in 96% samples according to the method of Willis and in 21.5% samples according to the technique of Faust. This study also indicated divergence between these techniques as to detection *Toxocara* eggs (43.1% by Willis and 9.8% by Faust) and *D. caninum* ovigerous capsules (19.6% by Willis and 5.8% by Faust (Coelho et al., 2009).

Thus, there is the need of associating different coproparasitological techniques in the laboratorial routine in order to increase the efficiency of the diagnosis of helminths and protozoa (Huber et al., 2004; Coelho et al., 2009).

Our group has worked to established an automated standard diagnosis method named Modified TF-Test®, which allows 3D computer analysis of parasitic structures present in the feces of animals by means of image recombination, leading thus to an important diagnostic innovation concerning helminths and protozoa affecting pets.

8. Treatment

Although parasitic resistance to certain anthelmintics have been reported, the mebendazole, albendazole (Amato Neto et al., 1983) and ivermectin (Machado & El Achkar, 2003) remain showing good efficacy.

9. Agents

Cryptosporidium spp. *and Giardia* spp.

10. Epidemiology

Similarly to giardiasis, cryptosporidiosis is a cosmopolitan gastrointestinal disease caused by protozoa of the genus *Cryptosporidium*, widely distributed all over the world (Smith et al., 2006; Xiao& Fayer, 2008; Ballweber et al., 2009). It is considered a neglected disease of great public health importance due to its frequent occurrence (Alves et al., 2006; Savioli et al., 2006; Carvalho, 2009), difficult treatment (Schnyder et al., 2009; Rossignol, 2010) and singular epidemiological aspects such as its transmission mode, zoonotic potential (Mtambo et al., 1996; Monis & Thompson, 2003; El-Sherbini et al., 2006), and variation in subtypes with the geographical region (Hunter et al., 2008; Xiao, 2010).

On account of their low host selectivity, *Cryptosporidium felis* (Huber et al., 2007) and several other *Cryptosporidium* species have been described in cats, including *Cryptosporidium parvum* (Sargent et al., 1998) and *Cryptosporidium muris* (Pavlasek & Ryan, 2007).

Infection prevalence rates of 8.1% (19/235) for *Cryptosporidium* spp. were reported by Mtambo et al. (1992) in the United Kingdom. In Brazil, different *Cryptosporidium* infection rates were found in different states by Funada et al. (2007), 11.3% (37/327), Huber et al. (2002), 12.5% (6/48), and Coelho et al. (2009), 3.9% (2/51), using different coproparasitological techniques.

In Australia, Palmer et al. (2008) used molecular analyses and verified that *Giardia* Assemblages F and D are present in the feces of domestic cats. This is important since infection by *Giardia duodenalis* assemblages are frequent in humans by assemblage B, while in pets assemblages C and D occur in dogs and assemblage F in cats (Monis & Thompson, 2003; Souza et al., 2007; Xiao & Fayer., 2008), there is also the possibility of cross infection by *Giardia* assemblages between animals and humans (Traub et al., 2004; Palmer et al., 2008; Feng & Xiao, 2011).

In our study, *Giardia* spp. was detected in 5.9% (3/51) fecal samples from domestic cats. Also in Brazil, Gennari et al. (1999) noted that 16.04% of 187 fecal samples from cats were positive for *Giardia* spp. In Australia, MacGlade et al. (2003) analyzed fecal samples from 40 cats and observed approximately 60% positivity prevalence for *Giardia*.

A similar occurrence was detected in Germany between 1999 and 2002, when fecal samples from 3164 cats were analyzed indicating that 51.6% had cysts of *Giardia* spp. (Barutzki & Schaper, 2003).

11. Physiopathogenesis

The pathophysiological mechanism of cryptosporidiosis consists in its intraenterocytic stage. This enteroinfection causes atrophy, fusion of intestinal villi and inflammation, which result in absorptive surface loss and unbalanced nutrient transport. It is not clear yet whether the parasite interferes with the cell function but it seems capable of inducing or inhibiting cell apoptosis (Chen et al., 1998; Dagci et al., 2002; Buret et al., 2003; Leav et al., 2003).

Histopathological analyses have revealed that cryptosporidiosis may lead to minimal inflammatory infiltration and villus blunting, while changes are more pronounced in immunosuppressed individuals, including greater inflammatory changes, epithelial cell barrier rupture with more extensive and intense inflammatory cell infiltration. Massive parasite infection in the enterocytes stimulates local inflammatory reaction, increasing the levels of prostaglandins, several cytokines, especially interferon. These inflammatory mediators change solute transport in the intestinal epithelial cell, leading to osmotic diarrhea (Leav et al., 2003).

Diarrhea due to poor absorption results of the interaction between parasitic products such as proteinases, which rupture the epithelial barrier, and the immune/inflammatory responses of the host, favoring deficient absorption of electrolytes and nutrients, combined with the hypersecretion of chlorine and water (Argenzio et al., 1990; Huang & White, 2006), inducing intestinal abnormalities, especially due to the activation of CD8+ lymphocytes in the intraepithelial compartment, with increased cytotoxic activity (Chai et al., 1999; Buret, 2009).

Cryptosporidium infection is auto-limiting for immunologically normal individuals. In immunodepressed humans, however, this disease is associated with high mortality and morbidity indexes (Hunter & Nichols, 2002), especially in HIV-positive (Cama et al., 2007), transplanted individuals (Dekinger et al., 2007) and children (Glaeser et al., 2004) showing deficient global count of T CD4+ lymphocytes (Assefa et al., 2009).

Parasitic infection by *Giardia intestinalis* is most frequently reported all over the word. It causes several intestinal, nutritional and general development disorders (Botero-Garcés et al., 2009; Singh et al., 2009).

Although giardiasis is an auto-limiting disease, it manifests in individuals mainly by means of acute diarrhea; however, asymptomatic chronic infections may occur, leading to malabsorption of vitamin A, B12 (Springer et al., 1997) and anemia due to iron deficiency (Ertan et al., 2002).

Children are most affected by this protozoan disease (Tellez et al., 1997; Thompson et al., 2000), especially in developing countries where hygienic-sanitary conditions are not adequate (Guimarães et al., 1995; Savioli al., 2006), and domestic animals may produce cysts potentially infective for humans (Eligio-García et al., 2008).

In Colombia, Botero-Garcés et al. (2009) verified that 27.6% of the 2035 studied children were infected by *G. intestinalis* and part of them had significant body development deficit.

12. Biology

As to *Cryptosporidium* biology, sporulated oocysts are ingested by the host and, following exposure to the gastric juice and pancreatic enzymes, excystation occurs in the duodenum releasing four sporozoites. The latter are covered by microvilli located in a parasitophorous vacuole and start the asexual reproduction. In this event, they develop successive merogonies, releasing eight and four sporozoites, respectively (Fortes et al., 2004).

The four merozoites released from the second merogony originate the sexual stages, resulting in the genesis of microgametes and macrogametes, which unite to form the zygote. Sporulation occurs inside the oocyst, developing four sporozoites. In this event, oocysts of thin (capable of starting a new cycle inside the same host by means of retroinfection) and thick wall (highly resistant under environmental conditions and released in the feces) are formed. In healthy people, the infection generally remains in the gastrointestinal tract (TZIPORI & GRIFFTHS, 1998).

Considering the biological cycle of *Giardia*, we must highlight that in addition to producing trophozoites and cysts, this flagellate protozoan is capable of infecting a large number of domestic animals (Geurden et al., 2010), as well as men (Thompson & Monis, 2004); this microorganism is also highly evolved and with the capacity for recombination among their Assemblages (Cacciò & Sprong, 2010).

13. Clinical signs

In general, the clinical signs of parasitized animals consist in diarrhea (Fortes, 2004). Gastrointestinal disorders may manifest severely in immunosuppressed individuals (Assefa et al., 2009), while clinical manifestation variation, infection persistence and severity of symptoms are directly correlated to TCD4+ lymphocyte count (Gupta et al., 2008).

Similarly to cryptosporidiosis, giardiasis may develop varied symptoms, especially acute diarrhea, abdominal pain (Springer et al., 1997; Cimerman et al., 1999), anemia and loss in the energetic and protein values (Ertan et al., 2002; Gendrei et al., 2003).

14. Diagnosis

The diagnosis of *Cryptosporidium* spp. and *Giardia* spp. must always be made by associating two or more techniques in order to increase the diagnosis efficacy (Mtambo et al., 1992; Huber et al., 2004; Coelho et al., 2009).

The intermittent release of *Cryptosporidium* oocysts requires that coproparasitological tests be repeated, including new sample collection, even after a negative result (Huber et al., 2002; Brook et al., 2008; Huber et al., 2005).

15. Treatment

To treat cryptosporidiosis, nitazoxanide, trimethoprim-sulfamethoxazole and pyrimethamine can be used with certain efficacy once there is no immunosuppression associated. The treatment of giardiasis has included metronidazole, nitazoxanide, furazolidone, quinacrine and paramomycin (Petri Jr., 2003).

16. Agents

Toxoplasma gondii.

17. Epidemiology

In Brazil, Dalla Rosa et al. (2010) and Bresciani et al. (2007) proved by means of serological methods the occurrence of anti-*T. gondii* antibodies in 14.33% (43/300) and 25% (100/400) of the analyzed cats, respectively. Also in Brazil, prevalence rates of 35.4% (84/237) were found by Silva et al. (2002) and 26.3% (132/502) by Pena et al. (2006).

Lucas et al. (1998) and Garcia et al. (1999) suggested that toxoplasmic infection is predominantly more frequent among younger animals, confirming that the prenatal stage is predominant for acquiring this infection.

This was confirmed in our study, in which 15.7% (11/70) cats were seroreactive for *T. gondii*, which occurred mainly in young animals (Coelho et al., 2011b). Association between sex and breed with occurrence of infection by *T. gondii* was not verified by Bresciani et al. (2007); Pinto et al. (2009) and Dalla Rosa et al. (2010).

18. Physiopathogenesis

Soon after the ingestion of environmental oocysts or tissue cysts, the parasite causes systemic infection, resulting in bradyzoite production (Dubey, 2010). It must be highlighted that toxoplasmosis manifests more severely in immunosuppressed individuals, especially those showing TCD4 lymphocyte count lower than 100 cells per mm^3 (Hoffmann et al., 2007).

19. Biology

As to *T. gondii* biology, it is important to emphasize that this parasite has zoonotic potential (Dubey, 2010), showing oocysts capable of contaminating the environment and remaining infective for long periods (Elmore et al., 2010).

The occurrence of these protozoan diseases has been correlated to management, environment (Modolo et al. 2008), livestock by-products (Hiramoto et al., 2001) and even dissemination through water (Jones & Dubey, 2010).

20. Clinical signs

Infection by *T. gondii* can cause several lesion levels in the host, including the asymptomatic forms, in addition to retinochoroiditis (Alves et al., 2010), cerebral lesions, psychiatric disorders (Torrey & Yolken, 2003; Youken et al., 2009) and disseminated forms (Barbosa et al., 2007).

It is an opportunistic infection, common in immunosuppressed patients, being the most common cause of secondary infection of the central nervous system, causing the occurrence of severe encephalitis (Collazos, 2003; Pradhan et al., 2007).

Experimental infections in cats are often asymptomatic, few animals get sick and deaths rarely occur (Omata et al., 1990; Sato et al., 1993). However, Dubey et al. (1996) and Elmore et al. (2010) report the occurrence of some lesions in neonates.

Experimental infections in cats are frequently asymptomatic, a few animals become ill and deaths are rare (Omata et al., 1990; Sato et al., 1993). Abortion and neonatal mortality have been described for pregnant cats orally inoculated with *T. gondii* tissue cysts (Powell et al., 2001).

21. Diagnosis

In addition to clinical manifestations, fecal analyses and molecular techniques (Elmore et al., 2010), several serological techniques have been the main methods employed for toxoplasmosis diagnosis (Camargo, 1964; Lappin et al., 1989; Dubey et al., 2004; Coelho et al., 2011b).

In humans, behavioral changes (Zhu, 2009), encephalic lesions (Zajdenweber et al., 2005) and ocular (Alves et al., 2010) may indicate presence of infection.

22. Treatment

Toxoplasmosis treatment includes sulfonamides, trimethoprim, pyrimethamine, ponazuril, clindamycin and their associations can be successfully employed (Mitchell et al., 2006; Dabritz et al., 2007).

23. Agents

Leishmania spp.

24. Epidemiology

The occurrence of leishmaniasis in domestic cats has been reported in a large number of countries (Mancianti, 2004; Maia et al., 2008; Silva et al., 2008). In our study, only the species *Leishmania (L.) chagasi* was found in the analyzed cats (Coelho et al., 2011c), which could be associated or not with other diseases (Coelho et al. 2010). Also in Brazil, Savani et al. (2004) and Silva et al. (2008) found *Leishmania (L.) infantum*. The latter has been equally described in cats in France (Ozon et al., 1998), Italy (Pennisi et al.., 2004), Spain (Ayllon et al., 2008) and Iran (Hatan et al., 2010).

The cutaneous form of *Leishmania (V.) braziliensis* was described in two cats from Rio de Janeiro State, Brazil (Schubach et al., 2004), while *Leishmania (L.) amazonensis* was described in Mato Grosso do Sul State (Souza et al., 2005). Craig et al. (1986) detected the occurrence of *L. mexicana* in cats from Texas, USA.

Studies of animal epidemiology have evidenced several infection prevalence levels according to the employed method and the study site. In our study, the analyzed tissue samples were from 52 domestic cats with 5.76% positivity. Similarly, Rossi et al. (2007) detected 6.7% positivity for *Leishmania* spp. among 200 analyzed cats.

Percentages superior to those obtained in our study were found in Portugal by Maia et al. (2008), who observed 30.4% (7/23) felines carrying leishmaniasis. In Greece, Diakou et al. (2009) verified that 3.87% (11/284) cats had anti-*Leishmania* antibodies. Similarly, in Spain, Solano-Galego et al. (2007) analyzed anti-*Leishmania infantum* antibodies from 445 cats and observed seroreactive prevalence in 6.29% of these animals.

25. Physiopathogenesis

After parasite replication, there is formation of perivascular congestion, mononuclear and neutrophil inflammatory infiltrate (Schubach et al., 2004) with secondary bacterial (Coelho et al. 2010) and fungal infections (Ozon et al., 1998) at the lesion sites. Lesions may be localized or systemic, affecting different organs, and may be associated with FIV/ FeLV; in these cases, the most severe form of the disease occur (Pennisi et al. 2002; 2004).

26. Biology

This heteroxenic protozoan has mammals as its definitive hosts and dipterans of the genera *Lutzomyia* and *Phlebotomus* as intermediate hosts and vectors (Fortes, 2004). As the dog is considered the main urban reservoir of this disease although there are frequent reports of this infection in cats, the role of felines in the biological cycle of this parasite is not well defined yet (Dantas-Torres et al. 2006).

However, xenodiagnosis studies carried out by Maroli et al. (2007) proved that sand flies are capable of acquiring the infection from naturally infected cats.

27. Clinical signs

Skin lesions are more frequent among felines. Infected animals may show vegetative lesions, dermatitis and ulcers (Coelho et al. 2010a); healthy animals may also carry this parasite (Coelho et al., 2010b), and in some cases the disseminated form may occur (Ozon et al., 1998).

Weight loss, pale mucosae, dehydration, systemic lymphadenomegaly and hepatomegaly, and ocular lesions are the main manifestations (Pennisi et al. 2004).

Laboratorial changes are irregular and may include pancytopenia (Marcos et al., 2009), hyperleukocytosis (Ozon et al., 1998), and discreet or no biochemical alteration (Souza et al., 2009).

28. Diagnosis

Diagnosis is based especially on serological (Mancianti , 2004), parasitological (Bresciani et al., 2010), molecular analyses (Coelho et al. 2010b), isolation in culture medium (Simões-Matos et al., 2004), and clinical manifestations (Dantas-Torres et al., 2006).

Clinical tests in places where the disease is endemic have shown that some infected animals remain seronegative (Ferrer et al., 1999). The serological titer shown by the animal is not related to the presence of symptoms and their intensity (Lima et al., 2003). On the other hand, PCR sensitivity and specificity are very high and this technique can detect the DNA of parasites in patients that remain clinically healthy for many years (Ferrer et al., 1999).

In a previous study, our research group suggested that antibody production in response to *Leishmania* spp. in felines is very low, which led to no serological reactions by means of IFA and ELISA (Serrano et al., 2008).

29. Treatment

Treatment may be based on allopurinol, meglumine antimoniate and ketoconazole (Pennisi et al., 2004). Rüfenacht et al. (2005) reported the use of griseofulvin, itraconazole, ketoconazole, selamectin, lufenuron, cephalexin and prednisolone for leishmaniasis treatment in cats.

30. Final considerations

The high occurrence of endoparasites observed among domestic and stray animals evidences the zoonotic potential of these helminth and protozoan diseases, suggesting greater concern about the therapeutic and prophylactic measures feasible to the feline population.

31. References

Abu-Madi, M.A., Behnke, J.M., Prabhaker, K.S., Al-Ibrahim, R. & Lewis, J.W. (2010). Intestinal helminthes of feral cat populations from urban and suburban districts of Qatar. *Veterinary Parasitoogy*. Vol.168, No.3-4, (Mar 2010), pp. 284-292, ISSN 0304-4017.

Acha, P.N. & Szyfres, B. (2003). *Zoonoses and communicable diseases common to man and animals: parasitoses* (terceira), PAHO, ISBN 92-75-11991-0, Washington, D.C.

Alves, J.M., Magalhães, V. & Matos M.A.G (2010). Toxoplasmic retinochoroiditis in patients with AIDS and neurotoxoplasmosis. *Arquivo Brasileiro de Oftalmologia*. Vol.73, No.2, (Apr 2010), pp. 150-154, ISSN 0004-2749.

Alves, M., Xiao, L., Antunes, F. & Matos, O. (2006). Distribution of *Cryptosporidium* subtypes in humans and domestic and wild ruminants in Portugal. *Parasitology Research*. Vol.99, No.3, (Aug 2006), pp. 287-292, ISSN 0932-0113.

Amato Neto, V., Moreira, A.A., Campos, R., Lazzaro, E.S., Chiaramelli, M.C., Pinto, P.L., Silva, G.R., Nishioka, S.A. & Leite, R.M. (1983). Tratamento da ancilostomíase, ascaridíase e tricocefalíase por meio do albendazol ou do mebendazol. *Revista do Instituto de Medicina Tropical de São Paulo*, Vol.25, No.6, pp. 294-299, ISSN 0036-4665.

Apelbee, A.J., Thompson, R.C.A. & Olson, M. (2005). *Giardia* and *Criptosporidium* in mammalian wildlife. The current status and future needs. *Trends in Parasitology*. Vol.21, No.8, (Aug 2005), pp.370-376, ISSN 1471-4922

Araújo, A., Reinhard, K.J., Ferreira, L.F. et al. (2008). Parasites as probes for prehistoric human migrations?. *Trends in Parasitology.*, Vol.24, No.3, (Mar 2008), pp. 112-115, ISSN 1471-4922.

Argenzio, R.A., Liacos, J.A., Levy, M.L., Meuten, D.J, Lecce, J.G. & Powell, D.W. (1990). Villous atrophy, crypt hyperplasia, cellular infiltration, and impaired glucose-NA absorption in enteric cryptosporidiosis of pigs. *Gastroenterology*, Vol.98, No.5, (May 1990), pp. 1129-1140, ISSN 0016-5085.

Assefa, S., Erko, B., Medhin, G., Assefa, Z., Shimelis, T. (2009). Intestinal parasitic infection in relation to HIV/AIDS status, diarrhea and CD4 T-cell count. *BMC Infectious Diseases*, Vol.18, No.9, (Sep 2009), pp. 155, ISSN 1471-2334.

Ayllon, T. et al. (2008). Serologic and molecular evaluation of *Leishmania infantum* in cats from central Spain. *Annals of The New York Academy Science*. Vol.1149, (Dec 2008), pp. 361-364, ISSN 0077-8923.

Baker, M.K., Lange, L., Vester, A. & van deer Plaat, S (1989). A survey of helminths in domestic cats in the Pretoria areaof Transvaal, Republic of South Africa. Part 1: The prevalence and comparison of burdens of helminths in adult and juvenile cats. *Journal of the South African Veterinary Association,* Vol.60, No.3, (Sep 1989), pp. 139-42, ISSN 0038-2809.

Ballweber, L.R., Panuska, C., Huston, C.L., Vasilopulos, R., Pharr, G.T. & Mackin, A. (2009). Prevalence and risk factors associated with shedding of Cryptosporidium felis in domestic cats of Mississippi and Alabama. *Veterinary Parasitology*, Vol.160, No.3-4, (Mar 2009), pp. 306-310, ISSN 0304-4017.

Barbosa, C.J., Molina, R.J., De Souza, M.B., Silva, A.C.A., Micheletti, A.R., Reis, M.A., Teixeira, V.P.A. & Silva-Vergara, M.L. (2007). Disseminated toxoplasmosis presenting as sepsis in two AIDS patients. *Revista do Instituto de Medicina Tropical de São Paulo*. Vol.49, No.2, (Mar-Apr 2007), pp. 113-116, ISSN 0036-4665.

Barutzik, D., Schaper, R. (2003). Endoparasites in dogs and cats in Germany 1999-2002. *Parasitology Research*, Vol.90, No.3, (Jul 2003), pp. 148-150, ISSN 0932-0113.

Bittencourt, V.R.E.P., Bittencourt, A.J., Perez, A.D.Q. (1996). Freqüência de parasitoses no setor de pequenos animais do Hospital Veterinário da Faculdade de Medicina Veterinária "Prof. Antônio Secundino de São José". *Revista Ecossistema*, Vol.21, (Outubro–Dezembro 1996), pp. 32-35, ISSN 0100-4107.

Blazius, R.D., Sheila, E., Prophiro, J.S., Romão, P.R.T. & Silva, O.S. (2005). Ocorrência de protozoários e helmintos em amostras de fezes de cães errantes da cidade de Itapema, Santa Catarina. *Revista da Sociedade Brasileira de Medicina Tropical*, Vol.38, No.1, (Janeiro-Fevereiro, 2005), pp. 73-74, ISSN 0037-8682.

Botero-Garces, J.H., Garcia-Montoya, G.M., Grisales-Patino, D., Aguirre-Acevedo, D.C. & Alvarez-Uribe, M.C. (2009). *Giardia intestinalis* and nutritional status in children participating in the complementary nutrition program, Antioquia, Colômbia, May to October 2006. *Revista do Instituto de Medicina Tropical de São Paulo*, Vol..51, No.3, (May-Jun 2009), pp. 155-162, ISSN 0036-4665.

Bresciani et al., (2010). Ocorrência de *Leishmania* spp. em felinos do município de Araçatuba, SP. *Revista Brasileira de Parasitologia Veterinária*. Vol.19, No.2, (Abr-Jun 2010), pp.127-129, ISSN 1984-2961.

Bresciani, K.D.S., Ishizaki, M.N., Kaneto, U.K.Y., Montano, T.R., Perri, S.H.; Vasconcelos, R.O. & Nascimento, A.O. (2008). Frequency and intensity of gastrointestinal helminths in domestic cats from Brazil, *Proceedings of The 83rd Annual Meeting of the American Society of Parasitologists*, pp. 81, Arlington, Texas, June 27-30, 2008.

Bresciani, K.D.S., Gennari, S.M., Rodrigues, A.A.R., Ueno, T., Franco, L.G., Perri, S.H.V. & Amarante, A.F.T. (2007). Antibodies to *Neospora caninum* and *Toxoplasma gondii* in domestic cats from Brazil. *Parasitology Research,* Vol.100, No.2, (Jan 2007), pp. 281–285, ISSN 1432-1955.

Brook, E.J., Christley, R.M.; French, N.P. & Hart, C.A. (2008). Detection of *Cryptosporidium* oocysts in fresh and frozen cattle feces: comparison of three methods. *Letters in Applied Microbiology,* Vol.46, No.1, (Jan 2008), pp. 26-31, ISSN 1472-765X.

Brooker, S., Bethony, J. & Hotez, P.J. (2004). Human hookworm infection in the 21st Century. *Advances in Parasitology,* Vol.58, (Mar 2004), pp. 197-288, ISSN 0065-308X.

Buret, A.G. Pathogenic mechanisms in giardiasis and cryptosporidiosis. In: Ortega-Pierres, G. et al. *Giardia* and *Cryptosporidium*: from molecules to disease, *CAB international,* 2009. cap.35, p. 428-441.

Cacciò, S.M. & Sprong, H. (2010). *Giardia duodenalis*: Genetic recombination and its implication for taxonomy and molecular epidemiology. *Experimental Parasitology.* Vol.124, No.1, (Jan 2010), pp. 107-112, ISSN 1090-2449.

Calvete, C., Lucientes, J., Castilho, J.A., Estrada, R., Gracia, M.J., Peribáñez, A. & Ferrer, M. (1998). Gastrointestinal helminth parasites in stray cats from the mid-Ebro Valley, Spain. *Veterinary Parasitology.* Vol.75, No. 2-3, (Feb 1998), pp. 235-240, ISSN 0304-4017.

Cama, V.A., Ross, J.M., Crawford, S.; Kawai, V., Chavez-Valdez, R., Vargas, D., Vivar, A., Ticona, E., Navincopa, M., Williamson, J., Ortega, Y., Gilman, R.H., Bern, C., Xiao, L. (2007). Differences in clinical manifestations among *Cryptosporidium* species and subtypes in HIV-infected persons. *Journal of Infectious Diseases,* Vol..196, No.5, (Sep 2007), pp. 684-691, ISSN 0022-1899.

Campos, D.M.B., Garibaldi, I.M., Carneiro J.R. (1974). Prevalência de helmintos em gatos (*Felis catus domesticus*) de Goiânia. *Revista de Patologia Tropical.* Vol.3, pp. 355-9, ISSN 1980-8178.

Camargo, M.E. (1964). Improved technique of indirect immunofluorescence for serological diagnosis of toxoplasmosis. *Revista do Instituto de Medicina Tropical,* Vol. 3, No.6, pp. 117-118, ISSN 00364665.

Carvalho, T.T.R. (2009). Estado atual do conhecimento de *Cryptosporidium* e *Giardia. Revista de Patologia Tropical,* Vol.38, No.1, pp. 1-16, ISSN 1980-8178.

Caumes, E. & Danis, M. (2004). From creeping eruption to hookworm-related cutaneous larva migrans. *The Lancet Infectious Diseases.* Vol.4, No.11, (Nov 2004), pp. 659-660, ISSN 1473-3099.

Caumes, E. (2006). It's time to distinguish the sign "creeping eruption" from the syndrome "cutaneous larva migrans". *Dermatology,* Vol.213, No.3, pp. 179-181, ISSN 1018-8665.

Chai, J.Y., Guk, S.M., Han, H.K. & Yun, C.K. (1999) Role of intra-epithelial lymphocytes in mucosal immune responses of mice experimentally infected with *Cryptosporidium parvum*. *Journal Parasitology,* Vol.85, No.2, (Apr 1999), pp. 234-239, ISSN 1937-2345.

Chen, X.M., Levine, S.A., Tietz, P., Krueger, E., Jefferson, M.A., Jefferson, D.M., Mahle, M. & LaRusso, N.F. (1998). *Cryptosporidium parvum* is cytopathic for cultured human biliary epithelia via an apoptotic mechanism. *Hepatology*, Vol.28, No..4, (Oct 1998), pp. 906-913, 1998, ISSN 1527-3350.

Cimerman, S., Cimerman, B. & Lewi, D.S. (1999). Avaliação da relação entre parasitoses intestinais e fatores de risco para o HIV em pacientes com AIDS. *Revista da Sociedade Brasileira de Medicina Tropical*.Vol.32, No.2, (Mar-Apr 1999), pp.181-185, ISSN 0037-8682.

Coelho, W.M.D., Amarante, A.F.T., Apolinário, J.C.A., Coelho, N.M.D. & Bresciani, K.D.S. (2011a). Occurrence of Ancylostoma in dogs, cats and public places from Andradina city, São Paulo State, Brazil. *Revista do Instituto de Medicina Tropical de São Paulo*. Vol.53, No.4, (July-August 2011), pp. 181-184, ISSN 0036-4665.

Coelho, W.M.D., Amarante, A.F.T., Apolinário, J.C.A., Coelho, N.M.D., Lima, V.M.F., Perri, S.H.V. & Bresciani, K.D.S. (2011b). Seroepidemiology of *Toxoplasma gondii, Neospora caninum* and *Leishmania* spp. infections and risk factors for cats from Brazil. *Parasitology Research*, Vol.109, No.4, pp. 1009-1013, ISSN 1432-1955.

Coelho, W.M.D., Richini-Pereira, V.B., Langoni, H. & Bresciani, K.D.S. (2011c). Molecular detection of *Leishmania* sp. in cats (Felis catus) from Andradina municipality, São Paulo State, Brazil. *Veterinary Parasitology*, Vol.176, No.2, (Mar 2011), pp. 281-282, ISSN 1873-2550.

Coelho, W.M.D., Lima, V.M.F., Amarante, A.F.T, Richini-Pereira, V.B., Langoni, H., Abdelnour, A. & Bresciani, K.D.S. (2010). Occurrence of *Leishmania (Leishmania) chagasi* in a domestic cat (Felis catus) in Andradina, São Paulo, Brazil: case report. *Revista Brasileira de Parasitologia Veterinária*, Vol.19, No.4, (Out-Dez 2010), pp. 256-258, ISSN 1984-2961.

Coelho, W.M.C., Amarante, AF.T., Soutello, R.V.G., Meireles, M. V. & Bresciani, K. D. S. (2009). Ocorrência de parasitos gastrintestinais em amostras fecais de felinos no município de Andradina, São Paulo. *Revista Brasileira de Parasitologia Veterinária*, Vol.18, No.2, (Abr-Jun 2009), pp. 46-49, ISSN 1984-2961.

Collazos, J. (2003). Opportunistic infectious of the CNS in patients with AIDS: diagnosis and management. *CNS Drugs*. Vol. 17, No.12, pp. 869-887, ISSN 1537-3458.

Côrtes, V.A., Paim, G.V. & Alencar Filho, R.A.A. (1998). Infestação por ancilostomídeos e toxocarídeos em cães e gatos apreendidos em vias públicas, São Paulo (Brasil). *Revista de Saúde Pública*, Vol.22, No.4, (Ago 1988), pp. 341-343, ISSN 0034-8910.

Craig et al. (1986 Am J Trop Med Hyg 35: 1100-1102) identified as Leishmania mexicana, the parasite isolated from dermal lesions of a cat from Texas, USA and JC Barnes et al. (1993 JAVMA 202: 416-418) described a case of disseminated cutaneous leishmaniasis by the same species in another cat from Texas.

Croese, J., Loukas, A., Opdebeeck, J. & Prociv, P. (1994). Occult enteric infection by Ancylostoma caninum: a previously unrecognized zoonosis. *Gastroenterology*, Vol.106, No.1, (Jan 1994), pp. 3-12, ISSN 0016-5085.

Dabritz, H.A., Miller, M.A., Atwill, E.R., Gardner, I.A., Leutenegger, C.M., Melli, A.C. & Conrad, P.A. (2007). Detection of Toxoplasma gondii-like oocysts in cat feces and estimates of the environmental oocyst burden. *Journal of the American Veterinary Medical Association*, Vol.231, No.11, (Dec 2007), pp. 1676-1684. ISSN 0003-1488.

Dagci, H.; Uston, S. & Taner, M.S. (2002). Protozoan infections and intestinal permeability. *Acta Tropica*. Vol.81, No.1, (Jan 2002), pp. 1-5, ISSN 0001-706X.

Dalla Rosa, L., De Moura A.B, Trevisani, N., Medeiros, A.P., Sartor, A.A., De Souza, A,P., Bellato, V. (2010) *Toxoplasma gondii* antibodies on domiciled cats from Lages municipality, Santa Catarina State, Brazil. *Revista Brasileira de Parasitologia Veterinária,* Vol.19, No.4, (Oct-Dec 2010), pp. 208–269, ISSN 1984-2961.

Dantas-Torres, F. et al. Leishmaniose felina: revisão de literatura. *Clínica Veterinária.* No.61, pp.32-40, 2006.

Diakou, A., Papadopoulos, E.; Lazarides, K (2005). Specific anti-*Leishmania* spp. antibodies in stray cats in Greece. *Journal of Feline Medicine and Surgery,* Vol.11, No.8, (Mar 2005), pp. 728-730, ISSN 1098-612X.

Dowd, A.J., Dalton, J.P., Loukas, A.C., Prociv, P. & Brindley, P. J. (1994). Secretion of cysteine proteinase activity by the zoonotic hookworm Ancylostoma caninum. *The American Journal of Tropical Medicine and Hygiene,* Vol.51, No.3, (Sep 1994), pp. 341-347, ISSN 0002-9637.

Dubey, J.P. (2010). Toxoplasmosis of animals and humans. *Parasites & Vectors.* Vol.3, No.112.

Dubey, J.P., Navarro, I.T., Sreekumar, C., Dahl, E., Freire, R.L., Kawabata, H.H., Vianna, M.C., Kwok, O.C., Shen, S.K., Thulliez, P. & Lehmann, T. (2004). *Toxoplasma gondii* infections in cats from Paraná Brazil: seroprevalence, tissue distribution, and biologic and genetic characterization of isolates. *Journal Parasitology.* Vol.90, No.4, (Aug 2004), pp. 721–726, ISSN 0022-3395.

Dubey, J.P., Mattix, M.E., Lipscomb, T.P. (1996). Lesions of neonatally induced toxoplasmosis in cats. *Veterinary Pathology.* Vol.33, No. 3, p.290-295, ISSN 1544-2217

Ederli, B.B., Ederli, N.B., Oliveira, F.C.R., Quirino, C.R. & Carvalho, C.B. (2008). Fatores de risco associados à infecção por *Cryptosporidium* spp. em cães domiciliados na cidade de Campos dos Goytacazes, Estado do Rio de Janeiro, Brasil. *Revista Brasileira de Parasitologia Veterinária,* Vol.17, No.1, pp. 250-266, ISSN 1984-2961.

Eligio-García, L., Cortes-Campos, A., Cota-Guajardo, S., Gaxiola, S. & Jiménez-Cardoso, E. (2008). Frequency of *Giardia intestinalis* assemblages isolated from dogs and humans in a community from Culiacan, Sinaloa, Mexico using β-giardin restriction gene. *Veterinary Parasitology.* Vol.153, No.6-4, (Oct 2008), pp. 205-209, ISSN 0304-4017.

Elmore, S.A., Jones, J.L., Conrad, P.A., Patton, S., Lindsay, D.S. & Dubey, J.P. (2010). *Toxoplasma gondii*: epidemiology, feline clinical aspects, and prevention. *Trends Parasitology.*Vol.26, No.4, (Apr 2010), pp. 190-196, ISSN 1471-4922.

El-Sherbini, G.T., Mohammad, K.A. (2006). Zoonotic cryptosporidiosis in man and animal in farms, Giza Governorate, Egypt. *Jounal of The Egyptian Society of Parasitology.* Vol.36, No.2, (Aug 2006), pp.49-58, ISSN 0253-5890.

Ertan, P., Yereli, K., Kurt, O., Balcioglu, I.C. & Onag, A. (2002). Serological levels of zinc, copper and iron elements among *Giardia lamblia* infected children in Turkey. *Pediatrics International,* Vol.44, No.3, (Jan 2002), pp. 286-288, ISSN 1442-200X.

Feng, Y. & Xiao, L. (2011). Zoonotic potential and molecular epidemiology of *Giardia* species and giardiasis. *Clin. Microbiol. Rev.* Vol.24, No.1, (Jan 2011), pp.110-140, ISSN 0893-8512.

Ferrer, L.M. Clinical aspects of canine leishmaniasis. In: Proceedings of the International Canine Leishmaniasis Forum. Barcelona, Spain. Canine leishmaniasis: an update. Wiesbaden: *Hoeschst Roussel Veterinary,* 1999. p.6-10.

Fortes, E. (2004). *Parasitologia Veterinária.* (quarta), Ícone, 114-115 p. São Paulo, SP.

Funada, M.R., Pena, H.F.J., Soares, R.M., Amaku, M. & Gennari, S.M. (2007). Freqüência de parasitos gastrintestinais em cães e gatos atendidos em hospital-escola veterinário da cidade de São Paulo. *Arquivo Brasileiro de Medicina Veterinária e Zootecnia*, Vol.59, No.5, pp. 1338-1340, ISSN 0102-0935.

Garcia, J.L., Navarro, I.T., Ogawa, L. & Oliveira, R.C. (1999). Seroprevalence of *Toxoplasma gondii* in swine, bovine, ovine and equine, and their correlation with human, felines and canines, from farms in north region of Paraná State, Brazil. *Ciência Rural.* Vol.29, No.1, (Jan-Mar 1999), pp. 91–97, ISSN 0103-8478.

Gatei, W., Barrett, D., Lindo, J.F., Eldemire-Shearer, D., Cama, V. & Xiao, L. (2008). Unique *Cryptosporidium* population in HIV-infected person, Jamaica. *Emerging Infectious Diseases*, Vol.14, No.5, (May 2008), pp. 841-843, ISSN 1080-6059.

Gendrei, D., Treluyer, J.M. & Richard-Lenoble, D. (2003). Parasitic diarrhea in normal and malnourished children. *Fundamental & Clinical Pharmacology.* Vol.17, No.2, (Apr 2003), pp.189-197, ISSN 1472-8206.

Gennari, S. M., Pena, H. F. J., Blasques, L. S (2001). Freqüência de ocorrência de parasitos gastrintestinais em amostras de fezes de cães e gatos da cidade de São Paulo. Vet News. Vol. 8, No. 52, pp. 10-12.

Gennari, S.M., Kasai, N., Pena, H.F.J. & Cortez, A. (1999). Ocorrência de protozoários e helmintos em amostras de fezes de cães e gatos da cidade de São Paulo. *Brazilian Journal of Veterinary Research and Animal Science*, Vol.36, No.2, pp. 87-91, ISSN 1413-9596.

Geurden, T.; Vercruysse, J. & Claerebout, E. (2010). Is *Giardia* a significant pathogen in production animals? Experimental Parasitology, Vol.124, No.1, (Jan 2010) pp. 98-106, ISSN 1090-2449.

Glaeser, C., Grimm, F., Mathis, A., Weber, R., Nadal, D. & Deplazes., P. (2004). Detection and molecular characterization of *Cryptosporidium* spp. Isolated from diarrheic children in Switzerland. *The Pediatric Infectious Disease Journal,* Vol.23, No.4, (Apr 2004), pp. 359-361, ISSN 1532-0987.

Guimarães, S. & Sogayar, M.I. (1995). Occurrence of *Giardia lamblia* in children of municipal day-care centers from Botucatu, São Paulo state, Brazil. *Revista do Instituto de Medicina Tropical de São Paulo*, Vol.37, No.6, (Nov-Dec 1995), pp. 501-506, ISSN 1678-9946.

Gupta, S., Narang, S.; Nunavath, V. & Singh, S. (2008). Chronic diarrhea in HIV patients: prevalence of coccidian parasites. *Indian Journal of Medical Microbiology,* Vol.26, No.2, (Apr-Jun 2008), pp. 172-175, ISSN 1998-3646.

Hanslik, T. (1998). Metastasis or visceral larva migrans? *Annales de Médecine Interne*, Vol.149, No.8, (Dec 1998), pp. 533-535, ISSN 0003-410X.

Hatam, G. R. et al. (2010). First report of natural infection in cats with *Leishmania infantum* in Iran. *Vector Borne Zoonotic Diseases.* Vol. 10, No.3, (Apr 2010), pp. 313-316, ISSN 1557-7759.

Hiramoto, R.M., Mayrbaurl-Borges, M., Galisteo, A.J. Jr., Meireles, L.R., Macre, M.S. & Andrade, H.F.Jr. (2001). Infectivity of cysts of the ME-49 *Toxoplasma gondii* strain in bovine milk and homemade cheese. *Revista de Saúde Pública.* Vol.35, No.2, (Abr 2001), pp. 113–118, ISSN 1518-8787.

Hochedez, P. & Caumes, E. (2007). Hookworm-related cutaneous larva migrans. *Journal of Travel Medicine.* Vol.14, No.5, (Sep-Oct 2007) pp. 326–33, ISSN 1708-8305.

Hoffmann, C., Ernst, M., Meyer, P., Wolf, E., Rosenkranz, T., Plettenberg, A., et al. (2007). Evolving characteristics of toxoplasmosis in patients infected with human immunodeficiency virus-1: clinical course and Toxoplasma gondii-specific immune responses. *Clinical Microbiology and Infection*, Vol.13, No.5, pp. 510-515, ISSN 1198-743X.

Hoffmann, R.P. (1987). *Diagnóstico Parasitismo Veterinário*. Sulina, Porto Alegre, RS.

Huang, D.B. & White, A.C. (2006). An update review on *Cryptosporidium* and *Giardia*. *Gastroenterology Clinics of North America*. Vol.35, No.2, (Jun 2006), pp. 291-314, ISSN 0889-8553.

Huber, F., Da Silva, S., Bomfim, T.C., Teixeira, K.R. & Bello, A.R. (2007). Genotypic characterization and phylogenetic analysis of *Cryptosporidium* sp. from domestics animals in Brazil. *Veterinary Parasitology*, Vo.l.150, No.1, (Nov 2007), pp. 65-74, ISSN 0304-4017.

Huber, F., Bomfim, T.C.B. & Gomes, R.S. (2005). Comparison between natural infection by *Cryptosporidium* sp., *Giardia* sp. in dogs in two living situations in the West Zone of the municipality of Rio de Janeiro. *Veterinary Parasitology*, Vol.130, No.1, (Jun 2005), pp. 69-72, ISSN 0304-4017.

Huber, F., Bomfim, T.C. & Gomes, R.S. (2004). Comparação da eficiência da coloração pelo método da safranina a quente e da técnica de centrífugo-flutuação na detecção de oocistos de Cryptosporidium em amostras fecais de animais domésticos. *Revista Brasileira de Parasitologia Veterinária*, Vol.13, No.2, pp. 81-84, ISSN 1984-2961.

Huber, F., Bomfim, T.C.B. & Gomes, R.S. (2002). Comparação entre infecção por *Cryptosporidium* sp. e por *Giardia* sp. em gatos sob dois sistemas de criação. *Revista Brasileira Parasitologia Veterinária*, Vol.11, No.1, pp. 7-12, ISSN 0103-846X.

Hunter, G.W. & Worth, C.B. (1945).Variations in response to filariform larvae of *Ancylostoma caninum* in the skin of man. *Journal Parasitology*. Vol. 31, No.6, (Dec 1945), pp. 366–372, ISSN 1937-2345.

Hunter, P.R. & Nichols, G. (2002). Epidemiological and clinical features of Cryptosporidium infection in immunocompromissed patients. *Clinical Microbiology Reviews*. Vo.l.15,No.1, (Jan 2002), pp. 145-154, ISSN 0893-8512.

Hunter, P.R. (2008). Geografic linkage and variation in Cryptosporidium hominis. *Emerging Infectious Diseases*, Vol.14, No.3, (March 2011), pp. 496-498, ISSN 1080-6059.

Ishizaki, M.N., Nascimento, A.A., Kaneto, C.N., Montano, T.R.P., Perri, S.H.V., Vasconcelos, R.O., & Bresciani, K.D.S. (2006). Frequência e intensidade parasitária de helmintos gastrintestinais em felinos da zona urbana do município de Araçatuba, SP. *ARS Veterinária*, Vol.22, No.3, 2006, pp. 212-216, ISSN 2175-0106.

Jacob, C.M.A, Pastorino, A.C., Peres, B.A., Melo, E.O., Okay, Y. & Oselka, G. (1994). Clinical and laboratorial features of visceral toxocariasis in infancy. *Revista do Instituto de Medicina Tropical de São Paulo*, Vol.36, No.1, (Jan-Feb 1994), pp. 19-26, ISSN 0036-4665.

Jones, J.L., Dubey, J.P. (2010). Waterborne toxoplasmosis - recent developments. *Experimental Parasitology*, Vol.124, No.1, (Jan 2010), pp. 10-25, ISSN 1090-2449.

Kalafalla, R.E. (2011). A survey study on gastrointestinal parasites of stray cats in Northern region of Nile Delta, Egypt. *PLos One*, Vol.6, No.7, (Jul 2011), ISSN 1932-6203.

Katagiri, S., Oliveira-Sequeira, T.C.G. (2007). Zoonoses causadas por parasitas intestinais de cães e o problema do diagnóstico. *Arquivos do Instituto Biológico*. Vol.74, No.2, (Abr-Jun 2007), pp. 175-184, ISSN 1808-1657.

Kwon, I.H., Kim, H.S., Lee, J.H., Choi, M.H., Chai, J.Y., Nakamura-Uchiyama, F., Nawa,Y. & Cho, K.H. (2003). A serologically diagnosed human case of cutaneous larva migrans caused by Ancylostoma caninum. *The Korean Journal of Parasitology*, Vol.41, No.4, (Dec 2003), pp. 233-237, ISSN 0023-4001.

Labarthe, N., Serrao, M., Ferreira, A., Almeida, N., Guerrero, J. (2004). A survey of gastrointestinal helminths in cats of the metropolitan region of Rio de Janeiro, Brazil. *Veterinary Parasitology*, Vol. 123, No.1-2, (Aug 2004), pp. 133–139, ISSN 0304-4017.

Landmann, J.K. & Prociv, P. (2003). Experimental human infection with the dog hookworm, *Ancylostoma caninum*. *The Medical Journal of Australia*, Vol.178, No.2, (Jan 2003), pp. 69-71, ISSN 0025-729X.

Lappin, M.R., Greene, C.E. Prestwood, A.K., Dawe, D.L.; Tarleton, R.L.(1989). Diagnosis of recent *Toxoplasma gondii* infection in cats by use of an enzyme-linked immunosorbent assay for immunoglobulin M. *American Journal of Veterinary Research*. Vol.50, No.9, (Sep 1989), pp. 1580-1585, ISSN 0002-9645

Leav, B.A., Mackay, M., Ward, H.D. (2003).*Cryptosporidium* species: new insights and old challenges. *Clinical Infectious Diseases*. Vol.36, No.7, (Apr 2003), pp. 903-908, ISSN 1058-4838.

Lima, F.G., Amaral, A.V.C., Oliveira Alves, R., Silva, E.B., Tassara, N., Freitas, P.H.O., Barbosa, V.T. (2006). Frequência de enteroparasitas em gatos no município de Goiânia-Goiás, no ano de 2004. *Enciclopedia Biosferera*. No.2, ISSN 1809-0583.

Lima, V.M.F., Gonçalves, M.E., Ikeda, F.A., Luvizotto, M.C.R. &Feitosa, M.M. (2003). Anti-leishmania antibodies in cerebospinal fluid from dogs with visceral leishmaniasis. *Brazilian Journal of Medical and Biolgical Research*. Vol.36, (Apr 2003), pp.485-489, ISSN 0100-879-X

Lucas, S.R.R., Hagiwara, M.K., Reche, A. Jr., Germano, P.M.L. (1998). Ocurrence of antibodies to *Toxoplasma* in cats naturally infected with feline immunodeficiency virus. *Braz J Vet Res Anim Sci*. Vol.35, No.1, pp.41–45, ISSN 1413-9596.

Mac Glade, T.R., Robertson, I.D., Elliot, A.D., Thompson, R.C.A. (2003). High prevalence of *Giardia* detected in cats by PCR. *Veterinary Parasitology*. Vol.110, No.3-4, (Jan 2003), pp.197-205, ISSN 0304-4017.

Machado, A.B., El-Achkar, M.E. (2003). Larva migrans visceral: relato de caso. *Anais Brasileiros de Dermatologia*., Vol.78, No.2, (Mar-Apr 2003), pp. 215-219, ISSN 0365-0596.

Maia, C., Nunes, M. & Campino, L. (2008). Importance of cats in zoonotic leishmaniasis in Portugal. *Vector Borne and Zoonotic Diseases*, Vol.8, No.4, (Aug 2008), pp. 555-559, ISSN 1557-7759.

Mancianti, F. (2004). Feline leishmaniasis: what´s the epidemiological role of the cat? *Parassitologia*, Vol.46, No.1-2, (Jun 2004), pp. 203-206, ISSN 0048-2951.

Marchioro, A.A., Colli, C.M., Mattia, S., Paludo, M.L., Melo, G.C., Adami, C.M., Pelloso, S.M., Guilherme, A.L.F. (2011). Eosinophilic count and seropositivity IgG antibodies to *Toxocara* spp. in children assisted at the public health service. *Revista Paulista de Pediatria*. Vol.29, No.1, (Jan-Mar 2011), pp.80-84, ISSN 0103-0582.

Marcos, R., Santos, M., Malhão F., Pereira, R., Fernandes, C.A, Montenegro, L., Roccabianca, P. (2009). Pancytopenia in a cat with visceral leishmaniasis. *Veterinary Clinical Pathology*. Vol.38, No.2, (Jun 2009), pp.201-202, ISSN 1939-165X.

Maroli, M. et al. (2007). Infection of sandflies by a cat naturally infected with *Leishmania infantum*. *Veterinary Parasitology*. Vol. 145, No. 3-4, (Apr 2007), pp. 357-360, ISSN 1984-2961.

McCarthy, J. & Moore, T.A. (2000). Emerging helminth zoonoses. *International Journal for Parasitology*, Vol.30, 2000, pp. 1351-1360, ISSN 0020-7519.

Mircean, V., Titilincu, A. & Vasile, C. (2010). Prevalence of endoparasites in household cat (*Felis catus*) populations from Transylvania (Romania) and association with risk factors. *Veterinary Parasitology*, Vol.171, No.1-2, (Jul 2010), pp. 163-166, ISSN 0304-4017.

Mitchell, S.M., Zajac, A.M., Kennedy, T., Davis, W., Dubey, J.P. & Lindsay, D.S. (2006). Prevention of recrudescent toxoplasmic encephalitis using ponazuril in an immunodeficient mouse model. *The Journal of Eukaryotic Microbiology*, Vol.53 (Suppl 1), pp. S164–165, ISSN 1550-7408.

Modolo, J.R., Langoni, H., Padovani, C.R., Barrozo, L.V., Leite, B.L.S., Gennari, S.M. & Stachissini, A.V.M. (2008). Occurrence of anti-*Toxoplasma gondii* antibodies in goat sera in the state of São Paulo, and its association with epidemiological variables, reproductive problems and risks on public health. *Pesquisa Veterinária Brasileira*, Vol.28, No.12, (Dec 2008), pp. 606–610, ISSN 0100-736X.

Monis, P.T. & Thompson, R.C. (2003). *Cryptosporidium* and *Giardia* zoonoses: fact or fiction?. *Infection Genetics and Evolution*, Vol.3, No.4, (Nov 2003), pp. 233-244, ISSN 1567-1348.

Mtambo, M.M.A., Nash, A.S.; Blewett, D.A., Wright, S. (1992). Comparison of staining and concentration techniques for detection of *Cryptosporidium* oocysts in cat faecal specimens. *Veterinary Parasitology*, Vol.45, No.1-2, (Dec 1992), pp. 49-57, ISSN 0304-4017.

Mtambo, M.M.A., Wright, S.E.; Nash, A.S. & Blewett, D.A. (1996). Infectivity of Cryptosporidium species isolated from a domestic cat (Felis domestica) in lambs and mice. *Research in Veterinary Science*, Vol.60, No.1, (Jan 1996), pp. 61-64, ISSN 0034-5288.

Mundim, T.C.D., Junior, S.D.O., Rodrigues, D.C., Cury, M.C. Freqüência de helmintos em gatos de Uberlândia, Minas Gerais. *Arq. Bras. Med.Vet. Zootec.* Vol.56, No.4, (Aug 2004), pp. 562-563, ISSN 0102-0935.

Ogassawara, S., Benassi, S., Larsson, C.E., Leme, P.T.Z., Hagiwara, M.K. (1986). Prevalência de infestações helmínticas em gatos na cidade de São Paulo. *Brazilian Journal of Veterinary Research and Animal Science.* Vol.23, No.2, (Nov 2011), pp. 145-9, ISSN 1413-9596.

Omata, Y, Oikawa, H., Kanda, M., Mikazuki, K., Nabayashi, T., Suzuki, N. (1990). Experimental feline toxoplasmosis: humoral immune responses of cats inoculated orally with *Toxoplasma gondii* cysts and oocysts. *The Japanese Journal of Veterinary Science.* Vol.52, No. 4, pp. 865-867, ISSN 0021-5295.

Overgaauw, P.A.M. (1997). Prevalence of intestinal nematodes of dogs and cats in the Netherlands. *The Veterinary Quartely.* Vol.19, No.1, (Mar 1997), pp.14-7, ISSN 0165-2176.

Overgaauw, P.A.M. & Boersema, J.H.A. (1998). Survey of *Toxocara* infections in cat breeding colonies in the Netherlands. *The Veterinary Quartely.* Vol.20, No.1, pp.9-11, ISSN 0165-2176.

Ozon, C., Marty, P., Pratlong, F., Breton, C., Blein, M., Lelievre, A. & Haas, P. (1998). Disseminated feline leishmaniosis due to Leishmania infantum in Southern France. *Veterinary Parasitology*, Vol.75, No.2-3, (Feb 1998), pp. 273-277, ISSN 0304-4017.

Palmer, C.S., Traub, R.J., Robertson, I.D., Devlin, G., Ress, R. & Thompson, R.C. (2008). Determining the zoonotic significance of *Giardia* and *Cryptosporidium* in Australian dogs and cats. *Veterinary Parasitology*, Vol.154, No.1-2, (June 2008), pp. 142-147, ISSN 0304-4017.

Pavlasek, I. & Ryan, U. (2007). The first finding of a natural infection of *Cryptosporidium muris* in cat. *Veterinary Parasitology*, Vol.144, No.3-4, (Marc 2007), pp. 349-352, ISSN 0304-4017.

Pradhan, S., Yadav, R., Mishra, V. N. (2007). *Toxoplasma* meningoencephalitis in HIV-seronegative patients: clinical patterns, imaging features and treatment outcome. *Transactions of the Royal Society of Tropical Medicine and Hygiene*. Vol.101, No. 1, (Jan 2007), pp. 25-33, ISSN 0035-9203.

Pena, H.F.J., Soares, R.M., Amaku, M., Dubey, J.P, Gennari, S.M. (2006). *Toxoplasma gondii* infection in cats from São Paulo State, Brazil: seroprevalence, oocyst shedding, isolation in mice, and biologic and molecular characterization. *Research in Veterinary Science*. Vol. 81, No.1, pp. 58-67, ISSN 0034-5288

Pennisi, M. G. et al. (2004). Case report of leishmaniasis in four cats. *Veterinary Research Communications*. Vol.28, No.1, (Aug 2004), pp. 363-366, ISSN 1573-7446.

Petri Jr, W. A. (2003). Therapy of intestinal protozoa. *Trends in Parasitology*. Vol.19, No.11, (Nov 2003), pp.523-526, ISSN 1471-4922

Pinto, L.D., Araujo, F.A.P., Stobb, N.S. & Marques, S.M.T. (2009). Seroepidemiology of *Toxoplasma gondii* in domestic cats treated in private clinics of Porto Alegre, Brazil. *Ciência Rural*. Vol.39, No.8, (Nov 2009), pp. 2464–2469, ISSN 0103-8478.

Powell, C.C., Brewer, M. & Lappin, M.R. (2001). Detection of *Toxoplasma gondii* in the milk of experimentally infected lactating cats. *Veterinary Parasitology*, Vol.102, No.1-2, (Dec 2001), pp. 29-33, ISSN 1984-2961.

Prociv, P. & Croese, J. (1996). Human enteric infection with Ancylostoma caninum: hookworms reappraised in the light of a "new" zoonosis. *Acta Tropica*, Vol.62, No.1, (Sep 1996), pp. 23-44, ISSN 0001-706X.

Ragozo, A.M.A., Muradian, V., Ramos e Silva, J.C., Caravieri, R., Amajoner, V.R., Magnabosco, C., & Gennari, S.M. (2002). Ocorrência de parasitos gastrintestinais em fezes de gatos das cidades de São Paulo e Guarulhos. *Brazilian Journal of Veterinary Research and Animal Science*, Vol.39, No.5, 2002, pp. 244-246, ISSN 1413-9596.

Rayes, A.A., Lanbertucci, J.R. (1999). A associação entre a toxocaríase humana e os abscessos piogênicos. *Revista da Sociedade Brasileira de Medicina Tropical*. Vol.32, No.4, (Jul-Ago 1999), pp.425-438, ISSN 0037-8682.

Rey, L. (2001). *Parasitologia: Ancilostomídeos e ancilostomíase: I. Os parasitos*. (terceira), Guanabara Koogan, Rio de Janeiro, pp.591-595.

Richey, T.K., Gentry, R.H., Fitzpatrick, J.E., Morgan, A.M. (1996). Persistent cutaneous larva migrans due to *Ancylostoma species*. *Southern Medical Journal*. Vol.89, No.6, (Jun 1996), pp. 609–611, ISSN 0038-2469.

Robertson, I.D. & Thompson, R.C. (2002). Enteric parasitic zoonoses of domestical dogs and cats. *Microbes and Infection*, Vol.4, No.8, (Jul 2002), pp. 867-873, ISSN 1286-4579.

Rossi, C. N. Ocorrência de *Leishmania* sp. em gatos do município de Araçatuba - São Paulo - Brasil. 2007. 87 f. Dissertação (Mestrado)–Universidade Estadual Paulista, Jaboticabal, 2007.

Rossignol, J.F. (2010). *Cryptosporidium* and *Giardia*: treatment options and prospects for new drugs. *Experimental Parasitology*, Vol.124, No.1, (Jan 2010), pp.45-53, ISSN 0014-4894.

Rüfenacht, S. et al. (2005).Two cases of feline leishmaniosis in Switzerland. *Veterinary Record*. Vol.156, No 17, pp.542-545, ISSN 0042-4900.

Santarém, V.A., Giuffrida, R. & Zanin, G.A. (2004). Larva migrans cutânea: ocorrência de casos humanos e identificação de larvas de *Ancylostoma* spp. em parque público do município de Taciba, São Paulo. *Revista da Sociedade Brasileira de Medicina Tropical*, Vol.37, No.2, (Março-Abril 2004), pp. 179-181, ISSN 0037-8682.

Sargent, K.D., Morgan, U.M., Elliot, A. & Thompson, R.C.A. (1998). Morphological and genetic characterization of *Cryptosporidium* oocysts from domestic cats. *Veterinary Parasitology*, Vol.77, No.4, (Jun 1998), pp. 221-227, ISSN 0304-4017.

Sato, K., Iwamoto, I. &Yoshiki, K. (1993). Experimental toxoplasmosis in pregnant cats. *The Journal of Veterinary Medical Science*. Vol.55, No.6, (Dec 1993), pp.1005-1009, ISSN 1347-7439.

Savani, E.S.M.M., Camargo,M.C.G.O., Carvalho,M.R., Zampieri,R.A. ,Santos, M.G., D'auria,S.R.N., Shaw,J.J., Floeter-Winter,L.M. (2004).The first record in the Americas of an autochthonous case of *Leishmania (Leishmania) infantum chagasi* in a domestic cat (*Felix catus*) from Cotia County, São Paulo State Brazil.*Veterinary Parasitology*. Vol.120, No.3, (Mar 2004), pp.229- 233, ISSN 1984-2961.

Savioli, L., Smith, H., Thompson, A. (2006). *Giardia* and *Cryptosporidium* join the "Neglected Diseases Initiative". *Trends in Parasitology*. Vol.22, No.5, (May 2006), pp.203-208, ISSN 1471-4922.

Schnyder, M., Kohler, L., Hemphill, A. & Deplazes, P. (2009). Prophylactic and therapeutic efficacy of nitazoxanide against Cryptosporidium parvum in experimentally challenged neonatal calves. *Veterinary Parasitology*, Vol.160, No.1-2, (Mar 2009), pp. 149-154, ISSN 0304-4017.

Schubach, T.M.P. et al. (2004). American cutaneous leishmaniasis in two cats from Rio de Janeiro, Brazil: first report of natural infection with *Leishmania (Viannia) braziliensis*. *Transactions of the Royal Society of Tropical Medicine and Hygiene*. Vol.98, No.3, (Mar 2004), pp.165-167, ISSN 0035-9203.

Şengür, G. & Öner, Y.A. (2005). The examination of intestinal flora and parasites in dogs and the role of the contamination of the playgrounds' sand with feces. *Turk Mikrobiyoloji Cemiyeti Dergisi*, Vol. 35, 2005, pp. 57-66, ISSN 0258-2171.

Serra, C.M.B., Uchôa, C.M.A. & Coimbra, R.A. (2003). Exame parasitológico de fezes de gatos (*Felis catus domesticus*) domiciliados e errantes da Região Metropolitana do Rio de Janeiro, Brasil. *Revista da Sociedade Brasileira de Medicina Tropical*, Vol.36, No.3, (Mai-Jun 2003), pp. 331-334, ISSN 1678-9849.

Serrano, A.C.M. et al. (2008). Leishmaniose em felino na zona urbana de Araçatuba - SP - relato de caso. *Clínica Veterinária*. No.76, pp.36-40.

Sharif, M., Daryani, A., Nasrolahei, M., Ziapour, S.P. (2010) A survey of gastrointestinal helminthes in stray cats in northern Iran. *Comparative Clinical Pathology*. Vol. 19, No.3, pp. 257–261, ISSN 1618-565X.

Shimizu ,T. (1993). Prevalence of *Toxocara* eggs in sandpits in Tokushima City and its Outskirts. *The Journal of Veterinary Medical Science*. Vol. 55, No.5, (Oct 1993), pp.807-811, ISSN 1347-7439.

Silva, A.V.M., Souza Cândido, C.D., Pita Pereira, D., Brazil, R.P. & Carreira, J.C. (2008). The first Record of American visceral leishmaniasis in domestic cats from Rio de Janeiro, Brazil. *Acta Tropica*, Vol.105, No.1, (Jan 2008), pp. 92-94, ISSN 0001-706X.

Silva, J. C. R. et al. (2002). Prevalence of *Toxoplasma gondii* antibodies in sera of domestic cats from Guarulhos and São Paulo, Brazil. *The Journal of Parasitology*. Vol. 88, No. 2, (Par 2002), pp. 419-20, ISSN 0022-3395

Silva, H. C. S., Castagnolli, K. C., Silveira, D. M., Costa, G. H. N., Gomes, R. A., Nascimento, A. A. (2001). Fauna helmíntica de cães e gatos provenientes de alguns municípios do Estado de São Paulo. *Semina: Ciênc. Agrár.* Vol.22, No.1, pp. 63-66, ISSN 1676-546X.

Simões-Mattos, L., Bevilaqua, C.M.L., Mattos, M.R.F. & Pompeu, M.M.L. (2004). Feline leishmaniasis: uncommon or unknown?. *Revista Portuguesa de Ciências Veterinárias*, Vol.99, No.550, pp.79-87, ISSN 0035-0389.

Singh, A., Janaki, L., Petri, W.A.Jr., Houpt, E.R. (2009). *Giardia intestinalis* assemblages A and B infections in Nepal. *American Journal of Tropical Medicine and Hygiene*. Vol.81, No.3, (Sep 2009), pp.538-539, ISSN 0002-9637.

Smith, H.V. & Nichols, R.A.B. (2010). *Cryptosporidium*: detection in water and food. *Experimental Parasitology*, Vol.124, No.1, (January 2010), pp. 61-79, ISSN 0014-4894.

Smith, H.V., Cacciò, S.M., Tait, A., McLauchlin, J. & Thompson, R.C.A. (2006). Tools for investigating the environmental transmission of *Cryptosporidium* and *Giardia* infections in humans. *Trends in Parasitology*, Vol.22, No.4, (Apr 2006), pp. 160-167, ISSN 1471-4922.

Solano-Gallego, L. et al. (2007). Cross-sectional serosurvey of feline leishmaniasis in ecoregions around the Northwestern Mediterranean. *American Journal of Tropical Medicine and Hygiene*. Vol .76, No.4,(Apr 2007), pp. 676-680, ISSN 0002-9637.

Sousa, V.R., Almeida, A.F.A., Cândido, A.C. & Barros, L.A., (2010). Ovos e larvas de helmintos em caixas de areia de creches, escolas municipais e praças públicas de Cuiabá, MT. *Ciência Animal Brasileira*, Vol.11, No.2, pp. 390-395, ISSN 1518-2797.

Souza, A.L. et al. (2005). Feline leishmaniasis due to *Leishmania (Leishmania) amazonensis* in Mato Grosso do Sul State, Brazil. *Veterinary Parasitology*, Vol.128, No.1-2, (Mar 2005), pp. 41-45, ISSN 1984-2961.

Souza, I.S., Martins, A.L.F., Moreira, W.S., Santurie, J.M. & Flores, M.L. (1982). Parasitos do estômago e intestino Delgado de Felis catis domesticus em Santa Maria, Rio Grande do Sul. Proceedings of the CONGRESSO BRASILEIRO DE MEDICINA VETERINÁRIA EM LÍNGUA PORTUGUESA, Camboriú, Brasil, 1982.

Souza, S.L., Gennari, S.M., Richtzenhain, L.J., Pena, H.F., Funada, M.R., Cortez, A., Gregori, F., Soares, R.M. (2007).Molecular identification of *Giardia duodenalis* isolates from humans, dogs, cats and cattle from the state of São Paulo, Brazil, by sequence analysis of fragments of glutamate dehydrogenase (gdh) coding gene. *Veterinary Parasitology*, Vol.149, No.3-4, (Nov 2007), pp. 258-264, ISSN 0304-4017.

Springer, S.C., Key, J.D. (1997). Vitamin B12 deficiency and subclinical infection with *Giardia lamblia* in an adolescent with agammaglobulinemia of Bruton. *Journal of Adolescent Health*. Vol.20, No.1, (Jan 1997), pp.58-61, ISSN 1054-139X.

Tellez, A., Morales, W., Rivera, T., Meier, E., Leiva, B., Linder, E. (1997). Prevalence of intestinal parasites in the human population of Leon, Nicaragua. *Acta tropica*. Vol.66, No.3, (Sep 1997), pp.19-125, ISSN 0001-706X

Thompson, R.C. (2000). Giardiasis as a re-emerging infectious disease and its zoonotic potential. *International Journal for Parasitology*. Vol.30, No. 12-13, (Nov 2000), pp. 1259-1267, ISSN 0020-7519.

Thompson, R.C.A. & Monis, P.T. (2004). Variation in *Giardia*: implications for taxonomy and epidemiology. *Advances in Parasitology,* Vol.58, No.4, pp. 69-137, ISSN 0065-308X.

Thompson, R.C.A., Palmer, C.S. & O´Handley, R. (2008). The public health and clinical significance of *Giardia* and *Cryptosporidium* in domestic animals. The *Veterinary Journal,* Vol.177, No.1, (July 2008), pp. 18-25, ISSN 1090-0233.

Tonelli, E. (2005). Toxocaríase e asma: associação relevante. *Jornal de Pediatria,* Vol.81, No.2, pp. 95-96, ISSN 1678-4782.

Torrey, E.F. & Yolken, R.H. (2003). *Toxoplasma gondii* and schizophrenia. *Emerging Infectious Disease,* Vol.9, No.11,(Nov 2003), pp. 1375-1380, ISSN 1080-6059.

Traub, R.J., Monis, P.T., Robertson, I., Irwin, P., Mencke, N. & Thompson, R.C.A. (2004). Epidemiological and molecular evidence supports the zoonotic transmission of *Giardia* among humans and dogs living in the same community. *Parasitology,* Vol.128, No.3, (Mar 2004), pp. 153-262, ISSN 0031-1820.

Tzannes, S., Batchelor, D.J., Graham, P.A., Pinchbeck, G.L., Wastling, J. & German, A.J. (2008). Prevalence of *Cryptosporidium, Giardia* and *Isospora* species infections in pet cats with clinical signs of gastrointestinal disease. *Journal of Feline Medicine and Surgery,* Vol.10, No.1, (Feb 2008), pp. 1-8, ISSN 1098-612X.

Tzipori, S., Angus, K.W., Campbell, I. & GRAY, E.W. (1980). *Cryptosporidium*: evidence for a single species genus. *Infection and Immunity*. Vol.30, No.3, (Dec 1980), pp. 884-886, ISSN 1098-5522.

Tzzipori, S. & Griffths, J.K. (1998). Natural History and Biology of *Cryptosporidium parvum. Advances in Parasitology,* Vol.40, pp. 5-36, ISSN 0065-308X.

Uga S. (1993). Prevalence of *Toxocara* eggs and number of faecal deposits from dogs and cats in sandpits of public parks in Japan. *Journal of Helminthology*. Vol.67, No.1, (Mar 1993), pp. 78- 82, ISSN 1475-2697.

Xiao, L. & Fayer, R. (2008). Molecular characterization of species and genotypes of *Cryptosporidium* and *Giardia* and assessment of zoonotic transmission. *International Journal for Parasitology,* Vol.38, No.11, (Sep 2008), pp. 1239-1255, ISSN 0020-7519.

Xiao, L. (2010). Molecular epidemiology of cryptosporidiosis: an update. *Experimental Parasitology,* Vol.124, No.1, (Jan 2010), pp. 80-89, ISSN 1090-2449.

Yoder, J. & Beach, M.J. (2010). *Cryptosporidium* surveillance and risk factors in the United States. *Experimental Parasitology,* Vol.124, No.1, (Jan 2010), pp. 31-39, ISSN 1090-2449.

Yolken, R.H. et al. (2001). Antibodies to Toxoplasma gondii in individuals with first-episode schizophrenia. *Clinical Infectious Diseases*. Vol.32, No.5, (Mar 2001), pp.842-844, ISSN 1537-6591

Zajdenweber, M., Muccioli, C. & Belfort Júnior, R. (2005). Acometimento ocular em pacientes com AIDS e toxoplasmose do sistema nervoso central: antes e depois do HAART. *Arquivos Brasileiros de Oftalmologia,* Vol.68, No.6, pp. 773-775, ISSN 0004-2749.

Zhu S. (2009). Psychosis may be associated with toxoplasmosis. *Medical Hypotheses,* Vol.73, No.5, (Nov 2009), pp. 799-801, ISSN 0306-9877.